Bone Marrow Pathology

3RD EDITION

Dedications

Kathryn Foucar:
To Elliott, Jim and Charlie Foucar and my mother Kathryn Brozovich

Kaaren Reichard:
To Ross, Vreni and Caroline Reichard and my parents

David Czuchlewski:
To Kristina, Abby and Talia; and to my parents, for letting a 10-year-old stay up late reading

Bone Marrow Pathology

VOLUME 1

3RD EDITION

Kathryn Foucar, MD
Professor and Vice Chair for Clinical Affairs
Department of Pathology
University of New Mexico Health Sciences Center
Medical Director, TriCore Reference Laboratories

Kaaren Reichard, MD
Associate Professor, Associate Chief
Department of Pathology
University of New Mexico Health Sciences Center
Medical Director, TriCore Reference Laboratories

David Czuchlewski, MD
Assistant Professor
Department of Pathology
University of New Mexico Health Sciences Center
Medical Director, TriCore Reference Laboratories

All of Albuquerque, New Mexico

PRESS

ASCP Press
American Society for Clinical Pathology
Chicago

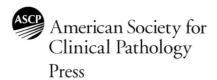
American Society for
Clinical Pathology
Press

Publishing Team

Erik N Tanck (editorial content/production)
Joshua Weikersheimer (publishing direction)

We welcome your feedback at
bonemarrowpathology@ascp.org

Printed in Singapore
14 13 12 11 10

Contents Volume 1

1: Hematopoiesis

2: Morphologic Review of Blood and Bone Marrow

3: Procurement and Indications for Bone Marrow Examination

4: Specialized Techniques in Bone Marrow Evaluation

5: Bone Marrow Reporting and Quality Assurance

6: Anemias

Tables by Chapter

15: Myeloid and Lymphoid Neoplasms with Eosinophilia (MLNE) and Abnormalities of PDGFRA, PDGFRB, or FGFR1

16: Myelodysplastic Syndromes

17: Myelodysplastic/Myeloproliferative Neoplasms

18: Acute Myeloid Leukemia

19: Blastic Plasmacytoid Dendritic Cell Neoplasms in Bone Marrow

20: Acute Leukemias of Ambiguous Lineage

Contents Volume 2 (abridged)

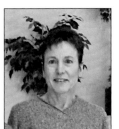

Kathryn Foucar

Acknowledgments

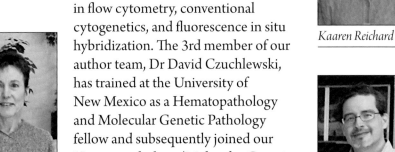

This 3rd edition represents a significant departure from previous editions in that 2 co-authors have played critical roles in this creation. Dr Kaaren Reichard has been my invaluable colleague for the last 7 of my 25 years at the University of New Mexico Health Sciences Center. Not only is she a superb diagnostician in hematopathology but she possesses remarkable expertise in flow cytometry, conventional cytogenetics, and fluorescence in situ hybridization. The 3rd member of our author team, Dr David Czuchlewski, has trained at the University of New Mexico as a Hematopathology and Molecular Genetic Pathology fellow and subsequently joined our Hematopathology/Molecular Genetic Pathology Division. The experience and unique expertise of each of these outstanding co-authors added immeasurably to the quality and diagnostic utility of this 3rd edition.

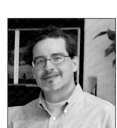

Kaaren Reichard

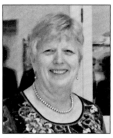

David Czuchlewski

Two other individuals at the University of New Mexico were stellar contributors to this creation and both warrant the sincerest gratitude of the authors. Linda Borgman worked tirelessly for over 18 months, providing all aspects of hands on and administrative support for each of the 36 chapters and appendix. Linda postponed her retirement to insure the successful completion of this work. This level of dedication and commitment is truly remarkable; the authors are honored to have had Linda at the "helm" of this project. Michael Grady provided outstanding artistic support for the sizable number of images and figures in every chapter. His talent is evident on virtually every page.

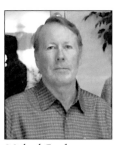

Linda Borgman

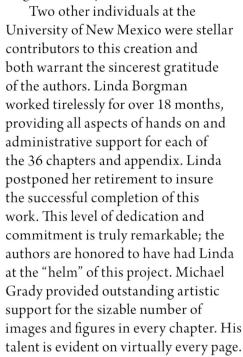

Michael Grady

Joshua Weikersheimer, ASCP Press, a friend, and colleague for all editions, has applied his unique artistic and publishing talents to this 3rd edition. Not only did Joshua provide strong support and guidance throughout this project, but he has contributed the many original and creative design features of this book.

Many pathologists kindly provided cases for illustration. These individuals include: J Anastasi, P Armell, M Benziger, AM Blenc, R Brynes, R Braziel, B Cabello-Inchausti, D Canioni, J Choi, L Contis, D Cornfield, S Deodare, T Elghentany, R Feddersen, W Finn, R Gascoyne, L Gates, S Geaghan, S Gheith, C Hanson, D Head, J Hussong, M Irani, J Jastram, J Jones, T Keith, C Kjeldsberg, S Kroft, C Leith, R Macaulay, I Maric, R McKenna, J Mo, D O'Malley, H Mooney, B Nelson, S Peiper, L Peterson, C Pitchford, L Rimsza, N Rosenthal, C Ross, J Said, C Sever, A Shrit, C Starkey, T Traweek, J Vardiman, A Vendrell, P Ward, W Williams, C Wilson, X Yao, QY Zhang.

In addition, P Izadi, MT(ASCP) provided many slides for photography of pediatric disorders. The authors sincerely thank all of these individuals. In particular, Cordelia Sever, Steve Kroft, and Parvin Izadi provided many cases for illustration.

Finally the authors would like to acknowledge other individuals in the Department of Pathology including our Chair, Thomas Williams who has provided strong leadership and support for each of the authors, while Nancy Risenhoover has provided executive administrative support for the faculty and staff involved in this project. The authors would also like to acknowledge the other members of the hematopathology/molecular pathology division including Carla Wilson MD, PhD, Mohammad Vasef MD, Qian-Yun Zhang MD, PhD, Heath Worcester MD, Barbara Masten PhD, and John Hozier PhD.

Foreword

The practitioner of diagnostic hematopathology may sometimes perceive the discipline as evolving in contradictory directions. Our increasing understanding promises ever more accurate and relevant diagnostic capabilities; yet each small advance seems to open another unsuspected chasm of mystery and uncertainty. To illustrate: the 2nd edition of this text, published in 2001, contained not a single mention of the gene *JAK2*. In the interim, some 3,600 peer-reviewed articles on *JAK2* have entered the literature—in addition to over 62,000 papers on leukemia, over 57,000 relevant to the bone marrow, and 760,000 relating to the blood.... One is reminded of Jorge Luis Borges' "garden of the forking paths," in which every turn in a labyrinth reveals but one small part of an infinite, incomprehensible whole.

Unlike the imaginary book in Borges' story, this text is not intended to encompass the entirety of a labyrinth. Rather, our goal in the 3rd edition has been to create a state of the art, highly practical "roadmap" to current best practices in blood and bone marrow diagnosis. We have structured the book to answer the types of questions that arise in day to day practice, emphasizing key features and providing relevant tips. We present differential diagnostic considerations and critical "clues and caveats" to help the reader avoid pitfalls. The book incorporates the full breadth of the 2008 World Health Organization (WHO) criteria—yet is intended to help the pathologist answer not only the question, "*What* are the possible diagnoses?" but also, "*How* will I proceed to find out?"

The morphologic, observational focus of hematopathology is fully embraced in this highly illustrated text. But, since morphology is often no longer the diagnostic endpoint, we present a multidisciplinary approach in which clinical and morphologic findings are integrated with immunophenotypic and molecular genetic features. Since we believe our shared responsibility extends to cost-effective patient care, we also delineate strategies for optimal utilization of these powerful techniques.

Even a brief comparison to the 2nd edition will reveal that all chapters have been extensively revised—often redone and re-illustrated entirely from scratch. Newly recognized benign and neoplastic disorders are thoroughly addressed. References have been comprehensively updated, as recently as a month or 2 prior to publication. Sidebars concentrating on molecular genetics are a new feature of this edition, providing greater depth of analysis without distracting the reader from matters of diagnosis and patient care.

The authors were committed to the creation of a practical, diagnostically relevant book, and we welcome your feedback at bonemarrowpathology@ascp.org. We hope you will find the book a valuable guide through the portions of the hematopathology labyrinth most relevant to you.

1

Hematopoiesis

Kathryn Foucar, MD

Adequate evaluation of bone marrow cannot occur without a basic understanding of hematopoiesis and normal bone marrow architecture/topobiology. However, the assessment of normal bone marrow is uniquely challenging for several reasons:

1. Neither stem cells nor progenitor cells are *morphologically* recognizable and, instead, are typically identified by either immunophenotypic characteristics or functional properties in cell culture systems.

2. All types of stem cells and progenitor cells are very rare in normal bone marrow, typically accounting for <0.001% of total nucleated cells.

3. Similarly, the functional unit of the bone marrow, the capillary venous sinus, is not readily apparent on light microscopic evaluation of either bone marrow aspirate smears or core biopsy sections.

4. Throughout the bone marrow, there are unique, submicroscopic, microenvironmental niches where stem/progenitor cells are selectively localized and subject to specific regulatory factor-induced lineage proliferation.

5. Numerous lineages are developing and maturing simultaneously, creating a "chaotic" appearance to bone marrow, especially on bone marrow aspirate smears.

6. Cell production rates for hematopoietic cells are astronomical, so these cell types predominate and can obscure other lineages that are also being produced in the bone marrow.

7. Significant age-related normal variations are seen in overall bone marrow cellularity as well as in the relative proportions of various cell types.

In this chapter, the basic features of hematopoiesis, including stem cells, bone marrow microenvironment, regulatory factors, and individual lineage production, will be presented, with an emphasis on those features either most relevant to bone marrow morphologic interpretation or most useful in terms of understanding abnormal bone marrow conditions. However, hematopoiesis is an area of intense investigation, and unique findings from current research will also be included, largely in brief synopsis format (see **sidebar 1.1**).

Beginning in midfetal development and extending throughout life, the bone marrow is the site of origin, maturation, and development of all peripheral blood hematopoietic elements [Foucar 2008, de Alarcon 2005, Wickramasinghe 2007]. In addition, widely dispersed macrophages, specialized dendritic cells (antigen-presenting cells) of the monocyte-macrophage lineage, lymphocytes, mast cells, and osteoclasts are also derived from hematopoietic stem cells (HSCs) **t1.1** [Bryder 2006].

Although highly variable, the life span of peripheral blood elements is relatively short, and consequently, astronomical production rates by the bone marrow are necessary to maintain homeostasis [Bryder 2006]. Estimated daily production rates for adults are as follows: neutrophils, $50\text{-}100/\mu L$ $(0.05\text{-}0.1 \times 10^9/L)$; platelets, $150\text{-}200 \times 10^3/\mu L$ $(150\text{-}200 \times 10^9/L)$; and erythrocytes, $150\text{-}200 \times 10^6/\mu L$ $(150\text{-}200 \times 10^9/L)$ [Bryder 2006, Kaushansky 2008, Lee 2004]. In addition, bone marrow mesenchymal stem cells (MSCs) are generally thought to produce the various endothelial, stromal, and chondro-osseous cells that constitute the bone marrow microenvironment **t1.1** [Dazzi 2006, Fox 2007, Gang 2007, Lakshmipathy 2005, Martinez 2007].

t1.1 Cell Types Produced by Hematopoietic and Mesenchymal Stem Cells

Hematopoietic Progeny	Mesenchymal Progeny
Erythrocytes	Endothelial cells
Neutrophils	Adipocytes
Eosinophils	Fibroblasts
Basophils	Osteoblasts
Monocytes/histiocytes	Osteocytes
Dendritic cells	Chondrocytes
Lymphocytes	Myofibroblasts
Natural killer (NK) cells	Reticular cells
Platelets	
Mast cells	
Osteoclasts	

References: [Bryder 2006, Dazzi 2006, Fox 2007, Gang 2007, Lakshmipathy 2005, Martinez 2007, Ng 2008]

[1.1] Bone Marrow Structure

The bone marrow is encased in cortical bone and traversed by trabecular bone. The surface of these bony trabeculae is lined by endosteum, which consists of a layer of endosteal lining cells with variable numbers of dispersed osteoblasts and osteoclasts [Wickramasinghe 2007]. The area between bony trabeculae consists of a highly organized meshwork of thin-walled capillary-venous sinuses with surrounding extracellular matrix [Wickramasinghe 2007]. The nutrient artery is the primary source of arterial blood for the marrow. By means of successive bifurcations, small branches of this nutrient artery ultimately form a plexus of sinusoids, the basic structural unit of the bone marrow [Wickramasinghe 2007].

The sinus lumen is contiguous with the extramedullary intravascular compartment, while all components outside this sinus lumen comprise the extravascular compartment. The sinus wall consists of an incomplete layer of flattened endothelial cells with little or no underlying basement membrane, while various mesenchymal (stromal) cells adhere to the abluminal surface of this sinus **f1.1** [Wickramasinghe 2007]. These mesenchymal cells produce both the

Mechanisms of Early Lineage Commitment in Hematopoiesis: Under the Shroud of the Progenitor Cell

[sidebar 1.1]

Hematopoietic stem cells and progenitor cells remain morphologically and immunophenotypically largely indistinguishable until quite late in their progression toward single lineage commitment. Yet, this outward homogeneity belies the extensive intracellular changes that characterize the early maturation of the stem cell. Although the subject of intensive investigation in both murine and human systems, the molecular correlates of the early stages of lineage commitment are only gradually being elucidated—a fact that reflects the extreme difficulty of studying exceedingly rare cells that shroud their developmental program under such bland morphologic cover. Consequently, both the field in general and the prevailing models of hematopoiesis are beset by a number of debates and controversies.

In both murine and human studies, the standard model of hematopoiesis holds that the initial stage of lineage differentiation is a decision point leading to either the myeloid or the lymphoid pathways, with no overlap or ambiguity once such a direction has been chosen (see **f1.2**). The myeloid pathway is then further subdivided in a subsequent choice between either granulocyte/monocyte (GM) or megakaryocytic/erythroid (ME) pathways. This model is supported by a wealth of experimental evidence, as pure populations representing each of these stages of commitment have been isolated and characterized [Akashi 2000, Kondo 1997].

Yet a peculiar feature of leukemias of ambiguous lineage (addressed in more detail in Chapter 20) suggests a potential problem with the model as outlined above. In short, if these leukemias arise from a simple "loss of control" of lineage commitment, one might expect that overlap between ME and lymphoid lineages would occur with equal frequency as overlap between GM and lymphoid pathways. In fact, while GM/lymphoid lineage overlap is commonly seen in these unusual leukemias, ME/lymphoid clones are relatively rare [Luc 2008b]. One might infer from this finding that the lymphoid lineage remains more closely tied to GM developmental pathways than to the ME program. In fact, much new evidence supports an "alternative" model of hematopoiesis that follows just such an outline.

Central to this hypothetical pathway is the so-called lymphoid-primed multipotent progenitor (LMPP) cell, which is characterized by high cell-surface expression of FLT3 and the capacity to produce *both* lymphoid and GM progeny [Adolfsson 2005, Yang 2005]; in contrast, LMPP cells seem to have only a limited capacity to produce cells of the ME pathway, although the precise degree and nature of this ME exclusion remain controversial. In particular, the transplantation of purified LMPP cells into mice depleted of hematopoietic cells results in reconstitution of full hematopoiesis—including erythropoiesis and megakaryopoiesis—suggesting that LMPP cells retain ME capacity and might, in

fact, represent true multipotent progenitor cells, a finding more compatible with traditional models of hematopoiesis [Forsberg 2006]. However, subsequent studies examining the expression of transcription factors including PU.1 and MPL have described the existence of a small distinct population of FLT3^high LMPP cells capable of ME differentiation, while the vast majority of LMPP cells retain the capacity to use only the GM and lymphoid pathways [Arinobu 2007, Luc 2008a].

How might such a cell fate decision be executed on the molecular level? Is there a discrete "restriction point" at which the decision is "made"? A recent study suggests that, in fact, lineage commitment may be a more gradual process, with cells arranged on a continuum of lineage fidelity. Looking at the LMPP population, Luc et al quantified the expression of transcription factors relating to ME, GM, and lymphoid programs (so-called transcriptional priming or lineage priming). They found that a gradual decrease in expression of ME transcription factors was followed by gradual decrease in GM transcription factors. Expression of the GM- and lymphoid-associated transcription factors was inversely proportional, so that as lymphoid priming increased, GM priming decreased, and vice versa. Moreover, the capacity of the cells to generate offspring of a given lineage correlated with their degree of priming for that lineage [Luc 2008a]. Taken together, the data support a model of hematopoiesis in which branch points are fluid, rather than rigid, boundaries that are crossed gradually in the course of maturation.

Much of the standard model of hematopoiesis was developed before microRNA (miRNA) was identified as an important cellular regulatory element [Baltimore 2008]. It is not surprising then that recent work examining the role of miRNA in hematopoiesis has yielded dramatic results. Briefly, miRNAs are RNA molecules targeted not for translation into peptides, but for incorporation into an RNA-induced silencer complex that uses the specific sequences of the miRNA to bind 3'-untranslated regions of various mRNAs, thus preventing translation of the latter. More than 30% of the human genome may be under translational regulation by miRNA [Schickel 2008]. Although our understanding of miRNA is truly in its infancy, already many lines of evidence point to a central role for miRNA in hematopoiesis—a function that may be unsurprising, given that levels of transcription factors and other proteins appear to be under exquisite control in these developmental pathways. CD34+ cells have high expression of 33 different miRNAs [Georgantas 2007], and although an in-depth consideration is beyond the scope of this discussion, a few examples will serve to illustrate the centrality that miRNA may play in lineage commitment. The miRNA miR-155 targets silencing PU.1, a transcription factor important in hematopoiesis, and enforced expression of miR-155 in a mouse model results in a myeloproliferative disorder [O'Connell 2008, Vigorito 2007]. Similarly, miR-150

overexpression induces megakaryocytic differentiation [Lu 2008]. The miRNAs of the so-called miR-17-92 complex form a mutual negative feedback loop with the transcription factor gene *RUNX1* [Fontana 2007]. In turn, the *RUNX1-RUNX1T1* fusion oncoprotein aims to silence the promoter region of miR-223, an miRNA shown to be important for granulocytic maturation (Chapter 18) [Fazi 2005, 2007]. In short, the crosstalk between transcription factors and miRNA increasingly seems to be a central trope in the regulation of hematopoiesis.

Yet another surprising development in our understanding of stem cell ontogeny relates to transcriptional activity within the long-term hematopoietic stem cell (HSC) compartment. Traditionally, these truly multipotent cells (from which all more differentiated progenitors and offspring are ultimately derived) have been thought to maintain some degree of simultaneous transcriptional priming for all of the possible lineages. It now appears that, in fact, true HSCs are predominantly primed for ME and GM, but *not* lymphoid, differentiation [Akashi 2003]. The lymphoid transcriptional program appears to be activated only in later stages of differentiation (ie, either the traditional common lymphoid progenitor or the LMPP) and appears to be mutually exclusive to ME priming [Adolfsson 2005, Luc 2008a, Mansson 2007].

Finally, data from T-cell precursors in the thymus have resulted in further challenges to the standard model of hematopoiesis, which postulates that a branch point between B- and T-cell pathways occurs after the loss of capacity to generate cells of the GM lineage **f1.2**. In fact, a subpopulation of precursor cells in the thymus is capable of producing both T cells and GM-lineage cells, but not B cells [Bell 2008, Wada 2008]. This putative GM/T-cell precursor may therefore represent yet another alternative to the canonical pathways of hematopoiesis.

It is worth remembering that the traditional model of hematopoiesis and some of the alternatives suggested by recent evidence are not mutually exclusive, and that very likely all of the possible pathways described herein are in use in different populations of progenitor cells. If true, this would lend a previously unappreciated element of redundancy to the process of hematopoiesis.

When considering the intricacies of early hematopoiesis at this level, one is tempted to regard the very subtle distinctions in lineage commitment and pathway development as academic, or even ultimately semantic. Yet, throughout the remainder of this textbook we will return repeatedly to this stage of development for clues and insights into the molecular derangements that may be driving the development of hematolymphoid malignancies. It is virtually certain that our advancing knowledge of normal hematopoiesis will pay huge dividends in our ability to understand, diagnose, and, hopefully, treat such diseases.

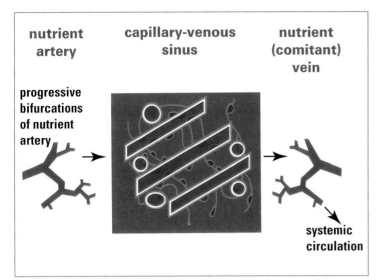

nutrient artery **capillary-venous sinus** **nutrient (comitant) vein**

progressive bifurcations of nutrient artery

systemic circulation

f1.1 *A capillary-venous sinus results from progressive bifurcations of the nutrient artery. Color code: pale blue, extracellular matrix; red, vascular lumen; blue, endothelium; green, stromal cell processes; and white, basement membrane.*

f1.2 *This schematic illustrates the properties of hematopoietic stem cells including self-renewal, lineage commitment, and apoptosis.*

stromal framework of the sinus wall and the intersinusoidal extracellular matrix, a proteinaceous "soup" maintained by a reticulin framework that contains numerous hematopoietic regulatory factors, adhesion molecules, and other proteins necessary for recruitment of precursor cells and stimulation of hematopoiesis [Dazzi 2006, Fox 2007, Gang 2007, Lakshmipathy 2005, Martinez 2007]. Mesenchymal cells, including endothelial cells, produce these regulatory factors.

All newly formed mature hematopoietic cells pass into bone marrow capillary-venous sinuses. These sinusoids drain into a system of collecting venules, which ultimately drain into the nutrient vein [Wickramasinghe 2007]. Passage of these hematopoietic elements through the sinus wall is not completely understood, but ultrastructural evidence suggests that mature cells, such as erythrocytes and granulocytes, pass directly through the cytoplasm of the endothelial cells (transcellularly) rather than between endothelial cells. In contrast, megakaryocytes reside adjacent to the capillary-venous sinuses and have cytoplasmic pseudopodia (proplatelet processes) that extend into the lumina of the sinuses [Geddis 2007, Junt 2007]. Fragmentation of these pseudopodia leads to release of platelets directly into the blood. Cell passage also occurs in the reverse direction in that some cells egress from the blood into the marrow via migration through the sinus wall.

Innervation of the marrow occurs via nerves that traverse the medullary cavity within nutrient canals adjacent to the arterioles and venules; evidence suggests that neuropeptides exert regulatory influence on hematopoiesis [Broome 2000]. The bone marrow does not contain lymphatic channels [Edwards 2008].

t1.2 Features of Mesenchymal Stem Cells (MSC)

Capable of self-renewal and differentiation into tissues of mesodermal origin

Influenced by numerous regulatory/stimulatory/inhibitory factors which control lineage differentiation

Proposed stages of maturation/differentiation include:
  pluripotent mesenchymal progenitor cells
  multipotent progenitor cell
  committed progenitor cells
  mature mesenchymal cell

Immunophenotype: CD90+ , CD105+ , CD106+ , CD76+ , SSEA-4+ , CD45− , HSC ag− , GD2+

Rare in bone marrow; 0.01% - 0.0001% of nucleated cells

Responsible for most cellular constituents of the bone marrow microenvironment, notably osteoblasts, reticular cells, adipocytes, chondrocytes, endothelial cells

Proposed capability of producing any mesodermal-derived lineage

Significant potential therapeutic role in tissue repair, regeneration, neoangiogenesis

Close association between HSC and MSC and progeny in bone marrow microenvironmental niches

References: [Anjos-Afonso 2007, Dazzi 2006, Fox 2007, Gang 2007, Martinez 2007, Ng 2008, Shiozawa 2008]

[1.2] **Mesenchymal Stem Cells and the Bone Marrow Microenvironment**

Similar to HSCs, MSCs are capable of both self renewal and multilineage differentiation **t1.2** [Dazzi 2006]. Although not identifiable morphologically and exceedingly rare in bone marrow, the immunophenotypic features, proposed stages of maturation, and role of MSCs in constituting the bone marrow microenvironment have been delineated **t1.2**

t1.3 Bone Marrow Microenvironment

Bone marrow stromal cells, extracellular matrix, and support matrix comprise the bone marrow microenvironment

Stromal cells regulate survival, self-renewal, migration, and differentiation of hematopoietic stem cells via cell-to-cell contact or production of regulatory factors and other molecules released into the extracellular matrix (molecular crosstalk between HSCs and bone marrow microenvironmental constituents)

Primary cellular components include osteoblasts, macrophages, reticular cells, fibroblasts, and adipocytes

Key role of osteoblasts in HSC survival via direct cell-to-cell contact/adhesion

Hematopoietic stem cells recruited to discrete spaces called "niches" to provide close contact with microenvironment

Hematopoietic stem cells may distribute along an oxygen gradient within the bone marrow microenvironment (lowest oxygen level adjacent to bony trabeculae)

Several niches described:

Bony HSC niche (adjacent to osteoblasts on endosteal surface of bony trabeculae)

Vascular stromal niche for committed progenitor cells (adjacent to reticular/endothelial cells along bone marrow sinuses)

HSC niches may also serve as a habitat for neoplastic cells which can promote both metastasis and chemo-resistance of hematogenous and/or solid tumors

HSC = Hematopoietic stem cell

References: [Dazzi 2006, Li 2006, Wilson 2006, Shiozawa 2008, Burger 2007, Parmar 2007, Dao 2007]

t1.4 Features of Hematopoietic Stem Cells (HSC)

Rare cells in bone marrow, not morphologically recognizable

Localize to specific microenvironmental niches where exposure to extracellular signals regulates self-renewal and differentiation

Usually noncycling (CD38–); facilitates survival and reduces exposure to mutagenic hazards

Identified by immunophenotype: Lin– , CD90+ , CD38- , CD34+ , CD117+

Identified by unique function of asymmetric cell division producing 1 HSC daughter and 1 daughter cell capable of multilineage differentiation

Successive stages of HSC maturation/differentiation include:

multipotent progenitor cells (all myeloid and lymphoid lineages)
oligopotent progenitor cells (common lymphoid progenitor and common myeloid progenitor cells)
lineage-restricted progenitor cells (enormous number of differentiated cells produced by single HSC)

Steady state, lifelong blood cell formation is achieved by the regulation of differentiation from HSC to more differentiated cell types and is controlled by activation and inactivation of specific genes as well as by the epigenetic status of the DNA; microRNAs also play role

References: [Blank 2008, Bryder 2006, Oakley 2007, Metcalf 2007b, Payne 2007]

[Anjos-Afonso 2007, Dazzi 2006, Fox 2007, Gang 2007, Martinez 2007, Ng 2008, Shiozawa 2008]. Factors that stimulate MSC growth and differentiation include transforming growth factor-β, platelet-derived growth factor, and fibroblast growth factor [Ng 2008].

The bone marrow microenvironment consists of diverse stromal/mesenchymal cells, extracellular matrix, and a reticulin support meshwork t1.3 [Burger 2007, Dao 2007, Dazzi 2006, Li 2006, Parmar 2007, Shiozawa 2008, Wilson 2006]. In recent years the concept of HSC niches has been proposed to explain the unique localization of HSCs within the bone marrow microenvironment [Shiozawa 2008, Wilson 2006]. Both endosteal and vascular hematopoietic stem cell niches have been proposed [Lataillade 2008]. Although incompletely understood, the bone marrow microenvironment constituents play an essential role in migration, localization, retention, proliferation, and differentiation of HSCs within these niches via molecular crosstalk [Dao 2007, Wilson 2006]. These microenvironmental niches protect HSCs and other early progenitor cells from toxic exposures. Neoplastic cells may localize to these same microenvironmental niches and consequently be protected from eradication by chemotherapeutic agents [Burger 2007, Li 2006, Shiozawa 2008]. Similarly, alterations in stem cell niches are linked to primary hematopoietic neoplasms [Lataillade 2008].

[1.3] Hematopoietic Stem Cells

Hematopoietic stem cells are the most well-studied of human stem cells and are the only stem cells in routine clinical use [Bryder 2006]. The concept of an HSC was proposed decades ago based on pioneering cell culture studies. Years of murine and human research have delineated many properties of these very rare, morphologically unrecognizable bone marrow cells t1.4 (see sidebar 1.1) [Blank 2008, Bryder 2006, Metcalf 2007b, Oakley 2007].

Hematopoietic stem cells possess the unique property of asymmetric cell division, producing one new HSC and another daughter cell capable of multilineage maturation [Metcalf 2007a]. The process of multilineage maturation and lineage commitment results in the production of enormous numbers of differentiated cells from a single HSC f1.2 [Bryder 2006, Ishikawa 2007, Metcalf 2007b]. Steady-state lifelong multilineage hematopoiesis and lymphopoiesis are achieved by the complex, intricate interrelationship between HSCs, MSCs, and the bone marrow microenvironment f1.3.

[1.4] Future Directions in Mesenchymal and Hematopoietic Stem Cell Therapy

The use of HSCs in either autologous or allogeneic bone marrow transplantation and stem cell engraftment is well established in the management of numerous neoplastic and non-neoplastic disorders. A new area of active investigation is the potential role of either MSCs or HSCs in the repair and/or regeneration of mesenchymal tissues. One key controversy

t1.5 Future Directions and Current Controversies: Regenerative Medicine

Hematopoietic stem cells best studied tissue-specific stem cells and only stem cells used in routine patient care (bone marrow transplantation, stem cell engraftment)

Mesenchymal vs hematopoietic stem cell derivation of nonhematopoietic (ie, mesenchymal) tissues not resolved

Stem cell "plasticity" controversy: putative role of hematopoietic stem cells in the production of normal and neoplastic nonhematopoietic lineages

Potential use of bone marrow-derived mesenchymal stem cells for tissue repair, regeneration, neoangiogenesis

Documented increase in circulating hematopoietic and endothelial progenitor cells after acute myocardial infarction; circulating angiogenic cells derived from hematopoietic progenitors

Pilot trials of intracoronary infusion of bone marrow progenitor cells following acute myocardial infarction

Potential use of bone marrow-derived mesenchymal stem cells for central nervous system injury, avascular osteonecrosis, other tissue injuries, and following bone marrow transplantation

Potential use of embryonic stem cells to create new tissues

References: [Abedi 2007, Brooke 2008, Bryder 2006, Fox 2007, Houghton 2004, Lakshmipathy 2005, Massa 2005, Muller 2008, Parr 2007, Ringden 2007, Schachinger 2006, Van Huyen 2008, Zeoli 2008, Zhang 2009]

relates to exactly which bone marrow stem cell (MSC vs HSC) is capable of mesenchymal and epithelial maturation [Abedi 2007, Parr 2007]. Current controversies, recent investigations, and potential new therapeutic opportunities are highlighted in **t1.5** [Abedi 2007, Brooke 2008, Bryder 2006, Fox 2007, Houghton 2004, Lakshmipathy 2005, Massa 2005, Muller 2008, Parr 2007, Ringden 2007, Schachinger 2006, Van Huyen 2008, Zeoli 2008, Zhang 2009].

[1.5] Hematopoietic Regulatory Factors

It has been known for decades that T lymphocytes, the monocyte-macrophage lineage, and other bone marrow stromal cells regulate hematopoiesis. However, the mechanisms underlying this regulation have been only recently at least partially delineated. Current evidence suggests that these disparate cell types regulate hematopoiesis via production of glycoproteins called cytokines that function as either inducers or inhibitors of hematopoiesis **t1.6** [Abbas 2007a, Hercus 2009, Lambert 2007, Metcalf 2008, Skubitz 2009, Slater 2003, Thomas 2004, Wickramasinghe 2007]. Over 30 hematopoietic cytokines have been characterized; some act primarily on hematopoietic cells, some act primarily on lymphoid cells, while others stimulate a wide variety of cell types [Abbas 2007a, Metcalf 2008]. Stimulatory cytokines include stem cell factor, colony-stimulating factors (CSFs), and various interleukins (ILs), while tumor necrosis factor (TNF)-β, transforming growth factor (TGF)-α, and macrophage inflammatory protein (MIP)-1α inhibit hematopoiesis **t1.6**. These cytokines were often named based on isolated properties that were typically detected from in vitro studies

t1.6 General Features of Hematolymphoid Growth Regulatory Factors (Cytokines)

Affect target cells by binding to cell surface receptor; when a cytokine does not bind to its receptor, the stem/progenitor cell undergoes apoptosis

Can affect target cells ranging from the most immature HSC to mature, differentiated cells

Significant synergy, overlap in function and redundancy among various cytokines

Steady state hematopoiesis is maintained by both stimulatory and inhibitory regulatory factors

Cells in a given lineage are responsive to more than one cytokine; simultaneous stimulation by a combination of cytokines may be required

Generally little overlap among cytokines that influence hematopoiesis and those that are lymphoid regulatory factors

Multiple different tissues (cells) produce the same cytokine (eg, CSFs, IL-6, IL-5 produced by many tissues)

A single cytokine can induce many different functions in target cell (eg, G-CSF has impact on proliferation, survival, differentiation commitment, and induction of maturation of immature granulocytic cells and functional activation of mature granulocytes)

A single cytokine can affect numerous different organs, tissues, and cell types demonstrating wide multisystem effects (eg, IL-11, IL-6, M-CSF)

Early acting cytokines: stem cell factor, GM-CSF, IL-1, IL-3, IL-6, and FLT3 ligand

Lineage-specific cytokines: G-CSF (granulocytes), EPO (erythroid cells), TPO (megakaryocytes), and IL-5 (eosinophils, basophils)

Inhibitory factors: TFG-β, IFN-α, TNF-α, MIP-1α, lactoferrin, transferrin, and platelet factor 4

CSF = colony-stimulating factor; IL = interleukin; M-CSF = monocyte colony-stimulating factor, GM-CSF = granulocyte-macrophage colony-stimulating factor; G-CSF = granulocyte colony-stimulating factor; FLT3 = fibroblast growth factor 3; EPO = erythropoietin; TPO = thrombopoietin; TFG = transforming growth factor; IFN = interferon; MIP = macrophage inflammatory protein

References: [Abbas 2007a, Hercus 2009, Lambert 2007, Metcalf 2008, Skubitz 2009, Slater 2003, Thomas 2004, Wickramasinghe 2007]

and may not reflect the major functions of these proteins in vivo.

Regulatory or growth factors exert their effects primarily within highly localized microenvironments of the bone marrow, and only on cells bearing specific membrane receptors. Receptor binding on immature "target" cells initiates a cascade of events that includes both cell proliferation and differentiation, while binding to mature cells characteristically enhances functional activity [Abbas 2007a, Metcalf 2008]. Most stimulatory cytokines exert their proliferative effects on committed progenitor cells (lineage-specific cytokines); early acting cytokines that influence HSC gene expression include stem cell factor, granulocyte macrophage (GM)-CSF, IL-3, and FMS-like tyrosine kinase 3 (FLT3) ligand **t1.6**.

t1.7 Selected Genes Involved in Hematopoiesis*

GATA1†	Crucial role in erythroid, megakaryocytic, mast cell, and dendritic differentiation
	Missense mutations in constitutional blood disorders
	Acquired mutations in Down syndrome-associated neoplasms
GATA2†	Maintenance and expansion of hematopoietic stem cells
	Mast cell development
SPI1/PU.1†	Positively or negatively interacts with GATA1
	Key role in mast cell, dendritic cell, granulocytic, monocytic and B-cell development
RAC1 (GTPase)	Role in hematopoietic stem cell localization
FOG1†	Friend of GATA1
	Role in erythropoiesis, megakaryopoiesis
	Essential co-regulator of GATA1
C/EBPA,E†	Crucial role in myeloid differentiation
	Mutated in various acute myeloid leukemias
	Development of megakaryocytes
CBFB†	Development of megakaryocytes, T cells, NK cells, and granulocytic cells
	Mutated in various acute myeloid leukemias
RUNX1†	Required for embryonic/fetal hematopoiesis/stem cells
	Required for granulocytic, monocytic, erythroid, megakaryocytic T- and B-cell development
	Mutated in various acute myeloid leukemias
RUNX2	Required for bone formation and osteoblast differentiation

*Both human and mouse studies
†Transcription factor

References: [Back 2004, Crispino 2005a,b, de Bruijn 2004, Elagib 2003, Fujiwara 2004, Ghiaur 2008, Gottgens 2004, Guo 2008, Gutierrez 2007, Johnson 2007, Lorsbach 2004, Metcalf 2007b, Schepers 2007, Sugiyama 2008, Tagata 2008, Talebian 2007]

[1.6] Overview of Hematopoiesis

All hematopoiesis is a developmental continuum that is regulated by the coordinated expression of many genes, some of which are presented in **t1.7**. Genes involved in hematopoiesis primarily include transcription factors. Some of these genes play a major role in the differentiation/development of multiple lineages. Mutations in these genes are linked to both constitutional disorders and neoplasms **t1.7** [Back 2004, Crispino 2005a, b, de Bruijn 2004, Elagib 2003, Fujiwara 2004, Ghiaur 2008, Gottgens 2004, Gutierrez 2007, Johnson 2007, Lorsbach 2004, Metcalf 2007b, Schepers 2007, Sugiyama 2008, Tagata 2008, Talebian 2007]. Hematopoietic cell development is characterized by the progressive loss of proliferative capacity and the gradual acquisition of biochemical, functional, and morphologic features of a specific lineage **f1.3, f1.4** [Wickramasinghe 2007].

[1.7] Hematolymphoid Lineages

[1.7.1] Granulopoiesis, Monopoiesis, and Mast Cell and Dendritic Cell Production

The granulocyte-monocyte progenitor cell is derived from the common myeloid progenitor cell and further differentiates into the monocyte/dendritic lineage, the granulocytic lineage, and the mast cell lineage **f1.3** [Bryder 2006, Metcalf 2007b, Ishikawa 2007]. The granulocytic-monocytic lineage predominates in the bone marrow; progeny of this lineage include neutrophils, eosinophils, basophils, monocytes/ macrophages, dendritic cells, and mast cells. Both early acting and lineage-specific stimulatory cytokines are essential for the production of these diverse mature cell types; specific bone marrow microenvironmental niches have been identified at least for the most numerous progeny, the neutrophil.

Neutrophils

Granulocytic precursors tend to reside adjacent to bony trabeculae, while maturing granulocytes are more centrally concentrated in the medullary cavity, forming the large maturation storage (reserve) compartment adjacent to bone marrow sinuses [Wickramasinghe 2007].

Binding of G-CSF to its surface membrane receptor triggers numerous intracellular signal transduction pathways that expand the granulocytic progenitor pool, support cell survival during differentiation, and stimulate phenotypic changes associated with maturation [Mermel 2006, Miranda 2007]. Granulocyte maturation occurs via a process of progressive nuclear segmentation with simultaneous acquisition of primary and, later, secondary (specific) cytoplasmic granules **t1.8** [Foucar 2008, Jacobsen 2007, Kierszenbaum 2002, Wickramasinghe 2007]. The earliest morphologically recognizable cell in the granulocytic lineage is the myeloblast, a cell with a large round nucleus, finely dispersed chromatin, variably prominent nucleoli, and scant to moderate amounts of pale blue cytoplasm **t1.8 i1.1, i1.2.**

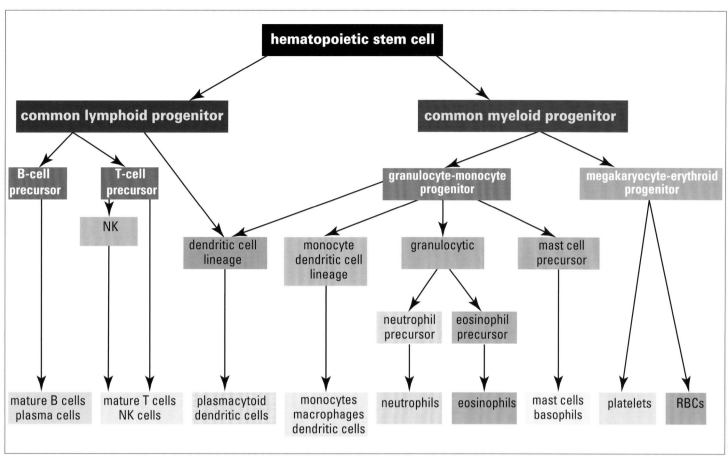

f1.3 *Stages of hematopoietic cell development starting at hematopoietic stem cell through common lymphoid and common myeloid progenitor cell stages illustrated. Note that dendritic cells may be derived from either common lymphoid or granulocyte/monocyte progenitors.* [Metcalf 2007b, Kierszenbaum 2002a, Ishikawa 2007]

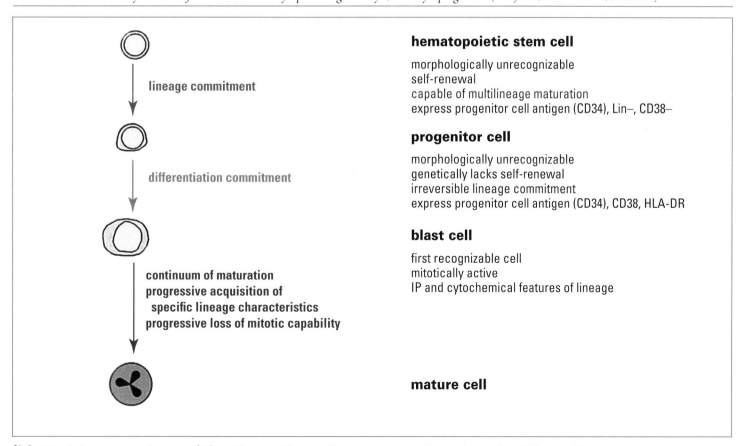

f1.4 *Morphologic, immunophenotypic (IP), and functional features of hematopoietic stem cells, progenitor cells, and blasts are illustrated.*

t1.8 Granulopoiesis

Stage of Maturation	Morphology		% in BM	Cytochemistry	Immunophenotype
Myeloblast		High nuclear-to-cytoplasmic ratio Blastic, dispersed chromatin Agranular/minimally granular cytoplasm	0-3%	MPO – to weakly + (up to 20 granules) α-naphthol chloroacetate esterase – to weakly +	CD34+, HLA-DR+, myeloid ag+
Promyelocyte		Eccentric nucleus with prominent paranuclear hof (pale zone) Sparse, concentrated primary granules	1%-4%	MPO+, lysozyme+, α-naphthol chloroacetate+	CD34–, HLA-DR–, myeloid ag+
Neutrophilic myelocyte		Round nucleus with condensed chromatin Moderate to abundant secondary (specific) granules, which produce a finely granular pink cytoplasm	12%-22%	MPO+, lysozyme+, α-naphthol chloroacetate+, leukocyte alkaline phosphatase+	CD34–, HLA-DR–, myeloid ag+
Neutrophilic metamyelocyte		Indented nucleus, condensed chromatin Cytoplasm packed with granules with predominance of secondary granules	12%-22%	MPO+, lysozyme+, α-naphthol chloroacetate+, leukocyte alkaline phosphatase+	CD34–, HLA-DR–, myeloid ag+
Band neutrophil		Horseshoe-shaped mature nucleus lacking discrete indentations Cytoplasm packed mostly with secondary granules; gelatinous (tertiary) granules also present	5%-14%	MPO+, lysozyme+, α-naphthol chloroacetate+, leukocyte alkaline phosphatase+	CD34–, HLA-DR–, myeloid ag+
Neutrophil		3-5 discrete nuclear lobes (joined by a thin chromatin strand) Highly condensed chromatin Cytoplasm packed with granules with predominance of secondary granules; gelatinous (tertiary) granules also present	9%-20%	MPO+, lysozyme+, α-naphthol chloroacetate+, leukocyte alkaline phosphatase+	CD34–, HLA-DR–, myeloid ag+

BM = bone marrow; MPO = myeloperoxidase

References: [Foucar 2008, Kierszenbaum 2002, Wickramasinghe 2007]

Variable, but sparse, primary cytoplasmic granules may be present i1.3. Although primary granules contain many enzymes, myeloperoxidase is the one most useful for cell identification i1.4. Myeloblasts express CD34, HLA-DR, CD117, myeloid antigens such as CD33, and CD13.

The subsequent morphologic stages of granulocytic maturation include promyelocyte, myelocyte, metamyelocyte, band, and the segmented granulocyte t1.8 i1.5, i1.6. The promyelocyte is the largest granulocytic cell and is characterized by a large, usually eccentric, nucleus with a prominent nucleolus, moderate amounts of cytoplasm containing easily recognizable azurophilic primary granules, and a paranuclear hof or Golgi region. The time of expression of granule proteins determines whether these proteins are primary granule constituents (proteins expressed during promyelocyte stage of maturation) or secondary granule constituents (proteins expressed at myelocyte/metamyelocyte stage) [Jacobsen 2007]. CD34 and HLA-DR expression is gradually lost, while promyelocytes retain CD13 and CD33.

Complex transcription programs govern terminal granulocyte maturation [Theilgaard-Monch 2005]. Progression of nuclear condensation leads to the development of the myelocyte; this is the last maturation stage with proliferative potential t1.8. Secondary granule formation is characteristic of this stage of maturation and is evidenced by the progressive acidophilia of the cytoplasm, beginning in the Golgi region i1.6, i1.7, i1.8. These neutrophil secondary granules contain lactoferrin, vitamin B_{12}-binding protein, proteases, and lysozyme.

Nuclear indentation is characteristic of a metamyelocyte. At this stage of maturation, secondary granules outnumber primary granules and the cytoplasm is uniformly acidophilic.

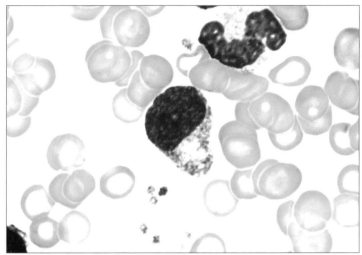

i1.1 *Myeloblast on bone marrow aspirate smear. (Wright)*

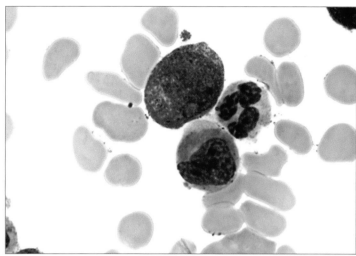

i1.2 *Myeloblast on bone marrow aspirate smear showing occasional cytoplasmic granules. (Wright)*

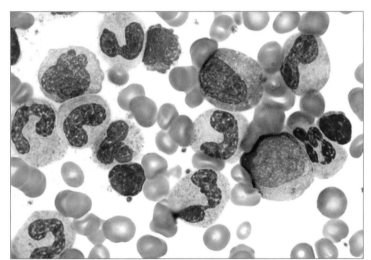

i1.3 *Myeloblast with primary granules in Golgi region (lower right) in conjunction with subsequent stages of granulocytic maturation on bone marrow aspirate smear. (Wright)*

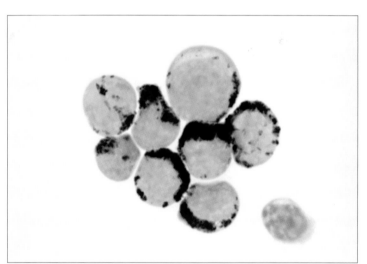

i1.4 *Myeloperoxidase cytochemical stain in maturing granulocytic cells illustrates spectrum of positivity linked to maturation. (cytochemical stain)*

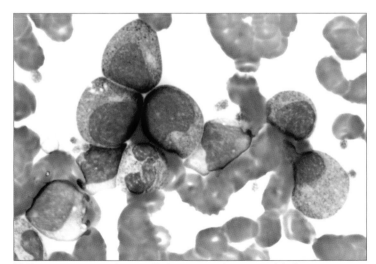

i1.5 *Immature granulocytic cells dominate in this region of the bone marrow aspirate smear. (Wright)*

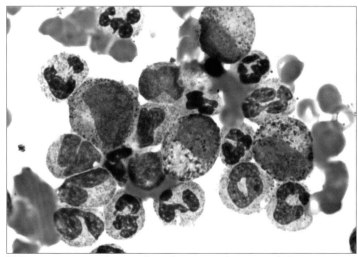

i1.6 *Maturing granulocytic cells predominate in this region of a bone marrow aspirate smear. (Wright)*

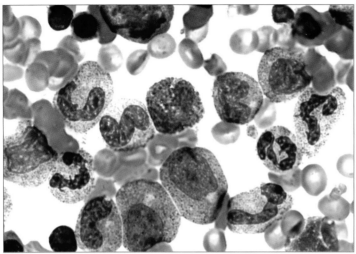

i1.7 *Bone marrow aspirate smear showing stages of granulocytic maturation. Note predominance of secondary granules in mature cells. (Wright)*

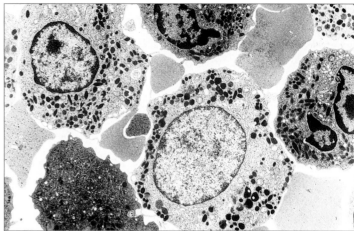

i1.8 *Electron micrograph illustrates the wealth of granules that fill the cytoplasm of developing myeloid cells. Although primary and secondary granules have slightly different ultrastructural features, in general, ultrastructural cytochemical stains are required for their delineation. Secondary granules predominate within the cytoplasm of myelocyte and segmented neutrophils.*

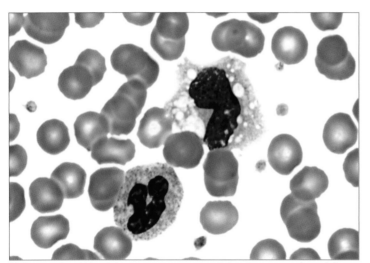

i1.9 *Peripheral blood showing mature neutrophil and monocyte. (Wright)*

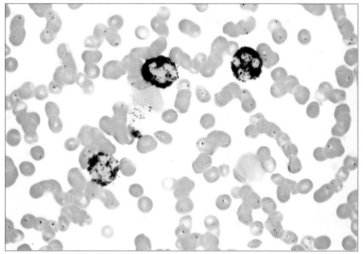

i1.10 *Myeloperoxidase cytochemical stain on peripheral blood shows strong positivity in neutrophils and very weak positivity in monocytes. (cytochemical stain)*

The nucleus assumes a horseshoe configuration at the band stage of maturation, while discrete nuclear segmentations define the mature segmented granulocyte. Morphologic distinction between a band and a mature granulocyte is arbitrary. During terminal maturation, tertiary granules form, which contain arginase and gelatinase [Jacobsen 2007].

Metamyelocytes, bands, and segmented granulocytes comprise the large maturation-storage compartment of the bone marrow, which can be released into the circulation in response to acute stress, infection, and other host challenges. Granulocytes pass through the bone marrow sinus wall, through endothelial cell cytoplasm, and into the circulation. Granulocytes and precursors are retained in the bone marrow by both surface chemokines and adhesion molecules. Downregulation of chemokine receptor expression is linked to neutrophil release into circulation [Eash 2009, Moser 2004,

Theilgaard-Monch 2005]. Other factors linked to neutrophil release include modulation of complement receptors, leukotriene, and adhesion molecule expression [Burdon 2005].

Segmented granulocytes circulate in the peripheral blood only a few hours before they egress into tissues **i1.9**, **i1.10**. Within the peripheral blood, neutrophils can reside in either the circulating or the marginated pools; these pools are of approximately equal size. Because the granulocytes of the marginated pool are attached to endothelial cells, only the cells in the circulating pool are acquired in venous blood samples. Following adherence to endothelial cells, neutrophils rapidly pass through the vessel wall and into tissues. The life span of these cells in tissues is unknown.

Maintenance of neutrophil homeostasis is critical, and blood neutrophil levels are maintained by release of the bone marrow maturation storage compartment and bone marrow

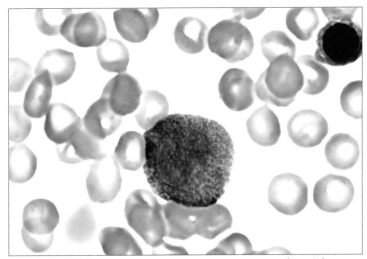

i1.11 *Eosinophilic myelocyte in bone marrow aspirate smear. (Wright)*

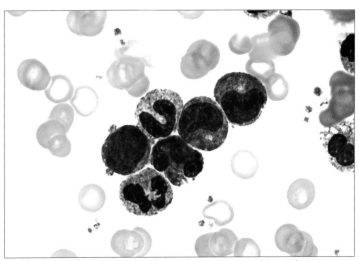

i1.12 *Eosinophil evident in bone marrow aspirate smear. (Wright)*

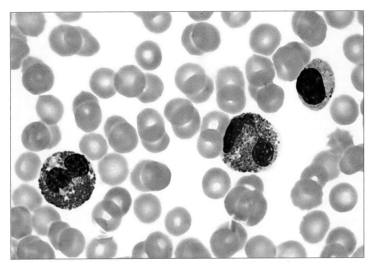

i1.13 *Peripheral blood showing mature eosinophilia. (Wright)*

neutrophil production [Mermel 2006]. In homeostatic states, the bone marrow produces $1\text{-}2 \times 10^9$ granulocytes per kilogram per day [Mermel 2006].

Eosinophils

Eosinophils provide the first line of defense against invading parasites and modulate immediate hypersensitivity reactions initiated by basophil/mast cell degranulation [Abbas 2007b]. Eosinophils are derived from a common granulocyte monocyte progenitor cell [Metcalf 2007a]. In addition to general multilineage proliferative factors such as IL-3 and GM-CSF, selective eosinophil growth factors include IL-5 [Tefferi 2006]. Eosinophils are recognized by their distinctive refractile secondary granules which contain major basic protein, eosinophil peroxidase, histaminase, arylsulfatase, and eosinophil cationic protein **i1.11**, **i1.12**, **i1.13** [Kierszenbaum 2002,

Wickramasinghe 2007]. Eosinophil cationic protein neutralizes heparin released from basophils, while histaminase and arylsulfatase also modulate immediate hypersensitivity reactions [Kierszenbaum 2002, Wickramasinghe 2007].

Basophils and Mast Cells

Although controversial, basophils and mast cells are thought by some investigators to be progeny of a common precursor cell that is derived from granulocyte/monocyte progenitor cells **i1.14**, **i1.15** [Metcalf 2007a]. Mast cells reside in tissues and play a prominent role in many biologic processes including initiation of allergic responses, activation during parasitic infections, and innate, protective immune responses to microbial pathogens **i1.16** [Obata 2007, von Kockritz-Blickwede 2008]. Mast cells may serve as a "hinge" between innate and adaptive immunity [Heib 2008]. Both cell types play a role in initiating allergic and hypersensitivity reactions by granule and mediator release [Abbas 2007b, Didichenko 2008, Obata 2007]. Granule contents include histamine, heparin, tryptase, and chymase **i1.17** [Heib 2008, Obata 2007]. Upon activation, mast cells produce IL-3, IL-5, and various lipid mediators, in addition to the release of granule contents [Abbas 2007b, Didichenko 2008]. Stem cell factor (the ligand for *c-kit*, CD117) is a key mast cell growth factor, while IL-3 plays a key role in basophil production and in prolonged basophil survival [Abbas 2007b, Didichenko 2008, Escribano 2006, Heib 2008, Obata 2007]. Basophil secondary granules are coarse, dark blue-black, and often overlay the segmented nucleus. Mast cell nuclei are round, and mast cell granules impart a dense purple-black appearance to the cytoplasm, often obscuring the nucleus (see **i1.15** and **i1.16**). Immunohistochemical stains useful in the identification of mast cells include CD117 and tryptase (see **i1.17**). Unlike mature basophils, mast cells are capable of mitosis [Obata 2007, Wickramasinghe 2007].

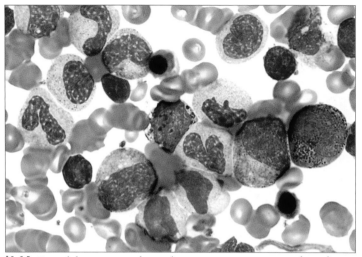

i1.14 *Basophil precursor evident on bone marrow aspirate smear (center). (Wright)*

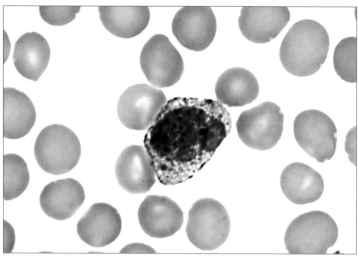

i1.15 *Basophil in peripheral blood. (Wright)*

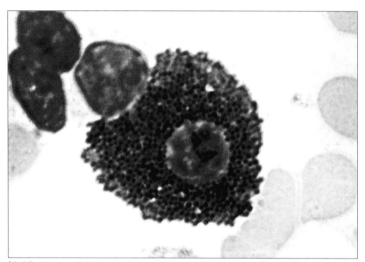

i1.16 *Mast cell present on bone marrow aspirate smear. (Wright)*

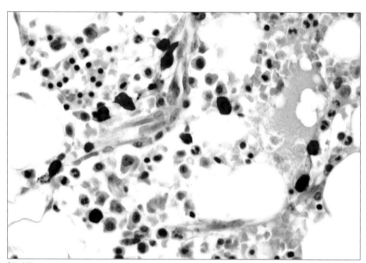

i1.17 *Mast cells adjacent to blood vessels and dispersed within bone marrow parenchyma highlighted by immunoperoxidase for tryptase on bone marrow core biopsy. (immunoperoxidase)*

Monocytes/Macrophages/Dendritic Cells

Monocytes are derived from granulocyte/monocyte progenitor cells. Monocyte CSF is instrumental in influencing these progenitor cells to differentiate into monocyte-macrophages [Sugimoto 2006]. In addition to phagocytic activity, mature monocytes and histiocytes (macrophages and dendritic, that is, specialized immune accessory cells) produce a plethora of cytokines that have potent regulatory activities in hematopoiesis, inflammatory states, and diverse immune reactions [Haller Hasskamp 2005]. The stages of monocyte maturation have been designated as monoblast, promonocyte, and mature monocyte, and are characterized by gradual nuclear folding and the acquisition of cytoplasmic granules that are positive for α-naphthyl acetate and α-naphthyl butyrate, both esterase stains **i1.18, i1.19, i1.20** [Taylor 2009]. However, monoblasts are not generally recognizable

in normal bone marrow, and promonocytes are present in low numbers and may overlap morphologically with the more predominant granulocytic cells [Wickramasinghe 2007]. Monocytes commonly express HLA-DR, CD14, and CD4 on their cell surface, in addition to other myeloid antigens such as CD13 and CD33. Immunohistochemical stains reasonably specific for monocytes/macrophages include CD163 and CD68 (PGM1 clone) [Lau 2004, Nguyen 2005]. Activated macrophages can express tartrate-resistant acid phosphatase [Janckila 2007]. The time required for monocyte maturation and development is not well understood. Mature monocyte-macrophage lineage cells remain as a major constituent of the bone marrow microenvironment and also migrate to all organs of the body. Within bone marrow, macrophages are concentrated in particles on bone marrow aspirate smears **i1.21**. On tissue sections, macrophages are dispersed throughout the medullary cavity.

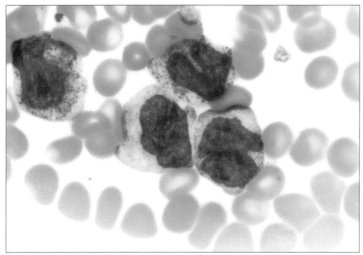

i1.18 *A cluster of monocytes within the bone marrow aspirate smear. Monocyte development is characterized by progressive maturation with condensation of nuclear chromatin and folding of the nucleus. The cytoplasm is abundant and blue-gray in appearance, and may be finely granulated or vacuolated. The 2 monocytes on the bottom of the cluster have a more finely dispersed nuclear chromatin pattern and are therefore less mature than the upper monocyte. (Wright)*

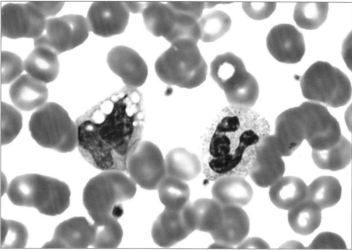

i1.19 *Monocyte with features of activation present in addition to neutrophil in peripheral blood smear. (Wright)*

Immunohistochemical techniques can highlight morphologically inconspicuous macrophages, which are often stellate **i1.22**. Monocytes circulate in the blood for approximately 20 hours before migrating to tissue to become fixed macrophages [Kierszenbaum 2002].

Myeloid dendritic cells are closely related to monocytes and are derived from a common stem/progenitor cell, while plasmacytoid dendritic cells are likely derived from either lymphoid or common myeloid precursors (see **sidebar 19.1**) [Ishikawa 2007, Manz 2001, Wu 2007, Zhang 2007]. Dendritic cells circulate in very low numbers (0.1%-1.0% of blood mononuclear cells)

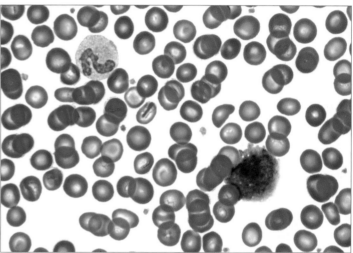

i1.20 *Nonspecific esterase cytochemical stain shows prominent cytoplasmic positivity in monocyte while neutrophil is negative. (cytochemical stain)*

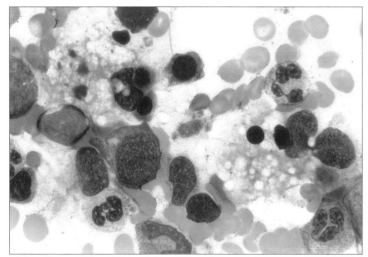

i1.21 *2 mature macrophages demonstrate the voluminous cytoplasm with ingested material that characterizes these cells on a bone marrow aspirate smear. Note the mature nuclear chromatin pattern of the nuclei of these 2 macrophages. (Wright)*

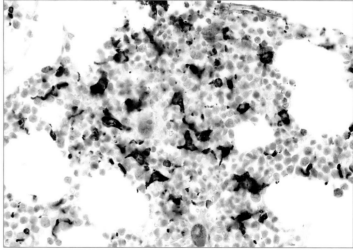

i1.22 *Immunoperoxidase for CD68 shows numerous macrophages with stellate cytoplasmic processes in bone marrow core biopsy section. (immunoperoxidase)*

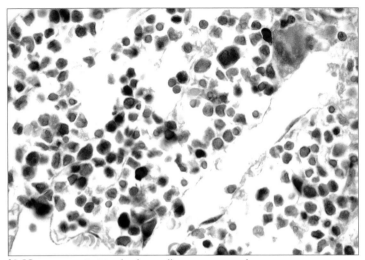

i1.23 *Very rare S100+ dendritic cells present on core biopsy section. (immunoperoxidase)*

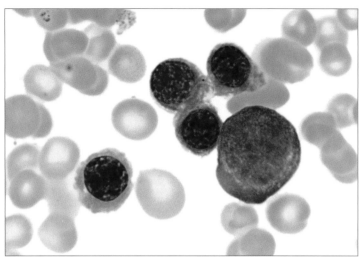

i1.24 *An erythroblast with both basophilic and orthochromic normoblasts is shown on this bone marrow aspirate smear. Note the large nuclear size, nuclear immaturity, and relatively high nuclear-cytoplasmic ratio of the erythroblast. (Wright)*

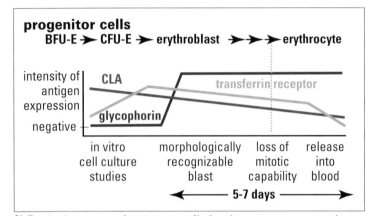

f1.5 *The changes in surface antigen profile that characterize maturation from erythroid progenitor cells to the mature erythrocyte are shown. Expression of common leukocyte antigen (CLA) progressively declines throughout this maturation process. Likewise, expression of the transferrin receptor also declines, while glycophorin expression increases dramatically with maturation from progenitor cells to the erythroblast stage of differentiation. BFU = burst-forming unit; CFU = colony-forming unit; E = erythroid.*

[Haller Hasskamp 2005, Merad 2009]. Dendritic cells migrate from blood to reside in all tissues. Because dendritic cells are inconspicuous on morphologic review, immunohistochemical techniques are required for cell identification **i1.23**. Common antigens expressed in dendritic cell subsets include CD1a, S100, CD123, CD23, and CD35 [Pileri 2002]. Dendritic cells are potent antigen-presenting cells capable of initiating a primary innate immune response [Merad 2009, Wu 2007, Zhang 2007].

Osteoclasts (see [1.7.5] "Bone Development" on page 22) and monocyte/macrophages have a common progenitor, confirming the hematopoietic stem cell derivation of these bone resorbing cells [Wickramasinghe 2007].

[1.7.2] **Erythropoiesis**

Erythrocyte production rates are remarkable; current estimates indicate that about 2 million reticulocytes are produced every second [Lee 2004]. As expected, exquisite control of RBC production is essential, and homeostasis is maintained by the balance between RBC production and RBC destruction [Chasis 2008, Rubiolo 2006, Testa 2004].

Megakaryocytes and erythroid cells are derived from a common bipotent progenitor [Klimchenko 2009]. In addition to early-acting cytokines (stem cell factor, FLT3 ligand), the lineage-specific cytokine responsible for erythropoiesis is erythropoietin (EPO), a protein that is produced both by renal cells in response to hypoxia and within the bone marrow (see **sidebar 9.1**) [Testa 2004]. Erythropoietin is a glycoprotein that is essential for the proliferation, differentiation, and survival of erythroid cells by delaying apoptosis (programmed cell death) [Chasis 2008, Rubiolo 2006, Testa 2004]. Like all growth factors, EPO activity is dependent on binding to specific cell surface receptors (EPOR); the binding of EPO to EPOR activates signal transduction pathways via JAK2 activation, resulting in a cascade of cytoplasmic and nuclear events. EPORs are present in highest numbers on erythroid progenitor cells and proerythroblasts, but are absent on mature erythrocytes [Rubiolo 2006]. Negative regulatory feedback is achieved via multiple pathways including heme (a major protein in mature erythrocytes) inhibition and actions of TNF-α and GATA1, while TGF-β also perturbs erythropoiesis in various ways [Chasis 2008].

The earliest morphologically recognizable cell in the erythroid lineage is the pronormoblast (also called erythroblast in this book) **i1.24**. These immature erythroid cells express transferrin receptors and glycophorin **f1.5**.

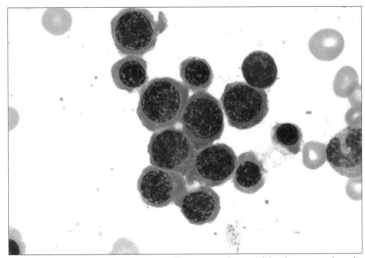

i1.25 *Bone marrow aspirate smear illustrates a cluster of developing erythroid precursors, including basophilic normoblasts, polychromatophilic normoblasts, and orthochromic normoblasts. Note the progressive decrease in overall nuclear size, and the gradual change from deeply basophilic to pink cytoplasm that characterizes gradual hemoglobin production within these cells. (Wright)*

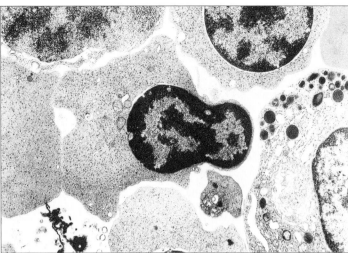

i1.26 *Ultrastructural photomicrograph shows ejection of the nucleus from an orthochromic normoblast. Once this ejection is complete, a reticulocyte will result.*

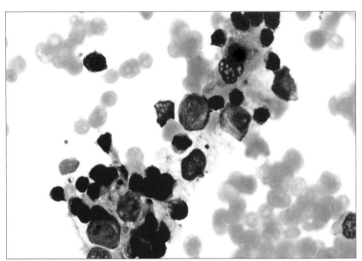

i1.27 *Attachment of developing erythroid cells to macrophages highlighted in this bone marrow aspirate smear. (Wright)*

The subsequent maturational process has been arbitrarily subdivided into the basophilic normoblast, polychromatophilic normoblast, orthochromic normoblast, reticulocyte, and mature erythrocyte stages **i1.25** [Wickramasinghe 2007]. This maturational process is characterized by progressive nuclear condensation with ultimate extrusion of the pyknotic nucleus at the end of the orthochromic normoblast stage **i1.26**. The process of erythroblast enucleation is complex requiring sorting of plasma membrane with formation of a plasma membrane around the pyknotic nucleus, while simultaneously maintaining the reticulocyte plasma membrane [Lee 2004]. These extruded nuclei bind to receptors on resident macrophages and subsequently undergo phagocytosis; the unique erythroid island configuration in bone marrow is the result of erythroblast-macrophage contact mediated by numerous adhesion molecules including CD163 expression on macrophages, which binds to an erythroid cell ligand **i1.27**, see also **i1.21** [Fabriek 2007, Rhodes 2008]. The essential role of this central macrophage in supporting erythropoiesis is well-documented [Chasis 2008]. Simultaneously with the nuclear changes described above, the cytoplasm gradually changes from a deeply basophilic, organelle-rich substance to one that consists almost entirely of hemoglobin. Adequate hemoglobin production is intimately linked to iron homeostasis, and the iron necessary for hemoglobin production can be acquired by developing normoblasts via surface transferrin receptors or via the direct transference of iron from the central macrophage to adherent normoblasts [Andrews 2008, Chasis 2008]. Expression of both common leukocyte and transferrin receptor antigens progressively declines with maturation, while glycophorin expression remains high throughout erythroid lineage maturation **f1.5**.

The erythroblast, basophilic normoblast, and early polychromatophilic normoblast are capable of mitotic division; erythroid cells normally exhibit the highest proliferation rate in the bone marrow [Testa 2004]. Once the nucleus has been extruded, only limited biochemical activity can occur, sufficient for the production of the final 20% of hemoglobin, degradation of internal organelles, reduction in plasma membrane, and maintenance of the cell membrane [Koury 2005]. Reticulocytes pass through the bone marrow sinus wall and endothelial cells into the circulating blood, where they mature and survive for approximately 120 days. Under steady-state conditions, approximately $2\text{-}4 \times 10^9$ erythrocytes are produced per kilogram per day [Lee 2004]. Under basal conditions, reticulocyte production rates range from 40,000-80,000/mL per day.

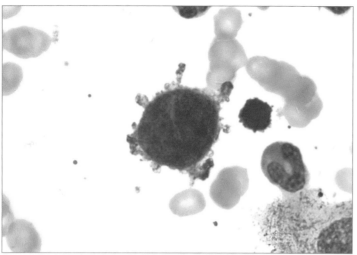

i1.28 *Bone marrow aspirate smear illustrates immature megakaryocytes. Note high nuclear/cytoplasmic ratio and cytoplasmic blebbing. (Wright)*

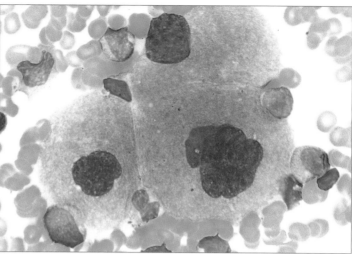

i1.29 *Mature megakaryocytes exhibit highly folded nuclei and voluminous, finely granular cytoplasm on this bone marrow aspirate smear. (Wright)*

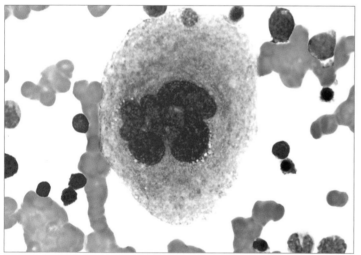

i1.30 *Hyperlobulation of megakaryocyte nuclei (endomytosis) is a characteristic feature of maturing megakaryocyte on bone marrow aspirate smear. (Wright)*

[1.7.3] **Megakaryocytopoiesis**

Although megakaryocytes comprise only 0.05% of nucleated cells in the bone marrow, more than a million platelets are produced every second [Italiano Jr 2008, Tomer 2004]. Furthermore, a normal adult produces 10^{11} platelets daily, and this can be increased 20-fold in response to physiologic demand [Deutsch 2006, Geddis 2007, Kaushansky 2008]. Megakaryocytes are derived from a megakaryocyte/erythroid progenitor cell that is the progeny of the common myeloid progenitor cell (see **f1.3**) [Deutsch 2006, Kaushansky 2008].

The regulatory factors that are currently recognized to influence megakaryopoiesis can be segregated into 2 general groups:

1. early-acting multilineage cytokines such as stem cell factor, GM-CSF, and IL-3

2. the megakaryocyte-specific cytokine, thrombopoietin (TPO) [Kaushansky 2008]

Thrombopoietin is produced by bone marrow stromal cells, hepatocytes, and proximal tubular epithelial cells in the kidney; regulation of TPO production is incompletely understood with mutually exclusive proposed models suggesting that TPO production is either constitutive or regulated [Kaushansky 2008, McCrann 2009]. TPO binds to c-Mpl receptors on platelets and megakaryocytes, so one model proposes that plasma levels of TPO are reduced when the platelet/megakaryocyte mass of c-Mpl receptors is increased, and vice versa [Kaushansky 2008].

The earliest stages of megakaryopoiesis have been determined largely through cell culture analyses, and such terms as burst-forming unit (BFU) and colony-forming unit (CFU) megakaryocyte have been applied to these cell cultures [Tomer 2004]. The earliest morphologically/immunologically recognizable megakaryocyte precursor, a megakaryoblast, is characterized by a high nuclear-to-cytoplasmic ratio, a non-lobulated nucleus, and surface antigen expression of platelet glycoproteins, CD41 and CD42b [Tomer 2004]. Cytoplasmic blebbing may be evident **i1.28**.

During maturation, megakaryocyte precursors switch from mitosis to endomitosis/polyploidization characterized by ongoing DNA synthesis with failure of cytokinesis, resulting in progressive nuclear lobulation with increasing DNA content and even greater increases in megakaryocyte cytoplasm [Lordier 2008, Deutsch 2006, McCrann 2009, Muntean 2007, Raslova 2006, Tomer 2004]. The nuclei do not separate into distinct separate lobes, but instead progressively fold and lobulate while remaining connected **i1.29**. The resulting amplification of the cytoplasm provides an efficient way to increase megakaryoctye mass and consequently increase platelet

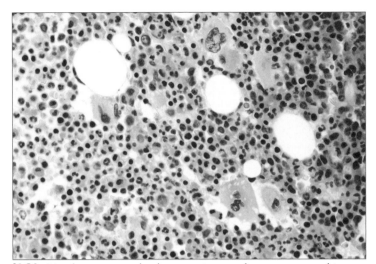

i1.31 *Megakaryocytes reside adjacent to sinuses on bone marrow core biopsy section. (H&E)*

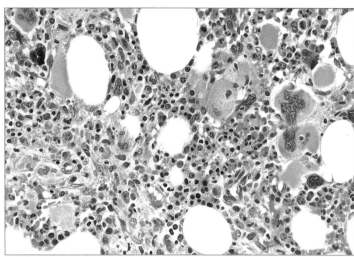

i1.32 *Neutrophils within megakaryocyte cytoplasm—so-called emperipolesis. (H&E)*

production **i1.30** [Raslova 2006]. Although not generally appreciated on routine biopsy sections, megakaryocytes reside adjacent to bone marrow sinuses and project pseudopodia (proplatelets) through these sinus walls, allowing for direct shedding of platelets into the circulation **i1.31**. Platelet shedding is achieved by expansion of the surface membrane and cytoskeletal rearrangements [Geddis 2007, Schulze 2006, Wickramasinghe 2007]. Because of this unique architectural localization, other cell types, especially neutrophils, may migrate through the megakaryocyte tubular systems to gain access to the peripheral circulation. This phenomenon has been termed "emperipolesis" **i1.32** [Wickramasinghe 2007].

Although multilobulated megakaryocytes are easily recognized on bone marrow aspirate smears and biopsy sections, the identification of megakaryoblasts and other immature megakaryocytes generally requires the application of immunophenotypic techniques. The 2 most useful techniques are immunophenotyping analyses for surface and cytoplasmic antigens unique to the megakaryocytic lineage and ultrastructural cytochemical studies for platelet peroxidase activity [Wickramasinghe 2007, Tomer 2004]. Megakaryoblasts, other immature forms, and megakaryocytes generally express surface and cytoplasmic CD31, CD41, CD42b, and CD61 **i1.33** [Tomer 2004]. However, caution should be exercised in the flow cytometric immunophenotyping of cells for expression of these antigens, since platelets adherent to blasts can give false-positive results [Betz 1992].

Subsequent maturation stages have been designated as basophilic megakaryocyte, granular megakaryocyte, and platelet-producing megakaryocyte. Megakaryocyte maturation occurs in 3 successive steps—proliferation, polyploidization, and cytoplasmic maturation, characterized by a progressive increase in overall cell size, increased nuclear lobulations, increased DNA content, and the development of

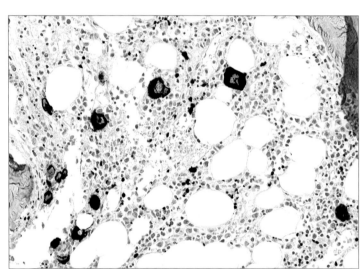

i1.33 *Normal megakaryocytes highlighted by immunoperoxidase staining for CD42b on bone marrow core biopsy section. (immunoperoxidase)*

demarcation membranes and multiple types of cytoplasmic granules (see **i1.28**, **i1.29**, **i1.30**) [Raslova 2007].

Successive megakaryocyte maturation is associated with the acquisition of additional surface platelet glycoproteins, such as Ib, IIb, and von Willebrand factor, as well as other proteins [Tomer 2004]. Within the cytoplasm, 4 types of granules (α, δ, γ, peroxisomes) are produced, each containing multiple enzymes and other types of proteins essential for platelet function [Wickramasinghe 2007]. As mentioned above, platelets fragment off of megakaryocyte pseudopods directly into the circulation [Geddis 2007]. Megakaryocytes may also circulate. Under physiologic conditions, increased numbers of circulating platelets are associated with increased binding of thrombopoietin (TPO), resulting in reduced TPO to stimulate bone marrow megakaryocytic precursor cells. Approximately $2\text{-}4 \times 10^9$ platelets per kilogram are produced daily, and platelet survival in the peripheral blood is approximately 10 days; platelet production can be increased 20-fold in accelerated platelet destruction states [Deutsch 2006, Geddis 2007, Kaushansky 2008]. Platelet factor 4 is a negative autocrine regulator of platelet production, key to platelet/megakaryocyte homeostasis [Lambert 2007].

[1.7.4] **Lymphopoiesis (B-, T-, Natural Killer Cells)**

Although a detailed review of the immune system is beyond the scope of this book, lymphopoiesis and the bone marrow factors that enhance B-cell, T-cell, or natural killer (NK) cell production will be reviewed briefly. In addition, the role of T/NK cells in the regulation of hematopoiesis will be highlighted. T, NK, and B lymphocytes are derived from the same stem cells that give rise to all hematopoietic elements after the maturation of these multipotent progenitors into common lymphoid progenitor cells [Hoebeke 2007, Haddad 2004, Luc 2008a, Mansson 2008]. Early B- and T-cell development is stimulated primarily by IL-7 [Abbas 2007c, Hoebeke 2007, Payne 2007]. Factors that influence B-cell proliferation, differentiation, and/or functional activities include IL-1, IL-2, IL-4, IL-5, IL-6, IL-7, IL-10, IL-11, adhesion molecules, and interferon gamma, while analogous T-cell factors include IL-1 to IL-10 and IL-15 [Abbas 2007c, Cornish 2006, Rossi 2003, Wickramasinghe 2007]. In addition, the Notch signaling pathway plays a key role in the production of T cells from common lymphoid progenitor cells [Maillard 2005]. Both stem cell factor and IL-15 are required for NK-cell development and differentiation [Benson 2009]. The bone marrow microenvironment serves as the "bursal equivalent" in humans, and is the primary site of postnatal B-cell development, while T/NK-cell precursors migrate from the marrow to the thymus for maturation and differentiation [Hao 2008, Schonland 2003, Veinotte 2008]. Antigenically mature T and B cells can proliferate in response to various cytokines [Jiang 2006, Peggs 2005]. T cells are long-lived and migrate among blood, bone marrow, thymus, and other solid organs throughout their life span [Wei 2006].

The stages of maturation of both B and T lymphocytes are generally defined by the surface antigen profile rather

t1.9 B-Cell Maturation

B-Cell Precursor Stages				Pre-B Cell	Mature B	Plasma Cell
TdT	TdT	TdT	vTdT	vTdT	HLA-DR	CIg
HLA-DR	HLA-DR	HLA-DR	HLA-DR	HLA-DR	CD19	CD38
CD34	CD34	vCD34	CD19	CD19	CD20	vCD79a
CD79a	CD19	CD19	CD10	CD10	SIg	vCD20
vCD45	vCD10	CD10	CD20	CD20	CD22	vCD45
CD43	cCD22	CD22	CD22	Cmu	CD79a	
	CD79a	CD79a	CD79a	CD22	CD79b	
	wCD45	wCD45	wCD45	CD79a	CD45	
	CD43	CD43	CD43	CD45		
				vCD43		

c = cytoplasmic expression; CIg = cytoplasmic immunoglobulin; SIg = surface immunoglobulin; TdT = terminal deoxynucleotidyl transferase; v = variable expression; w = weak expression

References: [Abbas 2007c, Hardy 2007, LeBien 2008, Rossi 2003]

t1.10 T-Cell Maturation

T-Cell Precursors in Bone Marrow*	Thymic Maturation Stages				Mature T Cell
CD34	CD34	vCD34	CD2	CD2	CD2
CD2	CD2	CD2	CD5	CD5	CD5
CD5	CD5	CD5	CD7	CD7	CD7
CD7	CD7	CD7	cCD3	CD3	CD3
CD38	CD38	CD38	CD1	CD1	CD4 or CD8
TdT	cCD3	cCD3	CD4,8	CD4,8	CD45
vCD3	TdT	CD1	CD45	CD45	
vcCD1	vCD1	CD4,8			
wCD45	wCD45	vTdT			
		wCD45			

*Represents 1% of CD34+ cells in pediatric bone marrow specimens
c = cytoplasmic expression; TdT = terminal deoxynucleotidyl transferase; v = variable expression; w = weak expression

References: [Abbas 2007c, Bendelac 2007, Zhu 2008]

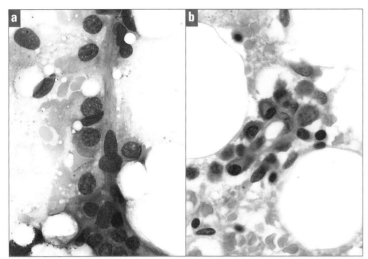

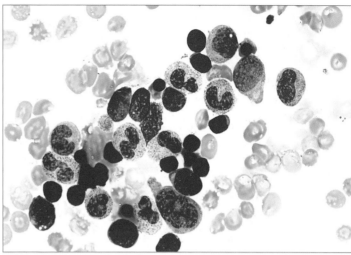

i1.34 *The perivascular localization of normal bone marrow plasma cells is evident on both aspirate smears* **a** *and biopsy sections* **b**. *(Wright; H&E)*

i1.35 *Abundant lymphoid cells with features of hematogones present on bone marrow aspirate smear from 13-day-old male infant. (Wright)*

than by morphologic features **t1.9, t1.10** [Abbas 2007c, Hardy 2007, Lucio 1999, Rossi 2003]. The earliest immunologically recognizable B cells express nuclear terminal deoxynucleotidyl transferase (TdT), surface CD34 (progenitor cell antigen), CD79a, and HLA-DR [Hardy 2007, Lucio 1999, Rossi 2003]. Many B-cell precursors also coexpress CD10. Further maturation is characterized by the acquisition of cytoplasmic mu heavy chain and, later, surface immunoglobulin. Under steady-state conditions, the B-cell precursors account for a very low percentage of the total bone marrow mononuclear cells in adults, even though they are physiologically much more numerous in very young children [Rossi 2003]. Plasma cells are the morphologically defined endpoint in the B-lymphocyte differentiation sequence; these terminally differentiated B cells are responsible for the humoral immune response [Medina 2002, Odendahl 2005]. Plasma cells are morphologically distinctive and typically comprise <5% of bone marrow cells. Plasma cells have eccentric round nuclei, abundant basophilic cytoplasm, and a paranuclear pale hof. Normally, plasma cells reside adjacent to vessels as well as individually dispersed in the medullary space **i1.34**.

A minority of the TdT-positive immature lymphocytes are T-cell precursors **t1.10**. T-cell maturation is characterized by the presence of cytoplasmic and, later, surface CD3, in conjunction with the expression of many other T-cell–associated antigens [Abbas 2007c, Bendelac 2007]. Terminal maturation is defined by the development of either a helper or a suppressor surface antigen profile.

Although the terms "lymphoblast" and "prolymphocyte" have been applied to developing lymphoid cells and are used in leukemia classification, these cell types are not recognized in normal bone marrow specimens. The term "lymphoblast" is used almost exclusively to describe neoplastic cells; therefore, alternate terms such as "lymphocyte precursor cells" are recommended for non-neoplastic cells.

As emphasized in Chapter 21, normal lymphoid precursors, so-called hematogones, can be morphologically identified in pediatric bone marrow specimens because of their highly condensed nuclear chromatin, inconspicuous nucleoli, and scant cytoplasm **i1.35**. However, distinct stages of lymphocyte maturation are not typically appreciated in normal bone marrow. Similarly, the time required for lymphopoiesis under steady-state conditions is not well-delineated. Lymphocytes migrate from blood to specific tissue sites throughout the body, selectively homing to B- or T-cell regions of lymph node, spleen, and widespread extranodal regions. T lymphocytes are characteristically long-lived and periodically recirculate.

Natural killer (NK) cells are thought to be closely related to T cells, and indeed, mature CD8+ cytotoxic suppressor T cells and NK cells are morphologically indistinguishable large granular lymphocytes [Bendelac 2007]. Similar to T cells, NK cells play a critical role in the regulation of hematopoiesis [Kotsianidis 2006]. NK cells are unique among mature hematopoietic cells in that they were initially defined by a functional activity, preceding a delineation of either morphologic or immunophenotypic characteristics [Caligiuri 2008]. This distinctive functional activity is major histocompatibility complex-nonrestricted cytotoxicity, but these cells were subsequently found to exhibit many other activities. For example, NK cells produce various cytokines (IL-1, IL-2, IL-4, CSFs, and interferons) that influence both hematopoiesis and many immune functions including innate immune responses to viruses and some other intracellular organisms [Bendelac 2007, Caligiuri 2008, Farag 2006, Karadimitris 2006, Kotsianidis 2006, Trotta 2005]. Although bone marrow-derived, NK cells mature in solid tissue sites such as lymph node after the migration of precursor cells in the circulation [Caligiuri 2008]. Some maturing NK cells recirculate while others remain in peripheral lymphoid organs.

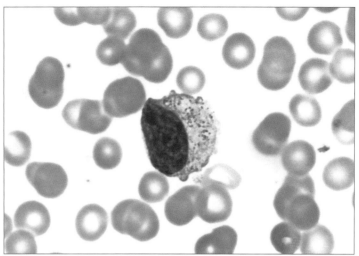

i1.36 *Peripheral blood smear shows a typical large granular lymphocyte. The nucleus exhibits condensed nuclear chromatin, while the abundant cytoplasm contains distinct azurophilic granules. (Wright)*

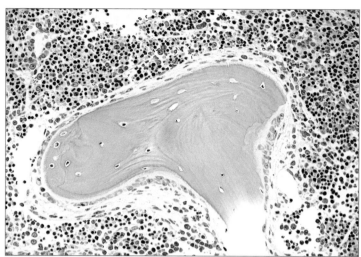

i1.37 *Prominent osteoblast rimming of bony trabeculae in bone marrow core biopsy section from a child. (H&E)*

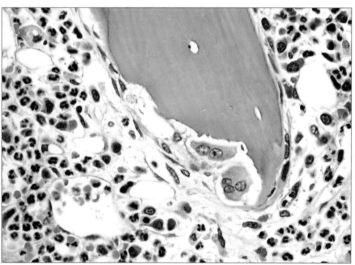

i1.38 *Osteoclasts within a Howship lacuna in bone marrow core biopsy specimen from a child. (H&E)*

Immunophenotyping studies reveal that NK cells can be identified by the expression of several NK-associated surface antigens now known to be adhesion molecules, including CD56 and CD16; while surface CD3 is absent, cytoplasmic CD3 epsilon is present [Trotta 2005, Oshimi 2007]. To avoid auto-aggression, NK cells express a diverse repertoire of inhibitory and activating receptors [Bendelac 2007, Grzywacz 2006]. If activating signals are unopposed by inhibitory signals, granzymes and perforin are released killing targets [Grzywacz 2006]. Immunoregulatory crosstalk between NK cells, monocytes, and dendritic cells is important in innate and adaptive immune responses [Nedvetzki 2007, Caligiuri 2008].

Cells with NK activity (both cytotoxic/suppressor T cells and true NK cells) are concentrated in the large granular lymphocyte population of peripheral blood mononuclear cells. These mature cells have round nuclei, condensed chromatin, inconspicuous nucleoli, and moderate to abundant amounts of pale blue cytoplasm, which contains a small number of prominent, coarse azurophilic granules **i1.36**. These granules contain cytolytic perforin and associated granule proteases (eg, granzyme) essential for the cytolytic activity of these cells [Grossman 2004, Grzywacz 2006]. It is estimated that 2 billion NK cells are in the circulation in adults [Caligiuri 2008].

[1.7.5]   **Bone Development**

The cortical bone outer framework with interlacing bony trabeculae provides structural support for the hematopoietic (medullary) cavity. The cellular components of this bony framework include osteoblasts, osteoclasts, and osteocytes. Osteoblasts are mesenchymal-derived cells that form a visible layer along bony trabeculae in specimens from children, while they are less conspicuous in adults **i1.37** [Canalis 2005, Li 2007]. Osteoblasts deposit osseous matrix (osteoid). As progressive amounts of osteoid are formed, osteoblasts become surrounded and internalized within bony trabeculae, becoming osteocytes, which reside in lacunar spaces [Wickramasinghe 2007]. Osteoclasts are hematopoietic stem cell derived and are closely related to monocytes and macrophages [Li 2007, Taichman 2005, Teitelbaum 2007]. Osteoclasts are multinucleated bone resorbing cells that reside in scattered Howship's lacunae visible along bony trabeculae of specimens from children and adolescents **i1.38** [Haylock 2006, Wickramasinghe 2007]. Cytokines such as RANK ligand and M-CSF induce monocyte/macrophage progenitors to differentiate into multinucleated osteoclasts [Teitelbaum 2007]. The mineralized bone itself is remodeled throughout life, but this is only morphologically apparent in specimens from children and adolescents. This remodeling is achieved through coordinated bone resorption by osteoclasts and bone formation by osteoblasts [Canalis 2005, Li 2007].

Because hematopoietic stem cells also reside preferentially along the endosteal surface of bony trabeculae, it is not surprising that studies in mice and humans have confirmed that osteoblasts play a key role in the maintenance of this hematopoietic stem cell niche, which directly regulates hematopoietic stem cell numbers and fate [Haylock 2006, Nilsson 2005, Taichman 2005, Mayack 2008]. Similarly, signal transduction molecules can regulate granulopoiesis indirectly by influencing the number of osteoblasts along the endosteum [Zhou 2008]. Very few osteoblasts can be detected in the blood; these cells are more readily apparent in blood during times of vigorous bone growth [Eghbali-Fatourechi 2005].

[1.8]   References

Abbas A, Lichtman A, Pillai S [2007a] In: *Cellular and Molecular Immunology*. 6th ed. Philadelphia: Saunders; 267-301.

Abbas A, Lichtman A, Pillai S [2007b] Immediate hypersensitivity. In: *Cellular and Molecular Immunology*. 6th ed. Philadelphia: Saunders; 441-461.

Abbas A, Lichtman A, Pillai S [2007c] Lymphocyte development and the rearrangement and expression of antigen receptor genes. In: *Cellular and Molecular Immunology*. 6th ed. Philadelphia: Saunders; 153-187.

Abedi M, Foster BM, Wood KD, et al [2007] Haematopoietic stem cells participate in muscle regeneration. *Br J Haematol* 138:792-801.

Adolfsson J, Mansson R, Buza-Vidas N, et al [2005] Identification of Flt3+ lympho-myeloid stem cells lacking erythro-megakaryocytic potential a revised road map for adult blood lineage commitment. *Cell* 121:295-306.

Akashi K, He X, Chen J, et al [2003] Transcriptional accessibility for genes of multiple tissues and hematopoietic lineages is hierarchically controlled during early hematopoiesis. *Blood* 101:383-389.

Akashi K, Traver D, Miyamoto T, Weissman IL [2000] A clonogenic common myeloid progenitor that gives rise to all myeloid lineages. *Nature* 404:193-197.

Andrews NC [2008] Forging a field: the golden age of iron biology. *Blood* 112:219-230.

Anjos-Afonso F, Bonnet D [2007] Flexible and dynamic organization of bone marrow stromal compartment. *Br J Haematol* 139:373-384.

Arinobu Y, Mizuno S, Chong Y, et al [2007] Reciprocal activation of *GATA1* and *PU.1* marks initial specification of hematopoietic stem cells into myeloerythroid and myelolymphoid lineages. *Cell Stem Cell* 1:416-427.

Back J, Dierich A, Bronn C, et al [2004] PU.1 determines the self-renewal capacity of erythroid progenitor cells. *Blood* 103:3615-3623.

Baltimore D, Boldin MP, O'Connell RM, et al [2008] MicroRNAs: New regulators of immune cell development and function. *Nat Immunol* 9:839-845.

Bell JJ, Bhandoola A [2008] The earliest thymic progenitors for T cells possess myeloid lineage potential. *Nature* 452:764-767.

Bendelac A, Savage PB, Teyton L [2007] The biology of NKT cells. *Annu Rev Immunol* 25:297-336.

Benson DM, Jr, Yu J, Becknell B, et al [2009] Stem cell factor and interleukin-2/15 combine to enhance MAPK-mediated proliferation of human natural killer cells. *Blood* 113:2706-2714.

Betz SA, Foucar K, Head DR, et al [1992] False-positive flow cytometric platelet glycoprotein IIb/IIIa expression in myeloid leukemias secondary to platelet adherence to blasts. *Blood* 79:2399-2403.

Blank U, Karlsson G, Karlsson S [2008] Signaling pathways governing stem-cell fate. *Blood* 111:492-503.

Brooke G, Rossetti T, Pelekanos R, et al [2009] Manufacturing of human placenta-derived mesenchymal stem cells for clinical trials. *Br J Haematol* 144:571-579.

Broome CS, Whetton AD, Miyan JA [2000] Neuropeptide control of bone marrow neutrophil production is mediated by both direct and indirect effects on CFU-GM. *Br J Haematol* 108:140-150.

Bryder D, Rossi DJ, Weissman IL [2006] Hematopoietic stem cells: the paradigmatic tissue-specific stem cell. *Am J Pathol* 169:338-346.

Burdon PC, Martin C, Rankin SM [2005] The CXC chemokine MIP-2 stimulates neutrophil mobilization from the rat bone marrow in a CD49d-dependent manner. *Blood* 105:2543-2548.

Burger JA, Burkle A [2007] The CXCR4 chemokine receptor in acute and chronic leukaemia: a marrow homing receptor and potential therapeutic target. *Br J Haematol* 137:288-296.

Caligiuri MA [2008] Human natural killer cells. *Blood* 112:461-469.

Canalis E [2005] The fate of circulating osteoblasts. *N Engl J Med* 352:2014-2016.

Chasis JA, Mohandas N [2008] Erythroblastic islands: niches for erythropoiesis. *Blood* 112:470-478.

Cornish GH, Sinclair LV, Cantrell DA [2006] Differential regulation of T-cell growth by IL-2 and IL-15. *Blood* 108:600-608.

Crispino JD [2005a] GATA1 in normal and malignant hematopoiesis. *Semin Cell Dev Biol* 16:137-147.

Crispino JD [2005b] GATA1 mutations in Down syndrome: implications for biology and diagnosis of children with transient myeloproliferative disorder and acute megakaryoblastic leukemia. *Pediatr Blood Cancer* 44:40-44.

Dao MA, Creer MH, Nolta JA, Verfaillie CM [2007] Biology of umbilical cord blood progenitors in bone marrow niches. *Blood* 110:74-81.

Dazzi F, Ramasamy R, Glennie S, et al [2006] The role of mesenchymal stem cells in haemopoiesis. *Blood* Rev 20:161-171.

de Alarcon P, Werner E [2005] Erythropoiesis, red cells, and the approach to anemia. In: *Neonatal Hematology*. Cambridge: Cambridge University; 40-57.

de Bruijn MF, Speck NA [2004] Core-binding factors in hematopoiesis and immune function. *Oncogene* 23:4238-4248.

Deutsch VR, Tomer A [2006] Megakaryocyte development and platelet production. *Br J Haematol* 134:453-466.

Didichenko SA, Spiegl N, Brunner T, Dahinden CA [2008] IL-3 induces a Pim1-dependent antiapoptotic pathway in primary human basophils. *Blood* 112:3949-3958.

Eash KJ, Means JM, White DW, Link DC [2009] CXCR4 is a key regulator of neutrophil release from the bone marrow under basal and stress granulopoiesis conditions. *Blood* 113:4711-4719.

Edwards JR, Williams K, Kindblom LG, et al [2008] Lymphatics and bone. *Hum Pathol* 39:49-55.

Eghbali-Fatourechi GZ, Lamsam J, Fraser D, et al [2005] Circulating osteoblast-lineage cells in humans. *N Engl J Med* 352:1959-1966.

Elagib KE, Racke FK, Mogass M, et al [2003] *RUNX1* and *GATA1* coexpression and cooperation in megakaryocytic differentiation. *Blood* 101:4333-4341.

Escribano L, Garcia Montero AC, Nunez R, Orfao A [2006] Flow cytometric analysis of normal and neoplastic mast cells: role in diagnosis and follow-up of mast cell disease. *Immunol Allergy Clin North Am* 26:535-547.

Fabriek BO, Polfliet MM, Vloet RP, et al [2007] The macrophage CD163 surface glycoprotein is an erythroblast adhesion receptor. *Blood* 109:5223-5229.

Farag SS, Caligiuri MA [2006] Human natural killer cell development and biology. *Blood* Rev 20:123-137.

Fazi F, Racanicchi S, Zardo G, et al [2007] Epigenetic silencing of the myelopoiesis regulator microRNA-223 by the AML1/ETO oncoprotein. *Cancer Cell* 12:457-466.

Fazi F, Rosa A, Fatica A, et al [2005] A minicircuitry comprised of microRNA-223 and transcription factors NFI-A and C/EBPalpha regulates human granulopoiesis. *Cell* 123:819-831.

Fontana L, Pelosi E, Greco P, et al [2007] MicroRNAs 17-5p-20a-106a control monocytopoiesis through AML1 targeting and M-CSF receptor upregulation. *Nat Cell Biol* 9:775-787.

Forsberg EC, Serwold T, Kogan S, et al [2006] New evidence supporting megakaryocyte-erythrocyte potential of flk2/flt3+ multipotent hematopoietic progenitors. *Cell* 126:415-426.

Foucar K, Viswanatha D, Wilson C [2008] Normal anatomy and histology of bone marrow. In: King D, Gardner W, Sobin L, et al, eds. *Non-Neoplastic Disorders of Bone Marrow (AFIP fascicle)*. Washington, DC: American Registry of Pathology; 1-40.

Fox JM, Chamberlain G, Ashton BA, Middleton J [2007] Recent advances into the understanding of mesenchymal stem cell trafficking. *Br J Haematol* 137:491-502.

Fujiwara Y, Chang AN, Williams AM, Orkin SH [2004] Functional overlap of *GATA1* and *GATA2* in primitive hematopoietic development. *Blood* 103:583-585.

Gang EJ, Bosnakovski D, Figueiredo CA, et al [2007] SSEA-4 identifies mesenchymal stem cells from bone marrow. *Blood* 109:1743-1751.

Geddis AE, Kaushansky K [2007] The root of platelet production. Science 317:1689-1691.

Georgantas RW, 3rd, Hildreth R, Morisot S, et al [2007] CD34+ hematopoietic stem-progenitor cell microRNA expression and function: a circuit diagram of differentiation control. *Proc Natl Acad Sci USA* 104:2750-2755.

Ghiaur G, Ferkowicz MJ, Milsom MD, et al [2008] Rac1 is essential for intraembryonic hematopoiesis and for the initial seeding of fetal liver with definitive hematopoietic progenitor cells. *Blood* 111:3313-3321.

Gottgens B [2004] Transcriptional regulation of haematopoiesis. *Vox Sang* 87(suppl):15-19.

Grossman WJ, Verbsky JW, Tollefsen BL, et al [2004] Differential expression of granzymes A and B in human cytotoxic lymphocyte subsets and T regulatory cells. *Blood* 104:2840-2848.

Grzywacz B, Kataria N, Sikora M, et al [2006] Coordinated acquisition of inhibitory and activating receptors and functional properties by developing human natural killer cells. *Blood* 108:3824-3833.

Guo Y, Maillard I, Chakraborti S, et al [2008] Core binding factors are necessary for natural killer cell development and cooperate with Notch signaling during T-cell specification. *Blood* 112:480-492.

Gutierrez L, Nikolic T, van Dijk TB, et al [2007] GATA1 regulates dendritic-cell development and survival. *Blood* 110:1933-1941.

Haddad R, Guardiola P, Izac B, et al [2004] Molecular characterization of early human T/NK and B-lymphoid progenitor cells in umbilical cord blood. *Blood* 104:3918-3926.

Haller Hasskamp J, Zapas JL, Elias EG [2005] Dendritic cell counts in the peripheral blood of healthy adults. *Am J Hematol* 78:314-315.

Hao QL, George AA, Zhu J, et al [2008] Human intrathymic lineage commitment is marked by differential CD7 expression: identification of CD7− lympho-myeloid thymic progenitors. *Blood* 111:1318-1326.

Hardy RR, Kincade PW, Dorshkind K [2007] The protean nature of cells in the B lymphocyte lineage. *Immunity* 26:703-714.

Haylock DN, Nilsson SK [2006] Osteopontin: a bridge between bone and blood. *Br J Haematol* 134:467-474.

Heib V, Becker M, Taube C, Stassen M [2008] Advances in the understanding of mast cell function. *Br J Haematol* 142:683-694.

Hercus TR, Thomas D, Guthridge MA, et al [2009] The granulocyte-macrophage colony-stimulating factor receptor: linking to its structure to cell signaling and its role in disease. *Blood* 114:1289-1298.

Hoebeke I, De Smedt M, Stolz F, et al [2007] T-, B- and NK-lymphoid, but not myeloid cells arise from human CD34(+)CD38(-)CD7(+) common lymphoid progenitors expressing lymphoid-specific genes. *Leukemia* 21:311-319.

Houghton J, Stoicov C, Nomura S, et al [2004] Gastric cancer originating from bone marrow-derived cells. *Science* 306:1568-1571.

Ishikawa F, Niiro H, Iino T, et al [2007] The developmental program of human dendritic cells is operated independently of conventional myeloid and lymphoid pathways. *Blood* 110:3591-3660.

Italiano Jr [2008] J. Megakaryocyte and platelet biology: getting your FAKs straight. *Blood* 111:482-483.

Jacobsen LC, Theilgaard-Monch K, Christensen EI, Borregaard N [2007] Arginase 1 is expressed in myelocytes/metamyelocytes and localized in gelatinase granules of human neutrophils. *Blood* 109:3084-3087.

Janckila AJ, Slone SP, Lear SC, et al [2007] Tartrate-resistant acid phosphatase as an immunohistochemical marker for inflammatory macrophages. *Am J Clin Pathol* 127:556-566.

Jiang H, Chess L [2006] Regulation of immune responses by T cells. *N Engl J Med* 354:1166-1176.

Johnson KD, Boyer ME, Kang JA, et al [2007] Friend of *GATA1*-independent transcriptional repression: a novel mode of *GATA1* function. *Blood* 109:5230-5233.

Junt T, Schulze H, Chen Z, et al [2007] Dynamic visualization of thrombopoiesis within bone marrow. *Science* 317:1767-1770.

Karadimitris A, Patterson S, Spanoudakis E [2006] Natural killer T cells and haemopoiesis. *Br J Haematol* 134:263-272.

Kaushansky K [2008] Historical review: megakaryopoiesis and thrombopoiesis. *Blood* 111:981-986.

Kierszenbaum AL [2002] Blood and Hematopoiesis. In: *Histology and Cell Biology: an Introduction to Pathology*. St. Louis: Mosby; 147-175.

Klimchenko O, Mori M, Distefano A, et al [2009] A common bipotent progenitor generates the erythroid and megakaryocyte lineages in embryonic stem cell-derived primitive hematopoiesis. *Blood* 114:1506-1517.

Kondo M, Weissman IL, Akashi K [1997] Identification of clonogenic common lymphoid progenitors in mouse bone marrow. *Cell* 91:661-672.

Kotsianidis I, Silk JD, Spanoudakis E, et al [2006] Regulation of hematopoiesis in vitro and in vivo by invariant NKT cells. *Blood* 107:3138-3144.

Koury MJ, Koury ST, Kopsombut P, Bondurant MC [2005] In vitro maturation of nascent reticulocytes to erythrocytes. *Blood* 105:2168-2174.

Lakshmipathy U, Verfaillie C [2005] Stem cell plasticity. *Blood Rev* 19:29-38.

Lambert MP, Rauova L, Bailey M, et al [2007] Platelet factor 4 is a negative autocrine in vivo regulator of megakaryopoiesis: clinical and therapeutic implications. *Blood* 110:1153-1160.

Lataillade JJ, Pierre-Louis O, Hasselbalch HC, et al [2008] Does primary myelofibrosis involve a defective stem cell niche? From concept to evidence. *Blood* 112:3026-3035.

Lau SK, Chu PG, Weiss LM [2004] CD163: A specific marker of macrophages in paraffin-embedded tissue samples. *Am J Clin Pathol* 122:794-801.

LeBien TW, Tedder TF [2008] B lymphocytes: how they develop and function. *Blood* 112:1570-1580.

Lee JC, Gimm JA, Lo AJ, et al [2004] Mechanism of protein sorting during erythroblast enucleation: role of cytoskeletal connectivity. *Blood* 103:1912-1919.

Li Y, Toraldo G, Li A, et al [2007] B cells and T cells are critical for the preservation of bone homeostasis and attainment of peak bone mass in vivo. *Blood* 109:3839-3848.

Li ZW, Dalton WS [2006] Tumor microenvironment and drug resistance in hematologic malignancies. *Blood Rev* 20:333-342.

Lordier L, Jalil A, Aurade F, et al [2008] Megakaryocyte endomitosis is a failure of late cytokinesis related to defects in the contractile ring and Rho/Rock signaling. *Blood* 112:3164-3174.

Lorsbach RB [2004] Megakaryoblastic disorders in children. Am J Clin Pathol 122 Suppl:S33-46.

Lu J, Guo S, Ebert BL, et al [2008] MicroRNA-mediated control of cell fate in megakaryocyte-erythrocyte progenitors. *Dev Cell* 14:843-853.

Luc S, Anderson K, Kharazi S, et al [2008a] Down-regulation of Mpl marks the transition to lymphoid-primed multipotent progenitors with gradual loss of granulocyte-monocyte potential. *Blood* 111:3424-3434.

Luc S, Buza-Vidas N, Jacobsen SE [2008b] Delineating the cellular pathways of hematopoietic lineage commitment. *Semin Immunol* 20:213-220.

Lucio P, Parreira A, van den Beemd MW, et al [1999] Flow cytometric analysis of normal B cell differentiation: a frame of reference for the detection of minimal residual disease in precursor-B-ALL. *Leukemia* 13:419-427.

Maillard I, Fang T, Pear WS [2005] Regulation of lymphoid development, differentiation, and function by the Notch pathway. *Annu Rev Immunol* 23:945-974.

Mansson R, Hultquist A, Luc S, et al [2007] Molecular evidence for hierarchical transcriptional lineage priming in fetal and adult stem cells and multipotent progenitors. *Immunity* 26:407-419.

Mansson R, Zandi S, Anderson K, et al [2008] B-lineage commitment prior to surface expression of B220 and CD19 on hematopoietic progenitor cells. *Blood* 112:1048-1055.

Manz MG, Traver D, Miyamoto T, et al [2001] Dendritic cell potentials of early lymphoid and myeloid progenitors. *Blood* 97:3333-3341.

Martinez C, Hofmann TJ, Marino R, et al [2007] Human bone marrow mesenchymal stromal cells express the neural ganglioside GD2: A novel surface marker for the identification of MSCs. *Blood* 109:4245-4248.

Massa M, Rosti V, Ferrario M, et al [2005] Increased circulating hematopoietic and endothelial progenitor cells in the early phase of acute myocardial infarction. *Blood* 105:199-206.

Mayack SR, Wagers AJ [2008] Osteolineage niche cells initiate hematopoietic stem cell mobilization. *Blood* 112:519-531.

McCrann DJ, Eliades A, Makitalo M, et al [2009] Differential expression of NADPH oxidases in megakaryocytes and their role in polyploidy. *Blood* 114:1243-1249.

Medina F, Segundo C, Campos-Caro A, et al [2002] The heterogeneity shown by human plasma cells from tonsil, blood, and bone marrow reveals graded stages of increasing maturity, but local profiles of adhesion molecule expression. *Blood* 99:2154-2161.

Merad M, Manz MG [2009] Dendritic cell homeostasis. *Blood* 113:3418-3427.

Mermel CH, McLemore ML, Liu F, et al [2006] Src family kinases are important negative regulators of G-CSF-dependent granulopoiesis. *Blood* 108:2562-2568.

Metcalf D [2007a] Concise review: hematopoietic stem cells and tissue stem cells: current concepts and unanswered questions. *Stem Cells* 25:2390-2395.

Metcalf D [2007b] On hematopoietic stem cell fate. *Immunity* 26:669-673.

Metcalf D [2008] Hematopoietic cytokines. *Blood* 111:485-491.

Miranda MB, Johnson DE [2007] Signal transduction pathways that contribute to myeloid differentiation. *Leukemia* 21:1363-1377.

Moser B, Wolf M, Walz A, Loetscher P [2004] Chemokines: Multiple levels of leukocyte migration control. *Trends Immunol* 25:75-84.

Muller I, Vaegler M, Holzwarth C, et al [2008] Secretion of angiogenic proteins by human multipotent mesenchymal stromal cells and their clinical potential in the treatment of avascular osteonecrosis. *Leukemia* 22:2054-2061.

Muntean AG, Pang L, Poncz M, et al [2007] Cyclin D-Cdk4 is regulated by *GATA1* and required for megakaryocyte growth and polyploidization. *Blood* 109:5199-5207.

Nedvetzki S, Sowinski S, Eagle RA, et al [2007] Reciprocal regulation of human natural killer cells and macrophages associated with distinct immune synapses. *Blood* 109:3776-3785.

Ng F, Boucher S, Koh S, et al [2008] PDGF, TGF-beta, and FGF signaling is important for differentiation and growth of mesenchymal stem cells (MSCs): Transcriptional profiling can identify markers and signaling pathways important in differentiation of MSCs into adipogenic, chondrogenic, and osteogenic lineages. *Blood* 112:295-307.

Nguyen TT, Schwartz EJ, West RB, et al [2005] Expression of CD163 (hemoglobin scavenger receptor) in normal tissues, lymphomas, carcinomas, and sarcomas is largely restricted to the monocyte/macrophage lineage. *Am J Surg Pathol* 29:617-624.

Nilsson SK, Johnston HM, Whitty GA, et al [2005] Osteopontin, a key component of the hematopoietic stem cell niche and regulator of primitive hematopoietic progenitor cells. *Blood* 106:1232-1239.

O'Connell RM, Rao DS, Chaudhuri AA, et al [2008] Sustained expression of microRNA-155 in hematopoietic stem cells causes a myeloproliferative disorder. *J Exp Med* 205:585-594.

Oakley EJ, Van Zant G [2007] Unraveling the complex regulation of stem cells: implications for aging and cancer. *Leukemia* 21:612-621.

Obata K, Mukai K, Tsujimura Y, et al [2007] Basophils are essential initiators of a novel type of chronic allergic inflammation. *Blood* 110:913-920.

Odendahl M, Mei H, Hoyer BF, et al [2005] Generation of migratory antigen-specific plasma blasts and mobilization of resident plasma cells in a secondary immune response. *Blood* 105:1614-1621.

Oshimi K [2007] Progress in understanding and managing natural killer-cell malignancies. *Br J Haematol* 139:532-544.

Parmar K, Mauch P, Vergilio JA, et al [2007] Distribution of hematopoietic stem cells in the bone marrow according to regional hypoxia. *Proc Natl Acad Sci USA* 104:5431-5436.

Parr AM, Tator CH, Keating A [2007] Bone marrow-derived mesenchymal stromal cells for the repair of central nervous system injury. *Bone Marrow Transplant* 40:609-619.

Payne KJ, Crooks GM [2007] Immune-cell lineage commitment: translation from mice to humans. *Immunity* 26:674-677.

Peggs KS, Allison JP [2005] Co-stimulatory pathways in lymphocyte regulation: the immunoglobulin superfamily. *Br J Haematol* 130:809-824.

Pileri SA, Grogan TM, Harris NL, et al [2002] Tumours of histiocytes and accessory dendritic cells: an immunohistochemical approach to classification from the International Lymphoma Study Group based on 61 cases. *Histopathology* 41:1-29.

Raslova H, Baccini V, Loussaief L, et al [2006] Mammalian target of rapamycin (mTOR) regulates both proliferation of megakaryocyte progenitors and late stages of megakaryocyte differentiation. *Blood* 107:2303-2310.

Raslova H, Kauffmann A, Sekkai D, et al [2007] Interrelation between polyploidization and megakaryocyte differentiation: a gene profiling approach. *Blood* 109:3225-3234.

Rhodes MM, Kopsombut P, Bondurant MC, et al [2008] Adherence to macrophages in erythroblastic islands enhances erythroblast proliferation and increases erythrocyte production by a different mechanism than erythropoietin. *Blood* 111:1700-1708.

Ringden O, Uzunel M, Sundberg B, et al [2007] Tissue repair using allogeneic mesenchymal stem cells for hemorrhagic cystitis, pneumomediastinum and perforated colon. *Leukemia* 21:2271-2276.

Rossi MI, Yokota T, Medina KL, et al [2003] B lymphopoiesis is active throughout human life, but there are developmental age-related changes. *Blood* 101:576-584.

Rubiolo C, Piazzolla D, Meissl K, et al [2006] A balance between Raf-1 and Fas expression sets the pace of erythroid differentiation. *Blood* 108:152-159.

Schachinger V, Erbs S, Elsasser A, et al [2006] Intracoronary bone marrow-derived progenitor cells in acute myocardial infarction. *N Engl J Med* 355:1210-1221.

Schepers H, Wierenga AT, van Gosliga D, et al [2007] Reintroduction of C/EBPalpha in leukemic CD34+ stem/progenitor cells impairs self-renewal and partially restores myelopoiesis. *Blood* 110:1317-1325.

Schickel R, Boyerinas B, Park SM, Peter ME [2008] MicroRNAs: Key players in the immune system, differentiation, tumorigenesis and cell death. *Oncogene* 27:5959-5974.

Schonland SO, Zimmer JK, Lopez-Benitez CM, et al [2003] Homeostatic control of T-cell generation in neonates. *Blood* 102:1428-1434.

Schulze H, Korpal M, Hurov J, et al [2006] Characterization of the megakaryocyte demarcation membrane system and its role in thrombopoiesis. *Blood* 107:3868-3875.

Shiozawa Y, Havens AM, Pienta KJ, Taichman RS [2008] The bone marrow niche: habitat to hematopoietic and mesenchymal stem cells, and unwitting host to molecular parasites. *Leukemia* 22:941-950.

Skubitz K [2009] Neutrophilic leukocytes. In: Greer JP, Foerster J, Rodgers G, et al, eds. *Wintrobe's Clinical Hematology*. 12th ed. Philadelphia: Lippincott Williams & Wilkins; 170-213.

Slater NJ, Yamaguchi M, Rothwell DG, et al [2003] The human granulocyte/macrophage colony-stimulating factor receptor alpha2 isoform influences haemopoietic lineage commitment and divergence. *Br J Haematol* 122:150-158.

Sugimoto Y, Katayama N, Masuya M, et al [2006] Differential cell division history between neutrophils and macrophages in their development from granulocyte-macrophage progenitors. *Br J Haematol* 135:725-731.

Sugiyama D, Tanaka M, Kitajima K, et al [2008] Differential context-dependent effects of friend of *GATA1* (*FOG1*) on mast-cell development and differentiation. *Blood* 111:1924-1932.

Tagata Y, Yoshida H, Nguyen LA, et al [2008] Phosphorylation of PML is essential for activation of C/EBP epsilon and PU.1 to accelerate granulocytic differentiation. *Leukemia* 22:273-280.

Taichman RS [2005] Blood and bone: two tissues whose fates are intertwined to create the hematopoietic stem-cell niche. *Blood* 105:2631-2639.

Talebian L, Li Z, Guo Y, et al [2007] T-lymphoid, megakaryocyte, and granulocyte development are sensitive to decreases in CBFbeta dosage. *Blood* 109:11-21.

Taylor G, Weinberg J [2009] Mononuclear phagocytes. In: Greer JP, Foerster J, Rodgers G, et al, eds. *Wintrobe's Clinical Hematology*. 12th ed. Philadelphia: Lippincott Williams & Wilkins; 249-280.

Tefferi A, Patnaik MM, Pardanani A [2006] Eosinophilia: Secondary, clonal and idiopathic. *Br J Haematol* 133:468-492.

Teitelbaum SL [2007] Osteoclasts: What do they do and how do they do it? *Am J Pathol* 170:427-435.

Testa U [2004] Apoptotic mechanisms in the control of erythropoiesis. *Leukemia* 18:1176-1199.

Theilgaard-Monch K, Jacobsen LC, Borup R, et al [2005] The transcriptional program of terminal granulocytic differentiation. *Blood* 105:1785-1796.

Thomas D, Vadas M, Lopez A [2004] Regulation of haematopoiesis by growth factors—emerging insights and therapies. *Expert Opin Biol Ther* 4:869-879.

Tomer A [2004] Human marrow megakaryocyte differentiation: multiparameter correlative analysis identifies von Willebrand factor as a sensitive and distinctive marker for early (2N and 4N) megakaryocytes. *Blood* 104:2722-2727.

Trotta R, Parihar R, Yu J, et al [2005] Differential expression of SHIP1 in CD56bright and CD56dim NK cells provides a molecular basis for distinct functional responses to monokine costimulation. *Blood* 105:3011-3018.

Van Huyen JP, Smadja DM, Bruneval P, et al [2008] Bone marrow-derived mononuclear cell therapy induces distal angiogenesis after local injection in critical leg ischemia. *Mod Pathol* 21:837-846.

Veinotte LL, Halim TY, Takei F [2008] Unique subset of natural killer cells develops from progenitors in lymph node. *Blood* 111:4201-4208.

Vigorito E, Perks KL, Abreu-Goodger C, et al [2007] microRNA-155 regulates the generation of immunoglobulin class-switched plasma cells. *Immunity* 27:847-859.

von Kockritz-Blickwede M, Goldmann O, Thulin P, et al [2008] Phagocytosis-independent antimicrobial activity of mast cells by means of extracellular trap formation. *Blood* 111:3070-3080.

Wada H, Masuda K, Satoh R, et al [2008] Adult T-cell progenitors retain myeloid potential. *Nature* 452:768-772.

Wei S, Kryczek I, Zou W [2006] Regulatory T-cell compartmentalization and trafficking. *Blood* 108:426-431.

Wickramasinghe S [2009] Bone marrow. In: Mills S, ed. *Histology for Pathologists*. 3rd ed. Philadelphia: Lippincott Williams & Wilkins; 799-836.

Wilson A, Trumpp A [2006] Bone-marrow haematopoietic-stem-cell niches. *Nat Rev Immunol* 6:93-106.

Wu L, Liu YJ [2007] Development of dendritic-cell lineages. *Immunity* 26:741-750.

Yang L, Bryder D, Adolfsson J, et al [2005] Identification of Lin(-)Sca1(+)kit(+)CD34(+)Flt3– short-term hematopoietic stem cells capable of rapidly reconstituting and rescuing myeloablated transplant recipients. *Blood* 105:2717-2723.

Zeoli A, Dentelli P, Rosso A, et al [2008] Interleukin-3 promotes expansion of hemopoietic-derived CD45+ angiogenic cells and their arterial commitment via STAT5 activation. *Blood* 112:350-361.

Zhang AL, Colmenero P, Purath U, et al [2007] Natural killer cells trigger differentiation of monocytes into dendritic cells. *Blood* 110:2484-2493.

Zhang ZL, Tong J, Lu RN, et al [2009] Therapeutic potential of non-adherent BM-derived mesenchymal stem cells in tissue regeneration. *Bone Marrow Transplant* 43:69-81.

Zhou L, Li LW, Yan Q, et al [2008] Notch-dependent control of myelopoiesis is regulated by fucosylation. *Blood* 112:308-319.

Zhu J, Paul WE [2008] CD4 T cells: fates, functions, and faults. *Blood* 112:1557-1569.

Morphologic Review of Blood and Bone Marrow

Kathryn Foucar, MD

2

Optimal bone marrow interpretation requires that the bone marrow aspirate smears, imprint, clot section, and core biopsy results be integrated with peripheral blood smear morphologic features, hemogram data, any specialized studies, other laboratory data, and clinical information [Hasserjian 2008]. Clinical information should include symptoms, duration of symptoms, physical findings, occupational and exposure history, travel history, and family/ personal medical history [Foucar 2008b].

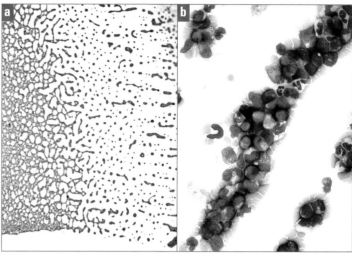

i2.1 *Composite of low **a** and high **b** magnification of peripheral blood smear demonstrating feather edge. Note that large cells are often dragged to the feather edge during blood smear preparation. (Wright)*

[2.1] Integration of Data

[2.1.1] Blood

Morphologic review of the blood smear requires integration with complete blood count (CBC) data; age-, sex-, and race-related normal ranges; and available clinical information **f2.1** [Foucar 2008b, Cheng 2004]. Because of the usefulness of the CBC and differential cell count in identifying significant pathologic disorders, it is imperative for each hematology laboratory to have robust and regularly assessed criteria for manual differential count/review and submission for senior technologist/pathologist review [Lantis 2003, Novis 2006].

Similarly, both the value and limitations of automated cell counters in the detection of blood abnormalities must be appreciated and factored into the development of manual blood smear review criteria [Buttarello 2008]. Because the CBC is a very common routine laboratory test used in screening

and basic health assessment, often a CBC abnormality is the catalyst for a bone marrow examination.

Blood smear review should begin with low-magnification scanning, focusing on the feather edge and sides, to identify large cells, microfilarial worms, and platelet clumps, which are often dragged to these regions of the smear during slide preparation **i2.1**. Next, the qualitative and quantitative features of platelets, erythrocytes, and all white blood cells (WBCs) must be assessed. The tabulation of blood findings provides essential evidence for the various hematologic disorders that will be reviewed in subsequent chapters.

[2.1.2] Age-Related Blood Findings

The most dramatic physiologic changes in blood occur in the period between birth and 1 month of age **t2.1, f2.1** [Proytcheva 2009]. At birth, hemoglobin levels frequently exceed 18 g/dL (180 g/L), and the mean corpuscular volume of these erythrocytes is

t2.1 Age/Gender-Related Physiologic Variations in Normal Blood Findings

Age	Finding
Newborn	Highest RBC, Hgb, Hct, reticulocyte count of any age
	Normoblastemia and prominent polychromasia*
	Highest WBC and absolute neutrophil count of any age
	Left shift with occasional blasts*
Infant/young child	Highest absolute lymphocyte count of any age
Adolescent	Higher RBC parameters in males
	Neutrophil predominance
Adult	Higher RBC parameters in males
	Neutrophil predominance

*Finding normal (physiologic) only in neonatal period
Hct = hematocrit; Hgb = hemoglobin; RBC = red blood cell;
WBC = white blood cell

References: [Foucar 2008a, Foucar 2008c, de Alarcon 2005]

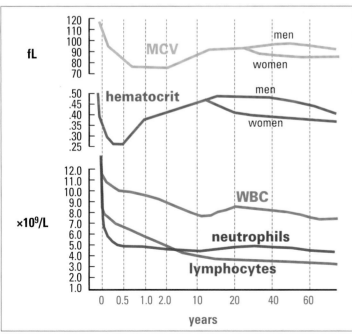

f2.1 *Approximate age-related normal ranges for various blood parameters are illustrated. MCV = mean corpuscular volume, WBC = white blood cell*

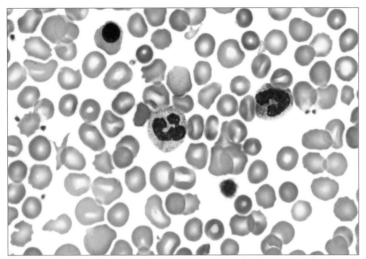

i2.2 *Blood smear of newborn showing prominent polychromasia and nucleated red blood cells. (Wright)*

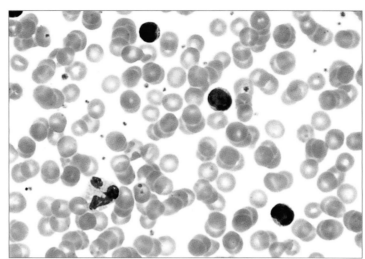

i2.3 *Mature lymphocytes predominate in the peripheral blood of a healthy 3-year-old child. (Wright)*

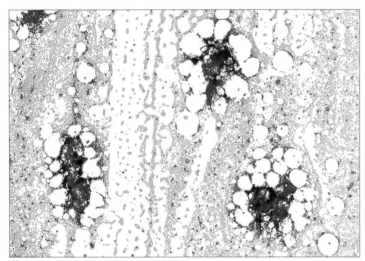

i2.4 *Bone marrow aspirate direct smear illustrates the proportion of fat and cells within widely spaced particles. (Wright)*

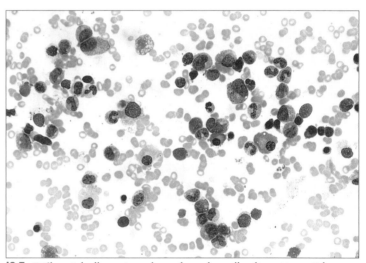

i2.5 *Differential cell counts can be performed on cells adjacent to particles on bone marrow aspirate direct smear. Note that cells are well-dispersed and uniformly stained. (Wright)*

substantially higher than is normal for any other age **i2.2**. The presence of both nucleated red blood cells and marked polychromasia is normal. After birth, the hematocrit progressively drops, until erythropoietin (EPO) production resumes at approximately 3-5 months of age [de Alarcon 2005, Proytcheva 2009]. The relative percentages and absolute cell counts for neutrophils and lymphocytes also show fairly pronounced age variations. Neutrophils predominate at birth, but by approximately 1-2 weeks of age, lymphocytes are more numerous in the blood of healthy neonates [Buescher 2005]. This physiologic predominance of lymphocytes persists throughout early childhood **i2.3** [Foucar 2008b]. During later childhood, there is a gradual shift, and by adolescence, the neutrophil has become the most numerous WBC and remains so throughout life. Likewise, red blood cell (RBC), hemoglobin, and hematocrit levels rise with adolescence

most predominantly in males; this sex-related disparity in normal RBC parameters persists throughout adult life. In contrast, platelet, eosinophil, basophil, and monocyte cell counts remain relatively stable throughout life and do not demonstrate significant physiologic age-related variations.

[2.1.3] **Bone Marrow Aspirate and Biopsy**

Morphologic review of the bone marrow aspirate smears includes a systematic evaluation of all hematopoietic and lymphoid lineages, as well as cytologic assessment of macrophages, plasma cells, and mast cells **i2.4**, **i2.5**. For each hematopoietic lineage, the maturation sequence and morphologic features should be assessed. Well-stained, good quality blood and bone marrow aspirate smears and imprint preparations are essential for this cytologic review

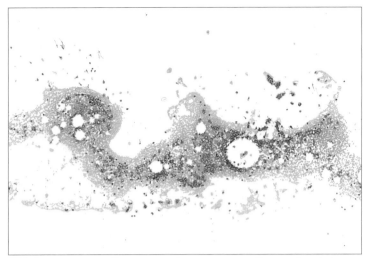

i2.6 *Imprint smears of bone marrow biopsy specimens illustrate the admixture of variably dispersed cells, fat, and erythrocytes that characterize these preparations. (Wright)*

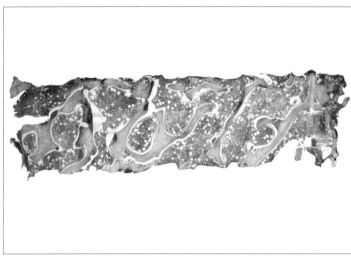

i2.7 *Low magnification of bone marrow core biopsy essential for evaluating bony trabeculae, overall cellularity, as well as possible focal infiltrates. (H&E)*

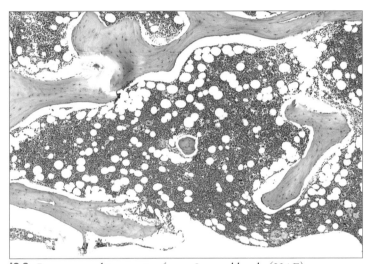

i2.8 *Bone marrow biopsy section from a 5-year-old male. (H&E)*

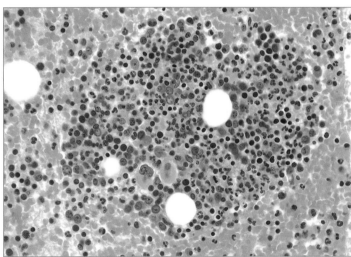

i2.9 *Clot section from a 5-year-old male illustrates normal cellularity and normal proportions of megakaryocytic, erythroid, and granulocytic cells. (H&E)*

i2.6. A suboptimal preparation often causes major problems in aspirate smear interpretation, making even differential counting unnecessarily difficult (see section 2.2, "Blood and Bone Marrow Artifacts," p 45) [Hasserjian 2008].

Likewise, thinly cut, step-sectioned, and well-stained sections of clotted aspirate and decalcified core biopsy specimens are essential for an integrated bone marrow evaluation **i2.7** [Hasserjian 2008]. Bone marrow biopsy is necessary for the evaluation of not only hematopoietic cells, but also blood vessels, bone, stromal elements, and any abnormal infiltrates **i2.8, i2.9, i2.10**. For optimal interpretation, all specimens, including blood smear, bone marrow aspirate smears, imprint preparations, clot sections, and core biopsies, should be available to the diagnostician for review and integrated reporting.

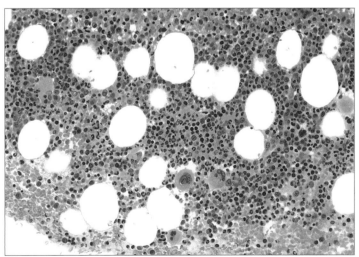

i2.10 *Clot section from a 45-year-old male illustrates normal cellularity and normal proportions of megakaryocytic, erythroid, and granulocytic cells. (H&E)*

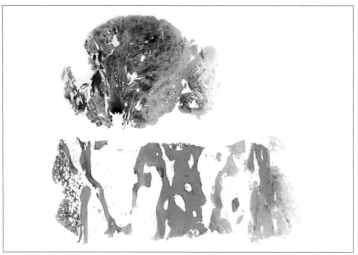

i2.11 *Bone marrow core biopsy (bottom) shows strikingly long subcortical hypocellular region with minimal hematopoietic elements for evaluation. (H&E)*

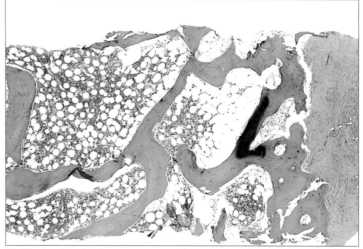

i2.12 *Good quality bone marrow core biopsy section showing cortical surface, small subcortical hypocellular zone, and significant amounts of intact bone marrow for evaluation. (H&E)*

[2.1.4] **Bone Marrow Cellularity and Differential Counts**

Although bone marrow aspiration and biopsy represent only a minute sample of the hematopoietic organ, specimens obtained from standard sites are generally representative of overall bone marrow activity. Therefore, in the vast majority of clinical situations, it is reasonable to make generalities about overall bone marrow cellularity and distribution of hematopoietic cell types within the marrow based on the aspirate and biopsy samples obtained from a single site. If aberrant cell distribution patterns of normal hematopoietic elements are suspected, radiographic studies, such as magnetic resonance imaging, can be used to assess the entire hematopoietic space. This has proven useful in some patients with presumed aplastic anemia, but a more cost-effective approach might include aspiration and biopsy of another site.

Bone marrow cellularity can be estimated from smears, but ideally it is determined on a good-quality biopsy section.

Because the subcortical region of the bone marrow is often hypocellular, especially in elderly patients, this area must be avoided in assessing cellularity. If a biopsy sample is small and consists largely of subcortical bone, it is inadequate for interpretation **i2.11**, **i2.12**. Biopsy sections with significant aspiration artifact are also inadequate for interpretation because the hematopoietic cavity is disrupted and filled with erythrocytes (see **[2.2]** "Blood and Bone Marrow Artifacts," p 45).

Bone marrow cellularity is highest at birth and in young children, and declines with age; broad ranges in normal cellularity by age are reported **t2.2**, **f2.2**, **i2.13**, **i2.14** [Wickramasinghe 2007]. Although gradual, the most significant decline in cellularity occurs in children followed by another significant decline in the elderly; cellularity is fairly stable throughout most of adulthood. These changes in cellularity correlate with an age-related decline in hematopoietic activity and thinning of bony trabeculae (elderly patients)

t2.2 Age-Related Normal Values in Bone Marrow

Age	% Cellularity	% Granulocyte	% Erythroid	% Lymphocytes	Comments
Newborn	80%-100%	40%-50%	40%	10%-20%	High EPO at birth; drops dramatically after birth; hematogones may be prominent*
1-3 months	80%-100%	50%-60%	5%-10%	30%-50%	Dramatic decline in erythroid precursors until EPO production resumes at 3-4 months; abundant lymphocytes with many hematogones*
Child	60%-80%	50%-60%	20%	20%-30%	Variable number of hematogones*; more numerous in young children
Adult (30-70 years)	40%-70%	50%-70%	20%-25%	10%-15%	Cellularity fairly stable throughout most of adulthood
Elderly (>70 years)	≤25%	50%-70%	20%-25%	10%-15%	Decline in cellularity in elderly may be linked to a reduction in bone volume with subsequent increase in volume of the hematopoietic cavity

*Hematogones are normal B-lymphocyte precursor cells (see text and Chapter 21)
EPO = erythropoietin

References: [Bain 1996, Friebert 1998, Gulati 1988, Hartsock 1965, Rimsza 2004, Trimoreau 1997, Wickramasinghe 2007, Zutter 1998]

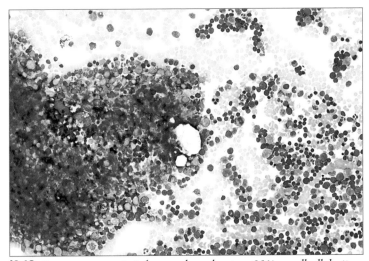

i2.13 *Bone marrow aspirate from newborn showing >98% overall cellularity. (Wright)*

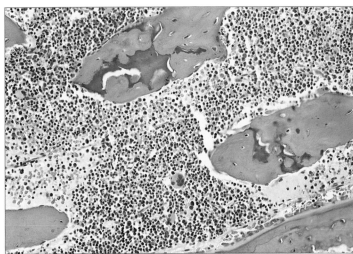

i2.14 *Bone marrow core biopsy from newborn showing 100% cellularity with prominent ossification of bony trabeculae. (H&E)*

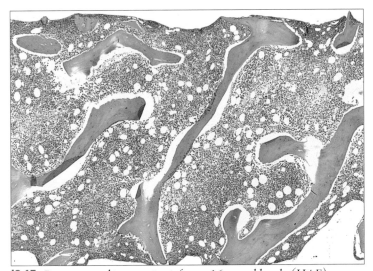

i2.15 *Bone marrow biopsy section is from a 16-year-old male. (H&E)*

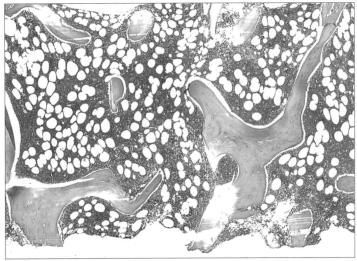

i2.16 *Bone marrow biopsy section is from a 35-year-old male. (H&E)*

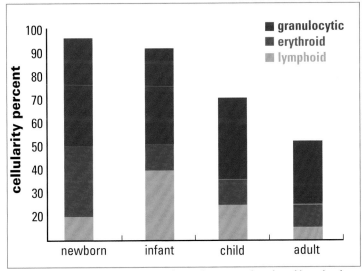

f2.2 *The approximate proportion of granulocytic, erythroid, and lymphoid cells in the bone marrow of newborns, 1-month-old infants, children, and adults is shown. Overall cellularity for these ages is illustrated by the combined height of each bar.*

[Wickramasinghe 2007]. As the cellularity declines, adipose cells become apparent i2.15, i2.16, i2.17, i2.18. Similarly, lineage proportions in bone marrow also vary by age; the erythroid lineage is much more abundant in newborn infants than in patients of any other age group, while lymphoid cells are physiologically uniquely abundant in infants and young children f2.2 [Rimsza 2004].

Along with assessment of nuclear and cytoplasmic features of cells, differential cell counts may be performed on bone marrow aspirate smears or touch preparations t2.2, t2.3 i2.19 [Aboul-Nasr 1999]. The total proportion of cells comprising each lineage, the maturation sequence for this lineage, and the myeloid-erythroid ratio are all determined from this differential cell count f2.2. Because the percentage of total bone marrow cells attributed to a given lineage is relative, this percentage must be correlated with overall cellularity to be meaningful. In addition,

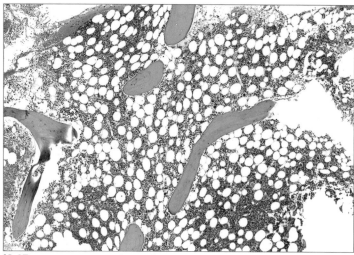

i2.17 *Bone marrow core biopsy from 52-year-old male showing overall cellularity approximating 30% to 40%. (H&E)*

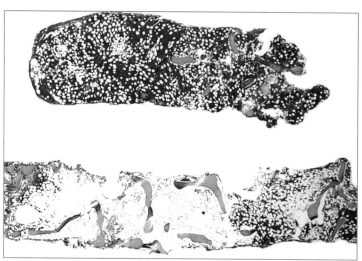

i2.18 *Two bone marrow core biopsy specimens obtained at the same time, one showing profound hypocellularity, while the other core specimen shows a generous proportion of hematopoietic elements highlighting sampling issues that can occur in bone marrow examination. (H&E)*

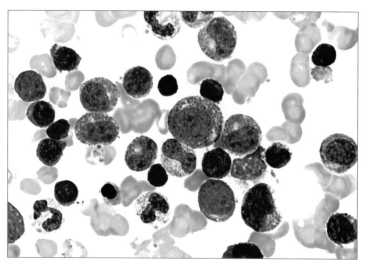

i2.19 *High magnification of bone marrow aspirate smear in area suited for differential cell counting. (Wright)*

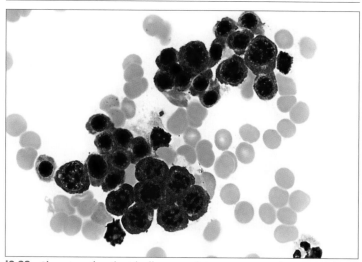

i2.20 *Clumping of erythroid cells can result in a spurious predominance of erythroid cells on differential count. Distinctive areas of cell clumping should be avoided when performing differential counts. (Wright)*

t2.3   Normal Adult Values for Bone Marrow Differential Cell Counts

Cell Type	Normal Range (%)
Myeloblasts	0%-3%*
Promyelocytes	1%-8%
Myelocytes	10%-15%
Metamyelocytes	10%-15%
Band/neutrophils	12%-25%
Eosinophils and precursors	1%-5%
Basophils and precursors	0-1%
Monocytes	0-2%
Erythroblasts	0-2%
Other erythroid cells	15%-25%
Lymphocytes	10%-15%†
Plasma cells	0-1%

*Percent myeloblasts higher in pediatric specimens (3%-4%), lower in specimens from adults, especially elderly (0-1%)
†Percent lymphocytes higher in specimens from young children due to abundant hematogones (benign lymphocyte precursor cells)

References: [Bain 1996, Wickramasinghe 2007]

these differential cell counts should be performed on several different preparations to avoid any focal cellular distribution anomalies. Erythroid cells are especially likely to be clustered, and these areas should be avoided in differential cell counts i2.20.

An assessment of the cytologic features of all hemato-lymphoid lineages is essential, based on an understanding of normal hematolymphoid cellular maturation stages. If morphologic abnormalities are detected, it is important to determine the significance and likely the cause, recognizing that minor dysplastic changes without clinical significance are commonly seen in bone marrow specimens, especially in elderly patients [Girodon 2001].

[2.1.5]   **Erythroid Lineage**

Because of the hypoxic intrauterine environment, EPO levels are initially very high, but promptly drop to nearly

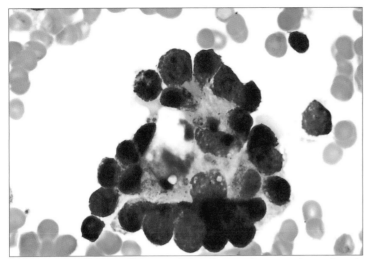

i2.21 *Erythroid lineage cells surround central macrophage secondary to ligand-ligand receptor interaction. (Wright)*

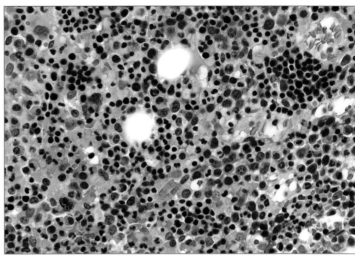

i2.22 *Bone marrow clot section at intermediate magnification showing prominent colonies of erythroid cells. (H&E)*

undetectable levels shortly after birth in normal neonates [de Alarcon 2005]. As a consequence, the number of erythroid cells in the bone marrow drops dramatically during the first few months of life. At their nadir, erythroid cells may constitute <5% of nucleated bone marrow cells, and hemoglobin levels may drop to 10 g/dL in a full-term neonate [de Alarcon 2005]. As the hematocrit progressively declines, the kidneys eventually sense hypoxia and EPO production resumes (see **sidebar 9.1** on oxygen sensing), resulting in an increase in the number of erythroid cells in the bone marrow to approximately 20% to 25% of nucleated cells under homeostatic conditions **f2.2** [Wickramasinghe 2007]. However, in response to severe sustained hypoxia, this cell line can increase remarkably (5-7 times the basal level) to become the most numerous bone marrow cell.

Under physiologic conditions relatively few immature erythroid cells (erythroblasts) are seen, with a progressive increase in the number of more mature forms. Prussian blue stain shows that approximately 20% of normoblasts characteristically contain several small iron granules; these cells are termed "sideroblasts." In pathologic states characterized by dyserythropoiesis, both morphologic and iron content abnormalities of erythroid cells may be present. Disorders associated with numeric, morphologic, and cytochemical abnormalities of erythroid cells will be detailed in subsequent chapters.

The normal collections of erythroid lineage cells surrounding a central macrophage is achieved by ligand-receptor interactions between antigens expressed on macrophages and ligands expressed on erythroid lineage cells **i2.21** [Chasis 2008, Fabriek 2007, Lee 2006]. Erythroid colonies can be readily identified on biopsy sections by their uniformly round nuclear contours, prominent cell membranes, and the dense homogeneous chromatin of the abundant orthochromic

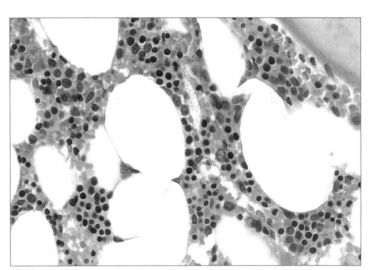

i2.23 *Small random islands of erythroid precursors are evident on this bone marrow biopsy section. The dense nuclear chromatin of orthochromic normoblasts highlights these islands. (H&E)*

normoblasts **i2.22, i2.23**. These erythroid colonies are generally small and nonparatrabecular [Foucar 2008c, Wickramasinghe 2007]. This colony formation can be highlighted by immunoperoxidase staining for hemoblobin A or glycophorin A **i2.24, i2.25**. In addition, nucleoli within erythroblast nuclei are distinctive on paraffin sections exhibiting an oblong to slightly bent configuration **i2.26** [Kass 1995]. Key blood and bone marrow checklist features of the erythroid lineage are listed on **t2.4**.

[2.1.6]   **Granulocytic Lineage**

The granulocytic lineage predominates in normal bone marrow specimens from patients of all ages, and accounts for approximately 50% to 70% of all nucleated cells **f2.2** [Wickramasinghe 2007]. The large maturation-storage compartment serves as a readily available reservoir of granulocytic cells necessary for host protection from infectious assaults and

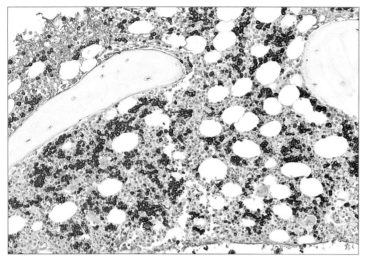

i2.24 *Low magnification of hemoglobin A staining of this bone marrow core biopsy highlights the colony formation of normal erythroid cells. (immunoperoxidase for hemoglobin A)*

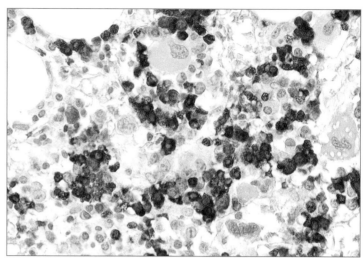

i2.25 *Immunoperoxidase staining for hemoglobin A highlights erythroid colony formation in this normal bone marrow core biopsy section. (immunoperoxidase for hemoglobin A)*

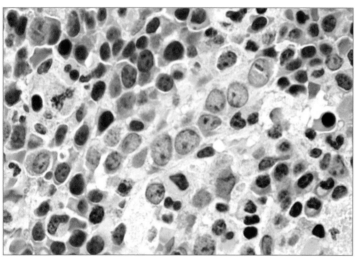

i2.26 *High magnification image of erythroblasts on bone marrow core biopsy illustrate oblong nucleoli characteristic of erythroblasts on tissue sections. (H&E)*

t2.4 Erythroid Lineage Checklist*

Blood	Bone Marrow
RBC indices	Overall cellularity
Morphology	Proportion of erythroid cells
Polychromasia, degree	Maturation pyramid
Abnormal forms, NRBC	Nuclear morphology (budding, karyorrhexis, nuclear bridging, megaloblastic changes)
RBC inclusions (HJ, Pappenheimer bodies, basophilic stippling)	
Organisms—within RBCs, other sites	Hemoglobinization of cytoplasm
	Vacuolization of cytoplasm
	Sideroblasts/siderocytes
	Size, number of iron granules
	Amount of storage iron
	Erythroid colony formation (islands) on clot, core biopsy highlighted by IHC for HgbA or glycophorin A

*Assess all lineages; assess for preservation of normal hematopoiesis
NRBC = nucleated red blood cells; HJ = Howell Jolly bodies;
IHC = immunohistochemical stain; HgbA = hemoglobin A

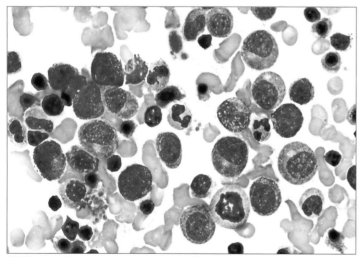

i2.27 *Abundant maturing granulocytic cells are evident on bone marrow aspirate smear. (Wright)*

other acute inflammatory conditions **i2.27**. More immature granulocytic cells are concentrated perivascularly and paratrabecularly, while mature forms are more centrally located **i2.28**. This cellular distribution can be highlighted by immunoperoxidase staining for myeloperoxidase [Foucar 2008c]. At low magnification, a distinctive paratrabecular distribution of bright myeloperoxidase positive cells is noted on core biopsies **i2.29**. In addition, normal selective perivascular localization of immature granulocytic cells is apparent at higher magnification **i2.30, i2.31**. Although mature neutrophils are also myeloperoxidase positive, these mature cells generally exhibit less intense positivity on immunohistochemical staining compared with more immature granulocytic cells **i2.32**. Abnormal localization of immature

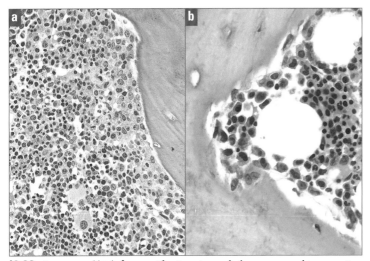

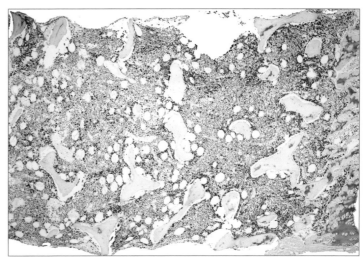

i2.28 *Low-* **a** *and high-* **b** *magnification views of a bone marrow biopsy section illustrate the paratrabecular localization of immature granulocytic cells. (H&E)*

i2.29 *Low magnification of bone marrow core biopsy stained with myeloperoxidase shows concentration of most brightly positive myeloperoxidase cells against bony trabeculae. (immunoperoxidase)*

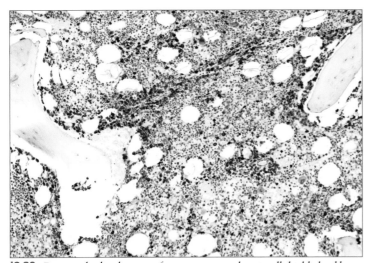

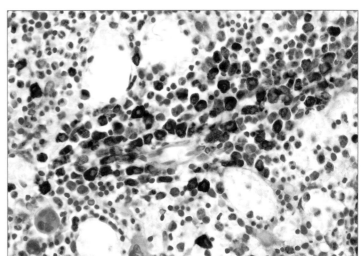

i2.30 *Perivascular localization of immature granulocytic cells highlighted by myeloperoxidase immunoperoxidase stain on bone marrow core biopsy section. (immunoperoxidase)*

i2.31 *Central vessel apparent surrounded by immature myeloperoxidase-positive granulocytic cells on high magnification of bone marrow core biopsy section. (immunoperoxidase)*

myeloid cells away from bony trabeculae can be identified on bone marrow biopsy sections in certain neoplastic processes that will be reviewed later in this book. Alterations in either the maturation pyramid or in the morphologic features of granulocytic cells can occur in a wide variety of neoplastic and non-neoplastic processes that will also be reviewed in subsequent chapters. Granulopoiesis can increase 10-fold in patients with sustained infections or other inflammatory conditions. A key checklist of blood and bone marrow features of the granulocytic lineage is listed in **t2.5**.

[2.1.7] **Megakaryocyte Lineage**

Megakaryocytes are the least numerous hematopoietic cell, accounting for substantially <1% of all nucleated cells. Although megakaryocytes can be assessed on aspirate smears, bone marrow sections are best for evaluating their morphology, quantity, and distribution. Megakaryocytes reside individually

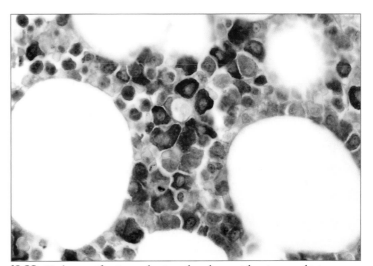

i2.32 *High magnification evaluation of myeloperoxidase immunohisto-chemical stain shows stronger positivity in immature granulocytic cells compared with neutrophils. (immunoperoxidase)*

t2.5 Granulocytic Lineage Checklist*

Blood	Bone Marrow
Absolute neutrophil count	Overall cellularity
Left shift	Proportion of granulocytic cells
Circulating blasts (Auer rods)	Maturation pyramid
Hypo/hypersegmentation of neutrophils	Proportion of myeloblasts (Auer rods)
Granularity of neutrophil cytoplasm: toxic granulation, hypogranular	Nuclear morphology of maturing cells (pseudo PH or megaloblastic changes)
Döhle bodies	Cytoplasmic morphology of maturing cells (granulation, Döhle bodies)
Organisms—intracellular, at feather	Cytochemical stains for blast identification
Basophilia	
Eosinophilia	Localization of immature and mature granulocytic cells on core biopsy
Nuclear and cytoplasmic features of eosinophils	ALIP on core biopsy (highlighted by MPO IHC)
Unique features of neutrophils and other granular cells in rare constitutional disorders such as Chédiak-Higashi syndrome, May-Hegglin anomaly, etc	CD34 staining on core biopsy: number, clustering

*Assess all lineages; assess for preservation of normal hematopoiesis
ALIP = abnormal localization of immature precursors;
MPO IHC = myeloperoxidase immunohistochemical stain; PH = Pelger Huët

t2.6 Megakaryocytic Lineage Checklist*

Blood	Bone Marrow
Number of platelets	Overall cellularity
Size, granularity of platelets	Number and distribution of megakaryocytes
Megakaryocyte nuclei (feather edge)	Overall megakaryocyte size, size range, and maturation pyramid
Platelet clumping	Megakaryocyte nuclear features: hypo/hyperlobation, pyknotic nuclei, uniformity of nuclear features
Platelet satellitism	
Pseudo platelets—RBC fragments, protein precipitate	Megakaryocyte clustering, intrasinusoidal localization on core biopsy
	Associated fibrosis and abnormal bony trabeculae
	Immature megakaryocytes by morphology, IHC: CD41, CD42b, CD31, CD61

*Assess all lineages; assess for preservation of normal hematopoiesis
IHC = immunohistochemical stain

adjacent to bone marrow sinusoids, but because these sinuses are normally inconspicuous, megakaryocytes appear to be randomly distributed individually on bone marrow biopsy sections i2.33 [Foucar 2008c, Geddis 2007, Wickramasinghe 2007]. In general, 2-4 megakaryocytes per high magnification (×40) field are noted on biopsy sections. Normal hematopoietic cells such as neutrophils may migrate through the megakaryocyte canalicular system, a phenomenon termed "emperipolesis" i2.34 [Wickramasinghe 2007]. In pathologic processes, megakaryocytes often cluster, exhibit morphologic abnormalities, and are increased in number (see Chapters 12 and 14). Although maturing megakaryocytes vary markedly

in size, the most readily identifiable megakaryocyte on tissue sections has multiple nuclear lobulations and is larger than all cells except fat cells. Immature megakaryocytes are much more difficult to recognize, because they are approximately the size of promyelocytes and have large immature nuclei and scant amounts of cytoplasm, similar to other hematopoietic precursor cells. Immunologic or ultrastructural techniques are required to identify these immature megakaryocytes i2.35, i2.36. A striking physiologic increase in megakaryocytes can occur in response to sustained thrombocytopenic states. A key blood and bone marrow checklist of features of platelets and megakaryocytes is listed in t2.6.

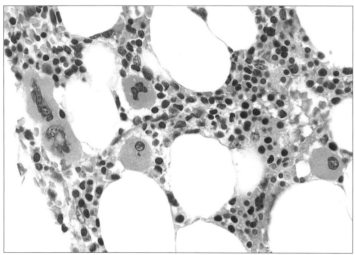

i2.33 *Several diffusely scattered megakaryocytes are shown. Although the megakaryocytes are located adjacent to the bone marrow capillary sinuses, this is generally not apparent on routine bone marrow biopsy sections. (H&E)*

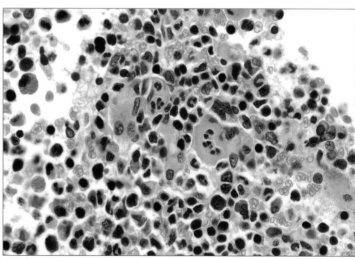

i2.34 *Many neutrophils are evident in the cytoplasm of megakaryocytes on this bone marrow clot section. (H&E)*

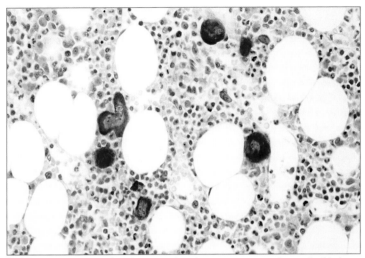

i2.35 *Immunoperoxidase for CD42b on bone marrow core biopsy highlights megakaryocytes at various stages of maturation. (immunoperoxidase)*

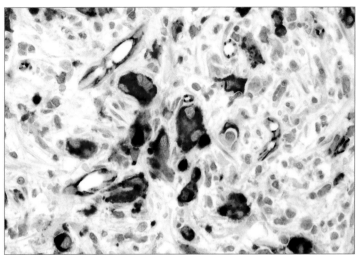

i2.36 *Abnormal megakaryocytic cells, including probably megakaryoblasts, highlighted by immunoperoxidase for CD42b on bone marrow core biopsy section. (immunoperoxidase)*

[2.1.8] **Lymphocytes and Plasma Cells**

Lymphocytes are more prominent in the bone marrow of children, especially very young children, in which lymphocytes can comprise up to 30% to 60% of cells on aspirate smears f2.2, i2.37 [Longacre 1989, Rimsza 2004]. These cells, designated as hematogones, may exhibit some nuclear immaturity and express either CD34 or the enzyme TdT, markers of immaturity, as well as B-cell antigens i2.38, i2.39 (see Chapter 21) [Rimsza 2000]. In adult patient specimens, lymphocytes generally comprise <20% of nucleated cells on differential counts and are morphologically mature with condensed nuclear chromatin [Foucar 2008b,b, Wickramasinghe 2007]. If hematopoiesis is reduced, both lymphocytes and plasma cells will be relatively more numerous.

On bone marrow biopsy sections, lymphocytes are generally inconspicuous and randomly admixed with

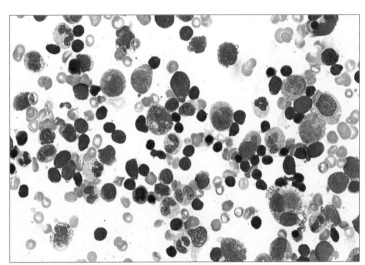

i2.37 *Abundant small, round lymphocytes evident on bone marrow aspirate smear from 13-day-old infant. (Wright)*

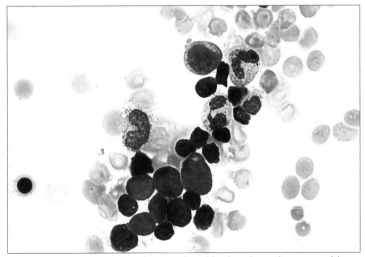

i2.38 *Bone marrow aspirate from 13-day-old infant shows that many of the lymphoid cells have the morphologic features of hematogones. (Wright)*

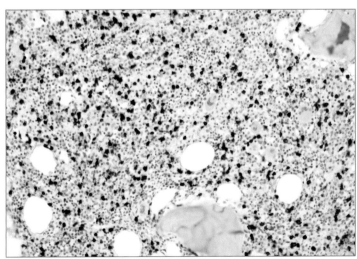

i2.39 *CD20 immunoperoxidase stain of bone marrow core biopsy in 14-month-old female shows abundant B cells. (immunoperoxidase)*

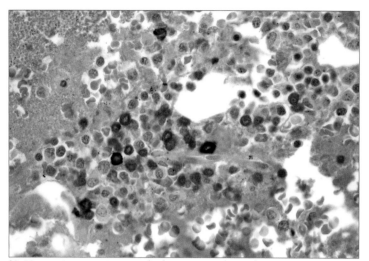

i2.40 *Dual staining for CD3 (red) and CD20 (brown) shows that T cells predominate in the bone marrow in adult patients.*

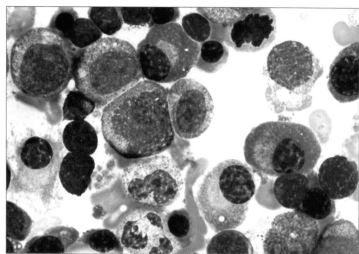

i2.41 *Increased plasma cells evident on bone marrow aspirate smear. (Wright)*

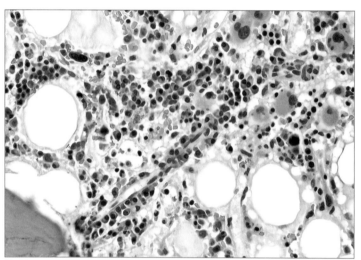

i2.42 *Distinct perivascular localization of plasma cells evident on bone marrow core biopsy section. (H&E)*

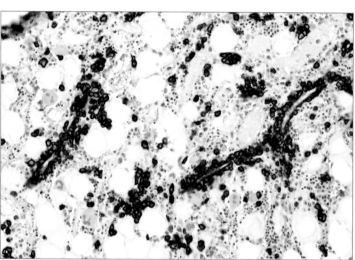

i2.43 *Perivascular localization of plasma cells highlighted by immunoperoxidase for CD138 on bone marrow core biopsy section. (immunoperoxidase)*

hematopoietic elements. Immunohistochemical studies show that T cells outnumber B cells in adults; these lymphoid cells are generally dispersed or occur in small collections i2.40. However, some patients, predominantly adults, develop benign lymphoid aggregates consisting of nonparatrabecular, dense collections of lymphocytes, with variable numbers of admixed histiocytes and plasma cells. These lymphoid aggregates and hematogones are discussed in detail in Chapter 21.

Abnormal lymphocytes can be identified on both bone marrow aspirate smears and biopsy sections. Cytologic features are best appreciated on aspirate smears, while the bone marrow biopsy section is essential for determining the pattern and extent of abnormal cell infiltration (see Chapters 22-26).

Plasma cells generally comprise <1% of all nucleated cells on aspirate smears, and these cells are concentrated within particles i2.41 [Wickramasinghe 2007]. If hematopoietic cells are reduced, the proportion of plasma cells increases. On histologic sections, normal plasma cells show a distinct perivascular localization i2.42. Dysplasia of plasma cells is best assessed on aspirate smears, while infiltrates of neoplastic plasma cells are more readily identified on biopsy sections (see Chapter 23). Plasma cells are highlighted by CD138 immunohistochemical staining on tissue sections, and plasma cell clonality can be assessed by immunoperoxidase/in situ hybridization staining for cytoplasmic kappa and lambda light chain expression i2.43. t2.7 includes a key blood and bone marrow checklist for assessment of features of lymphoid cells.

t2.7 Lymphoid Lineage Checklist*

Blood	Bone Marrow
Absolute lymphocyte count	Overall cellularity
Nuclear cytoplasmic ratio	Proportion of lymphoid cells; associated cell types (mast cells, histiocytes, eosinophils)
Uniformity vs heterogeneity	
Nuclear features including degree of chromatin condensation, presence of nucleoli, nuclear contours, nuclear size	Distribution of lymphoid cells on core biopsy; aggregates, interstitial or intrasinusoidal
	Morphologic features; nuclear and cytoplasmic
Cytoplasmic granules, vacuoles, crystals	Degree of preservation of hematopoietic bone marrow
Degree of preservation of hematopoiesis	Proportion, morphology, distribution of plasma cells
	Immunophenotype; flow cytometry, IHC

*Assess all lineages; assess for preservation of normal hematopoiesis
IHC = immunohistochemical stain

t2.8 Bone Marrow Stroma Checklist*

Bone Marrow Core Biopsy	Features Assessed/Comments
Overall core biopsy quality	Length of interpretable bone marrow core biopsy
	Subcortical region proportion, aspiration artifact, crush, fragmentation, other distortion
Overall cellularity	Exclude subcortical region
Reticulin fibers	Extent, fiber size, pattern (reticulin stain)
Collagen fibers	Extent (trichrome stain)
Sinuses	Dilated, intrasinusoidal cells
Number of vessels	Neoangiogenesis (CD34 stain)
Vessel walls	Thickened, amyloid deposition
Mast cells	Number, distribution, morphology, associated fibrosis, other associated cell types
Bony trabeculae	Osteosclerotic, anastomosing, bone remodeling, osteopenic, amount of osteoid, number of osteoblasts, osteoclasts, osteocytes
Amount of stroma	Characteristics of stroma
Smooth vs granular stroma	Gelatinous transformation vs fibrinoid necrosis
Interstitial deposits in stroma	Amyloid, fibrin
Evidence of necrosis of stroma/bone	Drop out of osteocyte nuclei; ghost cells
Macrophages	Number, dispersed or within granulomas, morphology, hemophagocytosis, organisms
Special stains	Selected use: reticulin, trichrome, Congo red, tryptase, other immunohistochemical, organism stains, other

*Blood picture highly variable

[2.1.9]   **Other Cell Types within Bone Marrow Stroma and Adjacent to Bone**

A variety of other cell types is evident on either bone marrow aspirate smears or biopsy sections; these include macrophages, mast cells, fibroblasts, fat cells, osteoblasts, and osteoclasts t2.8 [Wickramasinghe 2007]. Because many of these cells are concentrated in the stroma of bone marrow particles, the particle crush smear is useful in their assessment. Although macrophages may be increased in various pathologic conditions, normally they comprise <1% of cells on differential cell counts i2.44. Macrophages are highlighted by iron staining with Prussian blue i2.45, or by immunohistochemical stain for CD68. Both cytologic atypia of macrophages and hemophagocytosis are best appreciated on aspirate smears, while the pattern and extent of macrophage infiltration is ideally assessed using

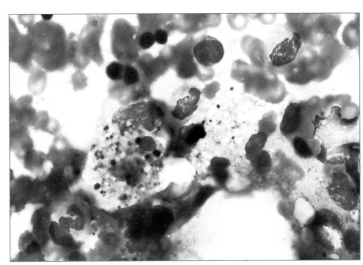

i2.44 *Macrophages evident on bone marrow aspirate smear containing abundant particles. (Wright)*

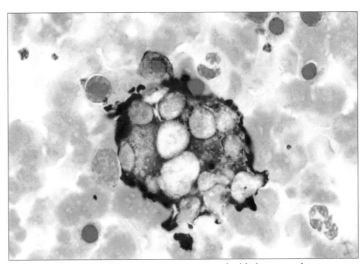

i2.45 *Iron staining of bone marrow aspirate can highlight macrophages containing increased storage iron. (Prussian blue)*

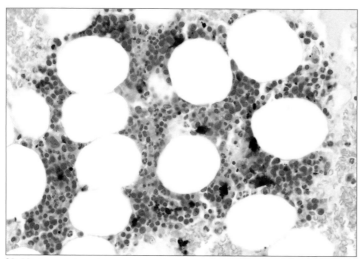

i2.46 *Iron stain on bone marrow clot section shows abundant iron-loaded macrophages with distinctive spindled appearance. (Prussian blue)*

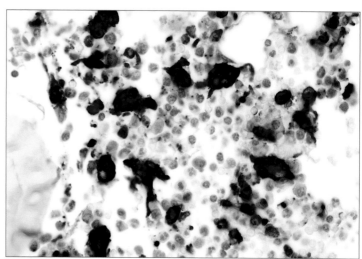

i2.47 *Immunohistochemical assessment for CD68 highlights abundant macrophages on bone marrow core biopsy section. (immunoperoxidase)*

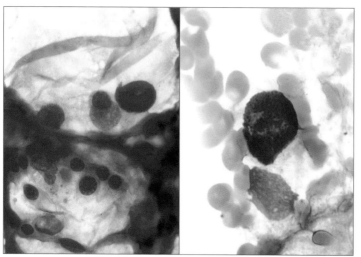

i2.48 *Because they are concentrated in darkly staining particles, mast cells are frequently inconspicuous on bone marrow aspirate smears. Intense cytoplasmic granulation obscures the nucleus. (Wright)*

morphology and immunohistochemical stains on core biopsy sections **i2.46**, **i2.47**. Disorders of this lineage are detailed in Chapter 27.

Mast cells are also concentrated within particles, and rarely are these cells counted in differential cell counts **i2.48**. Abnormal infiltrates of mast cells are best appreciated on biopsy sections. Under physiologic conditions, mast cells reside adjacent to blood vessels, but because of the prominent degranulation that occurs during tissue processing, normal mast cells are often very inconspicuous on biopsy sections. Both the number and distribution of mast cells on bone marrow biopsy sections can be highlighted with immunoperoxidase staining for either tryptase or CD117 **i2.49**, **i2.50** [Krokowski 2005, Patnaik 2007]. Despite degranulation, the abnormal mast cell infiltrates in systemic mast cell disease can generally be readily identified on biopsy sections, especially if discrete

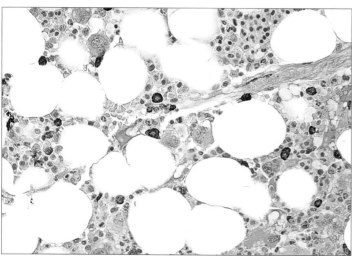

i2.49 *Medium magnification of a bone marrow biopsy section highlights both perivascular and individually dispersed mast cells. (immunoperoxidase for tryptase)*

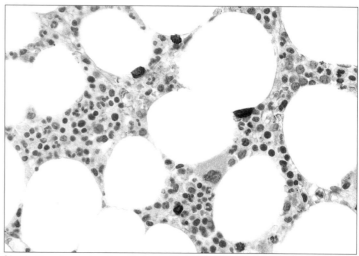

i2.50 *Randomly distributed mast cells are highlighted by immunoperoxidase staining for tryptase in this normal bone marrow core biopsy section. (immunoperoxidase for tryptase)*

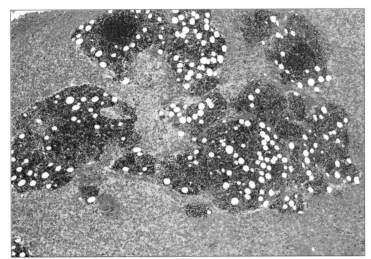

i2.51 *White globular fat cells evident on low magnification of bone marrow clot section. (H&E)*

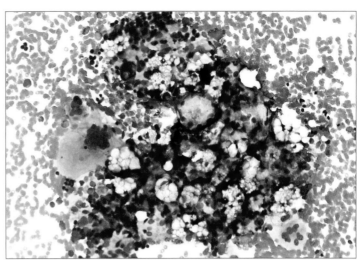

i2.52 *Both macrophages and fat cells are more prominent within bone marrow particles on aspirate smears following potent chemotherapy. (Wright)*

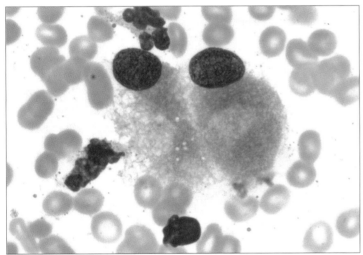

i2.53 *Bone marrow aspirate smear illustrates 2 osteoblasts exhibiting markedly eccentric nuclei and a Golgi region that is separate from the nucleus. (Wright)*

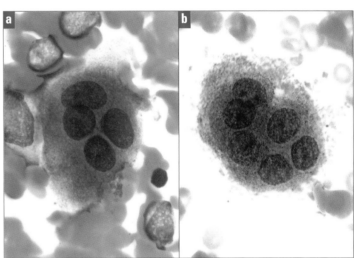

i2.54 *Bone marrow aspirate smears illustrate 2 osteoclasts, highlighting the range in cytoplasmic characteristics of these cells. Less mature osteoclasts have basophilic cytoplasm **a**, while brightly eosinophilic cytoplasm with coarse eosinophilic granules characterizes mature osteoclasts **b**. (Wright)*

lesions are present. Disorders of mast cells are reviewed comprehensively in Chapter 14.

Both fibroblasts and fat cells (adipocytes) are components of the bone marrow stroma. Except in 100% cellular specimens, adipocytes are readily apparent on aspirate and clot/core biopsy specimens **i2.51**. Fat cells become more prominent as the hematopoietic cellularity declines **i2.52**. Fat cells may show shrinkage in patients with severe starvation in conjunction with changes in the biochemical composition of the stroma, which characterizes gelatinous transformation (see Chapter 28). Fibroblasts are less conspicuous in normal marrow and are linked instead to pathologic conditions associated with collagen fibrosis (see Chapter 28).

Because visible active bony remodeling is minimal in normal adult specimens, osteoblasts and osteoclasts are only rarely seen on aspirate smears from normal patients older than

30 years, but these cells are commonly encountered in pediatric specimens **i2.53**, **i2.54** [Wickramasinghe 2007]. The osteoblast, characterized by a single, markedly eccentric nucleus and abundant blue-gray cytoplasm, can be seen in aspirate smears and touch imprints in specimens from young children in whom bony remodeling is physiologic. Multinucleated osteoclasts, characterized by multiple discrete small, round nuclei and abundant cytoplasm containing finely granular, variably eosinophilic material, may also occasionally be seen on pediatric aspirate and imprint smears. Both cell types are pathologic in samples from adults, and are generally associated with bone abnormalities (see next section). Both osteoblasts and osteoclasts are best appreciated on core biopsy sections. Both reside adjacent to bony trabeculae; osteoblasts form a more continuous layer along bony trabeculae specimens from children, while osteoclasts are intermittent and reside within lacunae [Foucar 2008c,

Wickramasinghe 2007]. **t2.8** provides a checklist for evaluation of bone marrow stromal cells and stroma.

[2.1.10] **Bone Marrow Stroma, Vessels, Bone, Abnormal Processes**

Evaluation of bone marrow stroma, vessels, and bone must all be performed on bone marrow biopsy sections. The bone marrow stroma, except for adipose cells, is quite inconspicuous in normal marrow. Only scattered thin reticulin fibers, often concentrated around vessels and identified by special stain, are normally present on bone marrow biopsy sections **i2.55**. A more prominent stroma is apparent in patients treated with some forms of chemotherapy, in patients with disorders inducing reticulin or collagen fibrosis, and in patients with gelatinous transformation (see Chapter 28) [Hasserjian 2008].

Blood vessels are generally inconspicuous on aspirate smears and biopsy sections; vessels can be highlighted using immunoperoxidase staining for CD34 **i2.56**. Although evidence of vasculitis or embolism is occasionally identified, blood vessels are generally thin-walled and infrequent on biopsy sections. Mild atherosclerotic changes may be evident in older patients. Increased vessel/sinusoidal density (neoangiogenesis) may be associated with primary and secondary neoplasms or with regeneration **i2.57**.

The eosinophilic bony trabeculae are evenly distributed throughout the bone marrow and contain dark-staining osteocytes in small lacunar spaces [Foucar 2008c, Wickramasinghe 2007]. In adults, bony trabeculae are generally thin and have smooth contours, while they are often thicker in children, especially teenagers and young adults **i2.58**. In pediatric biopsy sections, osteoclasts and osteoblasts can be identified, reflecting active

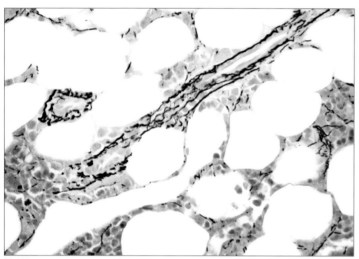

i2.55 *Reticulin fibers on bone marrow core biopsy from normal specimens show a concentration of fibers around blood vessels with only scanty reticulin fibers distributed diffusely throughout the medullary cavity. (reticulin stain)*

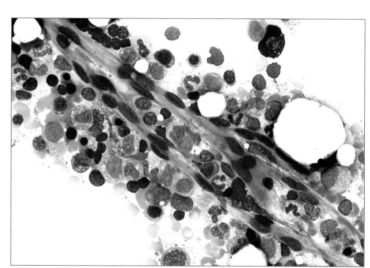

i2.56 *Capillaries evident within and adjacent to particles on bone marrow aspirate smear. (Wright)*

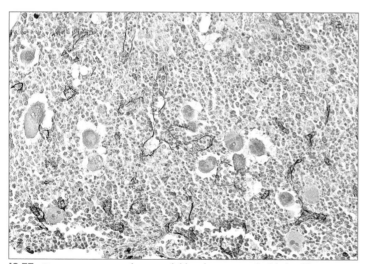

i2.57 *Prominent neovascularity and dilated sinuses are highlighted by CD34 staining in this neoplastic bone marrow core biopsy section. (immunoperoxidase)*

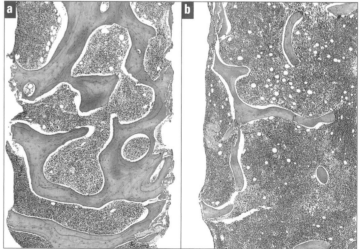

i2.58 *Age-related variations in size of bony trabeculae are highlighted on bone marrow biopsy sections from a 5-year-old male **a** and a 50-year-old male **b**. (H&E)*

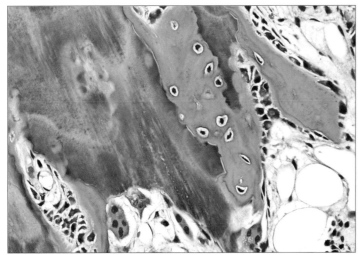

i2.59 *Bony trabeculae from bone marrow core biopsy from a 12-year-old male shows active bone formation with prominent rimming of osteoblasts and dispersed osteoclasts adjacent to bony trabeculae. (H&E)*

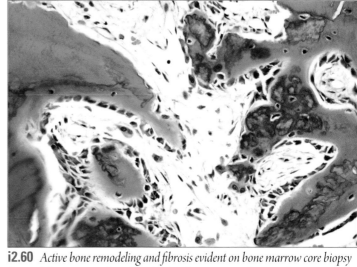

i2.60 *Active bone remodeling and fibrosis evident on bone marrow core biopsy from adult patient resulting from healing from previous biopsy of same region. (H&E)*

remodeling of bone, while in adult samples, prominent bony changes with increased osteoclasts or osteoblasts are usually indicative of a metabolic or neoplastic disorder **i2.59**. In addition, pronounced bony and stromal changes characterize previous biopsy sites, which are most likely to be sampled in patients who have undergone numerous prior bone marrow examinations **i2.60**. Marked variations in the thickness of bony trabeculae are often evidence of metabolic bone disorders, ranging from excessive bone production to excessive bone resorption (see Chapter 28). Pathologic bony changes, as well as other findings that may be apparent on the bone marrow biopsy such as necrosis, metastatic tumors, or amyloid deposition, are reviewed in Chapters 28 and 29. Key bone marrow assessment checklist features for bone marrow stroma are listed in **t2.8** (p 41).

[2.2] ## Blood and Bone Marrow Artifacts

A variety of artifacts may be apparent on blood smears and bone marrow preparations, which may either cause diagnostic challenges or interfere with interpretation. Common artifacts in both blood and bone marrow aspirate smears are spurious organisms resulting from contamination of stains **i2.61**. Major clues to the spurious nature of these organisms include both their abundance and their random extracellular distribution. Another more unique situation is the presence of intracellular bacteria on blood smears **i2.62**, **i2.63**. In rare circumstances, squamous cells with bacteria are encountered, presumably from the oval cavity of a slide handler **i2.63**. A more commonly encountered blood artifact is platelet satellitism, causing a spurious reduction in the platelet count **i2.64**. This phenomenon is linked to specific anticoagulants, notably ethylenediaminetetraacetic acid (EDTA).

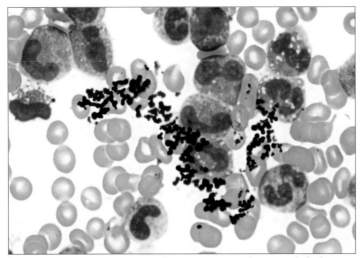

i2.61 *Abundant fungi growing within stain can cause diagnostic difficulties. Note that the organisms lay randomly throughout smears and are not within the cytoplasm of neutrophils. (Wright)*

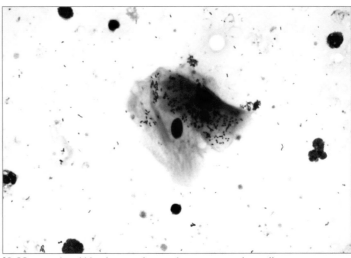

i2.62 *Peripheral blood smear showing large mononuclear cells containing intracytoplasmic bacteria on high magnification. (Wright)*

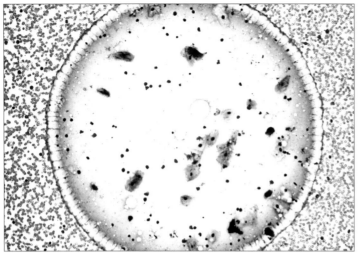

i2.63 *Low magnification of the same area as* **i2.62** *showing a distinctive lysing of red cells and numerous squamous cells with intracellular bacteria compatible with contamination from oral cavity of individual handling slide. (Wright)*

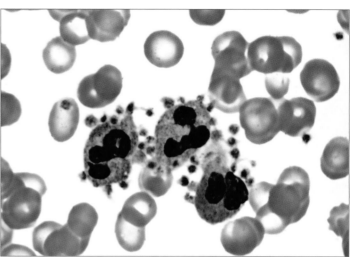

i2.64 *Prominent satellitism of platelets around neutrophils caused by specific types of anticoagulant used for complete blood count evaluation. (Wright)*

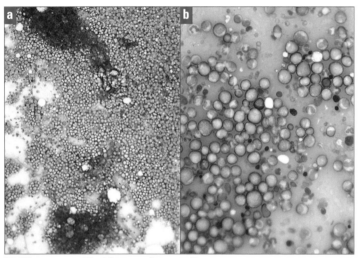

i2.65 *Low* **a** *and high* **b** *magnification of bone marrow aspirate smears illustrate a thick and poorly stained particle crush smear. (Wright)*

t2.9 Causes of Bone Marrow Artifacts

Overstaining or understaining of smears
Water contamination of staining solutions
Aspirate smears too thick
Excessive pressure for particle crush preparations
Small clots on aspirate smears
Aspiration of marrow from core biopsy sample
Core biopsy of previous biopsy site
Core biopsy consisting of hypocellular subcortical region
Crushed core biopsy specimen
Inadequate fixation of clot and biopsy specimens
Suboptimal sectioning and staining of clot and biopsy specimens
Excessive decalcification of bone marrow biopsy
Excessive exposure of biopsy to mercurial fixative
Failure to adequately wash B5-fixed specimens

References: [Bain 2001, Brown 1993, Salgado 1992]

Types of artifacts that may be encountered in aspirate smears and biopsy sections include those caused by sampling errors, poor technique at the bedside, and poorly performed laboratory procedures **t2.9** [Bain 2001, Salgado 1992]. As mentioned earlier, both understaining and overstaining of cells interfere with interpretation **i2.65**. Staining problems can also result from various causes, including water contamination of the staining solutions and organism overgrowth within solutions (see **i2.61**). In addition, on thick smears, cytologic detail is poor because cells are not evenly spread on the slides, and, consequently, staining is very uneven. Crush preparations often have very thick and, therefore, poorly stained areas. In addition, particle crush preparations can be subject to excessive pressure, resulting in extensive disruption and distortion of cells, making cell identification impossible **i2.66**, **i2.67**.

If the bone marrow aspirate begins to clot before smears are made, the result can be thick aggregates of agglutinated RBCs, platelets, and entrapped WBCs **i2.68**. It is impossible to identify WBCs in these thick areas, and differential cell counts on other areas of the slide may be unreliable because of the entrapment of cells in these clots. Prominent normoblast clumping mimicking particles may also occur in partially clotted specimens, interfering with cell counts **i2.69**. Extensive platelet clumping, especially common in aspirate smears from patients with essential thrombocythemia, also mimics particles and interferes with cell distribution and staining **i2.69**.

Various core biopsy artifacts can also be encountered. One common and major artifact is caused by aspiration of the marrow from the biopsy sample when the sample is taken from a site too close to the preceding aspiration site **i2.70**, **i2.71**. This common artifact can be avoided by performing the biopsy first. Other sampling artifacts include bone marrow biopsy specimens consisting of cartilage, cortical

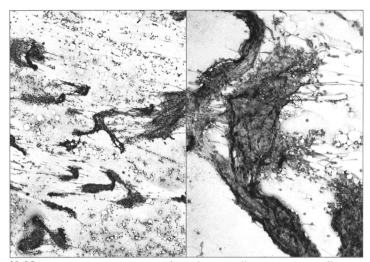

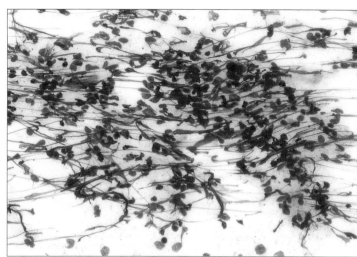

i2.66 *Bone marrow aspirate particle crush smears illustrate excessive cell crushing with streaking of nuclear material. (Wright)*

i2.67 *Virtually no intact cells are present on this excessively crushed bone marrow aspirate particle crush preparation. Note prominent nuclear streaking. (Wright)*

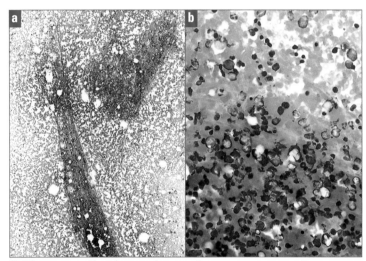

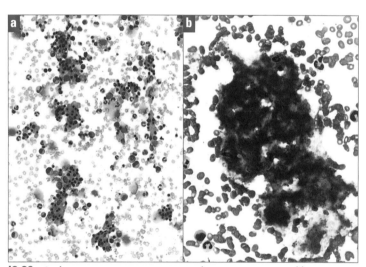

i2.68 *Low **a** and high **b** magnification of bone marrow aspirate direct smears illustrate several clots. Note marked cellular distortion. (Wright)*

i2.69 *On bone marrow aspirate smears, either prominent normoblast clumping from specimen clotting **a** or marked platelet clumping in a patient with essential thrombocythemia **b** can mimic particles and interfere with differential counting. (Wright)*

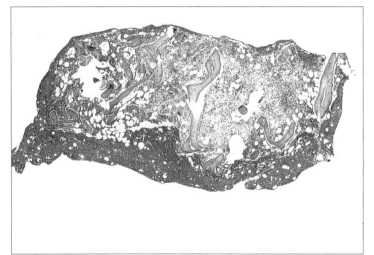

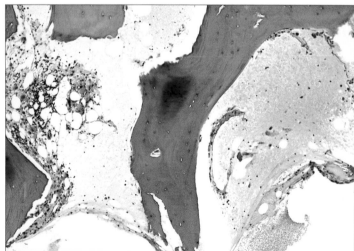

i2.70 *Extensive disruption of the hematopoietic cavity by aspiration is apparent at low magnification on this bone marrow biopsy section. (H&E)*

i2.71 *Bone marrow core biopsy showing extensive aspiration artifact. (H&E)*

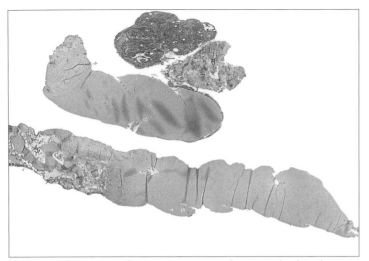

i2.72 *Core bone marrow biopsy section consists almost entirely of cartilage. (H&E)*

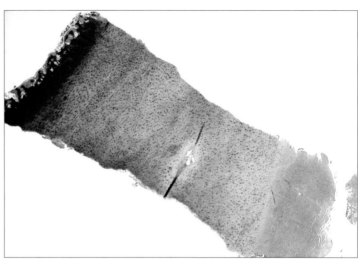

i2.73 *Bone marrow core biopsy specimen consisting exclusively of cortical bone and cartilage without hematopoietic cells. (H&E)*

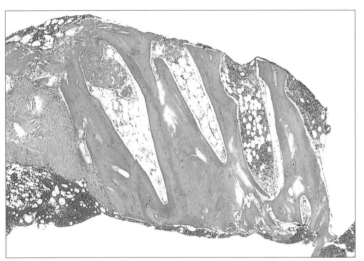

i2.74 *Core bone marrow biopsy section consists primarily of cortical and subcortical bone. Only a small area of hematopoiesis is present. (H&E)*

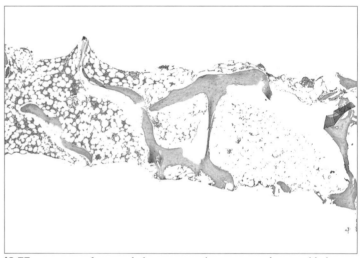

i2.75 *Low magnification of a bone marrow biopsy section from an elderly patient illustrates a large subcortical hypocellular zone that is not representative of the overall hematopoietic cavity. (H&E)*

bone, or subcortical bone (especially in older patients) that are not representative of the true hematopoietic cavity **i2.72**, **i2.73**, **i2.74**, **i2.75**. The bone marrow biopsy core can also be crushed, resulting in extreme cellular distortion **i12.76**, **i2.77**, **i2.78**. In patients with disorders that cause excessive bone resorption, such as multiple myeloma, the core biopsy can readily compress in an accordion-like fashion during the biopsy procedure, yielding a small crushed specimen. This artifact can be avoided by using a large-bore biopsy needle and by slowly advancing this needle during the procedure. Although much less common, the biopsy of a previous biopsy site can cause an erroneous diagnosis of metabolic bone disease or neoplasm (see **i2.60**) [Salgado 1992]. Bony remodeling, increased osteoblasts, increased osteoclasts, and stromal fibrosis are all identified in

these damaged fracture sites from previous biopsy (see Chapter 28). Sometimes bone marrow core biopsy specimens contain skin forced into the biopsy needle during the procedure **i2.79**. This is becoming more common because currently the skin is often not lanced before the core biopsy needle is inserted.

Finally, poor specimen processing techniques, including inadequate fixation, excessive fixation, or excessive decalcification, can all cause major difficulties in interpretation **i2.80**. Often, lymphocyte nuclei appear more irregular on these specimens. Plastic embedding techniques are also linked to irregularity of lymphocyte nuclei. Fixatives, notably B5, must be treated with Lugol iodine solution and washed out of tissue before slides are stained or a precipitate will cover cells **i2.80**.

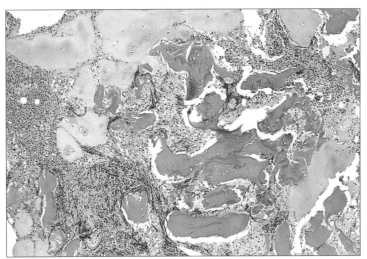

i2.76 *Bone marrow biopsy section illustrates pronounced crushing and cellular distortion of biopsy core from an infant with metastatic neuroblastoma. (H&E)*

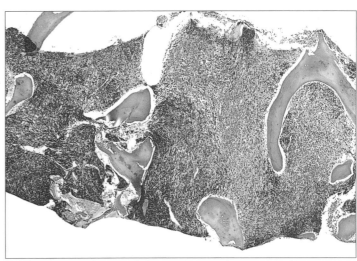

i2.77 *Low magnification of a bone marrow core biopsy section from a patient with acute leukemia demonstrates that half of the specimen is intact and half is crushed. (H&E)*

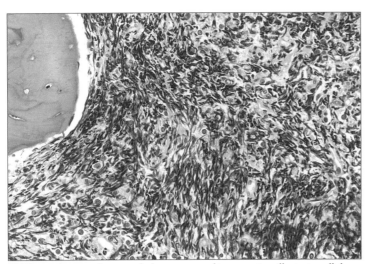

i2.78 *High magnification of a bone marrow biopsy section illustrates cellular distortion secondary to crush artifact. (H&E)*

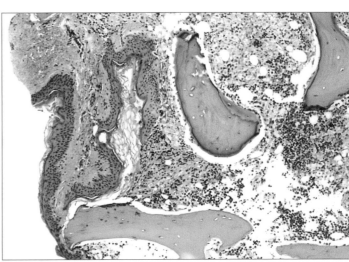

i2.79 *Bone marrow core biopsy containing segment of skin. This artifact is more common when the incision site is not lanced before the core biopsy needle is inserted. (H&E)*

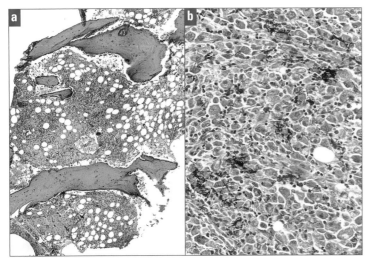

i2.80 *Low **a** and medium **b** magnification of bone marrow biopsy sections illustrate excessive B5 fixation with inadequate rinsing. Because of mercurial artifacts, the nature of the abnormal infiltrate is difficult to determine. (H&E)*

[2.3] Bone Marrow Report (see Chapter 5)

The bone marrow report must contain all relevant information obtained from review of the peripheral blood smear, laboratory data, and clinical data, as well as bone marrow features [Peterson 2002]. A well designed requisition form can optimize the availability of clinical, therapeutic, and physical examination information, although either review of electronic medical records or discussion with the clinician is essential to be certain that all relevant information is available to the diagnostician. Differential counts from both peripheral blood and bone marrow should be included in the report, as well as information regarding the types of samples obtained and morphologic abnormalities in any cell lineage within blood or bone marrow. Discrepancies between blood and bone marrow findings should be addressed, recognizing that specimen quality, sampling issues, ineffective hematopoiesis, splenic sequestration, and bone marrow fibrosis may be factors contributing to these discrepancies.

The results of all special studies must be delineated along with their significance in establishing the diagnosis (see Chapter 4). The comparison of the current bone marrow specimen to either previous bone marrow samples or extramedullary biopsy specimens is essential in some situations. For example, morphologic features of bone marrow lymphomatous infiltrates should always be compared with features of any previous biopsy specimens obtained from extramedullary sites of disease. The bone marrow report should contain information regarding morphologic concordance or discordance of the 2 sites of lymphoma. Likewise, any assessment of response to therapy generally requires side-by-side review of sequential bone marrow specimens.

When possible, the diagnosis should describe the cause of any pathologic processes identified, and a comment may be needed to recommend additional tests, list differential diagnostic possibilities, and highlight references pertinent to the bone marrow findings. A descriptive diagnosis is commonly rendered on bone marrow samples, because additional correlative studies are often necessary to determine the specific cause of a given abnormality. Additional tests should be recommended on an individual case basis with an explanation of the potential usefulness of the test in resolving diagnostic uncertainty. Coding of bone marrow reports for quality management/improvement programs is also highly recommended, along with any physician peer review data relevant to the quality of specimen obtained, appropriate indications for bone marrow examination, reporting turnaround time, and bone marrow interpretation (see Chapter 5).

[2.4]   Clues and Caveats

1. An understanding of normal age/sex-related blood parameters as well as normal hematopoiesis, bone marrow architecture, and age-related bone marrow changes are all essential for bone marrow interpretation.

2. A review of bone marrow aspirate, imprint, and biopsy preparations should include not only hematolymphoid elements but bone, stroma, vessels, and fat cells.

3. The subcortical hypocellular region becomes more prominent with advancing age and should be excluded from bone marrow cellularity determinations.

4. Immunoperoxidase staining for CD34, myeloperoxidase, hemoglobin A, and CD42b can complement the morphologic assessment of bone marrow architecture.

5. An interpretative, comprehensive bone marrow report should be generated that provides both the recommendation and rationale for additional diagnostic testing to resolve diagnostic uncertainty.

6. In my experience, poor specimen quality is the most common cause of diagnostic errors in bone marrow interpretation.

7. Cell identification on smears is hampered by poor stain quality, excessive pressure in preparing particle crush smears, and excessively thick smears.

8. Inadequate size, aspiration artifact, prolonged exposure to B5 fixative, or excessive decalcification can all compromise bone marrow biopsy interpretation.

9. Processing of bone marrow biopsy samples, including fixation and decalcification, often induces some nuclear irregularity of small benign lymphocytes that can mimic abnormal lymphoid infiltrates; processing also affects immunohistochemical studies.

10. With some fixatives, nucleated erythroid cells can be difficult to distinguish from lymphocytes, sometimes necessitating immunohistochemical assessment.

[2.5]   Acknowledgments

The authors are grateful to D Rospopo and L Owens, MT (ASCP), for preparing samples with artifacts.

[2.6]   References

Aboul-Nasr R, Estey EH, Kantarjian HM, et al [1999] Comparison of touch imprints with aspirate smears for evaluating bone marrow specimens. *Am J Clin Pathol* 111:753-758.

Bain BJ [1996] The bone marrow aspirate of healthy subjects. *Br J Haematol* 94:206-209.

Bain BJ, Clark DM, Lampert IA, Wilkins BS [2001] The normal bone marrow. In: *Bone Marrow Pathology*. 3rd ed. Edinburgh: Blackwell Science Ltd; 1-50.

Brown DC, Gatter KC [1993] The bone marrow trephine biopsy: a review of normal histology. *Histopathology* 22:411-422.

Buescher E [2005] Neutrophil function and disorders of neutrophils in the newborn. In: de Alarcon P, Werner E, eds. *Neonatal Hematology*. Cambridge: Cambridge University; 254-279.

Buttarello M, Plebani M [2008] Automated blood cell counts: state of the art. *Am J Clin Pathol* 130:104-116.

Chasis JA, Mohandas N [2008] Erythroblastic islands: niches for erythropoiesis. *Blood* 112:470-478.

Cheng CK, Chan J, Cembrowski GS, van Assendelft OW [2004] Complete blood count reference interval diagrams derived from NHANES III: Stratification by age, sex, and race. *Lab Hematol* 10:42-53.

de Alarcon P, Werner E [2005] Erythropoiesis, red cells, and the approach to anemia. In: *Neonatal Hematology*. Cambridge: Cambridge University; 40-57.

Fabriek BO, Polfliet MM, Vloet RP, et al [2007] The macrophage CD163 surface glycoprotein is an erythroblast adhesion receptor. *Blood* 109:5223-5229.

Foucar K, Viswanatha D, Wilson C [2008a] Laboratory evaluation of blood and bone marrow in non-neoplastic disorders. In: King D, Gardner W, Sobin L, et al, eds. *Non-Neoplastic Disorders of Bone Marrow (AFIP fascicle)*. Washington, DC: American Registry of Pathology; 57-73.

Foucar K, Viswanatha D, Wilson C [2008b] Non-neoplastic lymphoid and plasma cell disorders In: King D, Gardner W, Sobin L, et al, eds. *Non-Neoplastic Disorders of Bone Marrow (AFIP fascicle).* Washington, DC: American Registry of Pathology; 249-282.

Foucar K, Viswanatha D, Wilson C [2008c] Normal anatomy and histology of bone marrow. In: King D, Gardner W, Sobin L, et al, eds. *Non-Neoplastic Disorders of Bone Marrow (AFIP fascicle).* Washington, DC: American Registry of Pathology; 1-40.

Friebert SE, Shepardson LB, Shurin SB, et al [1998] Pediatric bone marrow cellularity: are we expecting too much? *J Pediatr Hematol Oncol* 20:439-443.

Geddis AE, Kaushansky K [2007] The root of platelet production. *Science* 317:1689-1691.

Girodon F, Favre B, Carli PM, et al [2001] Minor dysplastic changes are frequently observed in the bone marrow aspirate in elderly patients without haematological disease. *Clin Lab Haematol* 23:297-300.

Gulati GL, Ashton JK, Hyun BH [1988] Structure and function of the bone marrow and hematopoiesis. *Hematol Oncol Clin North Am* 2:495-511.

Hartsock RJ, Smith EB, Petty CS [1965] Normal variations with aging of the amount of hematopoietic tissue in bone marrow from the anterior iliac crest. a study made from 177 cases of sudden death examined by necropsy. *Am J Clin Pathol* 43:326-331.

Hasserjian RP [2008] Reactive versus neoplastic bone marrow: problems and pitfalls. *Arch Pathol Lab Med* 132:587-594.

Kass L, Strickland T [1995] Identification of proerythroblasts in tissue sections of bone marrow. *Hematol Pathol* 9:179-184.

Krokowski M, Sotlar K, Krauth MT, et al [2005] Delineation of patterns of bone marrow mast cell infiltration in systemic mastocytosis: value of CD25, correlation with subvariants of the disease, and separation from mast cell hyperplasia. *Am J Clin Pathol* 124:560-568.

Lantis KL, Harris RJ, Davis G, et al [2003] Elimination of instrument-driven reflex manual differential leukocyte counts. Optimization of manual blood smear review criteria in a high-volume automated hematology laboratory. *Am J Clin Pathol* 119:656-662.

Lee G, Lo A, Short SA, et al [2006] Targeted gene deletion demonstrates that the cell adhesion molecule ICAM-4 is critical for erythroblastic island formation. *Blood* 108:2064-2071.

Longacre TA, Foucar K, Crago S, et al [1989] Hematogones: a multiparameter analysis of bone marrow precursor cells. *Blood* 73:543-552.

Novis DA, Walsh M, Wilkinson D, et al [2006] Laboratory productivity and the rate of manual peripheral blood smear review: a College of American Pathologists Q-Probes study of 95,141 complete blood count determinations performed in 263 institutions. *Arch Pathol Lab Med* 130:596-601.

Patnaik MM, Rindos M, Kouides PA, et al [2007] Systemic mastocytosis: a concise clinical and laboratory review. *Arch Pathol Lab Med* 131:784-791.

Peterson LC, Agosti SJ, Hoyer JD [2002] Protocol for the examination of specimens from patients with hematopoietic neoplasms of the bone marrow: a basis for checklists. *Arch Pathol Lab Med* 126:1050-1056.

Proytcheva M [2009] Issues in neonatal cellular analysis. *Am J Clin Pathol* 131:560-573.

Rimsza L, Larson R, Winter S, et al [2000] Benign hematogone-rich lymphoid proliferations can be distinguished from B-lineage acute lymphoblastic leukemia by integration of morphology, immunophenotype, adhesion molecule expression, and architectural features. *Am J Clin Pathol* 114:66-75.

Rimsza LM, Douglas VK, Tighe P, et al [2004] Benign B-cell precursors (hematogones) are the predominant lymphoid population in the bone marrow of preterm infants. *Biol Neonate* 86:247-253.

Salgado C, Feliu E, Blade J, et al [1992] A second bone marrow biopsy as a cause of a false diagnosis of myelofibrosis. *Br J Haematol* 80:407-409.

Trimoreau F, Verger C, Praloran V, Denizot Y [1997] No sex-related difference in the myeloid:erythroid ratio in morphologically normal bone marrow aspirates. *Br J Haematol* 97:687.

Wickramasinghe S [2007] Bone marrow. In: Mills S, ed. *Histology for Pathologists.* 3rd ed. Philadelphia: Lippincott Williams & Wilkins; 799-836.

Wilson C [2008a] Laboratory evaluation of blood and bone marrow in non-neoplastic disorders. In: King D, Gardner W, Sobin L, et al, eds. *Non-Neoplastic Disorders of Bone Marrow (AFIP fascicle).* Washington, DC: American Registry of Pathology; 57-73.

Wilson C [2008b] Non-neoplastic granulocytic and monocytic disorders In: King D, Gardner W, Sobin L, et al, eds. *Non-Neoplastic Disorders of Bone Marrow (AFIP fascicle).* Washington, DC: American Registry of Pathology; 125-175.

Zutter MM, Hess JL [1998] Guidelines for the diagnosis of leukemia or lymphoma in children. *Am J Clin Pathol* 109:S9-22.

CHAPTER 3

Procurement and Indications for Bone Marrow Examination

Kathryn Foucar, MD

Although the information obtained from bone marrow examination is often essential for patient management, there are no "set rules" that determine which patients require this invasive procedure. Instead, the decision to perform a bone marrow examination is made on a case-by-case basis, after all available clinical and laboratory information has been analyzed. The frequency with which bone marrow examination is used in the clinical care of patients varies prominently based on practice site, extent of physician specialization, and institution at which the physician trained [Simpson 2008]. For this procedure to yield optimal information, discussions regarding procurement and types of specimens needed for routine and specialized testing are presented. Differential diagnostic considerations play a pivotal role in guiding initial specialized testing. Bone marrow examination is also a readily available means to monitor treatment response.

[3.1] Bone Marrow Examination

[3.1.1] **Indications**

General indications for bone marrow examination (BME) are listed in **t3.1** and **t3.2**; these include the investigation for hematolymphoid neoplasms, other blood abnormalities, assessment for possible infectious disease, staging for neoplasms, and further evaluation of abnormal lymphoid infiltrates initially detected in other sites [Foucar 2008,

Howell 2002, Simpson 2008, Vassilakopoulos 2005]. The relative number of patients undergoing bone marrow examination for these indications obviously varies in different practice settings and can vary over time [Simpson 2008]. In recent years, greater reliance has been placed on blood evaluation for assessing response to therapy for selected disorders, reducing the number of bone marrow examinations that some patients may undergo during disease diagnosis and management. In addition, the necessity of routine bone marrow examination in the staging of patients with such solid tumors as lymphoma, Hodgkin lymphoma, and certain carcinomas has been challenged, since bone marrow dissemination is generally very unlikely in those patients with localized disease by other assessments [Simpson 2008]. Furthermore, new radiologic techniques such as positron emission tomography (PET) scan may be useful in detecting bone marrow involvement by lymphoma [Pakos 2005].

For patients with peripheral blood abnormalities, several important variables must be factored into the decision-making process before bone marrow examination is performed. These variables include patient age, the type of blood abnormality, number of aberrant lineages, and clinical findings **t3.2**. In these patients, the decision to perform a bone marrow examination often depends on whether the abnormality can be "explained" by the overall clinical assessment of the patient. A decision to forego a bone marrow examination may be reversed at any time if the patient does not follow a clinical course predicted by the initial presumptive diagnosis.

Although exceptions exist, peripheral blood examination in conjunction with other laboratory studies is often sufficient

---

t3.1 Indications for Bone Marrow Examination*

Investigation of peripheral blood abnormality if cause cannot be determined by other means (see t3.2)

Primary diagnostic modality in patients with likely leukemia, myelodysplastic, myeloproliferative, or myelomatous disorder

Infectious disease assessment in which blood or other tissue sampling uninformative or extensive bone marrow effacement suspected

Evaluation for fever of unknown origin, systemic mast cell disease, metabolic bone disease, or unexplained splenomegaly

Evaluation for suspected constitutional hematologic disorder, storage disease,[†] or metastatic lesion

Staging and management of patients with certain types of neoplasms (eg, Hodgkin and non-Hodgkin lymphoma, some carcinoma types, other solid tumors)

Evaluation of patient with atypical but nondiagnostic lymphoid process in other sites

Unexplained radiographic lesions

Evaluation of patient who does not follow predicted course of initial diagnosis (eg, patient with presumed ITP who does not respond to therapy)

Ongoing monitoring of response to therapy in patients with hematolymphoid neoplasms and selected solid tumors

Bone marrow assessment prior to autologous SCT/BMT; rarely, possible donor for allogeneic SCT/BMT

*Decision to perform BME is made on an individual case basis after correlation of clinical and laboratory findings; in recent years, greater emphasis has been placed on using peripheral blood for both definitive diagnosis of leukemias and for monitoring response to therapy/BMT
[†]Definitive diagnosis of a storage disease is based on determination of actual biochemical defect rather than by morphologic assessment of bone marrow histiocytes; BME may not be necessary unless extent of histiocytic infiltration is clinically relevant
BME = bone marrow examination; SCT = stem cell transplant; BMT = bone marrow transplantation; ITP = immune thrombocytopenic purpura

References: [Foucar 2008, Howell 2002, Lee 2008, Simpson 2008, Vassilakopoulos 2005]

t3.2 Decision-Making Variables for Bone Marrow Examination in the Evaluation of Patients with Peripheral Blood Abnormalities*

Variable	Comments
Age	BME may be not necessary for either isolated neutropenia or thrombocytopenia in children; most significantly neutropenic adults undergo BME
	BME is generally not performed for infectious disease evaluation in children
Single vs multilineage aberrations	Multilineage abnormalities, especially combined dysplasia and numerical aberrations, generally necessitate BME
	BME is required for virtually all patients with unexplained pancytopenia
Anemia	BME is not required if etiology is apparent by RBC indices, morphologic review of blood smear, other laboratory tests, and clinical information
Erythrocytosis	BME is not required for secondary or relative erythrocytosis that can be explained by clinical situation (eg, chronic hypoxia)
Neutropenia	Transient isolated neutropenia is common in children; BME considered only if spontaneous remission does not occur
	In adults, unexplained, significant neutropenia often pursued with BME
Neutrophilia	BME is not necessary for toxic neutrophilia with obvious underlying etiology
	If toxic changes are absent or additional abnormalities such as basophilia are present, BME may be required, although both FISH and molecular assessment can be performed on blood[†]
Thrombocytopenia	Pretreatment BME may not be necessary in patients with a presumptive diagnosis of ITP
Thrombocytosis	BME is not required when clinical picture suggests reactive thrombocytosis
Blasts	With rare exceptions (severe infections in neonates and in patients receiving cytokine therapy) BME is generally required
Other abnormal cells	Evaluation of blood cells is sufficient for management in some patients; BME is necessary in others

*Decision to perform BME is made on an individual case basis after correlation of all clinical and laboratory findings
[†]Standard cytogenetic karyotyping can only be performed on blood samples with sufficient numbers of immature, ie, mitotically active cells; molecular analyses and FISH can utilize mature, ie, interphase cells
BME = bone marrow examination; FISH = fluorescence in situ hybridization; ITP = immune thrombocytopenia

References: [Foucar 1993, 2008]

for the diagnosis of an isolated anemia. For example, patients with iron deficiency anemia and a substantial proportion of patients with thalassemia, megaloblastic anemia, and various hemolytic anemias do not require bone marrow examination. Likewise, a patient with isolated erythrocytosis that can be explained by the clinical situation does not usually require a bone marrow examination.

Age is an important variable in assessing whether bone marrow examination should be performed on neutropenic patients. Because neutropenia is a common transient consequence of viral infections in children, bone marrow examination may not initially be warranted in an otherwise healthy child with isolated neutropenia [Foucar 1993]. Instead, the child's blood may be evaluated periodically for several weeks for evidence of spontaneous recovery. In contrast, because of the widely varied causes of neutropenia in adults, most of these patients with a significant, sustained neutropenia will require bone marrow examination early in their evaluation, especially if dysplasia or additional lineage abnormalities are also evident. For neutrophilia, either the presence or absence of toxic changes and clinical circumstances often discriminate between patients who require bone marrow examination and those in whom peripheral blood monitoring will suffice. The

identification of additional blood abnormalities in a patient with unexplained nontoxic neutrophilia will generally prompt investigation for a possible myeloproliferative or myelodysplastic neoplasm.

The role of bone marrow examination in the management of patients with isolated thrombocytopenia has changed over the years. Because immune thrombocytopenic purpura is almost always the cause of acquired, isolated thrombocytopenia in children, bone marrow examination is often necessary only in those patients who do not promptly respond to therapy [Segel 2009]. Although controversial, some authors recommend a similar therapeutic trial in adults with isolated thrombocytopenia; however, more differential diagnostic considerations and additional variables are often seen in adult patients which may necessitate upfront bone marrow examination.

Except in unique circumstances, such as life-threatening infections in infants, the presence of circulating blasts should prompt consideration of a bone marrow examination to assess for possible myelodysplasia, myeloproliferative neoplasms, leukemias, or infiltrative processes [Foucar 2008]. Likewise, bone marrow examination is also frequently required when other abnormal cells, including suspected lymphoma cells, are present in the peripheral blood. In these patients, factors that influence decisions regarding bone marrow examination include the extent of prior studies of extramedullary disease sites, results of flow cytometric immunophenotyping of blood, and anticipated treatment strategies. In some patients, definitive diagnosis can be made by means of peripheral blood specimens; specialized studies including comprehensive immunophenotyping, molecular analysis, and standard cytogenetics can all be performed on blood samples. However, the frequency of unsuccessful karyotyping is higher in blood samples than in bone marrow aspirate specimens [Weinkauff 1999].

[3.1.2] Special Considerations in Bone Marrow Examination

Before an initial bone marrow examination is performed, each case must be assessed to determine the types of samples required to provide the most comprehensive diagnostic information. For example, bilateral iliac crest biopsies or double core biopsies of the same iliac crest are optimal for staging in oncology patients, because the identification of focal carcinomatous or lymphomatous infiltrates increases with the amount of marrow examined [Barekman 1997, Jatoi 1999, Wang 2002]. If acute leukemia is a diagnostic consideration, preparation of numerous smears is essential to have sufficient material for a variety of cytochemical and/or FISH studies. In addition, unstained smears are often required for enrollment in study protocols. When the presumptive diagnosis is either leukemia or lymphoma, additional anticoagulated aspiration specimens should also be obtained for flow cytometric immunophenotyping, cytogenetic analysis, and possible molecular studies. Likewise, an extra aspirate for culture is indicated in patients with fevers and/or suppressed immune systems. Finally, in rare clinical situations an additional aspirate or biopsy may be necessary for electron microscopy. Likewise, special processing is required for those rare bone marrow core biopsies performed for metabolic bone disorder assessment.

[3.1.3] Contraindications to Bone Marrow Examination

Bone marrow examination, including both aspiration and biopsy sampling, can be safely performed on virtually any patient, including those with coagulation factor deficiencies or profound thrombocytopenia, as well as those receiving anticoagulant therapy. However, patients with coagulopathies such as hemophilia require factor transfusion to >50% of normal levels before this procedure. Similarly, diamino-d-arginine vasopressin (DDAVP) therapy may be useful in stimulating platelet function before bone marrow examination in patients with chronic renal failure. In contrast, platelet transfusions are generally not required, even for

t3.3 Complications of Bone Marrow Examination*

Complication	Comments
Hemorrhage	Most common complication; higher risk of significant hemorrhage in obese patients and patients with CMPN
	Rare reports of retroperitoneal hemorrhage; very rarely fatal
Local infection	Wound infections rare and generally require only topical medications
Broken needle	Very rare, complications usually minor
Neuropathy	Very rare, usually secondary to damage of lateral cutaneous thigh nerve
Osteomyelitis	Very rare, systemic therapy necessary
Cardiac tamponade	Perforation of posterior sternal plate is a very rare complication of sternal aspiration

*Overall complication rate is substantially <1%; serious complications are rare
CMPN = chronic myeloproliferative neoplasm

References: [Bain 2004, Devaliaf 2004, Le Dieu 2003, Marti 2004]

profoundly thrombocytopenic patients, unless prolonged oozing uncontrolled by pressure bandages occurs after the procedure.

Several unique clinical situations, such as prior irradiation to the region or overlying skin infection, may preclude posterior iliac crest examination. In adults, the sternum can be considered as an alternate site, but this is discouraged; sternal aspirations are generally not performed in children. Other alternate bone marrow sites in adults include the anterior iliac crest. In very young infants, the tibia can be considered an alternate site for bone marrow examination [Sola 1999].

[3.1.4] Complications of Bone Marrow Examination

When the posterior iliac crest site is used, complications of diagnostic bone marrow examination are exceedingly rare (<0.1-0.5%) and are generally minor, primarily consisting of either hemorrhage or infection at the site t3.3 [Bain 2004, Le Dieu 2003]. Bleeding can usually be controlled by manually applying pressure for several minutes to the site, but pressure bandages should be used on all thrombocytopenic patients to ensure hemostasis. Once these procedures are completed, the patient should be instructed to lie supine, and the biopsy site should be reevaluated within 10-15 minutes for any evidence of ongoing bleeding. The risk of more significant hemorrhage is greater in patients with underlying chronic myeloproliferative neoplasms and in obese patients [Bain 2004, Devaliaf 2004].

The rare wound infections that follow bone marrow examination are generally minor, requiring only topical medications. Other complications of diagnostic bone marrow examination are exceedingly rare and include neuropathy (usually transient) and osteomyelitis t3.3 [Bain 2004, Le Dieu 2003].

Although still <1%, the complication rate for bone marrow transplant donors is somewhat higher [Bortin 1983,

Buckner 1984]. In these individuals, life-threatening complications result almost exclusively from the general anesthesia. However, local complications from repeated iliac crest aspirations also occur. Both bleeding and neuropathy are relatively more common in these donors, while the rate of wound infections is very low. Studies comparing local anesthesia to conscious sedation for bone marrow examination show no differences in complication rates [Burkle 2004].

Complications of sternal aspiration, although rare, can be catastrophic [Bain 2004]. When the lower sternal plate is perforated during a sternal aspiration procedure, potentially fatal cardiac complications occur. For this reason, sternal aspiration should never be attempted by a novice. Also, this procedure should not be performed on patients with suspected myeloma or metastatic carcinoma, because these disorders cause bone erosion and thinning, increasing the likelihood of perforation [Marti 2004]. Similarly, sternal aspiration is also contraindicated in young children because of the higher potential for perforation of the sternal plate.

One additional consideration is the potential risk to the physician of contracting an infection from the patient. If bone marrow examination is necessary for the management of chronically infected patients, this procedure should be performed by an experienced physician. Depending on the patient's underlying infection, additional protective equipment could include eye protection, a specialized and custom-fit mask, protective coat/gown, and double gloves.

[3.2]   Bone Marrow Examination Sites

The distribution of hematopoietic bone marrow varies depending on patient age. In infants and young children, virtually all bones are hematopoietically active, while hematopoiesis is largely restricted to axial bones in adults. Although the anterior iliac crest (children and adults) and anterior tibial plateau (infants) can be used for bone marrow examination, the posterior iliac crest is by far the preferred site for both aspiration and biopsy. Because both aspiration and biopsy specimens are essential in the overall evaluation of bone marrow, this site should always be initially evaluated; alternate sites should be considered only if the posterior iliac crests are unacceptable. In infants, the anterior tibia can be used as an alternate aspiration site, if attempts to get specimens from the posterior iliac crest are unsuccessful. Methods to obtain intact clot specimens from the tibia in neonates have been described [Sola 1999]. Likewise, the anterior iliac crest is a suitable alternate site in patients in whom the posterior iliac crest cannot be used, because of local factors such as prior radiation therapy, morbid obesity, overlying skin disease, or incomplete ossification in neonates. As described earlier, sternal aspiration

should only be performed if there is no other suitable site; the procedure should be done by an experienced physician. A sternal aspiration is contraindicated in children and in adults with underlying conditions associated with bone resorption.

In most patients, generalizations regarding the overall hematopoietic cavity can be made from evaluation of a single site. Under physiologic conditions, diverse hematopoietic sites generally exhibit fairly uniform overall cellularity and cell lineage proportions. Also, with rare exceptions, primary hematopoietic neoplasms, such as leukemias, are thought to be uniformly dispersed throughout the hematopoietic cavities, so that the study of multiple sites generally does not improve diagnostic accuracy. However, bone marrow involvement in secondary neoplasms is random and focal. In these cases, bilateral or 2 unilateral core biopsies (>2 cm total) are necessary for optimal evaluation.

[3.3]   Bone Marrow Aspiration and Biopsy Procedures

The techniques used to obtain bone marrow aspiration and biopsy samples are fairly standardized, but efforts to improve the experience for patients should always be integrated into this procedure [Alberhasky 2004, Johnson 2008]. In this section, general techniques, suggestions to improve specimen quality and methods for obtaining specimens for both routine and specialized techniques will be reviewed. Because both aspiration and biopsy specimens are essential for overall bone marrow evaluation, this discussion will include both procedures. Likewise, because iliac crest is the preferred site for bone marrow aspiration and biopsy, this discussion will be restricted to this site. Several types of aspiration and biopsy needles are commercially available; a review of the advantages and disadvantages of each type is beyond the scope of this text. Instead, physicians within each institution must determine which types of commercial needles are optimal for obtaining good quality specimens.

The optimal sequence of performing bone marrow aspiration and biopsy procedures is controversial. Several authors recommend that the biopsy be performed first to eliminate any potential for aspiration artifact [Alberhasky 2004]. Others recommend that the aspiration be performed initially, because of the problem of rapid coagulation of the aspirated sample when aspiration follows biopsy. In my experience, if separate needles are used for each procedure, and if these needles are placed at different sites along the iliac crest, good quality aspirate and biopsy specimens can be obtained in either sequence. However, if aspiration artifact is a common specimen quality issue, core biopsies should be performed first.

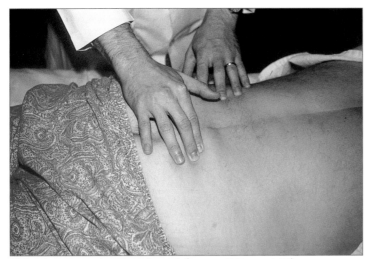

f3.1 *The posterior iliac crest is located. (courtesy R Brynes, MD)*

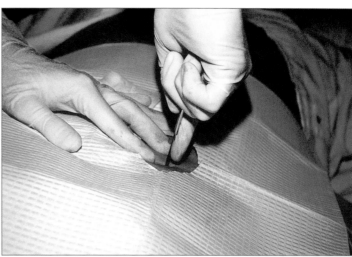

f3.2 *A larger needle is used for obtaining bone marrow biopsy specimens. Needle is held in the palm and is supported and directed by the index finger. (courtesy R Brynes, MD)*

After discussing with the patient the necessity of bone marrow examination for diagnosis, obtaining all necessary witnessed consent signatures, and administering any premedication, this procedure can begin. It is extremely important to carefully palpate the posterior iliac crest and locate landmarks **f3.1**. Once the posterior iliac crest is identified, this site can be highlighted by a fingernail mark to leave a slight depression. In heavier patients, it may be necessary for the patient to lie on his/her side and pull knees toward the chest to reduce the fat pad overlying the iliac crest. Throughout the procedure, a steady dialogue should be maintained with the patient, explaining each step, alerting the patient to discomfort, and reassuring and encouraging the patient.

Using appropriate sterile techniques and protective clothing and eyewear, the bone marrow tray should be opened and organized so those items can be located quickly. In addition, all needles should be checked to be sure they are intact and that the stylet can be easily locked into place and removed. Extra syringes for special studies, such as flow cytometry, cytogenetics, and molecular analyses, should be appropriately anticoagulated, and necessary media should be on hand before the procedure begins. Several large syringes should be available to ensure that maximum suction can be applied while aspirating. Once the skin has been sterilized, a local anesthetic is used first for the skin and subsequently the periosteum overlying the posterior iliac crest. A generous area of periosteum should be anesthetized because several different sites of entry into the iliac crest will be used during the procedure. Once local anesthesia has been achieved, a small skin incision is made.

If care is taken to use different entry sites along the posterior iliac crest, either bone marrow aspiration or biopsy can be performed first, although in general the biopsy should be performed first. With the central stylet of the core biopsy needle

appropriately locked in place, this needle is advanced through the skin incision down to the cortical bone **f3.2**. Because of the large size of the biopsy needle, a fair amount of pressure is required to advance the needle through the cortical bone using a rocking motion. The patient should be alerted to a possible sensation of pressure.

After the biopsy needle is firmly anchored in cortical bone, the central stylet should be removed and the needle slowly advanced at least 1-2 cm. The approximate length of the biopsy core within the biopsy needle should be evaluated by gently reinserting the central stylet, being careful not to apply any pressure that might force the core biopsy out of the needle. Continue advancing the biopsy needle with a steady twisting motion until an adequately sized sample is present within the needle. Before the needle is removed, it is essential that the biopsy specimen present within the needle be separated from surrounding bone marrow. To achieve this, the biopsy needle should be vigorously rotated in full circles in both directions. This rapid motion should be completed several times, and the needle should be advanced a small distance farther before removal. The biopsy needle should be slowly withdrawn using a slight twisting motion. Although some physicians use a small syringe to apply suction as the biopsy needle is being removed, this may inadvertently result in aspiration of this biopsy specimen, seriously compromising evaluation.

Once the bone marrow biopsy needle is removed, another stylet is inserted through the pointed end of the needle to slide the core biopsy out of the opposite end **f3.3**. Assess the biopsy for adequacy by careful examination. Cortical bone generally is homogeneous and white, while cartilage has a smooth, homogeneous, glistening appearance. If the biopsy specimen consists mostly of cortical bone or cartilage, or is very small, it is not satisfactory and repeated

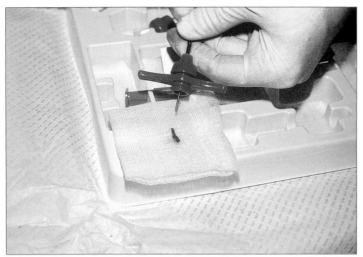

f3.3 *The biopsy sample is removed from the needle by inserting a probe (stylet) through the pointed end and pushing the sample out the opposite end. (courtesy R Brynes, MD)*

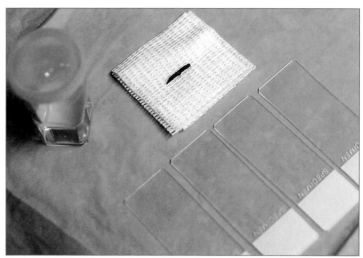

f3.4 *Preparation for imprint smears; core biopsy sample is gently touched to slides to make touch preparations, imprint smears.*

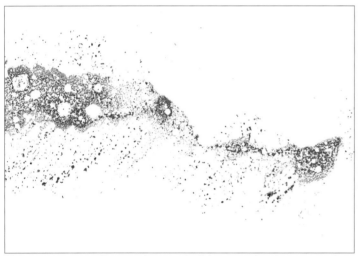

i3.1 *Imprint smear illustrates the typical cell dispersion that characterizes this touch preparation. Some cellular distortion may be present. (Wright)*

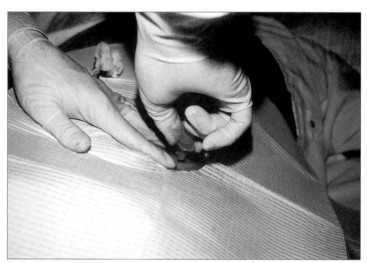

f3.5 *An aspiration needle is inserted into the iliac crest. (courtesy R Brynes, MD)*

attempts should be made to obtain a better biopsy specimen. A new biopsy needle should be used for a second biopsy attempt, because the beveled edge of the first needle is likely damaged by the process of inserting the first stylet. An adequate bone marrow biopsy specimen is red, and tiny bone flecks can be appreciated on gross examination. Many imprint smears should be made from this fresh biopsy specimen before its fixation for 1-2 hours **f3.4 i3.1**. This specimen is returned to the laboratory where it is decalcified for 1-2 hours before routine processing (see **appendix**).

If no biopsy specimen can be obtained after repeated attempts, imprint smears should be made from the bevel of the biopsy needle. Likewise, in those patients in whom biopsy is successful but aspiration is not, a second biopsy specimen can be obtained from which cells can be disaggregated for specialized studies, such as flow cytometry or cytogenetics [Novotny 2005].

To aspirate the bone marrow, a smaller needle is generally used **f3.5**. Using the same skin incision site, bone marrow aspiration can be performed by gently stretching this skin site to allow the needle to penetrate the iliac crest in a different region from that used for biopsy.

Once the iliac crest has been localized using the aspiration needle, a back and forth twisting motion is used to advance this needle through the cortical bone. Steady pressure is applied throughout this procedure, and the patient is alerted to possible sensations of pressure. Occasionally, a distinct "give" sensation is apparent to the physician, when the cortical bone is completely penetrated. Whether or not such a sensation is apparent, the needle must be advanced until it is solidly anchored in bone. Rapidly unlock and remove the central stylet, attach a large sterile syringe, alert the patient that aspiration possibly associated with pain is about to

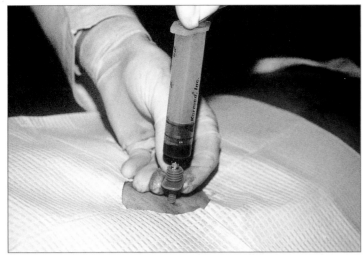

f3.6 *Bone marrow aspiration is performed by using a large syringe and applying rapid suction for a few seconds. (courtesy R Brynes, MD)*

occur, and rapidly apply maximal suction for 3-5 seconds or until 0.5-2.0 mL of bone marrow is aspirated **f3.6**. Small, rapidly collected aspirate specimens are optimal to reduce the amount of dilution by peripheral blood. Depending upon technical preferences, this aspirate may or may not be anticoagulated.

Non-anticoagulated specimens should be immediately handed to a technical assistant who will simultaneously prepare various smears and assess the quality of the aspirate. This initial aspirate should always be used for morphologic review and should ideally contain minimal peripheral blood contamination [Bain 2001]. Once sufficient particle crush and direct smears have been made **f3.7**, the remainder of the bone marrow aspirate will clot, which can be submitted for tissue sectioning, along with the bone marrow biopsy specimen. Anticoagulated aspirate specimens should be returned to the laboratory for further processing and smear preparation.

Subsequent aspirations may be obtained for flow cytometry, cytogenetics, culture, or molecular studies. Once again, the patient should be warned in advance of each additional aspiration, and the purpose of each aspiration should be explained to the patient.

If attempts at aspiration are unsuccessful, reinsert and lock the stylet and advance the needle a short distance. Repeat aspiration using a large syringe and rapidly applying suction. If multiple aspiration attempts are unsuccessful, remove the aspiration needle and make imprints from the beveled edge. An alternate site for aspiration, preferably the other posterior iliac crest, can be attempted using a new sterile needle.

Once the procedure is completed, steady pressure should be applied to the site for several minutes. After hemostasis has been achieved, a bandage should be applied, and the patient should be instructed to lie supinely. Pressure bandages may be

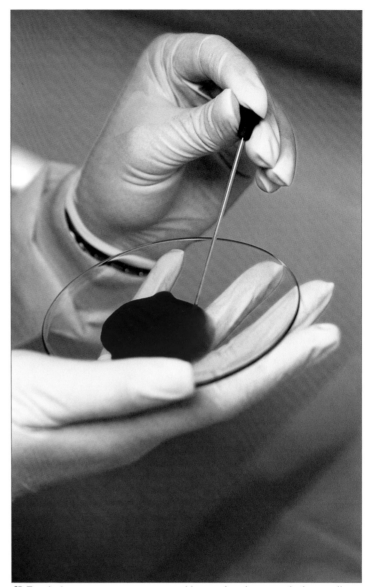

f3.7 *The bone marrow aspirate is quickly transferred to a watch glass to allow particles (white flecks) to be quickly identified and transferred to a slide for direct smear or particle crush preparations.*

required in thrombocytopenic patients, and the bone marrow site should be carefully evaluated shortly after this procedure to assess for prolonged bleeding. Explain to the patient what specimens have been obtained and when he or she can expect results from these studies. Several hours after the procedure, the patient should be contacted to assess status and answer any questions.

[3.4] Types of Preparations

Because aspiration and biopsy samples supply important diagnostic information, both bone marrow procedures are strongly recommended for all patients undergoing initial bone marrow examination [Foucar 2008, Wickramasinghe 2007]. Various smears and sections can be prepared from these bone marrow specimens **t3.4**. The aspirated marrow can be smeared directly

t3.4 Types of Routine Bone Marrow Preparations

Preparation	Procedure
Direct aspirate smears	Preparation is similar to that for a blood smear; place a few particles* at one end of a slide and spread with another slide
Buffy coat smear (after disruption of particles)	The bone marrow aspirate is anticoagulated; smears are prepared after particles are concentrated, then stirred extensively and mixed with plasma
Particle crush smear	A few particles* are placed on the center of the slide; excess blood is removed, after which 2 slides are gently compressed to spread and disperse particles as the slides are pulled apart
Imprint smears	The bone marrow biopsy sample is gently and repeatedly touched to the slide, or the slide is gently touched to the biopsy sample, which is held gently in place
Clot section	Remaining particles* from the aspiration are allowed to clot, then wrapped in paper, processed, and sectioned
	Particles may be concentrated and red blood cells either removed or lysed before processing
Bone marrow biopsy section	The bone marrow biopsy is fixed, decalcified, routinely processed, and cut into thin sections

*Bone marrow particles consist of a portion of blood vessel with adjacent stromal network and entrapped hematopoietic elements

References: [Brynes 1978, Foucar 2008, Wickramasinghe 2007, Lee 2008]

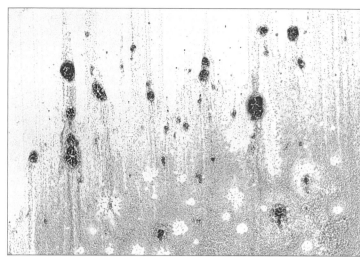

i3.2 *Low-power view of a bone marrow aspirate smear illustrates the dispersion of particles at the feather edge of a direct smear. (Wright)*

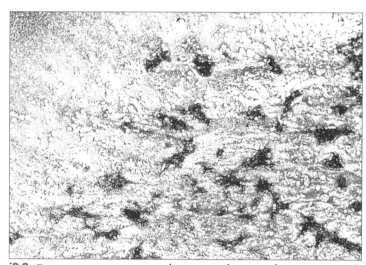

i3.3 *Bone marrow aspirate smear demonstrates how particles are concentrated in the center of a particle crush smear. Note thick and thin areas. (Wright)*

onto a slide (direct aspirate smears) or anticoagulated and smeared after centrifugation to concentrate the cells, followed by mixing with plasma (1 part buffy coat to 2 parts plasma [buffy coat smears]) i3.2 [Brynes 1978]. A third type of smear, the bone marrow particle crush preparation, is prepared by placing a few particles on the center of a slide, removing excess blood, and gently compressing these between 2 slides as these slides are pulled apart i3.3. After clotting, the remaining aspirated marrow can be routinely processed and sectioned i3.4. Erythrocytes can be lysed to concentrate the bone marrow particles in these clot specimens. Imprint smears are made either by gently touching the bone marrow biopsy to a stationary slide or by touching the stationary slide to the biopsy specimen (see i3.1). Although good imprint preparations can be obtained either way, care must be taken not to crush the biopsy specimen by holding it briefly in a gauze sponge. In addition, imprint smears can be made from the beveled edges of both the aspiration and biopsy needles if adequate specimens are not obtained. The bone marrow biopsy is then fixed, decalcified, routinely processed, and thin sectioned at several levels i3.5. Highly skilled technicians and well-maintained equipment are required to produce optimal sections.

The advantages and disadvantages of each of these bone marrow slide techniques are presented in t3.5. Morphologic detail is excellent on direct smears prepared from bone marrow aspirates, but dilution with peripheral blood may occasionally skew differential cell counts. Although morphologic detail is also good on buffy coat smears, the preparation of these smears requires substantial technical time, and there may be some distortion of cellular detail by the anticoagulant required, especially if delays in processing prolong the exposure of cells to the anticoagulant. Although the uniform dispersal of cells on these buffy coat smears is ideal for both differential cell counting and cytochemical/ immunostaining, rare reports suggest that the percentage of blasts may be underestimated in this preparation [Izadi 1993]. Even though particle crush smears are useful for assessing megakaryocytes, macrophages, and mast cells, significant

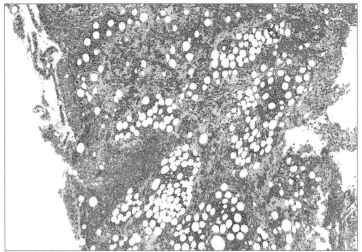

i3.4 *Bone marrow clot section was prepared after the bone marrow aspirate was allowed to clot and then processed. In this example, erythrocytes have not been removed, nor have the particles been concentrated. (H&E)*

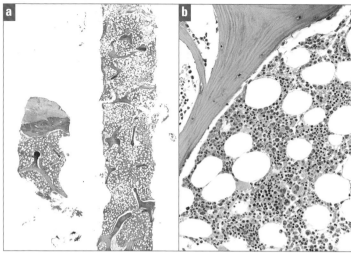

i3.5 *These bone marrow biopsy sections were prepared following optimal fixation and decalcification. On thin sections, cytologic detail is excellent. (H&E)*

t3.5 Comparison of Bone Marrow Preparations

Preparation	Advantages	Disadvantages
Direct smears	Morphology excellent Staining uniform Differential cell counts generally accurate	May be diluted with blood, causing skew in cell counts
Buffy coat smears after disruption of particles	Cells dispersed evenly over entire slide Morphology excellent Staining uniform	Aggregates of normoblasts may skew differential cell counts All cell-to-cell interrelationships lost Anticoagulant may distort morphology Percentage of blasts may be underestimated
Particle crush smears	Close concentration of particles useful for assessment of megakaryocytes, macrophages, mast cells, and cancer cells Best for assessing storage iron	Many cells may be broken or distorted Cell dispersal and staining very uneven (many areas on slide too thick for cell identification)
Imprint smears	Assess morphology of cells that do not aspirate because of fibrosis If aspirate unsuccessful, may be only way to assess cytology and perform differential count Rapid diagnosis of metastatic tumors in advance of biopsy section	Cells may selectively "touch off," and differential counts on imprint smears may not accurately reflect cell proportions in marrow, although these methods are generally comparable
Clot section	Assessment of cellularity and megakaryocyte numbers Since not decalcified, may be better than biopsy sections for those cytochemical stains that work on processed tissue Interrelationship of cell types can be evaluated	Reflects only cell types and lesions that were aspirable Some cytochemical stains (especially enzyme stains) do not work on processed tissue Mercurial fixation may inhibit other enzymes, such as chloroacetate esterase Granules in some cells, especially basophils and mast cells, lost in processing
Bone marrow biopsy sections	Ideal for determining involvement by focal processes such as carcinomas, lymphomas, granulomas, and other infiltrative processes (positive yield enhanced by bilateral biopsies and step sectioning) Best assessment of cellularity, interrelationships of cell types, and distribution of cells Best assessment of bone, blood vessels, stromal elements, lymphoid aggregates, and degree of fibrosis or necrosis Best for determining pattern of bone marrow infiltration by such diseases as chronic lymphoproliferative disorders, non-Hodgkin lymphoma, and mast cell disease	Some cytochemical stains (especially enzyme stains) do not work on processed tissue; decalcification further destroys some enzymes and antigens Mercurial fixation may inhibit other enzymes, such as chloroacetate esterase Granules in some cells, especially basophils and mast cells, lost in processing Plastic-embedded specimens not decalcified; retain most enzyme activity, but techniques time-consuming and not cost-efficient

References: [Aboul-Nasr 1999, Brynes 1978, Foucar 2008, Wickramasinghe 2007]

cellular distortion with many disrupted cells is consistently found on these smears. Also because the distribution of cells is highly variable with thick and thin areas, both overstained and understained regions are common on particle crush smears. As a result of distortion and uneven staining, only a limited area of a particle crush smear generally may be suitable for differential cell counting.

Imprint smears may be useful for assessing the morphologic characteristics of cells that do not readily aspirate, such as those associated with fibrosis. These smears become particularly valuable in bone marrow examinations in which the aspiration attempts have been unsuccessful. Review of these dry tap specimens reveals that hypercellularity or diffuse fibrosis accounts for the majority of unsuccessful aspirations. Even though differential cell counts obtained from imprint smears are generally comparable with other smears, cell counts may be occasionally skewed because cells that "touch off" during imprinting may not reflect overall cell proportions [Aboul-Nasr 1999]. The identification of neoplastic cells on imprint smears may expedite the diagnosis of bone marrow involvement by metastatic tumors.

Sections made from the clotted bone marrow aspirate are useful in evaluating cellularity, as well as in assessing megakaryocyte numbers and morphologic characteristics. However, because the clot section contains only those aspirable bone marrow elements, infiltrates associated with fibrosis are generally not present. Although paraffin section material can be used for many immunohistochemical stains, routine processing of both clot and biopsy tissue, in conjunction with decalcification of the core biopsy, results in degradation of some antigens and many enzymes. Clot sections do have an advantage over biopsy sections in that these cells have not been subjected to decalcification; consequently clot sections are much more suitable for molecular testing. Despite technical issues, many antigens are preserved in bone marrow clot section and core biopsy specimens. Ideally each laboratory should assess the success of various immunoperoxidase stains on specimens processed according to individual laboratory protocols (see Chapter 4).

Bone marrow biopsy sections that are at least 1 cm in length, well fixed, and sectioned, are ideal for determining involvement by a whole variety of focal processes, including carcinomas, lymphomas, granulomas, and other infiltrative lesions. Cytologic detail is best when mercurial-based fixatives are used, but cost and environmental issues have led many laboratories to switch to alternate fixatives such as azide zinc formalin [Bonds 2005]. Several studies indicate that the yield of positive diagnoses for focal processes increases with both the amount of bone marrow sampled (ie, bilateral specimens) and with step sectioning of individual bone marrow biopsy specimens [Wang 2002].

The bone marrow biopsy section is also the preferred specimen for evaluating overall bone marrow cellularity, interrelationships between cell types, and the distribution of cells. The pattern of bone marrow infiltration by chronic lymphoproliferative disorders and non-Hodgkin lymphoma can only be determined on bone marrow biopsy sections. Similarly, bone marrow biopsy sections are required for the evaluation of bony trabeculae and identification of fibrosis. Finally, the assessment of blood vessels, bone marrow stromal elements, lymphoid aggregates, and pathologic processes such as necrosis is ideally performed on bone marrow biopsy sections. For patients undergoing chemotherapy, the bone marrow biopsy is the best specimen for assessment of the distribution of residual malignant cells and evaluation of regenerating hematopoietic cells. Despite their value, bone marrow biopsy specimens have several disadvantages, the most important of which are the substantial loss of enzyme activity, cytoplasmic granules, and antigens that occurs during fixation, decalcification, and processing. Also, even in ideal sections, cytologic features of individual cells are not as well appreciated as they are with aspirate smears.

[3.5] Specialized Techniques

An extensive array of specialized techniques that enhance diagnostic accuracy and offer prognostic information can now be performed on bone marrow samples. Because of the significant contribution of these specialized studies for diagnosis and disease monitoring, a separate chapter is devoted to this discussion (see Chapter 4). Consequently, discussion of specialized techniques in the current chapter will focus only on the general types of specialized techniques that can be performed on bone marrow specimens and the acquisition of appropriate specimens t3.6, t3.7. Many cytochemical stains and fluorescence in situ hybridization (FISH) can be performed on air-dried smears including blood and bone marrow aspirate and imprint smears, while viable anticoagulated aspirate or blood samples are required for flow cytometric immunophenotyping, conventional karyotyping, and many molecular tests (see Chapter 4) t3.6, t3.7. If a suitable aspirate sample cannot be obtained for these specialized studies, cells can be disaggregated from a fresh extra bone marrow biopsy sample [Novotny 2005]. The cell yields from these biopsy specimens are greatly increased by flushing cells out of the core biopsy specimen using alternating Hank's balanced salt solution injections and aspirations all along the core through a very small-gauge needle, such as a tuberculin skin test needle. An extensive panel of immunohistochemical and in situ hybridization techniques can be performed on formalin-fixed, paraffin-embedded bone marrow biopsy core and clot sections. Similarly, many molecular techniques

t3.6 Specialized Techniques in Bone Marrow Evaluation*

Technique	Type of Specimen	Comments
Enzyme cytochemical stains (see t3.7)	Aspirate smears or plastic-imbedded biopsy sections	Enzyme identification critical in the diagnosis of acute leukemia and useful in some chronic lymphoproliferative disorders; immunohistochemical techniques available for some enzymes
Nonenzymatic cytochemical stains (see t3.7)	Aspirate smears or biopsy	Required for assessing iron stores, glycogen, mucin, and identifying organisms (in conjunction with bone marrow cultures) Note: Storage iron cannot be reliably assessed on decalcified specimens
Immunophenotyping: immunoperoxidase flow cytometry	Aspirate smears/clot and biopsy† sections Aspirate‡ or cells teased from unfixed biopsy sample	Useful in diagnosis of all types of leukemia, carcinoma, lymphoma, myeloma, as well as reactive lymphoid infiltrates
Cytogenetics	Aspirate‡ or cells teased from unfixed bone marrow biopsy	Yield prognostic and diagnostic information in hematolymphoid neoplasms
Fluorescence in situ hybridization	Aspirate smears, touch preparations	Valuable in detecting minimal residual disease Can assess metaphases and interphase cells
Molecular analyses	Aspirate‡ or cells teased from unfixed bone marrow biopsy§; paraffin-embedded specimens (PCR) on clot sections	Useful in determining B- and T-cell clonality, as well as other gene rearrangements, amplifications, and mutations
Electron microscopy	Aspirate‡ or cells teased from unfixed bone marrow biopsy	Although useful for cell identification and selected cytochemical stains, largely supplanted by immunologic techniques
Plastic imbedding	Biopsy	Biopsy not decalcified Sections suitable for enzyme as well as other cytochemical stains Ideal for very thin sectioning

*See Chapter 4 for complete discussion of specialized techniques
†Mercurial fixatives and decalcification may destroy antigens; others may be destroyed in processing. Therefore, paraffin immunoperoxidase techniques may not work for all antibodies
‡Sterile, anticoagulated bone marrow aspirate (4-5 mL)
§Some molecular techniques can be performed on formalin-fixed, paraffin-embedded tissue; cells can also be scraped from air-dried smears for molecular studies
PCR = polymerase chain reaction techniques

t3.7 Cytochemical Stains Commonly Used in Bone Marrow Examination*

Cytochemical Stain	Specimen Requirement	Comments
Myeloperoxidase	Air-dried smears (blood, aspirate, imprint)	Myeloid primary granule enzyme; immunoperoxidase antibody available for processed specimens
Sudan black B	Air-dried smears (blood, aspirate, imprint)	Lipid in myeloid primary granules
Naphthol-chloroacetate esterase	Air-dried smears (blood, aspirate, imprint) Formalin-fixed clot section†	Myeloid primary granule enzyme; also in mast cells; can be performed on formalin-fixed paraffin-embedded nondecalcified specimens
α-Naphthyl acetate esterase	Air-dried smears (blood, aspirate, imprint)	Enzyme in monocytes/macrophages is inhibited by fluoride; enzyme in megakaryoblasts is fluoride-resistant; also reacts with T-cell subsets
α-Naphthyl butyrate esterase	Air-dried smears (blood, aspirate, imprint)	Enzyme in monocytes/macrophages (diffuse positivity); also in T lymphocytes (focal, paranuclear positivity)
Acid phosphatase	Air-dried smears (blood, aspirate, imprint)	Ubiquitous enzyme; tartrate-resistant acid phosphatase useful in diagnosis of HCL; immunoperoxidase antibody available for processed specimens
Giemsa/toluidine blue	Air-dried smears (blood, aspirate, imprint) Clot and biopsy sections	Metachromatic stains useful in identifying mast cells and basophils
Periodic-acid Schiff	Air-dried smears (blood, aspirate, imprint) Clot and biopsy sections	Glycogen stain; glycogen present in many other cells, so must assess pattern of reactivity
Prussian blue	Air-dried smears (blood, aspirate, imprint) Clot and biopsy sections	Essential for evaluation of normoblastic and storage iron; usually accurately reflects total body iron stores Smears must contain particles to assess iron stores; normoblast iron can only be evaluated on smears Because iron may be leached out during decalcification, biopsy not optimal specimen for assessing either iron stores or erythroid iron

*See Chapter 4 for comprehensive discussion
†Naphthol chloroacetate esterase does not work on decalcified tissue
HCL = hairy cell leukemia

References: [Foucar 2008, Wickramasinghe 2007]

also can be performed on these types of specimens (see Chapter 4). The sensitivity, specificity, specimen limitations, and diagnostic usefulness of these techniques are included in Chapter 4. These specialized test results must be integrated with clinical, hematologic, and morphologic features for accurate interpretation.

[3.6] Clues and Caveats

1. Many clinical and laboratory parameters must be assessed in decision-making regarding if and when to perform a bone marrow examination.

2. Dialogue between pathologists and clinicians is essential in ensuring that all necessary bone marrow specimens are obtained correctly during the procedure.

3. Although rare, there are significant potential complications of bone marrow examination.

4. A large syringe is optimal for rapidly obtaining bone marrow aspiration samples with minimal blood contamination, because the stronger vacuum maximizes particle aspiration and reduces the total time needed to withdraw 1-2 mL of sample.

5. In cases in which neither aspiration nor biopsy samples can be obtained, imprint smears of the beveled edge of the needles may be valuable.

6. Variable results of paraffin immunoperoxidase studies on decalcified bone marrow biopsy specimens require that each laboratory determine antibody reaction patterns on specimens processed using its own laboratory procedures (see Chapter 4).

7. Improved yield of viable cells from bone marrow core biopsy specimens can be achieved by repeatedly injecting Hank's balanced salt solution into the fibrotic or hypercellular marrow with a small-gauge needle to gently flush out cells for specialized studies.

[3.7] Acknowledgments

Illustrations of bone marrow aspiration and biopsy techniques are courtesy of R Brynes, MD.

[3.8] References

Aboul-Nasr R, Estey EH, Kantarjian HM, et al [1999] Comparison of touch imprints with aspirate smears for evaluating bone marrow specimens. *Am J Clin Pathol* 111:753-758.

Alberhasky M [2004] Sure-handed sampling: easing the trauma of bone marrow collection. *CAP Today* 2004:85-87.

Bain BJ [2001] Bone marrow aspiration. *J Clin Pathol* 54:657-663.

Bain BJ [2004] Bone marrow biopsy morbidity and mortality: 2002 data. *Clin Lab Haematol* 26:315-318.

Barekman CL, Fair KP, Cotelingam JD [1997] Comparative utility of diagnostic bone-marrow components: a 10-year study. *Am J Hematol* 56:37-41.

Bonds LA, Barnes P, Foucar K, Sever CE [2005] Acetic acid-zinc-formalin: A safe alternative to B-5 fixative. *Am J Clin Pathol* 124:205-211.

Bortin MM, Buckner CD [1983] Major complications of marrow harvesting for transplantation. *Exp Hematol* 11:916-921.

Brynes RK, McKenna RW, Sundberg RD [1978] Bone marrow aspiration and trephine biopsy. An approach to a thorough study. *Am J Clin Pathol* 70:753-759.

Buckner CD, Clift RA, Sanders JE, et al [1984] Marrow harvesting from normal donors. *Blood* 64:630-634.

Burkle CM, Harrison BA, Koenig LF, et al [2004] Morbidity and mortality of deep sedation in outpatient bone marrow biopsy. *Am J Hematol* 77:250-256.

Devaliaf V, Tudor G [2004] Reply to: bone marrow examination in obese patients: CAT or not to CAT! *Br J Haematol* 125:538-539.

Foucar K, Duncan MH, Smith KJ [1993] Practical approach to the investigation of neutropenia. *Clin Lab Med* 13:879-894.

Foucar K, Viswanatha D, Wilson C [2008] Procurement and interpretation of the bone marrow specimen. In: King D, Gardner W, Sobin L, et al, eds. *Non-Neoplastic Disorders of Bone Marrow (AFIP fascicle)*. Washington, DC: American Registry of Pathology; 41-55.

Howell SJ, Grey M, Chang J, et al [2002] The value of bone marrow examination in the staging of Hodgkin's lymphoma: a review of 955 cases seen in a regional cancer centre. *Br J Haematol* 119:408-411.

Izadi P, Ortega JA, Coates TD [1993] Comparison of buffy coat preparation to direct method for the evaluation and interpretation of bone marrow aspirates. *Am J Hematol* 43:107-109.

Jatoi A, Dallal GE, Nguyen PL [1999] False-negative rates of tumor metastases in the histologic examination of bone marrow. *Mod Pathol* 12:29-32.

Johnson H, Burke D, Plews C, et al [2008] Improving the patient's experience of a bone marrow biopsy - an RCT. *J Clin Nurs* 17:717-725.

Le Dieu R, Luckit J, Sundarasun M [2003] Complications of trephine biopsy. *Br J Haematol* 121:822.

Lee SH, Erber WN, Porwit A, et al [2008] ICSH guidelines for the standardization of bone marrow specimens and reports. *Int J Lab Hematol* 30:349-364.

Marti J, Anton E, Valenti C [2004] Complications of bone marrow biopsy. *Br J Haematol* 124:557-558.

Novotny JR, Schmucker U, Staats B, Duhrsen U [2005] Failed or inadequate bone marrow aspiration: a fast, simple and cost-effective method to produce a cell suspension from a core biopsy specimen. *Clin Lab Haematol* 27:33-40.

Pakos EE, Fotopoulos AD, Ioannidis JP [2005] 18F-FDG PET for evaluation of bone marrow infiltration in staging of lymphoma: a meta-analysis. *J Nucl Med* 46:958-963.

Segel GB, Feig SA [2009] Controversies in the diagnosis and management of childhood acute immune thrombocytopenic purpura. *Pediatr Blood Cancer* 53:318-324.

Simpson CD, Gao J, Fernandez CV, et al [2008] Routine bone marrow examination in the initial evaluation of paediatric Hodgkin lymphoma: the Canadian perspective. *Br J Haematol* 141:820-826.

Sola MC, Rimsza LM, Christensen RD [1999] A bone marrow biopsy technique suitable for use in neonates. *Br J Haematol* 107:458-460.

Vassilakopoulos TP, Angelopoulou MK, Constantinou N, et al [2005] Development and validation of a clinical prediction rule for bone marrow involvement in patients with Hodgkin lymphoma. *Blood* 105:1875-1880.

Wang J, Weiss LM, Chang KL, et al [2002] Diagnostic utility of bilateral bone marrow examination: significance of morphologic and ancillary technique study in malignancy. *Cancer* 94:1522-1531.

Weinkauff R, Estey EH, Starostik P, et al [1999] Use of peripheral blood blasts vs bone marrow blasts for diagnosis of acute leukemia. *Am J Clin Pathol* 111:733-740.

Wickramasinghe S [2007] Bone marrow. In: Mills S, ed. *Histology for Pathologists*. 3rd ed. Philadelphia: Lippincott Williams & Wilkins; 799-836.

Specialized Techniques in Bone Marrow Evaluation

Kaaren Reichard, MD

Specialized techniques in bone marrow evaluation are a vital component in the workup and diagnosis of hematolymphoid processes. In fact, as we have become more accustomed to the routine use of these methods and the data they generate, one could argue that they are not so specialized anymore. These techniques include cytochemistry, immunohistochemistry (IHC), flow cytometric analysis, conventional cytogenetics, fluorescence in situ hybridization, molecular methods, and others (see **t3.6**). Using these specialized tests, pathologists classify and risk-stratify hematolymphoid neoplasms according y updated 2008 World Health Organization classification [Swerdlow 2008] . Additional techniques, still largely restricted to the research arena, such as gene expression profiling, array-based comparative genomic hybridization, and microRNA analysis, will also be discussed.

In this chapter, each of the specialized techniques has its own section for ease of discussion; however, there is generous cross reference to the other tests as appropriate. For example, IHC cannot be adequately addressed without concomitant reference to flow cytometry. An overview of each technique, indications for use, key quality assurance issues, and interpretation clues/pitfalls is presented.

[4.1] Cytochemistry

Cytochemical stains used in routine bone marrow evaluation include those that are enzymatic (eg, myeloperoxidase) and those that are nonenzymatic (eg, Prussian blue for iron (see **t3.7**), and reticulin and trichrome for reticulin and collagen fibrosis). These stains are routinely available and provide pertinent information in bone marrow evaluation.

Enzymatic cytochemical stains must be performed on unfixed/unstained specimens (eg, unstained peripheral blood smear, bone marrow aspirate smear, touch prep, and cytospin prep from flow specimen), and are useful in diagnosing and assigning lineage in acute myeloid leukemias (AML) (see **t3.7** for a list of cytochemical stains that can be used). Cytochemistries have been useful for decades and remain so in everyday routine clinical practice [Yam 1971]. Myeloperoxidase (MPO) or Sudan black B staining is useful in identifying cells of granulocytic lineage (see **appendix** for MPO staining protocol). MPO highlights granules of maturing and mature granulocytic cells with a distinctive green/blue appearance. Blasts contain relatively few granules, while neutrophils and promyelocytes are heavily granulated, rendering them readily identifiable **i4.1a**. MPO will also highlight Auer rods if present.

In a case of morphologic acute leukemia, a positive MPO stain in the blasts indicates AML or mixed phenotype acute leukemia (eg, B/myeloid, T/myeloid). The specificity is 100%; however, sensitivity is <100%. In AML with monocytic differentiation, approximately 5% to 10% of cases may show MPO positivity, but the blasts are also nonspecific esterase (NSE) positive (see next paragraph). A negative MPO stain does *not* exclude AML or equate with acute lymphoblastic leukemia. Several AML subtypes are characteristically MPO negative (AML with minimal differentiation, AML with monocytic differentiation, acute erythroid leukemia, and acute megakaryoblastic leukemia). A robust immunohistochemical MPO stain is also available for use in fixed tissue.

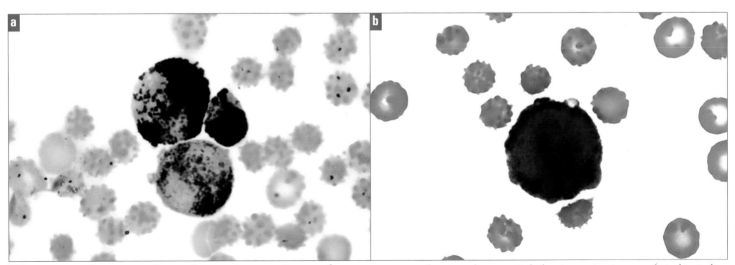

i4.1 *Composite illustrating myeloperoxidase* **a** *and non-specific esterase* **b** *positivity in a case of acute myelomonocytic leukemia on cytospin smear. (cytochemical stains for myeloperoxidase and non-specific esterase)*

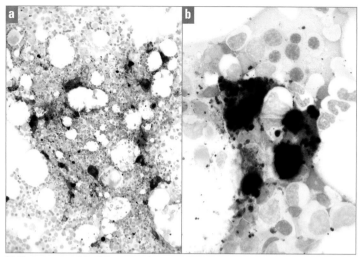

i4.2 *Low **a** and high **b** magnification of Prussian blue showing increased storage iron on bone marrow aspirate smear. (Prussian blue)*

Alpha naphthyl butyrate esterase (aka NSE) is an enzymatic cytochemical stain useful in identifying cells of monocytic lineage. Characteristic NSE positivity appears as a variably intense cytoplasmic tan/brown blush i4.1b. In contrast to MPO, this stain is technically trickier; therefore, close attention must be paid to ensure adequate internal (if possible) positive control cells (see **appendix** for staining protocol). A negative NSE test result does not definitely exclude a diagnosis of a monocytic leukemia, but, in our experience, is unusual.

To highlight bone marrow storage and erythroid iron, a nonenzymatic Prussian blue stain may be used (see **appendix** for staining protocol). Technically, this stain detects crystalline ferric ions. Such staining provides information about the availability of iron in macrophages and transferability to developing red cells. The Prussian blue stain is preferably performed on an aspirate smear containing ≥3 particles, as variability in storage iron can be seen and background artifact may hinder interpretation i4.2. Storage iron may be semiquantitatively assessed as normal, none, increased, or decreased. Alternatively, it may be graded on a scale from 0-6+ t4.1 [Fong 1977,

Gale 1963, Lundin 1964, Rath 1948]. Although a grade of 0 generally connotes possible iron deficiency, correlation with trephine biopsy/clot section iron, peripheral blood smear and red cell indices, and iron laboratory studies should be performed. Assessment of iron stores is also frequently performed on the core biopsy/clot section, which may be more accurate in evaluating iron stores than the aspirate smear [Krause 1979]. However, both may be indicated as prolonged exposure to dilute acids (as for core biopsies) will dissolve ferritin and thus lead to a falsely low/negative interpretation [Fong 1977]. Recently, it has been reported that using an intensive bone marrow iron grading method (assessment of iron in fragments [particles], in macrophages around fragments, and in erythroblasts) greatly improves overall bone marrow iron evaluation [Phiri 2009]. Key tips when interpreting bone marrow storage iron are listed in **t4.2**.

Assessing erythroid/sideroblastic iron is different from storage iron because it requires a cytologic preparation (aspirate smears or touch preparations). In the normal situation, precursor red cells are recognized by their dark, round and/or homogeneous nuclei (bright red on counter stain). Approximately 20%-50% of precursor red cells will contain anywhere from 1-7 small, randomly distributed cytoplasmic granules. With a good stain, increased or decreased sideroblastic iron can be reproducibly assessed. In addition, one may readily identify the presence of abnormal granule size or shape (large, irregular, chunky) or abnormal granule localization (forming a ring around the nucleus, so-called ring sideroblast). Such a finding alerts the diagnostician to pathologic red cell iron morphology. The definition of a ring sideroblast varies among experts, but typically 5 or more granules encircling at least 1/3 of the nucleus can be considered a ring sideroblast i4.3 [Lee 2008].

Reticulin and trichrome stains are used to evaluate bone marrow core biopsy specimens for increased reticulin and/or collagen fibrosis (see **appendix** for staining protocols). Increased deposition of reticulin fibers may be of varying severity and may

t4.1 Histologic Grading of Storage Iron

0	No visible iron using oil objective
1+	Small iron particles just visible in histiocytes using oil objective
2+	Small, sparsely distributed iron particles generally visible at low magnification (normal)
3+	Numerous small particles in histiocytes throughout the marrow particles
4+	Large particles that aggregate into clumps
5+	Dense, large clumps of iron
6+	Very large clumps of iron, intra- and extracellular

References: [Gale 1963, Rath 1948]

t4.2 Key Tips When Assessing BM Storage Iron

Good quality (≥3 BM particles) aspirate smear

Confirm positive control or repeat stain on second BM aspirate if suboptimal

Storage iron deposition may be heterogeneous in BM aspirate particles; therefore, concurrent correlative assessment of BM core biopsy/clot section stain may be useful

If no BM storage iron is suspected, an additional slide should be stained for confirmation before suggesting iron deficiency without supporting clinical/laboratory data

Formalin fixation may dissolve ferritin; therefore, a falsely low interpretation of storage iron may be rendered

BM = bone marrow

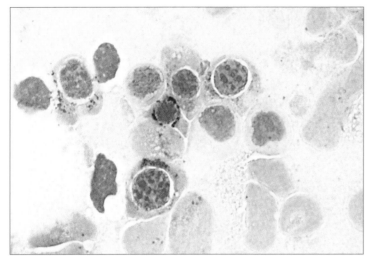

i4.3 *Prussian blue staining of bone marrow aspirate smear showing numerous ring sideroblasts. (Prussian blue)*

be seen in various non-neoplastic and neoplastic conditions [Kuter 2007]. On the other hand, detection of collagen fibrosis most often correlates to the presence of a neoplastic marrow disease process [Bauermeister 1971, Beckman 1990, Kuter 2007]. Two similar grading systems of reticulin fiber deposition are currently in use **t4.3**. Using the grading scale of 0-4, grades from 0-2 can be seen in marrows from normal subjects [Kuter 2007], whereas grades of 3 or 4 connote involvement by a pathologic disorder **i4.4**. Collagen fibrosis is graded using the same 5- or 4-grade scale **t4.3**; however, the presence of collagen fibrosis is clinically significant. It correlates with more severe underlying disease and is unlikely to be reversed with treatment of the inciting disease [Kuter 2007, Thiele 2005].

t4.3 Bone Marrow Reticulin and Collagen Fiber Grading Systems

Modified from [Bain 2001]		Modified from [Buesche 2006, Kuter 2007, Thiele 2005]	
0	No reticulin fibers demonstrable	Grade 0 (normal)	Scattered thin fibers concentrated around blood vessels
1	Occasional fine individual fibers and foci of a fine fiber network	Grade 1 (mild)	Patchy increase in fibers that are generally thin
2	Fine fiber network throughout most of the section; no coarse fibers	Grade 2 (moderate)	Diffuse increase in fibers throughout core biopsy, often coarse fibers; lacking significant overt collagen or osteosclerosis
3	Diffuse fiber network with scattered thick coarse fibers but no mature collagen	Grade 3 (marked)	Diffuse marked increase in fibers, usually coarse with areas of collagen fibrosis and osteosclerosis
4	Diffuse, often coarse fiber network with areas of collagenization		

Caveats: technical factors that influence stain include fixative, decalcification method, tissue processing, thickness of sections, and manual vs automated stains

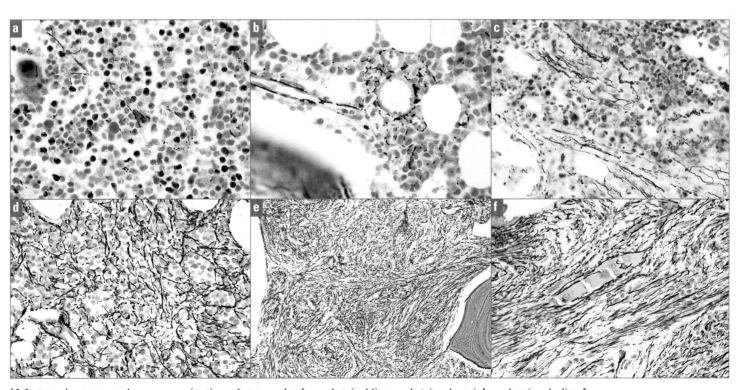

i4.4 *Reticulin staining in bone marrow (0-4): grade 0 **a**, grade 1 **b**, grade 2 (mild) **c**, grade 3 (moderate) **d**, grade 4 (marked) **e**, **f**.*

t4.4 Key Tips When Evaluating and Reporting BM Fibrosis

Variability occurs in reticulin staining; exercise caution with overinterpretation

Reticulin fibrosis may be seen in both non-neoplastic and neoplastic disorders; nonspecific

Care should be taken to mention specifically if reticulin and/or collagen fibrosis is present, as collagen fibrosis is considered to be irreversible

Prestaining technical factors may significantly impact the quantification of fibrosis, tissue fixative, decalcification, and thickness of BM sections

BM = bone marrow

References: [Buesche 2006, Kuter 2007, Thiele 2005]

t4.5 Indications for Immunohistochemistry in BM Evaluation

"Dry tap" yielding minimal BM elements for reliable morphologic review or flow cytometry: perform stains on core biopsy

Bland BM appearance but unexplained cytopenias or cytoses (eg, CD3, CD20, CD34)

Evaluation of BM hematopoietic architecture (CD34, myeloperoxidase, hemoglobin A, CD42b)

Evaluation of unexplained hypocellular BM (rule out hairy cell leukemia [CD20], hypocellular acute leukemia/myelodysplasia [CD34], etc)

Assessment of the extent of BM involvement by a neoplastic process

Characterization of a morphologically-atypical process (possibly focal, fibrotic) and not further characterized by other ancillary techniques

Evaluation for subtle involvement by known or unknown process (eg, CD3, CD20, CD30, CD138, CD34, myeloperoxidase, EBER)

BM = bone marrow

References: [Bacher 2005, Kremer 2005]

Key tips when interpreting reticulin and trichrome results are presented in **t4.4**.

[4.2] Immunohistochemistry

Immunohistochemistry is a valuable addition to the evaluation of bone marrow specimens. It is performed on fixed, paraffin-embedded (clot), and decalcified (trephine biopsy) materials. IHC should be performed on bone marrow when the diagnosis cannot be reasonably established with morphologic and other ancillary techniques **t4.5**. IHC is often very helpful in uncovering focal or subtle (eg, interstitial) lesions in the marrow and delineating marrow architecture. In addition, IHC is useful for categorizing fibrotic lesions or lesions associated with fibrosis that may not aspirate well for morphologic or flow cytometric evaluation.

Numerous antibodies are currently used in the routine clinical evaluation of hematolymphoid processes. **t4.6** lists some of the more common antibodies and their typical lineage

t4.6 Common Antibodies in BM Immunohistochemistry

Lineage	Antibodies
B-cell	CD19, CD20, CD79a, PAX5
T-cell	CD2, CD3, CD4, CD5, CD7, CD8
NK-cell	CD2, CD7 (weak), CD56
Plasma cell	CD38, CD138, cytoplasmic κ and λ, EMA, MUM1
Granulocytic	Myeloperoxidase, CD33
Monocytic/histiocytic	CD4 (weak), CD33, CD163, CD68
Megakaryocytic	CD31, CD41, CD42, CD61
Erythroid	Hemoglobin A, glycophorin, α-spectrin, CD117 on pronormoblasts
Immature	CD34, CD117, TdT, CD1a
Mast cell	Tryptase
Dendritic	CD1a (Langerhans cell), CD21 and CD35 (follicular dendritic cell), CD123 (plasmacytoid dendritic cell)
Germinal center	CD10, BCL6

BM = bone marrow; EMA = epithelial membrane antigen

t4.7 Selected Immunohistochemical Antibodies with Diagnostic/Prognostic Significance

Antigen	Tumor Positivity	Normal Cell Positivity
ALK-1	ALK+ ALCL and rare cases of DLBCL	Rare neuronal cell
Cyclin D1	Mantle cell lymphoma, hairy cell leukemia and plasma cell myeloma	Heterogeneous in endothelial cells (fibroblasts and dendritic cells) (nuclear)
CD2 and/or CD25	Aberrant if present on mast cells	CD2 and CD25+ T-cells (membrane)
ZAP70	If positive in CLL/SLL, more aggressive disease	Mature T cells (nuclear and cytoplasmic)
TCL-1	T-PLL, and blastic plasmacytoid dendritic cell neoplasm	CD3–/CD4–/CD8– T-cell precursors, pDCs, nongerminal center B cells (nuclear)

ALCL = anaplastic large cell lymphoma; ALK = anaplastic lymphoma kinase; CLL = chronic lymphocytic leukemia; DLBCL = diffuse large B-cell lymphoma; pDCs = plasmacytoid dendritic cells; SLL = small lymphocytic leukemia; TCL-1 = T-cell leukemia 1; T-PLL = T-prolymphocytic leukemia

References: [Higgins 2008, Olson 2008]

associations. Many disease states are categorized based on their expression of lineage-associated markers and lack of expression of other lineage-associated markers. Several antibodies used commonly in flow cytometry are, at the time of this writing, not routinely available for paraffin IHC. These antibodies include CD11b, CD13, CD14, CD16, CD36, and CD64 for evaluating granulocytic and monocytic maturation. On the other hand, IHC antibodies are available against transcription factors and cell cycle regulatory proteins, which help categorize certain neoplastic processes **t4.7** [Higgins 2008, Olsen 2008]. Although kappa and lambda immunostains are available for paraffin IHC, in our experience they are generally insufficiently sensitive to detect surface light chain expression on mature B lymphocytes.

t4.8 Comparison of Immunophenotypic Testing Modalities

Immunohistochemistry	Flow Cytometry
Fixed/archival tissue	Requires fresh tissue
Architectural preservation	Limited to cytologic review
Fibrotic/hypocellular specimen retains lesional cells	Lesional cells from fibrotic/hypocellular speciman may not be adequately represented in the analysis
No significant risk of antigen degradation in fixed and paraffin-embedded tissues	Increased risk of cell loss/diminished viability depending on specimen preservation/transport
	Cell viability drops within 24 hours in highly proliferative neoplasms
Generally uniparametric (2-color at best)	Multiparametric (4-6 color is current standard)
Some antibody limitation compared with flow cytometry	Broader antibody panel (CD13, CD14, CD36, CD64, surface kappa/lambda)
Markers of proliferative activity (Ki-67) oncogenes (p53), cell cycle proteins (cyclin D1), and viruses (HSV, CMV, EBV)	Not currently assessed by flow cytometry
At least half- to one-day turnaround time	Fast; 2-4 hour turnaround time can be achieved
Lineage of necrotic tumor cells may be established in some instances	Nonviable cells excluded from analysis
Limited detection sensitivity despite marked improvement in antigen retrieval techniques	Increased sensitivity for antigen detection and subtle changes compared to normal cell populations

HSV = herpes simplex virus; CMV = cytomegalovirus; EBV = Epstein-Barr virus

References: [Craig 2008, Dunphy 2004]

Although immunohistochemical antibodies are used daily for diagnosis and generally are put into clinical use after a clinical translational research project, neither the sensitivity nor specificity of antibodies, individually and in panels, has been generally reliably studied. In addition to observer interpretation variation, other parameters that contribute to varying IHC results include tissue procurement, fixation, antibody clones, dilutions, and antigen retrieval methods (or lack thereof) [Kirkegaard 2006]. Given these caveats throughout this book, the markers mentioned as detectable (positive) in disease states/ entities have been reported in most cases. The immunostain interpreter should also be aware of reactivity/cross-reactivity of antibodies with other cell types/tumors which could lead to an erroneous interpretation. For example, CD20 has been rarely seen in a subset of T-cell lymphomas, T/NK cell markers in pancreatic ductal carcinoma, and plasma cell antigens in a variety of carcinomas [Chu 2003, Rahemtullah 2008].

The decision to perform IHC and/or flow cytometry in bone marrow evaluation is not always straightforward. Each technique has its own set of advantages, disadvantages, and potential pitfalls, each of which must be known and considered when evaluating a particular case t4.8 [Craig 2008, Dunphy 2004]. When presented with a dry tap or markedly hemodilute bone marrow specimen, IHC rather than flow cytometry on the core biopsy is warranted. If additional core biopsy specimens are obtained at the time of the bone marrow procurement, several may be submitted for disaggregation for flow cytometry and/or cytogenetic/molecular studies as needed. Also, technical issues may interfere with the proper performance of IHC (improper antigen preservation or too robust antigen retrieval methods)

with possible erroneous interpretation t4.9. Pitfalls in interpretation and reporting (postanalytical error) are most often related to quality assurance issues and may result in a delayed diagnosis [Taylor 2002]. Key IHC quality issues are listed in t4.9. Careful attention to proper tissue procurement, decalcification, fixation, processing, sectioning, and antigen retrieval methods is necessary for optimal performance of ancillary studies. Different fixatives are available to process hematolymphoid specimens (formalin, B5, acetic acid zinc formalin, decalcification solution followed by formalin). Therefore, it is crucial to know the reactivity of particular antibodies depending on the fixative used. In addition, antigen retrieval techniques may be used for some antibodies, but not others. Careful review of appropriately chosen control tissues is critical to ensure ongoing immunohistochemical antibody hybridization success.

[4.3]   **Flow Cytometry**

Flow cytometry is a technique by which physical or chemical attributes of cells or particles are measured in a fluid (flow) stream. Current notable applications of flow cytometry include monitoring T-cell counts in patients with HIV infection, determining tumor DNA content, sorting specific populations, assessing hematolymphoid neoplasms, and determining nucleated cell differentials in routine peripheral blood CBC assessment.

Multiparametric flow cytometric analysis is a powerful tool in the diagnosis of myeloid and lymphoid disorders. "Multiparameteric" analysis uses a 3- to 6-color (or more) fluorescence testing method, in conjunction with forward

t4.9 Key Quality Control Issues in Decalcified Bone Marrow Immunohistochemistry (IHC)

Preanalytical

Inappropriate specimen handling may affect tissue antigen preservation (see Chapter 2)

B5 fixative less optimal than formalin-based fixatives for many IHC stains

Analytical

Daily positive and negative controls for each antibody

Positive control should be on the same slide as the test case if possible

If no internal control is present in the test case, the concurrent positive control slide should be from a similar tissue that was fixed, decalcified, and processed identically

Positive and negative control slides reveal instrumentation errors, particularly if test tissue resides on same slide as positive control (eg, aliquotting error, inadequate dispensing of antibody over tissue, etc)

Postanalytical

Recognize potential pitfalls of preanalytical and analytical variables, troubleshoot accordingly

Despite robust antigen retrieval methods, IHC remains less sensitive than flow cytometry—thus weak expression of aberrant antigens may be missed, particularly in decalcified tissue

Confirm correct tissue is on slide

Confirm correct antibody is applied by checking positive control and assessing for predicted positive internal cells within patient bone marrow

Interpretation of a single antibody may be misleading if not integrated with the complete morphologic and immunophenotypic context:

　　CD34 is positive on blasts, but not all blasts are CD34+
　　CD117 stains a variety of cell types, not just blasts (eg, erythroid precursors and mast cells)
　　Cyclin D1 is seen in multiple tumors
　　CD30 is present on a wide variety of cells including non-neoplastic activated lymphoid cells
　　BCL2 expression is normal in naive B-cells

Diagnostician must be aware of potential cross reactivities and full spectrum of cell types that may express a given antigen

Diagnostician would ideally assess a panel of antigens on a neoplastic population including those predicted to be *positive* based on differential diagnostic considerations as well as selected antibodies that are predicted to be *negative* in a given neoplasm

---

t4.10 Indications for Flow Cytometry in Blood/Bone Marrow Evaluation

Determine lineage of new acute leukemia

Evaluate for blood involvement by chronic lymphoid disorders

Evaluate for increased blasts in cases of MDS and/or MPN

Detect aberrant antigen expression (eg, MDS)

Evaluate for plasma cell dyscrasia

Monitor for minimal residual disease

MDS = myelodysplastic syndrome; MPN = myeloproliferative neoplasm

and side light scatter characteristics, allowing at least 5-8 different parameters (or more) to be evaluated simultaneously on cell populations. The terms "3- or 6-color" indicate the number of different antibodies that can be combined together simultaneously.

Given the diagnostic benefit imparted by multiparametric analysis, the indications for flow cytometry are broad **t4.10**. However, as with any single test, it is crucial to know the limitations of the study to make a full and accurate evaluation **t4.8** [Stetler-Stevenson 2007]. For instance, the cells of interest may not be represented or detectable in the flow sample, and IHC may be required for complete interpretation. Moreover, the same fresh specimen submitted for conventional cytogenetics or

fluorescence in situ hybridization (FISH) studies may *not* be adequate for these genetic tests.

From start to finish, the technique of flow cytometry is complex and heavily reliant on a viable specimen and adequate instrumentation [Stetler-Stevenson 2007]. It follows therefore that all components of the analytic process (specimen quality, technical, and interpretative issues) play key roles in the quality assurance of this technique **t4.11**. Knowledge of these quality issues is paramount to continued success in evaluating and reporting flow cytometric specimens. In addition, correlation with cytospin morphology ensures that the cells of interest were present for evaluation. Furthermore, knowledge of normal antigenic patterns on cell populations is mandatory to identify abnormalities [Craig 2008, Stetler-Stevenson 2007, 2009]. Clues to identifying abnormal populations in bone marrow specimens are detailed in **t4.12**.

Representative histograms illustrating some typical features of flow cytometry are shown in **f4.1**. **f4.1a** demonstrates how cell populations can be preliminarily identified based on cell size (forward scatter, displayed on the x-axis) and cytoplasmic complexity (side scatter, displayed on the y-axis). As cells enlarge and/or contain more cytoplasmic vacuoles/granules, they will be seen in the flow histograms as

t4.11 Key Quality Control Issues for Flow Cytometry

Preanalytical

Use of proper anticoagulant (Heparin, ACD, EDTA) or RPMI if solid tissue

Heparin is preferable if anticipating cytogenetic/FISH studies

2-3mm tissue aliquots preserves viability

Room temperature or cold pack preserves viability and antigenicity

Add tissue culture media if specimen to be shipped to referral laboratory

Process as quickly as possible particularly for highly proliferative tumors (eg, Burkitt lymphoma, acute leukemia)

Analytical

Check alignment of the laser paths, signal strength (detector output), detector sensitivity, fluorescent calibration, compensation

Reagent stability and appropriate reactivity

Consistency in specimen preparation, staining, incubation, washing

Consistency in gating technique, setting of markers or quadrants to determine positivity or negativity for a particular antigen

Postanalytical

Check for accurate gating, aberrant antigen expression

Check that all populations are reliably accounted for

Maintain competency with proficiency testing

Verify accuracy of numerical results

Correlate findings with cytospin slide from sample

t4.12 Flow Cytometric Clues to Help Identify an Abnormal Population

Light chain restriction in mature B-cells

Changes in antigen intensity (loss, gain, weak) relative to the comparable normal background population

Increased number of "normal" cells (eg, CD34+ blasts)

Lack of surface immunoglobulin expression on mature B-cells (bright CD45 population)

Aberrant expression of an antigen(s) not typically present on a particular population

Lack of predicted maturation of a population (eg, hematogones vs B-lymphoblasts, myelodysplasia)

further to the right on the x-axis or further up on the y-axis, respectively. Granulocytes normally exhibit high side scatter because of the presence of numerous cytoplasmic granules in contrast to lymphoid cells which are predominantly small in size with minimal cytoplasmic complexity. f4.1b demonstrates how CD45 may be combined with side scatter to further and more accurately identify cell populations. For example, normal lymphoid cells typically show the brightest expression of CD45 (furthest to the right on the x-axis) as compared with granulocytes, which are weaker for CD45 (shifted to the left of lymphoid cells) but still show characteristic high side scatter. Blasts may be identified as weak CD45+ cells, which have minimal side scatter (not shown). Cell populations are further evaluated by gating on certain populations and assessing for specific surface and/or intracellular antigen expression. f4.1c illustrates the lymphoid gate, which is

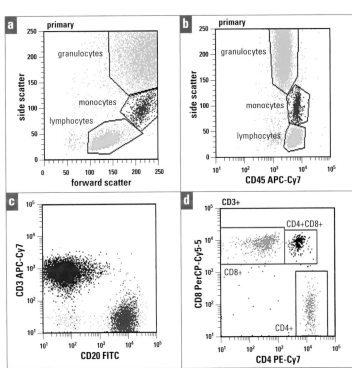

f4.1 Flow cytometry identifies specific cell populations based on scatter properties and antigen expression. a Different cell populations can be preliminarily identified based on their forward (x-axis) and side scatter (y-axis) properties. b CD45 vs side scatter further enhances the more specific cell populations present in a sample. c Lymphoid cells are separated into B-cell (CD20+) and T-cell groups (CD3+). A few CD3– and CD20– cells (grey) are seen in the lower left-hand corner and likely represent natural killer cells. d Further subclassification of the CD3+ T-cell gate reveals T-helper (CD4+) (cyan) and T-cytotoxic (CD8+) (pink) subsets. In the representative histogram, another small population of T-cells co-expressing CD4 and CD8 are noted (black).

Key: yellow = granulocytes, maroon = monocytes, grey = all lymphoid cells, dark blue = CD20+ B cells, green= CD3+ T cells, cyan = CD4+ T cells, pink = CD8+ T cells, black = CD4+CD8+ T cells separated into B-cell and T-cell groups predominantly, as determined by CD20 and CD3 expression, respectively. Further subclassification of the CD3+ T-cell gate reveals T-helper (CD4+) and T-cytotoxic (CD8+) subsets f4.1d.

Flow cytometry, along with polymerase chain reaction (PCR)-based molecular techniques, plays a significant role in minimal residual disease (MRD) testing. MRD is prognostic in several diseases, including pediatric precursor B-cell acute lymphoblastic leukemia (ALL), chronic myelogenous leukemia *BCR-ABL1+*, acute promyelocytic leukemia, and other myeloid neoplasms (see Chapter 36). Flow cytometry has a reported sensitivity of approximately $1/10^4$ cells and is most useful when an aberrant immunophenotypic fingerprint is present. However, over time, phenotypic "shifts" may occur, although at a reportedly low frequency [Borowitz 2005, Chen 2007].

[4.4] Conventional Cytogenetics

Conventional cytogenetic analysis plays an integral role in both diagnosing and predicting the prognosis of many neoplastic hematolymphoid disorders, particularly those with specific recurring abnormalities [Rowley 2008]. In some cases, cytogenetics may be the single most significant factor in determining risk stratification and overall response to therapy (eg, *BCR-ABL1* translocation in precursor B-cell

ALL). Although historically it was the role of board-certified cytogenetists, it is pathologists who now must integrate morphologic, immunophenotypic, and genetic data into a final interpretation.

t4.13 Indications for Conventional Cytogenetic Studies in Bone Marrow

Acute leukemia at diagnosis

CML and other myeloproliferative neoplasms at diagnosis

MDS at diagnosis for prognosis

Monitor response to therapy (evaluate ablation of abnormal clone)

Relapse of acute leukemia (evaluate for clonal evolution)

Progression of myelodysplastic and myeloproliferative neoplasms

Evaluate aplastic anemia vs hypoplastic MDS

Assess engraftment after other-sex bone marrow transplant

Lymphoproliferative disorders if specific subtype is difficult to determine (case by case basis)

Multiple myeloma for prognosis

Lymphomas with known recurring cytogenetic abnormalities (eg, Burkitt, mantle cell, anaplastic large cell, follicular, etc)

Therapy-related myeloid neoplasms

Involvement by nonhematopoietic tumor which would reveal diagnostic abnormality (eg, Ewing sarcoma, neuroblastoma, alveolar rhabdomyosarcoma)

CML = chronic myelogenous leukemia, *BCR-ABL1+* ; MDS = myelodysplastic syndrome

t4.14 Basic Components of Chromosomal Analysis

Specimen indication	Specify disease/disorder—important for culture set-up (eg, addition of mitogens or IL-4 to stimulate lymphoid or plasma cell proliferation, respectively)
Specimen collection and preservation	>1.0 mL of cellular, sterile bone marrow anticoagulated with *small* amount of sodium heparin
	Minimize peripheral blood contamination of bone marrow by rapid aspiration techniques
	7-10 mL of peripheral blood in sodium heparin tube
	Blood has higher culture failure rate unless significant percent blasts
	Lymph node most appropriate for lymphoma (small diced portions of representative lymph node in sterile transport media)
Specimen transport to the laboratory	Enhance preanalytical processes to reduce transit time so that specimen is processed as quickly as possible
	Maintain specimen at room temperature or refrigerate; do not freeze or expose to high temperature
	Add tissue culture media to sustain viability if shipping specimen to referral laboratory
Processing and analysis	Multiple methods for bone marrow: direct and culture (24 and 48 hour typically)
	Staining:
	G-banding: most common, Wright or Giemsa after trypsin treatment
	Q-banding: quinacrine mustard, fluorescence microscope, useful if metaphases are few or spreading is poor
	Analyze 20 metaphase spreads
	Document karyograms using computer images
Interpretation: What is a clone? *(Use strict standardized criteria to define a clone)*	At least 2 metaphases with the same additional chromosome or structural aberration
	At least 3 metaphases with the loss of the same chromosome (monosomy)
	If a single metaphase is identified with a potentially significant clone, this may be mentioned in the interpretation "as information"; however, it does not meet the definition of a clone
	Evaluate 10-30 more mitotic spreads for the abnormality to potentially confirm a clone
	Use ISCN 2009 nomenclature for karyotype reporting

t4.15 Key Quality Control Issues in Cytogenetic Analysis

Preanalytical

Suboptimal communication with cytogenetic laboratory about key diagnostic considerations

Improperly completed requisition form: with time-sensitive specimens, needed test may not be performed expeditiously

Nonspecific indication listed on requisition form (eg, "leukemia"): no tailored culture set-up is performed

Inadequate specimen:

    suboptimal anticoagulant such as EDTA limits cell growth in culture

    clotted blood or bone marrow

    hemodilution of bone marrow

    paucicellular (no significant neoplastic cells, fibrotic marrow, dry tap)

    poor viability (prolonged transport time)

Analytical

Staining problems, inadequate trypsinization

Suboptimal culture conditions in laboratory

Postanalytical

Resolution is ~5-10 Mb of DNA; small, submicroscopic or cryptic abnormalities will not be detected; perform FISH and/or molecular genetic studies as needed

The specific genes involved in an abnormality are not definitively known based solely on chromosomal breakpoint regions; need FISH or molecular genetics for definitive determination; however the involved genes may be "inferred" in certain situations [eg, in *PML-RARA* in t(15;17) and *BCR-ABL1* in t(9;22)]

Suboptimal chromosome spreads; pay extra attention for particular subtle abnormalities (eg inv 16) or perform targeted FISH

False-negative "normal" karyotype; karyotypes are based on dividing cells, the lineage of which is unknown; particularly in bone marrow, often have background "normal" dividing hematopoietic precursors, so tumor cells may not be well represented

Sensitivity for detecting a clonal abnormality is ~10% in 20 metaphases (if previous abnormality known, 5% for residual disease detection)

The indications for bone marrow cytogenetic analysis are listed in **t4.13**. Also occasionally, cytogenetics may provide support for a diagnosis in a morphologically ambiguous case (eg, presence of a cytogenetic abnormality in suspected low-grade myelodysplastic syndrome). Peripheral blood (PB) may be used in situations in which a bone marrow biopsy is not feasible or contraindicated; in general, however, PB cytogenetic analysis is associated with a >5% to 10% failure rate compared with bone marrow [Dewald 2002a]. Better success has been reported as the percentage of blasts in the PB increases [Hussein 2008a, 2008b]. In cases of bone marrow aspirate failure, submission of a trephine biopsy sample may provide metaphases for analysis [Fyfe 2009].

Conventional cytogenetic analysis is a highly complex technique that is significantly dependent on manual labor and interpretation for success [Dewald 2002a]. Automation is available for a small component of cytogenetic processing; however, the bulk of the technical work continues to require hands-on efforts by cytotechnologists and cytogenetists. Important components of the cytogenetic process applicable to bone marrow pathology are outlined in **t4.14** [Dewald 2002a]. Key quality control issues relevant to the success of a cytogenetic study are seen in **t4.15** [Shaffer 2005, Watson 2007]. Although this table highlights some of the limitations of conventional

t4.16 Advantages of Conventional Cytogenetic Testing

Entire chromosome complement is visualized

Provides a baseline assessment for future comparison, as needed

Will detect clonal evolution

Detection of a clone may help distinguish a neoplastic from non-neoplastic disorder

Characteristic abnormalities provide diagnostic and/or prognostic information (see **t4.13**)

cytogenetics, advantages still predominate and are listed in **t4.16**. In fact, routine cytogenetics is standard of care in most, if not all, newly diagnosed myeloid disorders.

Examples of common types of cytogenetic abnormalities are shown in **f4.2**. Metaphase cytogenetics has revealed many recurring cytogenetic aberrations in hematologic disorders [Rowley 2008]. Common cytogenetic abnormalities in myeloid neoplasms are listed in the **appendix** [Dewald 2002a, Dingli 2005, Mesa 2005, Mrozek 2007, Rowley 2008, Steensma 2002, Swerdlow 2008]. A suggested practical approach to the use of cytogenetic techniques in the workup of selected hematolymphoid neoplasms is also provided in the **appendix**.

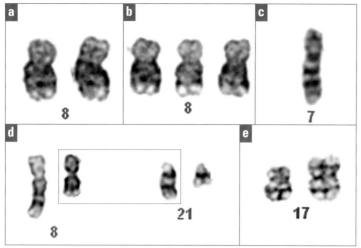

f4.2 *Partial karyogram appearance of various chromosomal configurations encountered in bone marrow pathology:* **a** *diploid (normal),* **b** *triploid (+8),* **c** *monosomy (−7),* **d** *translocation [t(8;21)] (abnormals boxed),* **e** *isochromosome [iso(17q) (abnormal right)].*

t4.17 Comparison of FISH with Conventional Karyotyping

FISH	Cytogenetics
Fast (24-48 hours) results	>3 days for most results
Straightforward set-up	Sterile culture technique
Use metaphase and/or interphase cells	Requires dividing (metaphase) cells
Analyze 200-500 cells quickly (<1 hour)	An abnormal marrow, 3-5 hours
May use paraffin-embedded and fresh tissues	Requires viable and dividing cells
Can use air-dried, unfixed specimens on slides	
1%-5% analytic sensitivity	5%-10% analytic sensitivity
Detects submicroscopic (small deletions, translocations) abnormalities (eg, t(12;21) in B-ALL, *FIP1L1-PDGFRA* fusion in eosinophilia)	Miss small genomic abnormalities
Specific genes are known	Specific genetic targets unknown

B-ALL = B-cell acute lymphoblastic lymphoma

[4.5] Fluorescence In Situ Hybridization

Fluorescence in situ hybridization has greatly enhanced our ability to use cytogenetics to study disease [Dewald 2002b]. FISH focuses on small genomic regions and/or single genes, which comprise on average 0.5-1.5 kB of DNA. This perspective is thus markedly different from conventional cytogenetics, which allows resolution in routine bone marrow evaluation of approximately 5 mB of DNA. Stated another way, FISH allows us to further define the genes/small genetic regions that correspond to a particular cytogenetic abnormality. Importantly, one must recognize that FISH only provides data about the specific genetic regions that are interrogated. There is no information about the remainder of the chromosomes as there is with conventional karyotyping. A comparison of FISH vs karyotyping is seen in **t4.17**. A suggested practical approach to the use of cytogenetic techniques in the workup of hematolymphoid neoplasms is shown in the **appendix**.

Validation of FISH probes is an important part of the clinical laboratory quality control process. It has recently been formally updated to ensure accurate probe performance in normal and abnormal conditions and to ensure FISH reader consistency and reproducibility [Wiktor 2006]. The general approaches to the FISH technique and quality control issues are listed in **t4.18** and **t4.19**, respectively. Undoubtedly, given the ongoing advancements in FISH testing and probes available, additional modifications of these quality control procedures will be put forth.

[4.5.1] Types of FISH Probes

There are 4 types of FISH probes, targeting
1. whole chromosomes
2. centromeric regions
3. specific loci
4. telomeres

In routine clinical practice, the latter 3 are used most often. Whole chromosome paints consist of chromosome-specific segments of DNA that span the entire chromosome and are differentially colored to distinguish amongst the 22 autosomes and 2 sex chromosomes. They may rarely be used on metaphase spreads to evaluate for a cryptic translocation or reveal the chromosomal origin of unidentifiable genetic material in the form of a marker or ring chromosome, or attached to an otherwise recognizable chromosome. Centromere-specific probes are used to detect aneuploidy. These probes are composed of highly repetitive alpha satellite DNA sequences associated with the centromere. Locus-specific probes are aimed at detecting loss or gain (including amplification) abnormalities of a particular genetic region without a concomitant loss of the whole chromosome. These probes may also span both sides of a gene's breakpoint region and aid in the identification of translocations. Telomere probes detect subtle abnormalities involving telomeric regions.

[4.5.2] FISH Probe Strategies

There are several routinely used FISH probe strategies. The probe strategies generally involve 2 different genetic loci, 1 of which may be a second gene region of interest, control locus, or centromeric region. Such combinations allow for the detection of deletions, gene duplication or amplification, aneuploidy, and translocations **f4.3**. Each of these probe detection strategies has its own analytical sensitivity, and each probe set (even if the same strategy) has a different reference range. Dual fusion probes have the best analytical sensitivity of <1%, while gene deletions, duplications, amplification, monosomy, and trisomy are roughly 8%-10%, 8%, 3%, 6%-8%, and 4%-5%, respectively, in our experience. These percentages are based on 2-color FISH, in which the control probe may not be located on the same chromosome.

The most sensitive probe strategy is the dual color-dual fusion to detect translocations. In this strategy, the fluorescent probes span the breakpoints of both genetic loci, thereby creating a typical abnormal 2-fusion pattern (orange and

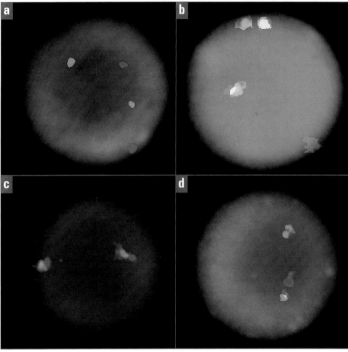

f4.3 *Fluorescence in situ hybridization (FISH) patterns in interphase cells using dual color–dual fusion (DCDF)* **a**, **b** *and break apart (BA)* **c**, **d** *probe strategies. Interphase nuclei are shown by DAPI (blue) staining. Composite illustrating* **a** *typical normal (2 orange, 2 green signals), and* **b** *abnormal (translocated) FISH pattern (2 fusion signals [orange and green overlapping], 1 orange and 1 green) for a DCDF probe. Composite illustrating* **c** *typical normal (2 fused signals), and* **d** *abnormal (gene rearrangement) FISH pattern (1 fused signal, 1 orange, 1 green) for a BA probe.*

t4.18 Basic Components of FISH Analysis

Specimen collection	Fresh cells in anticoagulant or sterile media, touch preparation, bone marrow aspirate smear (unfixed or stained), paraffin-embedded tissue
Specimen processing	Prepare the sample (interphase or metaphase) for probing and place on glass slide
	Denature target sample DNA and probe DNA
	Hybridize fluorescently labeled probe to target
	Wash away unbound and weakly homologous probe DNA
Interpretation	Read fluorescent signal patterns (manual or automated)
	Manual reading is generally 200 interphase cells (100 cells/reader)

t4.19 Key Quality Control Issues in FISH Testing

Preanalytical

Neoplastic cells should be present (cytologic evaluation is not performed in the cytogenetics laboratory)
% neoplastic cells should exceed analytic sensitivity of probe used based on individual probe validation studies

Analytical

Appropriate probe set is utilized (concurrent positive control)
Instrument quality control (temperature accurate, fixatives fresh, etc.)
Proper training of FISH technicians regarding:
    scoring criteria
    quality of specimen/hybridization/background/cell density
    biologic and technical factors that interfere with signal patterns (incomplete probe hybridization saturation, probe cross hybridization, non-condensed interphase DNA resulting in signal splitting, occasional random overlap of signals)

Postanalytical

Must know your individual laboratory's established reference ranges (analytical sensitivities) for each probe in each tissue site
Analytical sensitivities for 200 cells (established by each laboratory individually, varies by each probe and by site) but in general:
    dual color dual fusion strategy, <1%
    break-apart, ~4%
    monosomy, ~8%
    trisomy, ~4%-5%
Must evaluate fluorescence morphology/hybridization scores to determine if repeat hybridization is necessary
If abnormal value is within 5% of positive upper limit, additional cells should be read
If no neoplastic population is present to begin with, a negative result is meaningless

green overlap) in addition to the background residual loci (1 orange and 1 green signal) in a positive cell. The typical normal pattern is 2 separate orange and 2 separate green signals. Typical examples of the normal and abnormal patterns are shown in **f4.3a,b**.

The break-apart probe strategy was developed to detect rearrangements (most often translocations) in genes that have multiple partners (eg, *MLL, ALK, IGH@, MYC*). This probe strategy only reveals a rearrangement for the gene tested; it does not provide any data on the partner gene. The normal pattern is 2 fused signals reflecting 1 orange and 1 green signal that flanks the breakpoint region of the gene of interest. When rearranged/translocated, the pattern appears as separate orange and green signals along with the remaining background normal fused signal **f4.3c,d**.

[4.5.3] **FISH and MRD Detection**

FISH, for the most part, has limited usefulness in MRD testing. This is because the analytical sensitivity of most of the probe systems is >1%. One exception is the dual color-dual fusion probe, but in routine testing of 200 interphase nuclei is still only capable of detecting approximately 1 neoplastic cell/100 cells (1%) at best. Alternatively, if 6,000 nuclei are examined, the detection of 3 cells with the abnormal pattern leads to a positive diagnosis for MRD (0.05%) [Dewald 2002b]. In contrast to FISH, molecular genetic studies and flow cytometry are better equipped to detect MRD at reported levels of $1/10^{4-5}$ and $1/10^4$, respectively.

[4.6] **Molecular Studies**

Molecular studies are useful in the evaluation of both lymphoid and myeloid malignancies in bone marrow **t4.20** [Sen 2002, Viswanatha 2007]. The rationale for using molecular testing depends on the case, the suspected diagnosis, evaluation for possible submicroscopic abnormality(ies) with prognostic significance, and the need for follow-up MRD testing. Because of its high sensitivity, molecular technology is most often used in MRD testing, along with flow cytometry. Although it may appear that these techniques perform duplicate testing, they are in fact complementary to one another and require knowledge of analytical sensitivities, specimen requirements, testing limitations, and disease phase (at presentation vs during or after therapy) for the most effective use. MRD testing is further discussed in Chapter 36.

Currently, the vast majority of molecular tests use PCR-based methodology, rather than traditional Southern blot technique, for reasons outlined in **t4.21**. The decision to use PCR or the Southern blot method depends on several

t4.20 Indications for Molecular Testing

To assist in diagnosis (neoplastic vs reactive) when other modalities not informative

To assist in classification [eg, *CBFB-MYH11* fusion in acute myeloid leukemia with inv(16)]

To aid in prognostication (eg, *FLT3* ITD in acute myeloid leukemia)

On therapy, post-therapy or pretransplant monitoring

t4.21 Comparison of Polymerase Chain Reaction (PCR) and Southern Blot Methods

	PCR	Southern blot
Time	<5 days	2-3 weeks
Labor	Minimal	Labor intensive
Cost	Less	More
Materials	Fresh, frozen, fixed	Fresh or frozen only
Amount of DNA	≤1 µg	5-10 µg
Radioactivity	Not used	Used
Automatable	Yes	No
MRD detection	Increased sensitivity	Poor sensitivity

factors, including type of material available (ie, fresh vs fixed), disorder being investigated, sensitivity of the test, and false-positive and false-negative rates. PCR has become the more popular of the 2 tests because it is faster, can be performed on fixed material, and requires less material than Southern blot. As with all testing methodologies, PCR DNA- and RNA-based tests are not without limitations. Key quality assurance issues that should be considered are listed in **t4.22**.

In bone marrow evaluation, the application of these techniques is highly dependent on the type of case. **t4.23** provides a limited synopsis of the strengths of the various molecular techniques available to identify prognostically and diagnostically relevant molecular alterations. In practice, a combination of the most "global" test (eg, cytogenetics) should be partnered with a more sensitive molecular test to include/exclude certain recurring abnormalities that are significant yet possibly cryptic (eg, *BCR-ABL1* in CML). The identification of such molecular fingerprints is becoming increasingly important for not only predicting a particular disease entity or its overall prognosis, but also targeted therapy. As the list of recurring abnormalities elongates, these specialized testing techniques will become even more routine, and thus our knowledge of each of their strengths and weaknesses and interpretative pitfalls is crucial.

t4.22 Key Quality Control Issues in Polymerase Chain Reaction (PCR)-Based Testing

Preanalytical

RNA-based assays

Fresh, well-preserved tissue

Fixed tissue may be used but has a higher rate of failure due to RNA degradation and/or inhibitors of the PCR process

DNA-based assays

Certain fixatives (eg, B5) and decalcification of bone marrow markedly impede the quality of DNA and isolation

Analytical

Daily positive and negative controls to ensure method validity

False-positive results

Meticulous attention paid to control contamination

IGH@ and *TRG@* (~5%-10% of cases)

Minute biopsy with amplification of small number of cells

TRG@:
Limited exon diversity, similarly sized PCR products
Selectively skewed reactive population

False negative (*IGH@* 35%, *TRG@* 20%)

Precautions to avoid DNA and RNA degrading enzymes

Insufficient tissue/cells of interest

Minor DNA/base pair alterations that abrogate binding of the PCR primers (hence no amplification and PCR failure); more common in tumors that have undergone somatic hypermutation (eg, FL, some DLBCLs, BL, post germinal center lymphomas) (up to 50% false negative)

Postanalytical

False-positive and false-negative results, suggest additional tests/close follow-up as warranted

Experienced analyst

Expertise with testing methods to troubleshoot problems

Knowledge of current literature to effectively communicate the result

BL = Burkitt lymphoma; DLBCL = diffuse large B-cell lymphoma; FL = follicular lymphoma

t4.23 Comparison of 4 Specialized Techniques

	Flow Cytometry	Conventional Cytogenetics	FISH	Molecular
Turnaround time	<24 h	At least 3 d	24-48 h	PCR (3-5 d)
Requirement for fresh/viable cells	Yes	Yes	No	No[‡]
Requirement for dividing cells	No	Yes	No	No
Analytical sensitivity	$1/10^4$	5%	1%-5%	$1/10^5$
Global evaluation of chromosomes	No	Yes	No	No
Capability of detecting "cryptic" chromosomal abnormalities	No	No	Yes	Yes
Capability of detecting nucleotide alterations such as mutations, internal tandem duplications	No	No	No	Yes
Capable of detecting chromosomal numerical abnormalities	No	Yes	Yes*	No
Useful in minimal residual disease detection	Yes[†] ($1/10^3$ - $1/10^4$ cells)	No	Maybe ($1/10^2$ - $1/10^3$ cells)	Yes[†] ($1/10^5$ cells)

*FISH is only capable of detecting numerical abnormalities if the probe targets that specific abnormality
[†]Phenotypic shifts do occur—may alter original immunophenotypic and/or molecular profile
[‡]Yes for most RNA-based assays

FISH = fluorescence in situ hybridization

[4.7] Additional Ancillary Techniques: GEP, Array CGH, MicroRNA

[4.7.1] Gene Expression Profiling

Gene expression profiling (GEP) is a technique that measures gene expression (mRNA), and in conjunction with the availability of the entirely sequenced human genome, provides a high throughput approach to unraveling previously unrecognized genetic aberrations in cancer. It centers on the simultaneous assessment of hundreds to thousands of gene expression levels in a single experiment. These experiments most often evaluate the relative amount of mRNA expressed in normal vs abnormal cells. Altered levels of some mRNAs (compared with normal) suggest a change in cellular needs and indicate a possible pathologic state. The large amount of information generated has led to the development of many computer-based information management (software) tools to analyze, interpret, and catalog the data t4.24. Such information may impart to us knowledge about the pathogenesis at work in tumor types. The routine use of gene expression profiling is still, however, currently limited for clinical use due to expense and technical complexity. Gene expression profiling is a technically complex and challenging technique that includes specimen preparation, analysis, and statistical output. Knowledge of the intricacies of these various steps and potential quality control issues is essential for accurate interpretation t4.25.

Gene expression profiling has been performed on a wide variety of tissue and tumor types, including hematolymphoid neoplasms. GEP is able to identify new subgroups within a known disease entity, may predict a certain type of tumor, and provides biological insight into tumors with its characteristic detection of gene deregulation. Identification of signature profiles and putative genetic targets sets the stage for better predicting outcome, response to therapy, and identification of specific targeted therapies. It is well beyond the scope of this text to discuss in detail all the recent works in this field; however, a brief sampling of recent achievement is presented in t4.26.

In AML, GEP studies have also identified prognostically relevant subgroups. These may prove particularly useful in the ~50% of adult AML cases that are cytogenetically normal and show a diverse range of outcomes with current management (see Chapter 18). GEP studies are not limited to these areas and have been done in various hematolymphoid tumors and other solid tumors [Alizadeh 2000, Mrozek 2009, Savage 2003].

[4.7.2] Array-Based Comparative Genomic Hybridization (Array CGH)

Comparative genomic hybridization (CGH) is a technique dating from the early 1990s used to characterize copy number changes in genetic regions across the entire genome. This technique is not capable of detecting translocations unless they are unbalanced and result in a loss of material. The aim of CGH studies is to elucidate gene regions that are likely involved in the pathogenesis of a particular disease state (constitutional or neoplastic). Ultimately, further refinement of the gene regions to identify particular gene(s) that play a role in that disease may lead to targeted treatment, as well as prediction of tumor progression, therapeutic response, and overall outcome.

The CGH method involves labeling genomic normal and abnormal DNA with 2 different fluorochromes and then hybridizing this DNA to normal metaphase chromosomes.

---

t4.24 Basic Components of Gene Expression Profiling

DNA microarrays are constructed by arraying or spotting PCR-amplified cDNA (from normalized cDNA libraries, clones, or gene fragments) or synthetic oligonucleotides selected to represent as many previously identified unique gene transcripts as possible, at a high density in gridded patterns onto glass slides, silicon wafers, or nylon membrane supports; the microarrays are used in a cohybridization process involving 2 or more fluorescently labeled probes prepared from mRNA samples obtained from cell or tissue samples representing different experimental treatments, disease states, developmental stages, or phenotypes of interest

Kinetic analysis allows gene expression levels to be determined from the locations on the array and level of hybridization (measured as fluorescence) detected for each probe

A heat map of the gene expression profiling patterns is generated with green representing relatively reduced levels of expression relative to baseline, where red represents upregulation

Cluster analysis places certain groups together based on the gene expression profiles

---

t4.25 Key Quality Assurance Issues in Gene Expression Profiling

Preanalytical

Study population background (cellularity, ethnicity)—diverse or not

Analytical

Processing and mRNA isolation

Hybridization differences

% background nontumor cells possibly diluting expression data

Postanalytical

Data normalization

Clustering techniques

Gene filtering

Complex statistical analysis

Differences between the normal and abnormal cells along the metaphase chromosomes are quantified and thus display alterations in copy number (gain or loss) in the tumor cells. As may be seen, this is a time-consuming process and requires technical experience in dealing with cytogenetic specimens.

To avoid some of these technical difficulties, array-based CGH was established in which the metaphase chromosome spread is replaced by genomic targets in the form of bacterial artificial clones, cDNA clones, or oligonucleotides. As such, this new technique has been applied to human genetic (eg, constitutional studies) and cancer research [Li 2009, Savage 2003].

Multiple CGH studies have focused on hematolymphoid neoplasms; a few examples are mentioned to illustrate the benefit gained. In plasma cell myeloma, array CGH was able to identify specific subgroups that had different clinical outcomes [Carrasco 2006]. Tyybakinoja et al identified cryptic gene copy alterations in cytogenetically normal AML [Tyybakinoja 2007].

t4.26 Selected Gene Expression Profiling Findings in Hematolymphoid Disorders

Disorder	Finding
AML	An 86-probe set predicts overall survival in cytogenetically normal AML
AML	New subgroups which could be diagnostically relevant
ALL	Small sets of genes are an independent predictor of patient outcome or relapse
T-LGL	Deregulation of apoptotic and sphingolipid-mediated signaling
Immature myeloid/ T-cell leukemia	New subgroup of acute leukemia

AML = acute myeloid leukemia; ALL = acute lymphoblastic leukemia; T-LGL = T-cell large granular lymphocyte leukemia

References: [Bullinger 2004, Catchpoole 2007, Flotho 2007, Metzeler 2008, Mrozek 2009, Shah 2008, Valk 2004, Wilson 2006, Wouters 2008]

Distinct mantle cell lymphoma genotypes may be identified, which may predict leukemic spread and patient outcome [Rubio-Moscardo 2005]. Finally, genomic profiling is finding new genetic lesions in acute leukemia that contribute to further understanding of disease pathogenesis [Mullighan 2009].

[4.7.3] MicroRNAs

What are microRNAs? MicroRNAs (miRNAs) are 19- to 25-nucleotide noncoding single-stranded RNA molecules capable of regulating gene expression [Fabbri 2008, Kato 2008, Vasilatou 2009]. Present studies show that miRNAs can act either as oncogenes or as tumor suppressor genes or sometimes as both. miRNAs are involved in a wide spectrum of biologic processes, including cell cycle regulation, differentiation, development, metabolism, neuronal patterning, and aging. **t4.27** illustrates known examples of miRNAs in hematopathologic disease and their putative functions. miRNA-based subclassifications of diseases may yield clinically relevant prognostic information [Visone 2009]. Despite the fact that knowledge of miRNAs is still emerging, it is postulated that putative therapeutic targets against miRNAs will be identified.

[4.7.4] Nonrandom X-Chromosome Inactivation (HUMARA Assay)

The human androgen receptor gene (HUMARA) assay is also used to establish clonality in a variety of neoplastic hematopoietic diseases [Busque 2009, Busque 1996, Willman 1994]. Interestingly, skewing of X-inactivation ratios has been detected in the blood of elderly women, but may not implicate overt clonality [Busque 2009, Swierczek 2008]. The HUMARA assay is not routinely available and requires experience to interpret [Agarwal 2009].

t4.27 microRNAs in Selected Hematolymphoid Tumors

MicroRNA	Genomic Locus	Expression in Tumors	Function
miR-15a/miR-16-1	13q14	Downregulated in CLL	Regulates BCL2
miR-181a	1q31	Downregulated in CLL and AML with MLD	Regulates TCL1
miR-204	9q21	Downregulated in *NPM1* mutated AML, normal karyotype AML	
miR-155	21q21	Upregulated in DLBCL, Hodgkin, pediatric Burkitt lymphoma, and AML with FLT3 ITD	Activates lymphoproliferation and myeloproliferation
miR-17~92 cluster	13q14 vs31-q32	Upregulated in lymphomas	May develop lymphoproliferative disease, downregulation of proapoptotic gene Bim, MYC binds and activates the expression of this miRNA cluster region

AML = acute myeloid leukemia; CLL = chronic lymphocytic leukemia; DLBCL = diffuse large B-cell lymphoma; ITD = internal tandem duplication; MLD = multilineage dysplasia

References: [Calin 2005, Cimmino 2005, Costinean 2006, Dixon-McIver 2008, Kluiver 2005, Marcucci 2008, Mendell 2008, Neilson 2007, Nicoloso 2007, O'Donnell 2005, Pekarsky 2006, Xiao 2008]

[4.8] Clues and Caveats

1. Integration of specialized testing data with the clinical and morphologic findings is required for accurate bone marrow interpretation.

2. Knowledge of the analytical sensitivities, diagnostic capabilities, and interpretation pitfalls of IHC, flow cytometry, cytogenetics, FISH, and molecular studies in the evaluation of hematolymphoid disorders is critical.

3. MPO and NSE cytochemical stains help identify AMLs with granulocytic or monocytic differentiation, respectively.

4. Special stains for erythroid and storage iron help identify altered iron utilization states.

5. Increased fibrosis may be of varying severity and significance. Collagen fibrosis tends to be irreversible.

6. IHC is mainly performed on fixed tissues with architectural preservation. Simultaneous evaluation of multiple antigens is rarely done and low-level residual disease may be missed.

7. Flow cytometric analysis is fast, with a reported analytic sensitivity of up to $1/10^4$, but requires a fresh specimen with viable tumor cells. Paucicellular, poorly viable specimens may yield false-negative results. Certain disease states may be missed on flow cytometric analysis (Hodgkin lymphoma, some T-cell lymphomas).

8. Conventional cytogenetics provides a global view of the entire chromosomal complement. It requires viable and dividing cells of interest, has a relatively low resolution (5-10 mB), and small or submicroscopic aberrations go undetected.

9. FISH is fast, does not require dividing tumor cells, but only answers the specific question(s) asked. The status of the remainder of the chromosomal complement is unknown.

10. PCR-based molecular studies are highly sensitive and specific (on the order of $1/10^4$-10^5) but must be rigorously controlled to avoid contamination. The reasons for false-negative and -positive results must be recognized and additional studies performed as necessary.

[4.9] References

Agarwal N, Nussenzveig RH, Swierczek SI, et al [2009] Does HUMARA assay for assessment of clonal hematopoiesis have shortcomings? *Blood* 114:2357-2358; author reply 2358-2359.

Alizadeh A, Eisen M, Davis R, et al [2000] Distinct types of diffuse large B-cell lymphoma identified by gene expression profiling. *Nature* 403:503.

Bacher U, Haferlach T, Kern W, et al [2005] Conventional cytogenetics of myeloproliferative diseases other than CML contribute valid information. *Ann Hematol* 84:250-257.

Bain BJ, Clark DM, Lampert IA, Wilkins BS [2001] Special techniques applicable to bone marrow diagnosis. In: *Bone Marrow Pathology*. 3rd ed. Oxford: Blackwell Science; 51-89.

Bauermeister DE [1971] Quantitation of bone marrow reticulin—a normal range. *Am J Clin Pathol* 56:24-31.

Beckman EN, Brown AW, Jr [1990] Normal reticulin level in iliac bone marrow. *Arch Pathol Lab Med* 114:1241-1243.

Borowitz MJ, Pullen DJ, Winick N, et al [2005] Comparison of diagnostic and relapse flow cytometry phenotypes in childhood acute lymphoblastic leukemia: implications for residual disease detection: a report from the children's oncology group. *Cytometry B Clin Cytom* 68:18-24.

Buesche G, Georgii A, Kreipe HH [2006] Diagnosis and quantification of bone marrow fibrosis are significantly biased by the pre-staining processing of bone marrow biopsies. *Histopathology* 48:133-148.

Bullinger L, Dohner K, Bair E, et al [2004] Use of gene-expression profiling to identify prognostic subclasses in adult acute myeloid leukemia. *N Engl J Med* 350:1605-1616.

Busque L, Mio R, Mattioli J, et al [1996] Nonrandom X-inactivation patterns in normal females: lyonization ratios vary with age. *Blood* 88:59-65.

Busque L, Paquette Y, Provost S, et al [2009] Skewing of X-inactivation ratios in blood cells of aging women is confirmed by independent methodologies. *Blood* 113:3472-3474.

Calin GA, Ferracin M, Cimmino A, et al [2005] A microRNA signature associated with prognosis and progression in chronic lymphocytic leukemia. *N Engl J Med* 353:1793-1801.

Carrasco DR, Tonon G, Huang Y, et al [2006] High-resolution genomic profiles define distinct clinico-pathogenetic subgroups of multiple myeloma patients. *Cancer Cell* 9:313-325.

Catchpoole D, Lail A, Guo D, et al [2007] Gene expression profiles that segregate patients with childhood acute lymphoblastic leukaemia: an independent validation study identifies that endoglin associates with patient outcome. *Leuk Res* 31:1741-1747.

Chen W, Karandikar NJ, McKenna RW, Kroft SH [2007] Stability of leukemia-associated immunophenotypes in precursor B-lymphoblastic leukemia/lymphoma: A single institution experience. *Am J Clin Pathol* 127:39-46.

Chu P, Arber D, Weiss L [2003] Expression of T/NK-cell and plasma cell antigens in nonhematopoietic epithelioid neoplasms. *Am J Clin Pathol* 2003:64-70.

Cimmino A, Calin GA, Fabbri M, et al [2005] miR-15 and miR-16 induce apoptosis by targeting BCL2. *Proc Natl Acad Sci USA* 102:13944-13949.

Costinean S, Zanesi N, Pekarsky Y, et al [2006] Pre-B cell proliferation and lymphoblastic leukemia/high-grade lymphoma in E(mu)-miR155 transgenic mice. *Proc Natl Acad Sci USA* 103:7024-7029.

Craig FE, Foon KA [2008] Flow cytometric immunophenotyping for hematologic neoplasms. *Blood* 111:3941-3967.

Dewald G, Keterling R, Wyatt W, Stupca P [2002a] Cytogenetic studies in neoplastic hematologic disorders. In: McClatchey K, ed. *Clinical Laboratory Medicine*. 2nd ed. Philadelphia: Lippincott Williams & Wilkins; 658-685.

Dewald GW [2002b] Cytogenetic and FISH studies in myelodysplasia, acute myeloid leukemia, chronic lymphocytic leukemia and lymphoma. *Int J Hematol* 76Suppl2:65-74.

Dingli D, Grand FH, Mahaffey V, et al [2005] Der(6)t(1;6)(q21-23;p21.3): a specific cytogenetic abnormality in myelofibrosis with myeloid metaplasia. *Br J Haematol* 130:229-232.

Dixon-McIver A, East P, Mein CA, et al [2008] Distinctive patterns of microRNA expression associated with karyotype in acute myeloid leukaemia. *PLoS ONE* 3:e2141.

Dunphy CH [2004] Applications of flow cytometry and immunohistochemistry to diagnostic hematopathology. *Arch Pathol Lab Med* 128:1004-1022.

Fabbri M, Croce CM, Calin GA [2008] MicroRNAs. *Cancer J* 14:1-6.

Flotho C, Coustan-Smith E, Pei D, et al [2007] A set of genes that regulate cell proliferation predicts treatment outcome in childhood acute lymphoblastic leukemia. *Blood* 110:1271-1277.

Fong TP, Okafor LA, Thomas W, Jr [1977] Westerman MP. Stainable iron in aspirated and needle-biopsy specimens of marrow: a source of error. *Am J Hematol* 2:47-51.

Fyfe AJ, Drummond M, Morris A [2009] Successful routine cytogenetic analysis from trephine biopsy speciments following failure to aspirate bone marrow. *Br J Haematol* 146(5):573-582.

Gale E, Torrance J, Bothwell T [1963] The quantitative estimation of total iron stores in human bone marrow. *J Clin Invest* 42:1076-1082.

Higgins RA, Blankenship JE, Kinney MC [2008] Application of immunohistochemistry in the diagnosis of non-Hodgkin and Hodgkin lymphoma. *Arch Pathol Lab Med* 132:441-461.

Hussein K, Ketterling RP, Dewald GW, et al [2008a] Peripheral blood cytogenetic studies in myelofibrosis: overall yield and comparison with bone marrow cytogenetic studies. *Leuk Res* 32:1597-1600.

Hussein K, Ketterling RP, Hulshizer RL, et al [2008b] Peripheral blood cytogenetic studies in hematological neoplasms: predictors of obtaining metaphases for analysis. *Eur J Haematol* 80:318-321.

Kato M, Slack FJ [2008] microRNAs: small molecules with big roles - C. elegans to human cancer. *Biol Cell* 100:71-81.

Kirkegaard T, Edwards J, Tovey S, et al [2006] Observer variation in immunohistochemical analysis of protein expression, time for a change? *Histopathology* 48:787-794.

Kluiver J, Poppema S, de Jong D, et al [2005] BIC and miR-155 are highly expressed in Hodgkin, primary mediastinal and diffuse large B cell lymphomas. *J Pathol* 207:243-249.

Krause JR, Brubaker D, Kaplan S [1979] Comparison of stainable iron in aspirated and needle-biopsy specimens of bone marrow. *Am J Clin Pathol* 72:68-70.

Kremer M, Quintanilla-Martinez L, Nahrig J, et al [2005] Immunohistochemistry in bone marrow pathology: a useful adjunct for morphologic diagnosis. *Virchows Arch* 447:920-937.

Kuter DJ, Bain B, Mufti G, et al [2007] Bone marrow fibrosis: pathophysiology and clinical significance of increased bone marrow stromal fibres. *Br J Haematol* 139:351-362.

Lee SH, et al [2008] ICSH guidelines for the standardization of bone marrow specimens and reports. *Int J Lab Hem* 30:349-364.

Li MM, Andersson HC [2009] Clinical application of microarray-based molecular cytogenetics: an emerging new era of genomic medicine. *J Pediatr* 155:311-317.

Lundin P, Persson E, Weinfeld A [1964] Comparison of hemosiderin estimation in bone marrow sections and bone marrow smears. *Acta Med Scand* 175:383-390.

Marcucci G, Radmacher MD, Maharry K, et al [2008] MicroRNA expression in cytogenetically normal acute myeloid leukemia. *N Engl J Med* 358:1919-1928.

Mendell JT [2008] miRiad roles for the miR-17-92 cluster in development and disease. *Cell* 133:217-222.

Mesa RA, Li CY, Ketterling RP, et al [2005] Leukemic transformation in myelofibrosis with myeloid metaplasia: a single-institution experience with 91 cases. *Blood* 105:973-977.

Metzeler KH, Hummel M, Bloomfield CD, et al. [2008] An 86 probe set gene expression signature predicts survival in cytogenetically normal acute myeloid leukemia. *Blood* 112(10):4193-4201.

Mrozek K, Marcucci G, Paschka P, et al [2007] Clinical relevance of mutations and gene-expression changes in adult myeloid leukemia with normal cytogenetics: are we ready for a prognostically prioritized molecular classification? *Blood* 109:431-448.

Mrozek K, Radmacher MD, Bloomfield CD, Marcucci G [2009] Molecular signatures in acute myeloid leukemia. *Curr Opin Hematol* 16:64-69.

Mullighan CG [2009] Genomic analysis of acute leukemia. *Int J Lab Hematol* 31:384-397.

Neilson JR, Zheng GX, Burge CB, Sharp PA [2007] Dynamic regulation of miRNA expression in ordered stages of cellular development. *Genes Dev* 21:578-589.

Nicoloso MS, Kipps TJ, Croce CM, Calin GA [2007] MicroRNAs in the pathogeny of chronic lymphocytic leukaemia. *Br J Haematol* 139:709-716.

O'Donnell KA, Wentzel EA, Zeller KI, et al [2005] c-Myc-regulated microRNAs modulate E2F1 expression. *Nature* 435:839-843.

Olsen RJ, Chang CC, Herrick JL, et al [2008] Acute leukemia immunohistochemistry: a systematic diagnostic approach. *Arch Pathol Lab Med* 132:462-475.

Pekarsky Y, Santanam U, Cimmino A, et al [2006] Tcl1 expression in chronic lymphocytic leukemia is regulated by miR-29 and miR-181. *Cancer Res* 66:11590-11593.

Phiri KS, Calis JC, Kachala D, et al [2009] Improved method for assessing iron stores in the bone marrow. *J Clin Pathol* 62:685-689.

Rahemtullah A, Longtine JA, Harris NL, et al [2008] CD20+ T-cell lymphoma: clinicopathologic analysis of 9 cases and a review of the literature. *Am J Surg Pathol* 32:1593-1607.

Rath CE, Finch CA [1948] Sternal marrow hemosiderin; a method for the determination of available iron stores in man. *J Lab Clin Med* 1948;33:81-86.

Rowley JD [2008] Chromosomal translocations: revisited yet again. *Blood* 112:2183-2189.

Rubio-Moscardo F, Climent J, Siebert R, et al [2005] Mantle-cell lymphoma genotypes identified with CGH to BAC microarrays define a leukemic subgroup of disease and predict patient outcome. *Blood* 105:4445-4454.

Savage KJ, Monti S, Kutok JL, et al [2003] The molecular signature of mediastinal large B-cell lymphoma differs from that of other diffuse large B-cell lymphomas and shares features with classical Hodgkin lymphoma. *Blood* 102:3871-3879.

Sen F, Vega F, Medeiros LJ [2002] Molecular genetic methods in the diagnosis of hematologic neoplasms. *Semin Diagn Pathol* 19:72-93.

Shaffer L, Slovak M, LJ C [2009] *ISCN 2009: An International System for Human Cytogenetic Nomenclature (2005)*. Unionville, CT: S Karger.

Shah MV, Zhang R, Irby R, et al [2008] Molecular profiling of LGL leukemia reveals role of sphingolipid signaling in survival of cytotoxic lymphocytes. *Blood* 112:770-781.

Steensma DP, Tefferi A [2002] Cytogenetic and molecular genetic aspects of essential thrombocythemia. *Acta Haematol* 108:55-65.

Stetler-Stevenson M [2007] Clinical flow cytometric analysis of neoplastic hematolymphoid cells (Guideline H43-A2). In: *clinical and Laboratory Standards Institute Approved Guidelines*. 2nd ed. Wayne, PA: Clinical and Laboratory Standards Institute; 1-80.

Stetler-Stevenson M, Yuan CM [2009] Myelodysplastic syndromes: the role of flow cytometry in diagnosis and prognosis. *Int J Lab Hematol* 31:479-483.

Swerdlow S, Campo E, Harris N, et al [2008] *WHO Classification of Tumours: Pathology and Genetics: Tumours of Haematopoietic and Lymphoid Tissues*. Lyon, France: IARC 2008.

Swierczek SI, Agarwal N, Nussenzveig RH, et al [2008] Hematopoiesis is not clonal in healthy elderly women. *Blood* 112:3186-3193.

Taylor C, Shi SR, Barr N, Wu N [2002] Techniques of immunohistochemistry: principles, pitfalls, and standardization. In: Dabbs D, ed. *Diagnostic Immunohistochemistry*. Philadelphia: Churchill Livingstone; 2002:3-44.

Thiele J, Kvasnicka HM, Facchetti F, et al [2005] European consensus on grading bone marrow fibrosis and assessment of cellularity. *Haematologica* 90:1128-1132.

Tyybakinoja A, Elonen E, Piippo K, et al [2007] Oligonucleotide array-CGH reveals cryptic gene copy number alterations in karyotypically normal acute myeloid leukemia. *Leukemia* 21:571-574.

Valk PJ, Verhaak RG, Beijen MA, et al [2004] Prognostically useful gene-expression profiles in acute myeloid leukemia. *N Engl J Med* 350:1617-1628.

Vasilatou D, Papageorgiou S, Pappa V, et al [2009] The role of microRNAs in normal and malignant hematopoiesis. *Eur J Haematol* epub ahead of print.

Visone R, Rassenti LZ, Veronese A, et al [2009] Karyotype specific microRNA signature in chronic lymphocytic leukemia. *Blood* epub ahead of print.

Viswanatha D, Larson R [2007] Molecular diagnosis of hematopoietic neoplasms. In: McPherson R, Pincus M, eds. *Henry's Clinical Diagnosis and Management by Laboratory Methods*. 21st ed. Philadelphia: Saunders Elsvier; 1295-1322.

Watson M [2007] Quality assurance and quality control in clinical cytogenetics. In: *Current Protocols in Human Genetics*: John Wiley & Sons; Unit 8.2.

Willman CL, Busque L, Griffith BB, et al [1994] Langerhans'-cell histiocytosis (histiocytosis X)—a clonal proliferative disease. *New Engl J Med* 331:154-160.

Wiktor AE, Van Dyke DL, Stupca PJ, et al [2006] Preclinical validation of fluorescence in situ hybridization assays for clinical practice. *Genet Med* 8:16-23.

Wilson CS, Davidson GS, Martin SB, et al [2006] Gene expression profiling of adult acute myeloid leukemia identifies novel biologic clusters for risk classification and outcome prediction. *Blood* 108:685-696.

Wouters BJ, Koss C, Delwel R [2008] Gene expression profiling for improved dissection of acute leukemia: a recently identified immature myeloid/T-lymphoid subgroup as an example. *Blood Cells Mol Dis* 40:395-400.

Xiao C, Srinivasan L, Calado DP, et al [2008] Lymphoproliferative disease and autoimmunity in mice with increased miR-17-92 expression in lymphocytes. *Nat Immunol* 9:405-414.

Yam LT, Li CY, Crosby WH [1971] Cytochemical identification of monocytes and granulocytes. *Am J Clin Pathol* 55:283-290.

Bone Marrow Reporting and Quality Assurance

Kaaren Reichard, MD

Bone marrow examination is essential for the diagnosis of primary hematopoietic disorders (congenital and acquired), for evaluating secondary processes (metastatic, infectious, metabolic), and for assessing response to therapy. In this regard, a comprehensive and accurate, yet succinct, bone marrow report is of paramount importance in communicating the key findings to clinicians. The final bone marrow report requires integration of all available clinical, laboratory, morphologic, and special techniques information. Despite these common goals, variability in the format, terminology, and content of bone marrow reports remains, which can interfere with the communication/interpretation of a diagnosis. In this chapter, we outline strategies for more uniform bone marrow reporting using data checklists, and discuss synoptic reporting as one method to achieve standardized reporting [Lee 2008, Murari 2006, Parwani 2008, Peterson 2002, Qu 2007, Wilkins 2009]. We also discuss the bone marrow "integrated report" as a useful tool for providing a final overall diagnosis with available prognostic information. Such a report is valuable given that some pieces of necessary data (eg, cytogenetics, molecular studies, serologic results) may not be available at the time of initial release of the bone marrow report.

[5.1] Components of Bone Marrow Examination

Indications prompting bone marrow examination have been presented in Chapter 3. Upon procurement of a bone marrow specimen, clinical and morphologic assessment begins. Suitable clinical information useful for interpretation includes patient age, gender, relevant clinical/pathologic history, surgical interventions, drug regimen, and laboratory data **t5.1** [Hasserjian 2008, Peterson 2002, Qu 2007, Foucar 2008]. These data are often difficult to obtain, but may be extremely useful in discriminating non-neoplastic from neoplastic conditions and in avoiding unindicated and potentially costly additional studies. After obtaining the clinical data, bone marrow morphologic assessment commences. Morphologic review of blood and bone marrow is thoroughly covered in Chapter 2, including recognition of potential artifacts.

The ideal components of a bone marrow examination include peripheral blood smear with concurrent complete blood count and differential, bone marrow aspirate smears with at least 3 particles per smear, adequately fixed clot section and trephine biopsy, touch preparation, and an iron-stained aspirate smear **t5.2**. In addition, some experts advocate performing a reticulin stain routinely on core biopsy sections to assess for potentially subtle alterations in the reticulin fibers, which may be associated with a pathologic process [Hasserjian 2008, Kuter 2007].

These various specimens provide both an "anatomic" and "cytologic" view of the bone marrow. Due to differences in expertise and organizational set-ups, some pathology services receive only the so-called "anatomic" portion of the biopsy (clot section and trephine biopsy) for examination, while others (often hematologists) review the "clinical" portion (peripheral blood smear, aspirate smears). Other institutions may receive and report all the components together. Regardless, since there are inherently different pathologic data to be gleaned from the different preparations, review of all the specimens with resultant integrated reporting should be attempted, if possible. For example, bone marrow aspirate smears/

t5.1 Desired Clinical Information for Complete BM Interpretation

Patient age and gender

Relevant clinical history (previous diagnosis, family history, therapeutic regimens with dates, transplantation, radiation exposure)

Pertinent current clinical history (indications for biopsy, weight loss, fever, night sweats)

Physical examination (mass lesions, adenopathy, splenomegaly, petechiae, phenotypic abnormalities)

Current and recent medication list

Social and work history (drug, alcohol, toxin, herbal medicine, and/or natural remedies exposure, occupation)

Travel history

Radiographic findings (X-ray, CT scan, MRI, PET scan, skeletal survey)

Laboratory studies (CBC, coagulation tests, Coombs test, urine/ serum protein electrophoresis, culture results, liver function tests, LDH , viral serologies, other)

BM = bone marrow; CBC = complete blood count; CT = computed tomography; LDH = lactate dehydrogenase; MRI = magnetic resonance imaging; PET = positron emission tomography

References: [Peterson 2002, Foucar 2008]

t5.2 Ideal Components for BM Examination

Peripheral blood smear with concurrent CBC and differential

Bone marrow aspirate smears with ≥3 particles/smear (5 total, 2-3 stained)

Clot section

Trephine biopsy

Touch preparation (3 slides, 1 stained)

Iron-stained aspirate smear

BM = bone marrow; CBC = complete blood count

t5.3 Obtainable Data from Different Components of Bone Marrow Examination

Component Being Evaluated	BM Aspirate	Touch Prep	BM Clot	Core Biopsy
Cellularity	+/−	−	+	+
Bony remodeling	−/+ *	−/+ *	−	+
Bony trabeculae	−	−	−	+
Sinuses	−	−	−	+
Marrow architecture	−	−	+/−	+
Lineage maturation	+	+	−/+	−/+
Erythroid/granulocytic lineage dysplasia	+	+	−	−
Megakaryocyte #, morphology	+	−/+	+	+
Megakaryocyte clustering	−/+	−	+	+
ALIP	−	−	−/+	+
M:E ratio	+	+	+/−	+/−
Fibrosis	−	−	−	+
Lymphoid aggregates	−/+	−/+	+	+
Infiltrates often with associated fibrosis[†]	−	−	−/+	+
Granulomas	−/+	−	+	+
Increased histiocytes[‡]	+	+	−/+	−/+
Plasma cells and cytology	+	+	+/−	+/−[§]
Plasma cell aggregates	−/+	−	+	+
Auer rods	+	+	−	−
Ancillary studies				
Cytochemistry	+	+	−	−
Immunohistochemistry	−	−	+	+
Flow cytometry	+	−	−	−[¶]
Cytogenetics	+	−	−	−[¶]
FISH	+	+	+/−	+/−
Molecular – DNA	+	+/−	+	−/+ [□]
Molecular – RNA	+	−	−	−

*May see osteoclasts or osteoblasts
[†]Mast cell aggregates, non-Hodgkin lymphoma, classical Hodgkin lymphoma, hairy cell leukemia
[‡]Distinguish hemophagocytosis from tumors, storage disease
[§]The number is enhanced by immunohistochemistry
[¶]Unless received in sterile RPMI for disaggregation
[□]Decalcification severely affects DNA quality
− = not obtainable; + = obtainable; ALIP = abnormal localization of immature precursors; BM = bone marrow; M:E ratio = ratio of myeloid to erythroid precursors; FISH = fluorescence in situ hybridization

Reference: Modified from [Cotelingam 2003]

touch preparations are ideal for clear-cut assessment of trilineage maturation and dysplasia, while the trephine biopsy illustrates overall architecture, status of bone and stroma, and degrees of fibrosis, lymphoid or granulomatous infiltrates t5.3. Additionally, the ability to perform ancillary studies is uniquely different between these types of marrow specimens t5.3. Flow cytometric and cytogenetic studies require fresh aspirate specimens or unfixed disaggregated core biopsies, while immunohistochemistry is best suited for paraffin-embedded tissues. t5.3 provides a comparative assessment of the various bone marrow specimen components to provide optimal cytologic and morphologic information and perform specialized testing.

[5.2] **Bone Marrow Reporting**

Bone marrow reports are notoriously lengthy, time-consuming, and variable in format even among pathologists at the same institution. This variation is not unexpected due to differences in personal style, training, and the different components of the bone marrow evaluation that require analysis. As a result, experts in this field have set forth guidelines to assist in the standardization of bone marrow reporting [Lee 2008, Parwani 2008, Peterson 2002, Qu 2007, Foucar 2008]. For the most part, these guidelines are presented as checklists for the pathologist, although synoptic reporting is becoming more widely used and encouraged [Murari 2006, Parwani 2008, Qu 2007]. An example of a checklist for evaluating

t5.4 Suggested Checklist for Evaluation of Bone Marrow Specimens

Header of Report

Patient data: name, date of birth, hospital, medical record #, social security #

Date of procedure

Referring physician(s)

Body of Report

Specimens	PB and/or BM aspirate, touch prep, clot section, trephine biopsy; site (left/right iliac crest/sternal)
Diagnosis	Use WHO 2008 classification of neoplastic tumors as appropriate
Comments	Mention relevant clinical, morphological, immunophenotypic, cytochemical, and/or genetic studies pertinent to diagnosis
	Suggest etiologies and/or additional workup (serology, culture, radiologic imaging, RT-PCR for MRD)
	Compare with previous bone marrow or other specimen; document similarities/differences
	Refer to additional testing that is pending
	Discuss discrepancies of PB versus BM findings
	Document communication with clinician
Clinical history	See t5.1
Peripheral blood	See t2.4, t2.5, t2.6, t2.7
Bone marrow (aspirate, touch prep)	If both aspirate/touch prep performed and show similar findings, can report together
	Adequacy of specimen: presence of particles, cellularity, hemodilution, quality of stain
	M:E ratio with accompanying differential counts (aspirate smear or touch prep)
	Hematopoiesis (see t2.4, t2.5, t2.6, t2.7)
	Other (see t2.8)
Bone marrow (clot, core biopsy)	If both performed and show similar features, can report together; mention minor differences (eg, LA in clot only)
	Adequacy of specimen
	Biopsy: aspiration artifact (mild, severe), crush artifact, fragmentation of specimen, interpretable length, presence of only subcortical marrow, quality of H&E stain, thickness of section
	Cellularity
	Hematopoietic architecture and bone marrow stroma (see t2.8)
Special studies	Cytochemistry results
	Iron stains, preferable on BM aspirate to detect ring sideroblasts and storage iron
	Organism stains on tissue section
	IHC: why performed (particularly if concurrent flow for similar markers); stains performed, results
	Flow cytometry
	Cytogenetics, FISH, molecular studies

BM = bone marrow; FISH = fluorescence in situ hybridization; IHC = immunohistochemistry; LA = lymphoid aggregate; M:E = myeloid:erythroid; MRD = minimal residual disease; PB = peripheral blood; RT-PCR = reverse transcriptase polymerase chain reaction

---

bone marrow specimens is shown in **t5.4**. This is a detailed, lengthy, and comprehensive checklist, which serves as a consistent reminder of the variety of pathologic alterations that may be encountered in the bone marrow and that may require further investigation. However, each of these details need not be mentioned in the final report if noncontributory to the overall case. One of the main advantages of having a checklist or template handy is that potentially subtle abnormalities are less likely to be overlooked.

Incorporating the salient checklist findings into a succinct final report is challenging and heavily dependent on the diagnostician. However, uniformity and standardization of a bone marrow report is beneficial for clinicians, pathology colleagues, and the other members of the health care management team (eg, trainees, technologists, persons inputting data for clinical trials, etc). These benefits include the use of uniform and up-to-date terminology, consistent location of particular information in the report, and potentially improved turnaround time. In addition, 4 items that have been shown to provide more effective communication include

1. use of diagnostic headers to highlight key issues
2. consistent report layout
3. optimization of information presentation
4. limit extraneous or repeated information [Valenstein 2008]

t5.5 Key Components of a Bone Marrow Written Report

Positive or negative results (eg, presence or absence of neoplasia)

Overall cellularity and adequacy of trilineage hematopoiesis

Comparison with previous pathologic material; if discrepancies arise, these should be addressed

Adequacy of the specimen(s)

Presence of bone marrow artifacts (see Chapter 2)

Pertinent special studies that support the diagnosis (eg, immuno-phenotypic results, cytogenetic abnormality)

If not a clear-cut diagnosis, suggested additional studies for further investigation

Document communication with clinician(s)

Key interpretative components that should be included in every bone marrow report are listed in **t5.5**. One need only mention those components that can be evaluated and/or are relevant to the case at hand. Several key issues include adequacy of the specimen and presence of artifacts that may hamper interpretation, as well as communicating clearly the presence or absence of a disease process. In most de novo evaluations of the bone marrow, if no specific alteration is identified to explain a peripheral blood or other systemic abnormality, referral to the cellularity of the bone marrow and overall hematopoietic function (eg, intact trilineage hematopoiesis) will suffice. In addition to issuing a report that clearly communicates the findings, it is advisable to directly notify clinicians, verbally if possible, about a new, potentially unsuspected diagnosis. This immediate communication should be followed as soon as possible by a finalized report.

Further enhancements of bone marrow reporting may incorporate standardized reporting templates using computer technology, so-called synoptic reporting. Synoptic reporting is an extension of standardized reporting, reliant on user-friendly laboratory information systems [Murari 2006, Parwani 2008, Qu 2007]. Such reporting is a valuable tool for pathologists, providing assurance that critical values are resulted and, for clinicians, providing a report that is clear and accurate for use in staging, treatment, etc. There are numerous benefits to such a reporting practice, not the least of which is the generation of a report in which all information is conveyed in a similar manner, with similar terminology, in a similar location in the text, in every case.

Although extremely useful and valuable, synoptic templates require a significant upfront time commitment to initially design the checklist, create the computer template, and perform a "back-end" assessment of the report to validate that the report printout is suitable for clinical use. An extensive series of drop-down tabs need to be instituted, as well as zones for free text, which are occasionally needed. Ultimately, a succinct yet thorough report is generated that communicates the "need to know" information quickly and easily to the clinician(s).

[5.3] Integrated Reports

Due to time constraints and turnaround time issues, the bone marrow report is often released before additional critical data are received (eg, serological studies, culture results, cytogenetics, fluorescence in situ hybridization [FISH], and molecular/genetic testing). As a consequence, these data are all released as individual reports and are not necessarily optimally correlated with the initial bone marrow report. Consequently, integrated reports, which incorporate all of these ancillary data points, are valuable. Such reports unify all the aspects of a case and provide not only diagnostic, but prognostic information to the clinician.

Logistically, integrated reports are difficult to do, as they requires the pathologist to keep track of the various specimens linked to a case until results are obtained. In the interim, each individual report (bone marrow morphology, flow cytometry, etc) is completed so that the clinician is aware and has documentation of the diagnosis and work in progress. As cytogenetic and molecular studies may take up to 10 days, these are the tests, in our experience, that are most typically delayed in reporting. Once available, prognostic information and/or refinements of the morphologic diagnosis should be issued in a final integrated report. Suggested components for an integrated report are listed in **t5.6**. Examples are shown in the **appendix**.

t5.6 Components of a Final Integrated Report*

Header of Report

Patient data: name, date of birth, hospital, medical record #, social security #

Date of procedure

Referring physician(s)

Body of Report

Specimens

Final integrated diagnosis

Comment	Mention all ancillary data used to arrive at ultimate diagnosis
	Submit prognostic information, as known
	Include references as appropriate
	Note suggested follow-up studies
	Document final discussion with clinician
Previously issued reports (copy and paste)	Initial BM morphology report
	Flow cytometric analysis
	Conventional cytogenetics
	FISH
	Molecular studies
	Serologic/culture results

*See examples of final integrated reports in **appendix**
BM = bone marrow; FISH = fluorescence in situ hybridization

[5.4]   Quality Assurance

The scope of a bone marrow quality assurance program includes not only technical and interpretative quality control issues, but also a global overview of the entire process. Key technical and interpretative quality control issues in bone marrow examination are listed in **t5.7** and **t5.8**. These quality control factors must be evaluated regularly, and defects corrected promptly. Quality assurance focuses on the overall functioning and success of the process, including patient outcomes, clinical decision-making, and pathologist/clinician interaction. Some of the variables of this process include ensuring appropriate indications for performing bone marrows, low complication rates, and adequate communication between clinician and pathologist **t5.9**. As the bone marrow examination quality assurance process involves the pathologist, clinicians, laboratory personnel, and potentially others, it serves as a good measure of the efficient interaction of clinical, laboratory, pathology, and patient services.

t5.7 Key Technical Quality Control Issues in BM Examination*

Requisition form	Indication(s) noted and legible
	Clinical data specified or available through electronic medical record (see **t5.1**)
Specimen collection	Procedure performed or overseen by experienced individual to ensure adequacy
BM aspirate	Drawn appropriately for slide preparations
	Drawn into appropriate medium for ancillary studies (eg, sodium heparin for cytogenetics)
	Real-time assessment of specimen adequacy
	verification of presence of particles absence of clotting
	Smears prepared at bedside to ensure sufficient material for evaluation (at least 5 air-dried smears each containing particles)
BM core	Perform biopsy prior to aspiration to avoid aspiration artifact
	Ensure adequacy by gross morphologic assessment (length, % bone, cartilage); at least 1 cm of intact BM for adequate biopsy
Specimen processing	Confirm properly functioning stain to ensure valid identification of nucleated cells
BM core	Prompt removal from decalcification to preserve antigenicity
	Standardized histologic processing to ensure consistent results
	Appropriate sectioning—not too thick or superficial

*See Chapter 2 for complete discussion of bone marrow artifacts and Chapter 3 for more information on specimen adequacy
BM = bone marrow

t5.8 Key Interpretative Quality Control Issues in BM Examination*

Recognize bone marrow artifacts that can impact morphology and ability to recognize cell lineages

Fixation variation may result in "halo" or balloon effect or nuclear changes rendering distinction among various cell types difficult

Verify validity of concurrent positive controls when interpreting cytochemistry, iron stains, IHC

Generous use of targeted IHC, flow, cytogenetics, or molecular as needed for specific differential diagnostic considerations

Utilize checklist for reporting to ensure thorough evaluation yet succinct final report

Utilize template, as applicable, to expedite reporting efficiency and reduce typographical and grammatical errors

Delineate suboptimal components in final report comment section, as appropriate, to prompt further workup or repeat biopsy

*See Chapter 2 for complete discussion of bone marrow artifacts
BM = bone marrow; IHC = immunohistochemistry

t5.9 Key Components of a Quality Assurance Program for BM Examination*

Documentation of informed consent of patient

Indications for bone marrow examination are appropriate

Complications of BM procedure are within acceptable range and rare

BM biopsies performed or overseen by experienced, credentialed personnel

Transit time of specimens to laboratory is acceptable

Monitor pathologist turnaround time to finalize case

Document interpretation accuracy using internal and external peer review process

Verify communication between clinicians and pathologists

Verify timely communication of diagnosis and/or need for additional studies with patient

*See Chapter 3 for bone marrow indications and complications
BM = bone marrow

[5.5] Clues and Caveats

1. Obtaining relevant clinical information, in conjunction with adequate bone marrow specimen materials, is optimal for bone marrow evaluation.

2. Generous use of templates and checklists enhances pathologist efficiency, promotes accuracy and clarity in printed reports, and provides easily identifiable diagnostic and/or prognostic information to the clinician(s).

3. Use integrated reports to provide up-to-date diagnostic and prognostic information based on clinical, morphologic, laboratory, culture, serologic, immunophenotypic, cytogenetic/FISH, and molecular studies (potentially from a variety of different laboratories/ institutions).

4. Monitor quality measures in all aspects of specimen management (collection, processing, interpretation) to troubleshoot as necessary and to maximize correct diagnostic interpretation.

5. Implement and use a bone marrow quality assurance program that consistently ensures appropriate use of bone marrow testing, appropriate communication of information to clinicians, appropriate therapy or follow-up for patients, and accurate pathologic diagnoses (internal and external peer review).

[5.6] References

Cotelingam JD [2003] Bone marrow biopsy: interpretive guidelines for the surgical pathologist. *Adv Anat Pathol* 10:8-26.

Foucar K, Viswanatha D, Wilson C [2008] Laboratory evaluation of blood and bone marrow in non-neoplastic disorders. In: King D, Gardner W, Sobin L, et al, eds. *Non-Neoplastic Disorders of Bone Marrow (AFIP fascicle)*. Washington, DC: American Registry of Pathology; 2008:57-73.

Hasserjian RP [2008] Reactive versus neoplastic bone marrow: problems and pitfalls. *Arch Pathol Lab Med* 132:587-594.

Kuter DJ, Bain B, Mufti G, et al [2007] Bone marrow fibrosis: pathophysiology and clinical significance of increased bone marrow stromal fibres. *Br J Haematol* 139:351-362.

Lee SH, Erber WN, Porwit A, et al [2008] ICSH guidelines for the standardization of bone marrow specimens and reports. *Int J Lab Hematol* 30:349-364.

Murari M, Pandey R [2006] A synoptic reporting system for bone marrow aspiration and core biopsy specimens. *Arch Pathol Lab Med* 130:1825-1829.

Parwani A, Mohanty S, Becich M [2008] Pathology reporting in the 21st centruy: the impact of synoptic reports and digital imaging. *LabMedicine* 39:582-586.

Peterson LC, Agosti SJ, Hoyer JD [2002] Protocol for the examination of specimens from patients with hematopoietic neoplasms of the bone marrow: a basis for checklists. *Arch Pathol Lab Med* 126:1050-1056.

Qu Z, Ninan S, Almosa A, et al [2007] Synoptic reporting in tumor pathology: advantages of a web-based system. *Am J Clin Pathol* 127:898-903.

Swerdlow S, Campo E, Harris N, editors, et al [2008] *WHO Classification of Tumours: Pathology & Genetics: Tumours of Haematopoietic and Lymphoid Tissues.* 4th ed. Lyon, France: IARC Press; 2008.

Valenstein PN [2008] Formatting pathology reports: applying 4 design principles to improve communication and patient safety. *Arch Pathol Lab Med* 132:84-94.

Wilkins BS, Clark DM [2009] Making the most of bone marrow trephine biopsy. *Histopathology* 55:631-640.

CHAPTER

6

Anemias

Kathryn Foucar, MD

Anemia is the most common hematologic disorder in both developed and undeveloped countries. Iron deficiency is the cause of anemia in an estimated 3 billion people worldwide [Andrews 2008, Angeles Vazquez Lopez 2006, Chen 2007, Moy 2006, Umbreit 2005]. Similarly, various constitutional anemias (notably those which often confer resistance to infection of erythrocytes by malaria) are prevalent in many parts of the world in which over half of the population may harbor anemia-associated genetic mutations [Ayi 2004, Calis 2008, Cooke 2004, Rund 2005]. There are numerous types and causes of anemia; pathophysiologic mechanisms range from inadequate hemoglobin production to reduced erythrocyte survival time to failed bone marrow production. Many anemias can be successfully diagnosed from complete blood count (CBC), findings on morphology review and other laboratory tests, in conjunction with clinical correlation. Bone marrow examination is not necessary in these patients. Although all categories of anemia will be highlighted in this chapter, the emphasis will be placed on those anemias typically requiring bone marrow examination. The expected bone marrow findings will be presented for those anemias in which bone marrow examination is not typically performed. The reader is referred to Chapter 7 for a discussion of aplastic anemia and other bone marrow failure disorders, while red cell aplasia is the focus of Chapter 8.

[6.1] **Erythropoiesis**

The production of sufficient numbers of morphologically normal RBCs is dependent on a bone marrow that contains an adequate number of stem cells and erythroid progenitor cells, an intact microenvironment, and sufficient regulatory factors (see Chapter 1). In addition, all nutrients necessary for hemoglobin production and cell division, such as iron, vitamin B_{12} (cobalamin), and folate, must be available to developing erythroid cells [Foucar 2008, Means 2009]. Early-acting cytokines induce multiple hematopoietic lineages, including erythroid cells, while erythropoietin is the major erythroid lineage growth factor (see Chapter 1 for detailed discussion of hematopoiesis). Erythropoiesis occurs within "islands" in the bone marrow in which erythroid precursors adhere to a central macrophage, providing the optimal microenvironmental niche for erythrocyte production [Chasis 2008, Rhodes 2008]. Erythropoiesis requires approximately 5 to 7 days for maturation from an erythroblast to a reticulocyte, which can then be released into the peripheral blood. However, this maturation interval can be reduced substantially in response to acute anemia (see Chapter 1).

Once released into the blood, reticulocytes acquire their final complement of hemoglobin and metabolic machinery becoming mature erythrocytes with a survival time of about 4 months [Means 2009]. Reticulocyte quantitation is a critical parameter in assessing erythrocyte production; multiple automated methodologies for reticulocyte quantitation are used in clinical practice [Buttarello 2002, Ivory 2007]. Under homeostatic conditions, mature RBCs exhibit a fairly uniform size (as measured by RBC distribution width [RDW] and mean corpuscular volume [MCV]) and normal hemoglobin content (as measured by mean corpuscular hemoglobin concentration [MCHC]). With aging, erythrocytes become progressively dense and are eventually removed by the spleen [Lew 2007]. Normal values for hemoglobin, hematocrit, RBC count, and MCV show substantial age-related and sex-related variations **t6.1, appendix**.

[6.2] **Definition**

Anemia is defined as decreased RBC count, hemoglobin, and hematocrit levels in relation to age/sex-adjusted normal ranges (see **appendix**) [Beutler 2006, Robins 2007, Wakeman 2007]. In addition to a reduction in these numerical parameters, other qualitative abnormalities of erythrocytes may be evident, often reflected by abnormalities in MCV, MCHC, and RDW. Some patients with constitutional microcytic RBC disorders (thalassemia minor, hemoglobin E) may have an elevated RBC count, while hemoglobin and hematocrit levels are reduced. Further subclassification of anemias is based on additional laboratory findings, genetic testing, and, occasionally, bone marrow features.

---

t6.1 Age- and Sex-Related Variations in Erythrocyte Normal Ranges

RBC count, hemoglobin, hematocrit, MCV, and reticulocyte count are higher at birth than at any other time during life

All RBC parameters normally decline after birth until erythropoiesis resumes at 2-4 months (so-called physiologic anemia or physiologic nadir)

Normal range RBC parameters, including MCV, are lower in toddlers and young children compared to older subjects

During adolescence RBC parameters increase more for males than females; this sex-related difference in normal ranges persists throughout adulthood

Race-related variations in erythrocyte normal ranges have been postulated based on documentation of lower RBC values in normal African American children and adolescents

MCV = mean corpuscular volume; RBC = red blood cell

References: [Beutler 2005, Cheng 2004, de Alarcon 2005, Robins 2007]

[6.3] Systematic Approach to Anemia

The evaluation of a patient for possible anemia should include a CBC with differential cell counts and RBC parameters, including RBC count, MCV, MCHC, and RDW t6.2. In addition, the reticulocyte count is essential for determining the status of bone marrow production of erythrocytes [Buttarello 2002, Ivory 2007]. Review of the peripheral blood smear is also necessary to identify morphologic clues to a specific etiology for the anemia that will direct further testing. These "clues" include distinctive sizes and shapes of erythrocytes, as well as features of other lineages [Bain 2005, Means 2009].

Numerous other laboratory tests are commonly used in the evaluation of selected patients with anemia, including Coombs' direct antiglobulin test, serum bilirubin (total, direct, and indirect), lactate dehydrogenase, serum iron, total iron-binding capacity (transferrin), serum ferritin, serum vitamin B$_{12}$, methylmalonic acid, homocysteine, serum folate, and erythrocyte folate. Many other tests, such as erythropoietin levels, serum transferrin receptor levels, tests for nonimmune RBC hemolysis, and measurements of RBC enzymes, are useful in selected patients [Foucar 2008, Means 2009]. The appropriate utilization of these tests depends on information obtained from CBC results, peripheral blood smear review, and clinical findings.

t6.2 Systematic Approach to Anemia Evaluation

Basic understanding of erythropoiesis, including factors that contribute to the regulation of RBC production

Appreciate that hemoglobin is composed of a porphyrin ring, iron, and globin chains (α and β in hemoglobin A), and that a defect in any of these components can cause a failure in adequate hemoglobin production, producing anemia

Apply of age- and sex-related normal ranges

Assess key clinical parameters:
  family history of anemia, other hematologic disorders
  onset, duration of anemia
  physical stigmata of constitutional disorders
  medications, toxic exposures, alcohol ingestion, homeopathic remedies
  underlying illnesses (cardiopulmonary, GI, collagen vascular disorders, etc)
  jaundice, spleen size, mucosa, nails, fingers, neurologic findings
  severity of anemia symptoms, other symptoms

Integrate CBC data with morphologic assessment:
  size, shape, hemoglobin content, uniformity of RBCs, nucleated RBCs
  degree of polychromasia
  abnormal RBC forms, inclusions, organisms
  agglutination, rouleaux
  assessment of platelets and WBCs

Distinguish isolated anemia from multilineage abnormalities

Develop differential diagnoses based on all information and pursue with targeted laboratory testing, bone marrow examination as appropriate

CBC = complete blood count; GI = gastrointestinal; RBC = red blood cell; WBC = white blood cell

References: [Bain 2005, Chen 2007, Latvala 2004, Means 2009, Means 2009]

t6.3 Overview of Classification of Anemias: Prototypic Features

Constitutional Anemia	vs	Acquired Anemia
Onset at birth or early infancy		Onset throughout life
Dysmorphic features may be present		Absence of dysmorphic features
Positive family history (variable)		Negative family history
Established somatic molecular genetic defects		No somatic genetic defects
Proliferation Defect	vs	**Survival Defect**
Low reticulocyte count		High reticulocyte count
Reduced erythroid lineage in BM		Increased erythroid lineage in BM
Normal morphology of RBCs		Distinctive RBC abnormalities based on type of survival defect (sickle cells, spherocytes, schistocytes, bite cells)
Nuclear Maturation Defect	vs	**Cytoplasmic Maturation Defect**
All proliferating cells effected		Only erythroid lineage effected
Multilineage hyperplasia in BM		Erythroid hyperplasia in BM
Macrocytic, normochromic anemia		Microcytic, often hypochromic anemia (usually)
Usually acquired (folate or cobalamin deficiency)		Iron deficiency-acquired, globin chain defects-constitutional, porphyrin ring defects-constitutional or acquired
Non-Neoplastic Anemia	vs	**Hematologic Neoplasm with Anemia**
Isolated anemia, typical		Multilineage abnormalities frequent
Other lineage abnormalities "explainable" by clinical findings		May see left shift, circulating blasts
		May see dysplastic forms of erythroid cells and other lineage cells

BM = bone marrow, CBC = complete blood count; GI = gastrointestinal; RBC = red blood cell; WBC = white blood cell

References: [Bain 2005, Chen 2007, Latvala 2004, Means 2009]

Bone marrow examination is generally reserved for patients in whom the cause of the anemia is not apparent from laboratory and clinical assessment, or in those patients developing an unexpected complication or exacerbation of the anemia. Likewise, anemic patients with other lineage abnormalities, suspected aplasia, or suspected bone marrow infiltration also generally require bone marrow examination. The morphologic features of erythropoiesis and iron status should be assessed in bone marrow specimens from anemic patients (see Chapter 2) [Foucar 2008].

[6.4] **Pathogenesis and Classification of Anemia**

In the evaluation of an anemia case, it is important to determine the pathophysiologic mechanisms responsible for the anemia (ie, proliferation, maturation, or survival defects), and to distinguish between inherited (constitutional, congenital) and acquired disorders **t6.3** p 94, **t6.4** p 95. In addition to patient age, a careful family history of blood disorders and past evaluations of the patient for hematologic disorders can provide evidence helpful in distinguishing congenital from acquired disorders. Congenital anemias include proliferation, maturation, and survival disorders, and range from congenital hypoproliferative anemias to various constitutional RBC enzyme, membrane, and hemoglobin defects. Certain types of constitutional anemia, such as the thalassemias, exhibit a broad range in severity secondary to the diversity of genetic defects found in these patients. Acquired anemias also include proliferation, maturation, and survival disorders **t6.3, t6.4**. The most common types of acquired anemia are

t6.4 Classification of Anemias

Mechanism	Congenital	Acquired
Proliferation defect	Fanconi anemia Diamond-Blackfan anemia Dyskeratosis congenita Shwachman-Diamond syndrome	Aplastic anemia Red cell aplasia (many types) Anemia of chronic disease* Bone marrow effacement disorders Paroxysmal nocturnal hemoglobinuria*
Nuclear maturation defect	Congenital dyserythropoietic anemia Congenital megaloblastic anemia (multiple types) Transcobalamin II deficiency Other rare constitutional disorders (orotic aciduria, methionine synthetase deficiency)	Vitamin B_{12} deficiency (megaloblastic anemia) Folate deficiency (megaloblastic anemia)
Cytoplasmic maturation defect	Thalassemia Congenital sideroblastic anemia Erythropoietic protoporphyria	Iron deficiency anemia Acquired sideroblastic anemia

Intrinsic survival defect	Membrane defects:
	  hereditary spherocytosis
	  hereditary elliptocytosis
	Enzyme deficiencies:
	  glucose 6-phosphate dehydrogenase deficiency
	  pyruvate kinase deficiency
	Hemoglobinopathy:
	  sickle cell anemia
		Paroxysmal nocturnal hemoglobinuria*

Extrinsic survival defect	Congenital TTP (ADAMTS13 deficiency)	Immune-mediated hemolytic anemia (many types) Micro/macro-angiopathies (many types including HUS, TTP, thermal injury, clostridial sepsis, cardiac valve dysfunction, vascular malformation)

*Pathogenesis of anemia multifactorial
TTP = thrombotic thrombocytopenic purpura; HUS = hemolytic uremia syndrome

References: [Foucar 2008, Means 2009]

those secondary to either nutritional deficiencies, especially iron deficiency, or chronic disease, a complex multifactorial anemia in which the primary underlying mechanism may be sustained inflammatory cytokine production (see Chapter 34). Additional causes of acquired anemias include autoantibody production, turbulent blood flow, microangiopathies, toxic exposures, potent chemotherapy, neoplasms, infections, and acute hemorrhage. The pathogenesis of these diverse acquired anemias range from proliferation defects (bone marrow suppression, parvovirus) to RBC survival defects (autoantibodies, all vessel abnormalities, hemorrhage).

Proliferation defects range from stem cell, bone marrow microenvironment, or regulatory factor disorders, to disorders that efface the bone marrow **t6.3** p 94, **t6.4** p 95. In patients with proliferation defects, the anemia is the result of a reduction in bone marrow erythroid elements. In some of these patients, erythropoiesis is basically intact but compromised by invading neoplasms. In other patients with proliferation defects, the erythroid lineage is markedly reduced with only rare erythroblasts (see Chapters 7 and 8).

The causes of RBC maturation defects are also heterogeneous, ranging from acquired nuclear or cytoplasmic defects to constitutional disorders such as congenital dyserythropoietic anemia. In RBC maturation defects, bone marrow erythroid hyperplasia is characteristically evident, although actual RBC production, as determined by reticulocyte count, is ineffective, indicating that most cells die within the bone marrow. In contrast, the erythroid hyperplasia in patients with erythrocyte survival defects is effective, and increased numbers of reticulocytes are released into the blood. Erythrocyte survival defects may be secondary to either intrinsic RBC abnormalities or extrinsic (environmental) abnormalities. In patients with intrinsic or extrinsic survival defects, anemia results when bone marrow erythrocyte production cannot compensate for increased RBC destruction causing reduced RBC survival time.

[6.4.1] Constitutional and Acquired Erythrocyte Proliferation Disorders

Although rare, several types of constitutional bone marrow disorders are associated with anemia secondary to proliferation defects **t6.4** p 95 (see Chapters 7 and 8 for discussion and illustrations). Those congenital disorders associated with evolving aplastic anemia include Fanconi anemia, dyskeratosis congenita, Shwachman-Diamond syndrome, amegakaryocytic thrombocytopenia, and familial aplastic anemia [Dokal 2008]. The specific phenotypic abnormalities seen in these patients, patterns of genetic transmission, and morphologic findings are detailed in Chapter 7. Although initial bone marrow hypercellularity

may be evident in infants with Fanconi anemia, affected patients characteristically develop progressive pancytopenia and gradual loss of hematopoietic elements within the bone marrow. In other congenital disorders, such as Shwachman-Diamond syndrome and amegakaryocytic thrombocytopenia, single-lineage aplasia initially predominates. However, complete trilineage bone marrow aplasia ultimately develops in a substantial proportion of these cases.

In contrast, in patients with Diamond-Blackfan syndrome, only the bone marrow erythroid lineage is initially affected (see Chapter 8) [Dokal 2008, Gazda 2006, Lipton 2006]. These infants have a normochromic, macrocytic anemia that is usually evident in the first few months of life. In addition to anemia, RBCs contain increased fetal hemoglobin and may express i antigen on their surface membrane. The bone marrow contains only scattered, morphologically normal, erythroid precursors, while other hematopoietic lineages are initially unremarkable (see Chapter 8 for illustrations and detailed discussion). Recent evidence suggests that eventual multilineage bone marrow failure is more common than was appreciated [Dokal 2008].

Proliferation defects resulting from either acquired aplastic anemia or acquired red cell aplasia are more common than their congenital counterparts **t6.4** p 95 [Sawada 2008, Skeppner 2002, Thompson 2006, Young 2004] (see Chapters 7 and 8 for complete discussions and illustrations). Even though the morphologic features of acquired aplastic anemias are variable, most patients develop profound trilineage hypoplasia with fairly unremarkable bone marrow stroma, bone, and lymphoid elements (see Chapter 7). Likewise, acquired red cell aplasia is characterized by a loss of erythroid lineage, while the megakaryocytic and granulocytic lineages are preserved **i6.1**. In these patients, the widely dispersed residual erythroblasts must be assessed for parvoviral inclusions (see Chapter 8) [Sawada 2008, Young 2004].

In addition to aplastic anemia and pure red cell aplasia, bone marrow infiltration by neoplasms, bone marrow fibrosis, and bone marrow suppression from chemotherapy or radiation are associated with acquired RBC proliferation defects. Although the bone marrow features in these disorders range from complete effacement to marked hypocellularity, normal hematopoietic elements, including the erythroid lineage, are consistently decreased. Other cases of acquired erythroid hypoplasia are uncommon and include endocrinopathies, renal disease (see Chapter 34), T-cell immune aberrations, and paroxysmal nocturnal hemoglobinuria (PNH), an acquired clonal hematopoietic disorder that usually manifests as a hemolytic anemia [see "Acquired Erythrocyte Survival Defects (Paroxysmal Nocturnal Hemoglobinuria)," p 118].

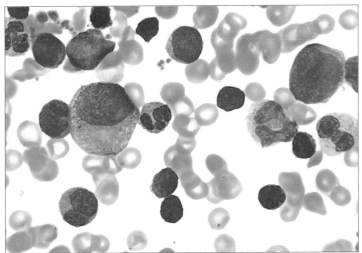

i6.1 *Bone marrow aspirate smear from a patient with acquired pure red cell aplasia shows only rare, isolated, normal-appearing erythroblasts (upper right) admixed with normal granulocytic cells. (Wright)*

Finally, anemia is very common in patients with chronic inflammatory and neoplastic disorders, so-called anemia of chronic disease. Although the cause of anemia in these patients is likely complex and multifactorial, sustained increased production of cytokines that mediate immune/inflammatory responses and altered iron metabolism caused by induction of hepcidin are the dominant factors inducing chronic anemia (see Chapter 34) [Andrews 2008, Dallalio 2006, Weiss 2005]. Features of anemia of chronic disease include impaired erythropoiesis due to blunted response to erythropoietin (proliferation defect), reduced iron for erythropoiesis (maturation defect), and modestly decreased erythrocyte survival time (survival defect). Sustained production of hepcidin, a master regulator of iron homeostasis and an antibacterial protein, is the likely cause of these defects [Andrews 2008]. Liver production of hepcidin is induced by cytokines and iron [Andrews 2008, Theurl 2008]. In anemia of chronic disease, a normocytic, normochromic anemia is typical, but hypochromia is occasionally identified. Bone marrow examination reveals generally normal numbers of erythroid elements, reduced numbers of sideroblasts (iron-containing erythroid precursors), and increased storage iron within histiocytes (see Chapter 34).

[6.4.2] **Erythrocyte Maturation Disorders**

Maturation defects in RBC production may result from either constitutional or acquired nuclear or cytoplasmic defects. Ineffective erythropoiesis, characterized by bone marrow erythroid hyperplasia and inappropriately low reticulocyte counts, is a feature of all types of maturation defects **t6.3** p 94, **t6.4** p 95 [Foucar 2008, Means 2009]. Nuclear maturation defects result in megaloblastic anemias, a single morphologic entity with multiple causes, either congenital or acquired, all resulting in defective DNA synthesis **t6.3** p 94, **t6.4** p 95. This defect is actually a decrease in DNA synthesis per unit time, in which an individual cell cannot readily double its DNA content to undergo mitosis. Because most cells are attempting to divide, the bone marrow in patients with megaloblastic anemia exhibits hypercellularity and a very high proliferative rate. However, most of these proliferating cells actually die in the bone marrow and fail to produce adequate hematopoietic progeny for the peripheral blood. This excessive intramedullary cell death results in high lactate dehydrogenase levels. In addition to bone marrow cells, all proliferating cells in the body are affected in patients with nuclear maturation disorders. Since all hematopoietic lineages are affected, the blood findings can range from anemia to severe pancytopenia.

In contrast, only erythroid elements are affected in cytoplasmic maturation defects. In these disorders, some aspect of hemoglobin production is impaired. The defect may involve globin chain synthesis, inadequate iron for heme, or impaired porphyrin synthesis. Any defect in hemoglobin production results in inadequate amounts of hemoglobin per RBC. The morphologic manifestations of this inadequate hemoglobin production are microcytosis and hypochromia of mature erythrocytes. In patients with cytoplasmic maturation defects, although the bone marrow shows erythroid hyperplasia, effective erythrocyte production as measured by the reticulocyte count is suboptimal for the degree of anemia. Other morphologic abnormalities may also be evident, depending on both the specific type of maturation defect and the duration of disease. However, the granulocytic and megakaryocytic lineages are intact and morphologically unremarkable.

[6.4.3] **Constitutional Erythrocyte Maturation Disorders**

Constitutional nuclear maturation disorders are rare and include congenital megaloblastic anemia **sidebar 6.1**, transcobalamin II deficiency, orotic aciduria, and methionine synthetase deficiency **t6.3** p 94, **t6.4** p 95 [Aminoff 1999, Diaz 1999, Fleming 1999, Foucar 2008, Labay 1999, Means 2009]. In some cases the genetic defects responsible for these constitutional disorders have been identified and include mutations in cubulin (intrinsic factor receptor) and mutations in the thiamine transporter gene **sidebar 6.1** [Aminoff 1999, Diaz 1999, Fleming 1999, Labay 1999]. All of these nuclear maturation defects are associated with prominent megaloblastic changes with nuclear-cytoplasmic dysynchrony in all hematopoietic lineages in the bone marrow (morphologic features of megaloblastic anemias are discussed in more detail in the section on acquired maturation defects) **i6.2**.

Congenital Megaloblastic Anemias

Folate and/or cobalamin (vitamin B$_{12}$) deficiencies and autoimmune disorders are more common causes of megaloblastic anemia than are inborn errors of metabolism. Practically speaking, then, the entities described in this sidebar will rarely be encountered in clinical practice and should only be considered after acquired causes of megaloblastic anemia are excluded. Nevertheless, genetic defects responsible for these constitutional disorders have been identified and offer fascinating insight into the intricate metabolic pathways permitting effective hematopoiesis.

Most of the implicated genes pertain to cobalamin and folate metabolism, reflecting the importance of these vitamins in the production of nucleic acid. The defects causing inherited cobalamin misutilization may be divided into 2 groups: those affecting cobalamin absorption and transport, and those affecting intracellular processing **fS6.1**, **tS6.1.1**. Congenital absence of intrinsic factor is similar in pathophysiologic consequence to acquired pernicious anemia, but the absence of intrinsic factor is due to inherited mutations in the *GIF* gene (gastric intrinsic factor) rather than to autoantibody-mediated attack; indeed, this rare syndrome is sometimes called "congenital pernicious anemia." Imerslund-Gräsbeck syndrome arises from defects in *CUBN* (cubulin) or *AMN* (amnionless), 2 essential components of the intestinal intrinsic factor receptor. Distinguishing between intrinsic factor deficiency and Imerslund-Gräsbeck syndrome may be difficult, though it

should be remembered that they will produce the same results in the Schilling test as their "typical" acquired analogues, pernicious anemia and intestinal malabsorption [Grasbeck 2006].

After successful intestinal absorption, cobalamin must then be conveyed to the cells that will utilize it metabolically. About 80% of cobalamin in the blood is bound by haptocorrin (also called R-binder and encoded by the gene *TCN1*, transcobalamin I). Carriage by haptocorrin targets a molecule of cobalamin specifically for hepatic delivery. Interestingly, while congenital haptocorrin deficiency results in low serum cobalamin levels, it does *not* appear to cause megaloblastic anemia, neurologic deficits, or other manifestations of cobalamin deficiency [Obeid 2006]. For this reason, haptocorrin deficiency is sometimes

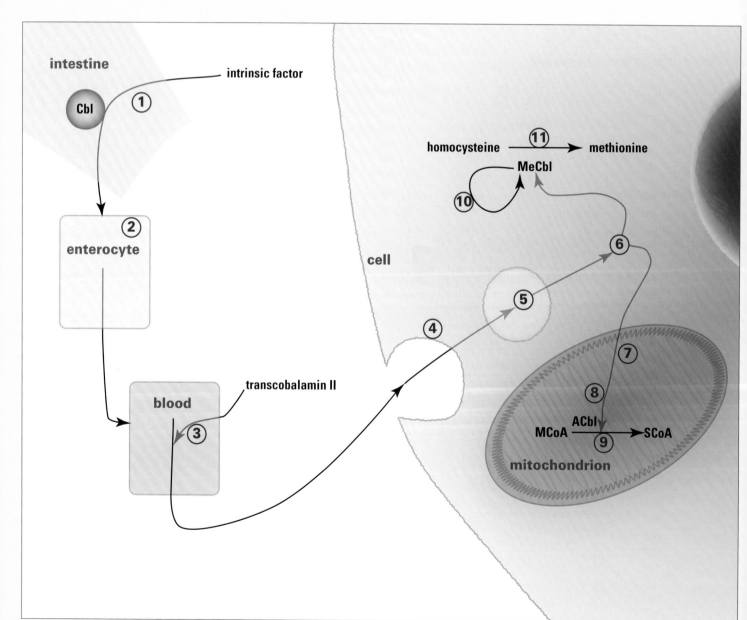

fS6.1 *ACbl=adenozylcobalamin; Cbl = cobalamin; MCoA = methylmalonyl coenzyme A; MeCbl = methylcobalamin; SCoA = succinyl coenzyme A*

termed "cobalamin pseudodeficiency," and this benign condition should be remembered as a potential cause of low cobalamin levels in a patient without evidence of megaloblastic changes. Transcobalamin II carries approximately 20% of cobalamin in the blood and targets delivery to every cell in the body. Congenital deficiency of transcobalamin II, in contrast to that of haptocorrin, is a cause of severe, early-onset congenital megaloblastic anemia and its attendant neurologic complications. Of extreme diagnostic importance is the realization that, since most circulating cobalamin is bound to haptocorrin and not to transcobalamin II, cobalamin levels in patients with transcobalamin II deficiency may actually be normal.

Once cobalamin has been successfully targeted to a somatic cell, it must be released from the intermediary endocytotic vesicle and chemically reduced; it may then remain in the cytosol, where it participates as the methylcobalamin cofactor of methionine synthase, or it may be shuttled into the mitochondrion, where it forms the adenosylcobalamin cofactor participating in methylmalonic acid metabolism **fS6.1**. Mutations may arise in genes coding for proteins involved in any of these steps. Inspection of **fS6.1** and **tS6.1.2** reveals 3 distinct groups of mutations with different biochemical consequences. Mutations that occur before the cytosolic/mitochondrial "split" in the pathway will result in elevated levels of both methylmalonic acid and homocyst(e)ine, while those mutations affecting individual arms of the pathway will result in elevated levels of either methylmalonic acid or homocyst(e)ine, but not both. Those cases with elevated methylmalonic acid levels are clinically described as methylmalonic aciduria, and megaloblastic anemia may be a prominent component of these multisystem syndromes.

Inherited abnormalities of folate metabolism have also been described. However, the folate processing defect most specifically tied to congenital megaloblastic anemia is the very rare syndrome of hereditary folate malabsorption. These patients develop megaloblastic anemia, mucositis, and neurologic deficits due to a defect in intestinal folate absorption. Very recently, a folate transporter that functions in the intestine was indeed identified, coded by the gene *SLC46A1* (suggested revised name *PCFT*, proton-coupled folate transport) [Nakai 2007]. As predicted, mutations in this gene have now been identified in a patient with hereditary folate malabsortion [Min 2008], neatly confirming the original hypothesis. Affected patients are completely dependent on parenteral folate administration, with which growth and development may be relatively normal. Tragic case reports exist of several successive children dying in a family before a diagnosis could be reached [Jebnoun 2001].

Finally, given that megaloblastic anemia is a *direct* consequence of deficiencies in DNA synthetic capacity, and only an *indirect* consequence of cobalamin and/or folate deficiency, it is not surprising that inborn metabolic errors affecting pathways completely unrelated to cobalamin and folate have been shown to produce the common phenotype of congenital megaloblastic anemia. For example, orotic aciduria is a rare cause of congenital megaloblastic anemia due to defective de novo pyrimidine biosynthesis; mutations in the *UMPS* gene (uridine monophosphate synthetase), the protein product of which catalyzes the final 2 steps of this metabolic pathway, have been identified [Suchi 1997]. Diagnosis is aided by detecting excess urinary orotic acid excretion. The peripheral blood demonstrates microcytic erythrocytes against the larger megaloblastic background, potentially suggesting an erroneous diagnosis of a mixed megaloblastic/iron deficiency anemia. Congenital megaloblastic anemia is also present in some cases of Lesch-Nyhan syndrome [van der Zee 1968]. Similarly, a congenital megaloblastic anemia responsive to thiamine administration has been identified. In this syndrome, the anemia coexists with diabetes mellitus and sensorineural deafness. Linkage analysis in affected families pinpointed mutations in the thiamine transport protein, encoded by the gene *SLC19A2* (solute carrier family 19 [thiamine transporter], member 2) [Labay 1999, Neufeld 1997, Raz 1998].

tS6.1.1   Inherited Abnormalities of Cobalamin Absorption and Transport

fS6.1 #	Syndrome	Gene(s) Affected	Defect	Consequence
1	Congenital pernicious anemia/ hereditary intrinsic factor deficiency	*GIF* (gastric intrinsic factor)	Inborn absence of IF prevents cobalamin absorption	Megaloblastic anemia Low serum cobalamin Absence of anti-intrinsic factor or anti-parietal cell antibodies Rare cases show adult onset
2	Megaloblastic anemia 1/ Imerslund-Gräsbeck syndrome	*CUBN* (cubulin) *AMN* (amnionless)	Cubulin and amnionless are both essential subcomponents of the intestinal receptor for the IF-cobalamin complex Pro1297Leu is most common *CUBN* mutation	Megaloblastic anemia Failure to thrive Neurologic deficits Often proteinuria
3	Transcobalamin II deficiency	*TCN2* (transcobalamin II)	Transcobalamin II carries ~20% of cobalamin in the blood, and targets delivery to all somatic cells	Megaloblastic anemia Failure to thrive Neurologic defects
—	Transcobalamin I (haptocorrin) deficiency	*TCN1* (transcobalamin I)	Haptocorrin carries ~80% of cobalamin in the blood, and targets delivery exclusively to the liver Specific mutations in *TCN1* have not yet been identified; diagnosis is based on absence of serum haptocorrin by immunoassay	Decreased serum cobalamin level with *no* apparent phenotypic consequence (aka "cobalamin pseudodeficiency")

IF = intrinsic factor

tS6.1.2 Inherited Abnormalities of Intracellular Cobalamin Metabolism

fS6.1 #	Complementation Type	Gene Affected	Defect	Consequence
Defects within Mitochondrial Adenosylcobalamin Metabolism (Methylmalonic Aciduria)				
7	cblA	*MMAA* [*methylmalonic aciduria* (Cbl deficiency) cbl*A* type]	Gene product thought to aid Cbl translocation into and/or stabilization within mitochondria About 40 mutations described, most commonly 433C→T	Methylmalonic aciduria/acidemia, developmental delay and early acidotic crisis; anemia may be seen as a component of pancytopenia, although not typically megaloblastic
8	cblB	*MMAB* [*methylmalonic aciduria* (Cbl deficiency) cbl*B* type]	Gene product is ATP:Cbl adenosyltransferase, which catalyzes synthesis of the active coenzyme adenosylcobalamin (ACbl)	Methylmalonic aciduria/acidemia, developmental delay and early acidotic crisis; more severe than cblA; anemia may be seen as a component of pancytopenia, although not typically megaloblastic
–	cblH	Unknown	Complementation analysis reveals that very rare cases of apparent cblA in fact represent mutations of a different, as yet uncharacterized gene	Similar to cblA
9	Methyl-malonyl-CoA mutase deficiency	*MUT* (methyl-malonyl Coenzyme A *mutase*)	Gene product is the enzyme methylmalonyl CoA mutase, which converts methlymalonyl-CoA to succinyl-CoA Mutations classified as complete [mut(0)] or partial [mut(–)]; the former is associated with more severe phenotype	Methylmalonic aciduria/acidemia, developmental delay and early acidotic crisis; more severe than cblA; anemia may be seen as a component of pancytopenia, although not typically megaloblastic
Defects Affecting Both AdenosylCbl and MethylCbl Metabolism				
4	cblF	*LMBRD1*	Very rare Unmetabolized Cbl is trapped in lysosomes	Megaloblastic anemia; failure to thrive; developmental delay; elevated methylmalonic acid and homocyst(e)ine
5	cblC	*MMACHC* [*methylmalonic aciduria* (Cbl deficiency) cbl*C* type, with *homocystinuria*]	Gene product is thought to be involved in intermediate steps of intracellular Cbl metabolism (post-uptake but before generation of the active coenzymes) Most common inborn error of Cbl metabolism 42 mutations, most commonly 271dupA	Megaloblastic anemia; failure to thrive; developmental delay; seizures; ophthalmologic abnormalities; thrombotic microangiopathy; elevated methylmalonic acid and homocyst(e)ine; late clinical onset may be seen (neurologic symptoms predominating)
6	cblD	*MMADHC* [*methylmalonic aciduria*, cbl*D* type, with *homocystinuria*]	Gene product is proposed to constitute a branch point between cytosolic and mitochondrial pathways of Cbl metabolism Responsible gene only recently identified Mutations cluster in 3 different domains, correlating with elevated methylmalonic acid or homocyst(e)ine, or both	Megaloblastic anemia; developmental delay; seizures; elevated methylmalonic acid and/or homocyst(e)ine, or isolated homocyst(e)ine, depending on site of mutation
Defects Affecting MethylCbl Metabolism				
10	cblE	*MTRR* (methionine synthase reductase, *aka* 5-methyltetrahydrofolate-homocysteine methyltransferase reductase)	Reactivates oxidized Cbl cofactor of MTR Multiple mutations are described; S454L is associated with milder, predominantly hematologic presentation	Megaloblastic anemia; developmental delay; ataxia; cerebral atrophy; seizures; blindness; elevated homocyst(e)ine
11	cblG	*MTR* (methionine synthase, *aka* 5-methyltetrahydrofolate-homocysteine methyltransferase)	Gene product converts homocysteine to methionine, the key Cbl dependent step in methionine synthesis Most patients carry the 3518C→T mutation	Megaloblastic anemia; developmental delay; ataxia; cerebral atrophy; seizures; blindness; elevated homocyst(e)ine

ATP = adenosine triphosphate; Cbl = cobalamin; CoA = coenzyme A

Reference: [Quadros 2010, Whitehead 2006]

Congenital Dyserythropoietic Anemia

Congenital dyserythropoietic anemias (CDAs) comprise another group of rare hereditary erythrocyte maturation disorders that are primarily the result of mitotic defects, resulting in ineffective erythropoiesis and marked dyserythropoiesis [Heimpel 2003, Heimpel 2006, Renella 2009, Wickramasinghe 2005]. Despite their rarity, CDAs have been intensely investigated, and multiple subtypes have been delineated which are linked to specific genetic defects sidebar 6.2, t6.5. In general, these patients have a mild to moderate anemia, often macrocytic, with prominent erythrocyte anisopoikilocytosis, punctate basophilic stippling, and a low reticulocyte count i6.3, i6.4, i6.5, i6.6. In one subtype, CDA II, increased hemolysis by the Ham (acidified-serum) test mimics PNH. Although there are some differences in peripheral blood morphology and

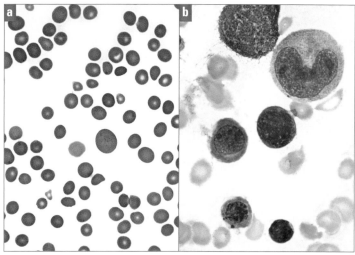

i6.2 *Possible congenital megaloblastic anemia in 7-month old infant showing peripheral blood features **a** and megaloblastic changes on bone marrow aspirate smear **b**. (Wright)*

t6.5 Peripheral Blood and Bone Marrow Findings in Patients with Congenital Dyserythropoietic Anemias (CDAs)*

	CDA I	CDA II†	CDA III, familial	Type III, sporadic
Inheritance	Autosomal recessive	Autosomal recessive	Autosomal dominant	Autosomal recessive
Genetic localization	15q15.1-15.3, codanin-1 mutations	20q11.2, likely genetic heterogeneity	15q21-25	None
Blood				
RBC size	Macrocytic	Normocytic	Normo-macrocytic	Macrocytic
RBC morphology	Anisopoikilocytosis	Anisopoikilocytosis	Anisopoikilocytosis	Anisopoikilocytosis
Anemia	Mild-moderate	Mild-severe	Mild	Mild-moderate
Bone marrow				
Erythroid hyperplasia	Prominent	Prominent	Prominent	Prominent
Erythroid morphology	Megaloblastic; internuclear chromatin bridging; nuclear budding; occasional binucleate forms	Normoblastic; bi/multinucleated normoblasts; nuclear karyorrhexis	Megaloblastic; "gigantoblasts" (up to 12 nuclei); nuclear karyorrhexis	Megaloblastic; "gigantoblasts"; nuclear karyorrhexis
Other lineages	Normal, usually	Normal, usually	Normal, usually	Not assessed
Other laboratory tests				
Acidified-serum test	− (rare+)	+	−	−
Sugar water test	− (rare+)	−	−	Not studied
Agglutination by anti-i and anti-I	variable	+	Variable	Not studied
				Not studied
SDS-PAGE	Normal	Abnormal	Normal	Not studied

*Reports describe proposed additional subtypes
†Designation HEMPAS (hereditary erythroblastic multinuclearity with positive acidified serum) (test) sometimes applied to patients with CDA II
+ = positive; − = negative; RBC = red blood cell; SDS-PAGE = sodium dodecyl sulfate-polyacrylamide gel electrophoresis

References: [Dgany 2002, Gasparini 1997, Heimpel 2003, Heimpel 2006, Lind 1995, Renella 2009, Tamary 2005, Wickramasinghe 2005]

[sidebar 6.2] # The Congenital Dyserythropoietic Anemias: *CDAN1* and Genetic Cartography

For the majority of the inherited syndromes described in this chapter and this book, we report the identity of the mutated gene and the known or hypothetical functional consequence of the change. Usually left undescribed, other than for a footnote or 2 directing the reader to the reference, is the difficult work that went into discovering the responsible gene amidst the vast background of the human genome. The congenital dyserythropoietic anemias (CDAs) present an excellent opportunity for describing this process in more detail. The mutations responsible for CDA type I have been discovered using painstaking linkage analysis, while other subtypes remain works in progress.

Briefly, linkage analysis relies upon the ability to "follow" the inheritance of specific genetic material from generation to generation, based on the patterns created by numerous polymorphisms throughout the genome. Such polymorphic markers and their neighboring genes are said to be linked when they are inherited together. Since chromosomes segregate independently, genes or markers that reside on the same chromosome will be more closely linked than those that occupy 2 different chromosomes. In a large family with a given phenotype, it might therefore be possible to discover (eg, assuming full penetrance and an absence of homologous recombination, or crossing over) that everyone with the phenotype carries a certain copy of a given chromosome—a finding that would implicate a gene somewhere on that chromosome.

The phenomenon of homologous recombination is critical to further refinement of linkage. If one individual with the phenotype in question receives a recombinant chromosome with only a small region derived from the putative "problem" chromosome, then it logically follows that the gene of interest is likely to be contained in that smaller region. Thus, linkage analysis for rare traits is ideally performed in extended affected families, since studying large numbers of individuals increases the likelihood of observing the informative recombination events that permit high-resolution mapping. Often, even the smallest implicated region will still contain a relatively large number of genes, necessitating guesswork and laborious sequencing in the quest for the final answer.

This process was applied to congenital dyserythropoietic anemia type I, yielding *CDAN1* as the mutated gene [Tamary 1998]. First, 25 affected individuals were identified in four large, consanguineous Bedouin families. (Consanguinous families are especially well-suited to linkage analysis for rare alleles.) Linkage analysis, as described before, was performed using markers on chromosome 15q to narrow the region of suspicion to a span of 1.3 to 1.6 million nucleotides on 15q15.1-15.3. Unfortunately, at least 17 genes are present in this region, 12 of which were of unknown function at the time. One of the genes is *EPB42*, the gene coding for erythrocyte membrane protein 4.2, mutations of which cause hereditary spherocytosis. Although there seemed no obvious connection between abnormalities of cytoskeletal/membrane dynamics and CDA, the presence of an erythroid-associated gene in the implicated region aroused the interest of investigators. Direct sequencing of *EPB42*, however, revealed no mutations in the affected CDA patients. Researchers went on to sequence 13 of the candidate genes before identifying, in multiple patients, homozygous mutations in a gene of unknown function, which they named *CDAN1* (codanin-1, for *c*ongenital *d*yserythropoietic *an*emia, type *I*) [Dgany 2002].

In assessing the function of unknown genes, often the first step is a kind of reasoning by analogy, in which known proteins with domains or sequences similar to those encoded by the novel gene point the way towards its potential role. Such analysis revealed similarities between domains of codanin-1 and proteins that associate with microtubules, actin, and spectrin [Dgany 2002]. Thus, given the prominence of nuclear changes in CDA type I, codanin-1 might be involved in maintaining nuclear integrity by connecting the nuclear membrane to the cytoskeleton. However, direct experimental evidence for the role of codanin-1 in normal or diseased cells remains to be gathered.

Linkage analysis has also identified a CDA type II-associated locus at 20q11.2 [Gasparini 1997]. However, the implicated region generates 90 transcripts, and sequencing has uncovered no mutations in the seven genes judged most likely, based on known function, to disrupt hematopoiesis when mutated [Lanzara 2003]. The remaining genes in the region remain incompletely characterized and have not been sequenced in affected individuals. Linkage analysis of CDA type III in a Swedish family has revealed that the causative gene lies within 15q21-25, a region sufficiently large to have hindered further investigation of specific genes [Lind 1995].

laboratory findings among the various subtypes, bone marrow morphologic findings are the most reliable way to subclassify CDAs t6.5 [Dgany 2002, Gasparini 1997, Heimpel 2003, 2006, Lind 1995, Tamary 2005, Wickramasinghe 2005]. The degree of erythroid multinucleation, presence of internuclear bridges, types of nuclear dyspoietic findings, and gigantic forms are all used to subclassify these disorders into types I to III, while prominent bone marrow erythroid hyperplasia is common to all CDAs i6.7, i6.8, i6.9, i6.10, i6.11, i6.12, i6.13, i6.14. Although less pronounced, cytoplasmic defects include vacuolization, ring sideroblasts, and basophilic stippling. On electron microscopy, defects in the nuclear membrane are prevalent, and cytoplasmic contents may actually spill through these defects into the nucleus i6.15, i6.16. In addition, electron-lucent areas in the heterochromatin create a "Swiss-cheese" appearance in many erythroblasts in CDA I [Renella 2009, Wickramasinghe 2005]. Single case reports of proposed new subtypes have also been published, and these new subtypes are often designated as CDA IV - VIII or variant type [Renella 2009, Wickramasinghe 2005]. The disease course is generally mild, but complications of iron overload may be major [Heimpel 2003, 2006]. The differential diagnosis of CDA includes other constitutional anemias with dyserythropoiesis including thalassemias, other hemoglobinopathies, hereditary sideroblastic anemias, congenital megaloblastic anemias, erythropoietic porphyria, and diverse acquired anemias including those secondary to myeloid neoplasms, toxins, and infections [Carpenter 2004, Phillips 2007, Renella 2009, Wickramasinghe 2005]. In the neonatal period, CDA I may manifest with jaundice, hepatomegaly, and thrombocytopenia, causing potential diagnostic problems, but this rare disease is well known in highly limited family kindreds [Shalev 2004].

Thalassemia

Due to increased malarial resistance, thalassemia is a common genetic disorder worldwide. In both α- and β-thalassemia, globin chain production is impaired; α-thalassemia results from defective α chain production, while β-thalassemias exhibit defective β-globin production. Thalassemias are prevalent in patients of African, Middle Eastern, Southeast Asian, and Asian descent. Defects in both α-chain production (α-thalassemia) and β-chain production (β-thalassemia) have been well characterized clinically, hematologically, and molecularly [Quek 2007, Rund 2005]. The genetic

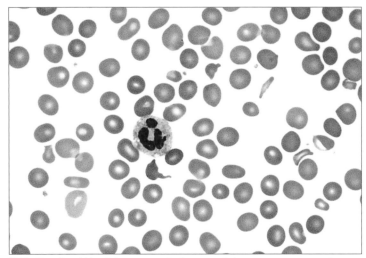

i6.3 *Peripheral blood showing marked anisopoikilocytosis in patient with congenital dyserythropoietic anemia I. (Wright) (courtesy P Izadi)*

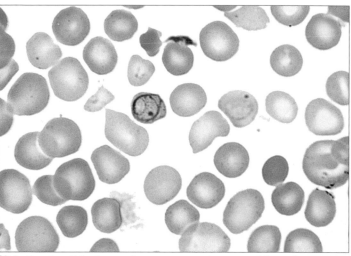

i6.4 *Peripheral blood smear from a patient with congenital dyserythropoietic anemia I shows a macrocytic anemia with moderate anisopoikilocytosis. Note Cabot ring. (Wright) (courtesy T Dutcher, MD)*

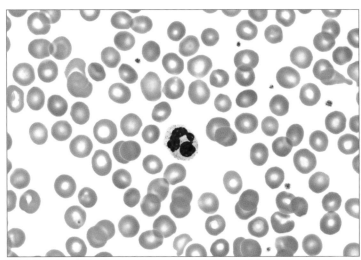

i6.5 *Peripheral blood smear showing modest anisopoikilocytosis in patient with congenital dyserythropoietic anemia II. (Wright) (courtesy R Brynes, MD)*

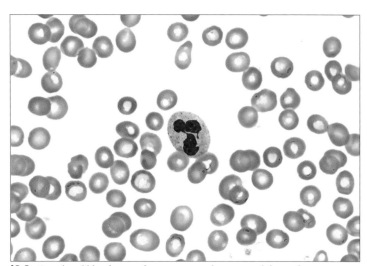

i6.6 *Peripheral blood smear from patient with congenital dyserythropoietic anemia III. (Wright) (courtesy R Brynes, MD)*

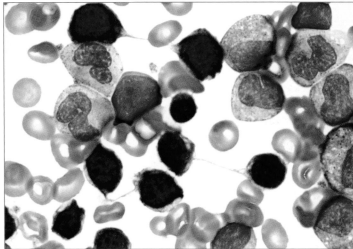

i6.7 *Bone marrow aspirate smear from patient with congenital dyserythropoietic anemia I showing internuclear bridging of erythroblasts. (Wright) (courtesy P Izadi)*

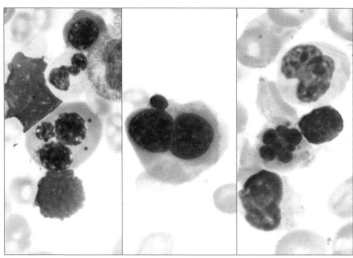

i6.8 *Bone marrow aspirate smear composite shows erythroid binucleation and nuclear budding in the bone marrow of a patient with congenital dyserythropoietic anemia I. (Wright)*

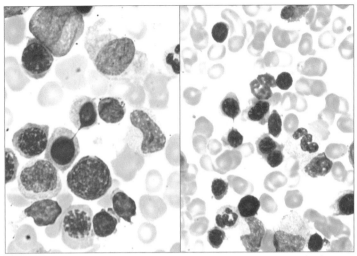

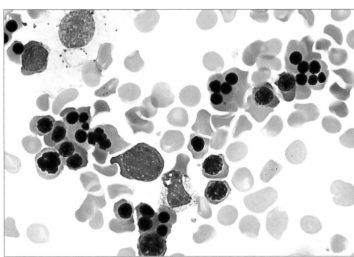

i6.9 *Bone marrow aspirate smear composite illustrates internuclear bridging in a case of congenital dyserythropoietic anemia I. (Wright) (courtesy T Dutcher, MD)*

i6.10 *Bone marrow aspirate smear showing striking multinucleation in patient with congenital dyserythropoietic anemia II. (Wright) (courtesy R Brynes, MD)*

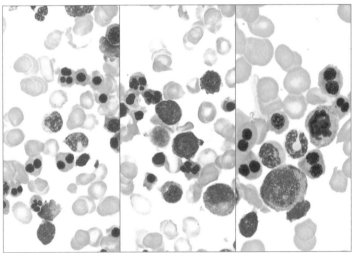

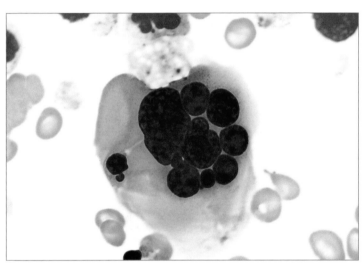

i6.11 *Bone marrow aspirate smear composite illustrates normoblastic erythroid hyperplasia with many binucleate and trinucleate orthochromic normoblasts, which characterizes this case of congenital dyserythropoietic anemia II. (Wright) (courtesy T Dutcher, MD)*

i6.12 *Bone marrow aspirate smear from patient with congenital dyserythropoietic anemia III showing strikingly enlarged and multinucleated erythroid precursor. (Wright) (courtesy R Brynes, MD)*

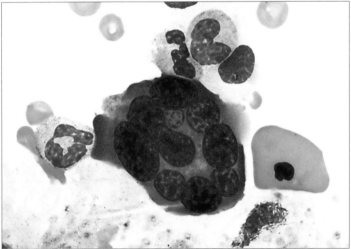

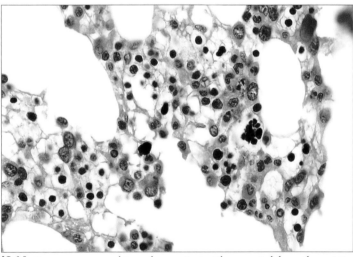

i6.13 *Bone marrow aspirate smear from patient with congenital dyserythropoietic anemia III showing striking multinucleation and marked macrocytosis of erythroid precursors. (Wright) (courtesy R Brynes, MD)*

i6.14 *Bone marrow core biopsy from patient with congenital dyserythropoietic anemia III showing marked multinucleation of erythroid precursors. (H&E) (courtesy R Brynes, MD)*

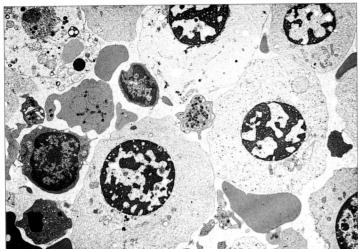

i6.15 *Defects in nuclear pores are evident by electron microscopy in a case of congenital dyserythropoietic anemia I.*

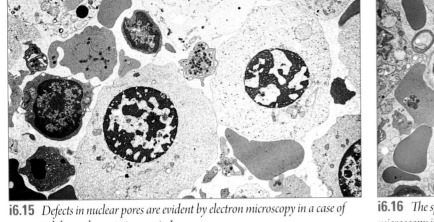

i6.16 *The spilling of cytoplasmic contents into the nucleus is evident by electron microscopy in a case of congenital dyserythropoietic anemia I. Also characteristic is the "Swiss cheese" appearance created by electron lucent "holes" in the heterochromatin.*

defects responsible for the thalassemias are complicated, and more than 200 different genetic abnormalities have been described, the majority of which are single nucleoside substitutions (point mutations) in β-thalassemia, while larger mutations predominate in α-thalassemias **sidebar 6.3** [Quek 2007, Repapinou 2007, Rund 2005].

Impaired hemoglobin production is linked to combined defective cytoplasmic maturation of RBCs and decreased

[sidebar 6.3] The Thalassemias and Sickle Cell Anemia: Classic Genetics and Recent Insights

Ever since Linus Pauling defined sickle cell anemia as the first "molecular disease" [Pauling 1949], inherited abnormalities at the α- and β-globin loci have been among the most closely studied in human genetics, so it is unsurprising that the genetic bases of the resulting diseases, including α-thalassemia and β-thalassemia, are well-understood. For each of these disorders we will present the classic description of the genetics along with additional insights into the complex changes that can produce and influence these phenotypes.

α-Thalassemia

The basic genetics of α-thalassemia are not complicated. Each chromosome 16 carries 2 copies of the α-globin gene (*HBA1* and *HBA2*), meaning there are normally four copies of the gene. α-thalassemia occurs when genetic lesions, typically large structural rearrangements, lead to decreased functionality at these loci. Loss of only one copy still permits adequate α chain production, leading to silent carrier status. Absence of 2 copies results in α-thalassemia trait, with mild anemia and thalassemic indices. Loss of 3 copies creates a significant excess of β-chains, which form unstable tetramers (hemoglobin H) and cause severe anemia. Fetal hydrops is the consequence of total absence of functional α-globin genes.

Our understanding of the α-globin locus, however, is now somewhat more comprehensive than this simplistic picture of four isolated potential targets of mutation. Indeed, a relatively large region of the surrounding genome is necessary for proper function of the α-globin gene. Comparative analysis of the α-globin region across many species reveals 24 widely spaced, evolutionarily-conserved sequences surrounding the gene [Hughes 2005]. Transfer of fully 135 kb (ie, 135,000 bases) surrounding the α-globin gene is necessary to support normal α-chain synthesis. Thus, regulatory elements essential to the function of the gene are located at some distance from the gene itself [Higgs 2005]. It appears that these distant upstream regulatory elements physically interact with the α-globin gene by "looping out" of the intervening sequence, so that alteration in chromatin structure is necessary for gene expression [Vernimmen 2007].

Alterations to these complex regulatory dynamics are rare causes of α-thalassemia, meaning that the disease can result in the setting of four perfectly normal copies of the gene itself [Higgs 2008]. For example, inherited mutations in the *ATRX* gene cause α-thalassemia with mental retardation. Acquired mutations of *ATRX* are also seen in α-thalassemia myelodysplastic syndrome (ATMDS), in which new-onset α-thalassemia occurs in the context of myelodysplastic syndrome.

β-Thalassemia

Classic β-thalassemia arises from mutations in the β-globin gene (*HBB*) on chromosome 11. Whereas α-thalassemia often involves large scale alterations and deletions, changes to the β-globin gene are more often point mutations. These changes lead to compromise of β-globin synthesis, ranging from complete absence to only mild decrease in β-globin production; the severity of the mutations in turn dictates the degree of anemia. The presence of a single mutated β-globin gene almost always produces an asymptomatic carrier state with only mild anemia and thalassemic indices (ie, β-thalassemia trait). However, in rare cases a mutation behaves in a dominant fashion, with symptomatic anemia resulting from inheritance of only one copy. These unusual alleles produce a β-globin variant so unstable that it overwhelms the cell's proteolytic machinery, leading to ineffective erythropoiesis [Thein 2008].

A more complete picture of the phenotypic variability in β-thalassemia also requires consideration of changes occurring away from the β-globin locus. Changes in the α-globin gene can profoundly affect the phenotype of β-thalassemia. When β-thalassemia is inherited together with α-thalassemia–associated mutations, the resulting deficit in α-chains reduces the α/β imbalance and blunts the effect of the β-globin mutations. Similarly, the severity of a given β-thalassemia mutation is heightened when rare duplications of the α-globin gene are also present. A distinct set of polymorphisms influences the individual's innate ability to upregulate the production of fetal hemoglobin (HgbF), which tends to ameliorate the severity of β-thalassemia. HgbF levels in normal adults differ by as much as 20-fold [Thein 1998], and up to half of this variability is explained by polymorphisms at 3 locations [Menzel 2007, Sankaran 2008, So 2008, Thein 1987, Uda 2008].

Yet another level of globin regulation occurs at the epigenetic level. The progression from embryonic to fetal to adult hemoglobin synthesis is facilitated by successive silencing via methylation of ε- and γ-globin promoters [Lavelle 2006]. As our knowledge of globin gene silencing becomes more specific, these epigenetic programs will likely prove attractive targets for therapeutic regulation of globin synthesis in sickle cell anemia and the thalassemias [Saunthararajah 2008].

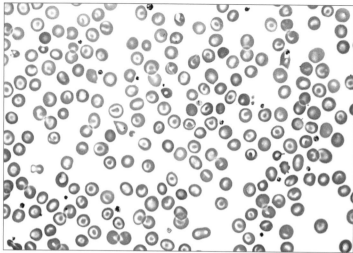

i6.17 *Peripheral blood from patient with β-thalassemia minor. (Wright)*

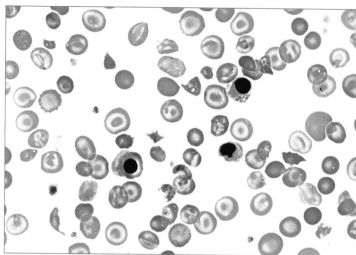

i6.18 *Peripheral blood from patient with β-thalassemia intermedia post-splenectomy showing nucleated reds and striking anisopoikilocytosis. (Wright)*

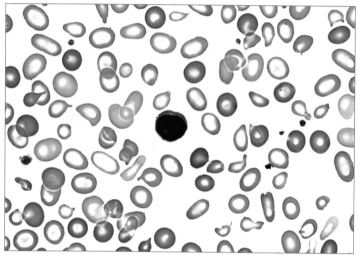

i6.19 *Peripheral blood from patient with β-thalassemia major showing marked anisopoikilocytosis and hypochromia. (Wright)*

RBC survival. The constitutional cytoplasmic maturation defect results from imbalanced globin chain production [Rund 2005]. Inadequate amounts of hemoglobin A that result from reduced production of either α or β chains lead to the production of hypochromic, microcytic erythrocytes [Rund 2005, Sirdah 2008]. Other mechanisms for anemia are also operative in patients with thalassemia, including decreased erythrocyte survival (the consequence of precipitation of excess unaffected globin chains) and ineffective erythropoiesis secondary to either increased intramedullary cell death of erythroid precursors [Libani 2008].

Depending on the type of genetic defect, patients with thalassemia have a variably severe microcytic, hypochromic anemia, relatively increased RBC count, variable reticulocyte count, and fairly normal RDW, at least in less severe cases **i6.17, i6.18, i6.19** [Rund 2005]. Qualitative abnormalities such as coarse basophilic stippling, targeting, and, rarely, Cabot rings may also be evident on blood smears.

Noninvasive prenatal screening techniques using fetal erythroblasts isolated from maternal blood have been developed [D'Souza 2008]. In patients with mild β-thalassemia, hemoglobin electrophoresis reveals an increase in hemoglobin A_2 $(\alpha_2\delta_2)$. Fetal hemoglobin may also be increased, more commonly in more severely affected patients, but occasionally in those with mild disease. Even though molecular testing is becoming a more common method, detection of α-thalassemia is more problematic, requiring complicated hemoglobin α- and β-chain synthesis rate studies not generally suitable for a screening test [Repapinou 2007]. Combined hemoglobinapathies such as either β-thalassemia/HgbE or α-thalassemia/HgbE are common in Southeast Asia [Sripichai 2008, Tritipsombut 2008]. In thalassemic patients with significant anemia, the bone marrow characteristically shows erythroid hyperplasia; iron overload may also be evident in long-term transfusion-dependent patients **i6.20, i6.21**. Other hematopoietic lineages are generally unremarkable. Iron overload is a major management problem in more severe cases of thalassemia [Rund 2005].

Other Constitutional Erythrocyte Maturation Disorders

The remaining types of constitutional RBC maturation defects are very rare, consisting primarily of congenital sideroblastic anemias, erythropoietic porphyrias, and other rare disorders that are not generally encountered in clinical practice. Like its acquired counterpart, congenital sideroblastic anemia is characterized by a dimorphic blood picture, increased bone marrow storage and sideroblastic iron, and numerous ring sideroblasts **i6.22, i6.23, i6.24** [Camaschella 2008, 2009]. Iron abnormalities and erythrocyte abnormalities may become more pronounced following splenectomy **i6.25, i6.26, i6.27**. The bone marrow is typically hypercellular with

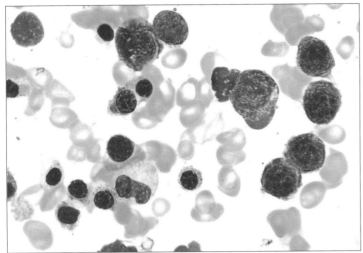

i6.20 *Bone marrow aspirate smear from a patient with severe thalassemia illustrates the erythroid hyperplasia that characterizes this genetic disorder. (Wright)*

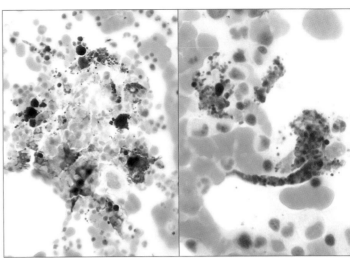

i6.21 *Macrophage iron overload (common in severely anemic, transfusion-dependent patients) is evident on these bone marrow aspirate smears from a patient with thalassemia. (Prussian blue)*

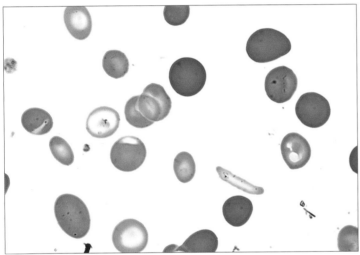

i6.22 *Peripheral blood smear from an infant with congenital sideroblastic anemia shows a prominent dimorphic picture. (Wright)*

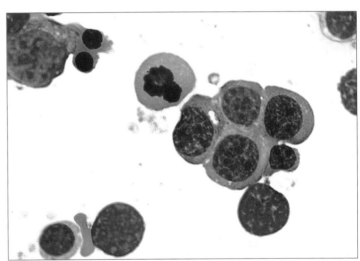

i6.23 *Striking erythroid hyperplasia is evident on this bone marrow aspirate smear from an infant with congenital sideroblastic anemia. (Wright)*

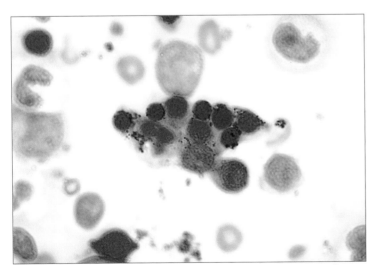

i6.24 *Iron stain documents the markedly increased sideroblastic iron with numerous ring forms on this bone marrow aspirate smear from an infant with congenital sideroblastic anemia. (Prussian blue)*

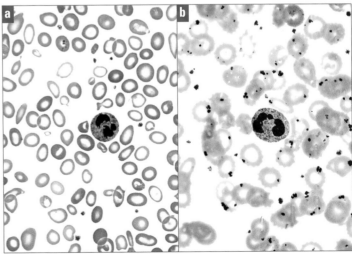

i6.25 *Peripheral blood composite from patient with congenital sideroblastic anemia comparing pre-* **a** *and post-splenectomy* **b** *picture. Note striking Pappenheimer bodies following splenectomy. (Wright) (courtesy C Starkey, MD)*

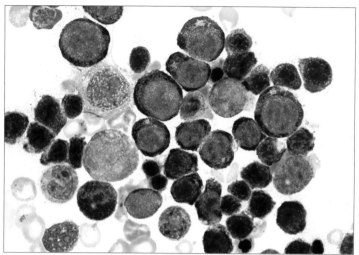

i6.26 *Bone marrow aspirate smear from patient with congenital sideroblastic anemia showing striking erythroid hyperplasia. (Wright) (courtesy C Starkey, MD)*

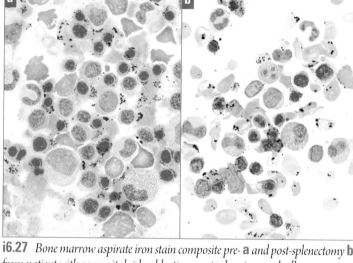

i6.27 *Bone marrow aspirate iron stain composite pre-* **a** *and post-splenectomy* **b** *from patient with congenital sideroblastic anemia showing markedly increased erythroid iron with numerous ring sideroblasts. Note abundance of Pappenheimer bodies postsplenectomy. (Prussian blue) (courtesy C Starkey, MD)*

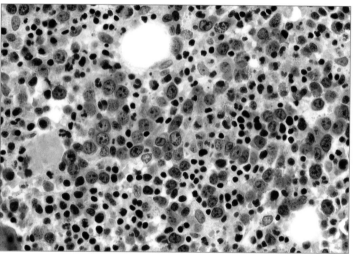

i6.28 *Bone marrow core biopsy from patient with congenital sideroblastic anemia showing striking erythroid hyperplasia with numerous erythroblasts. (H&E) (courtesy C Starkey, MD)*

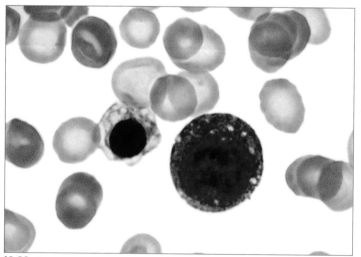

i6.29 *Bone marrow aspirate smear from child with Pearson syndrome. Note vacuolated myeloid and erythroid cells with numerous erythroblasts. (Wright) (courtesy L Contis, MD)*

marked erythroid hyperplasia **i6.28**. Various defects in heme synthesis or mitochondrial DNA account for these iron abnormalities in bone marrow erythroid elements and for the resulting hypochromic anemia or dimorphic erythrocyte picture. Although generally X-linked recessive, other patterns of inheritance of constitutional sideroblastic anemia have been described. Gene mutations in *ALAS2* (delta-aminolevulinic acid synthase) have been described in some cases of X-linked congenital sideroblastic anemia [Camaschella 2009]. Other mutations and other inheritance patterns have been described in various rare congenital sideroblastic anemias that include primary mitochondrial disorders as well as DNA mutation disorders [Camaschella 2008, 2009 Finsterer 2007]. In Pearson syndrome, a rare constitutional mitochondrial DNA microdeletion disorder, progressive bone marrow failure, sideroblastic anemia, and vacuolated hematopoietic precursors have been noted **i6.29**. Congenital erythropoietic porphyria is an autosomal recessive disorder caused by mutations in the *UROS* gene, which encodes uroporphyrinogen III synthesase. The blood picture resembles that of CDA I [Phillips 2007].

[6.4.4] **Acquired Erythrocyte Maturation Disorders**

Megaloblastic Anemia

Acquired nuclear maturation disorders, the megaloblastic anemias, are substantially more common than their constitutional counterparts **t6.3** p 94, **t6.4** p 95. Deficiency of either serum vitamin B₁₂ or folate, both essential for DNA synthesis, accounts for the vast majority of cases of megaloblastic anemia [Andres 2006, Carmel 2008a, Carmel 2009, Foucar 2010b, Solomon 2007, Wickramasinghe 2006]. Other causes include drugs that act as antagonists to folate, purine, or pyrimidine, as well as drugs that decrease the availability of

t6.6 Tests Useful in the Diagnosis and Distinction of Cobalamin and Folate Deficiencies

Disorder	Serum Cobalamin	Serum Folate	RBC Folate	Methylmalonic Acid (Serum)	Homocysteine (Serum)
Vitamin B$_{12}$ deficiency	↓	normal, ↑	↓, normal	↑	↑
Folate deficiency	normal	↓	↓	normal	↑
Combined cobalamin & folate deficiency	↓	↓	↓	↑	↑

References: [Carmel 2009, Foucar 2008, Foucar 2010b, Green 2005, Solomon 2005, Wickramasinghe 2006]

vitamin B$_{12}$ for DNA synthesis. Adequate vitamin B$_{12}$ and folate for hematopoiesis requires sufficient dietary intake, successful absorption in the gastrointestinal tract, and delivery to the bone marrow. A defect or abnormality at any of these steps will result in megaloblastic anemia. General categories of vitamin B$_{12}$ and folate deficiency include inadequate intake, defective absorption, defective transport, disorders of metabolism, and increased requirement (folate) [Foucar 2010b, Wickramasinghe 2006].

The most common cause of vitamin B$_{12}$ deficiency is inadequate absorption secondary to intrinsic factor deficiency, an autoimmune disorder termed *pernicious anemia*. In contrast, inadequate intake is the most common cause of folate deficiency; however, the increased requirement for dietary folate in pregnant women or patients with chronic hemolytic anemias also may lead to deficiency [Carmel 2008b].

t6.7 Blood and Bone Marrow Findings in Megaloblastic Anemias

Blood	Comments
Variable cytopenias, often pancytopenia	Ineffective hematopoiesis
Marked macrocytosis, oval macrocytes	Progeny of megaloblastic bone marrow; decreased reticulocytes
Red blood cell fragments, schistocytes, inclusions	Macrocytes damaged in circulation; may see tear drop forms; may see occasional Howell-Jolly bodies, basophilic stippling, and Cabot rings
Nuclear hypersegmentation of neutrophils	Reflection of mitotic defect in granulocytic lineage

Bone Marrow	Comments
Hypercellular	All cell lines proliferating; increased mitotic activity; karyorrhexis
Marked erythroid hyperplasia	Myeloid: erythroid ratio may be reversed; slight left shift in maturation pyramid
Nuclear-cytoplasmic dissociation	Nucleus "young-appearing" with finely stippled chromatin; cytoplasm more mature
Granulocytic hyperplasia	Blasts not increased; giant metamyelocytes and bands present

References: [Carmel 2008b, 2009, Foucar 2008, 2009b, Means 2009, Wickramasinghe 2006]

Various laboratory tests can be used to evaluate a patient for possible serum vitamin B$_{12}$ or folate deficiency **t6.6** [Carmel 2008b, Carmel 2009, Means 2009, Foucar 2010b, Moridani 2006, Wickramasinghe 2006]. The most "routine" of these tests include assays for serum vitamin B$_{12}$, serum folate, and RBC folate levels. Because serum folate levels fluctuate with dietary intake, the RBC folate level is considered to be a more accurate reflection of overall folate stores, but fasting serum folate measurement is also useful. Additional tests include homocysteine and methylmalonic acid levels, and measurement of antibodies to parietal cells or intrinsic factor [Carmel 2008b, Carmel 2009, Foucar 2010b, Moridani 2006, Wickramasinghe 2006].

Prominent peripheral blood and bone marrow abnormalities are characteristic of megaloblastic anemias, but a wide spectrum of blood findings can be seen in patients with documented cobalamin deficiency **t6.7** [Andres 2006]. In advanced megaloblastic anemia, pancytopenia is evident [Andres 2006]. As a reflection of the megaloblastic marrow, macrocytosis, giant bands, and hypersegmented neutrophils may all be present **i6.30**. A distinctive macrocyte with an oval cytoplasmic contour is characteristic of megaloblastic anemia. However, because macrocytes are readily damaged in the circulation,

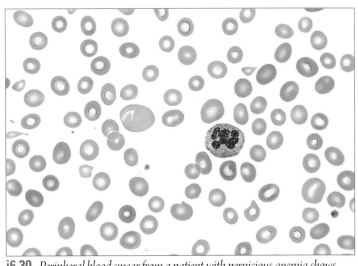

i6.30 *Peripheral blood smear from a patient with pernicious anemia shows a severe anemia with oval macrocytes as well as fragmented forms. A hypersegmented neutrophil is also present. (Wright)*

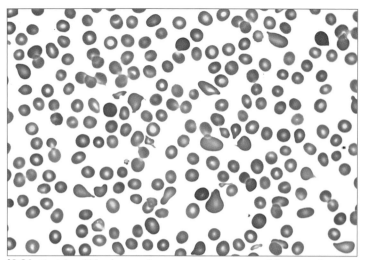

i6.31 *Peripheral blood smear showing oval macrocytes and fragmented erythroid cells in patient with megaloblastic anemia. (Wright)*

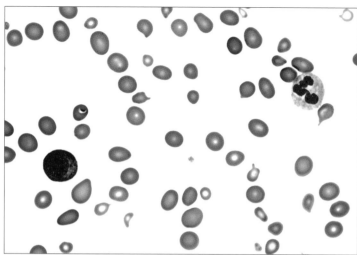

i6.32 *Peripheral blood showing marked normocytic anemia (MCV 99fL) in child with severe megaloblastic anemia. Note anisopoikilocytosis and fragmented erythroid cells. (Wright)*

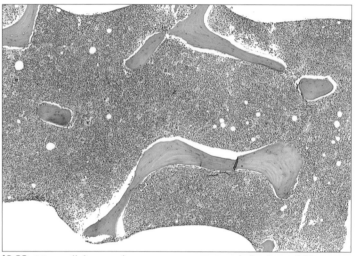

i6.33 *Hypercellularity is characteristic in patients with florid megaloblastic anemia, as seen on this bone marrow biopsy section from a 40-year-old woman. (H&E)*

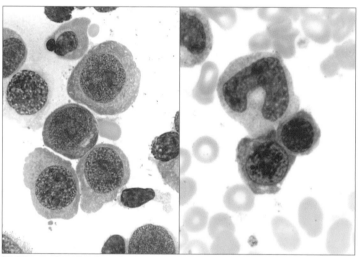

i6.34 *Erythroid and myeloid abnormalities in megaloblastic anemia are shown on this composite of bone marrow aspirate smears. (Wright)*

RBC fragments and schistocytes may also be evident **i6.31**. As a consequence, the RDW is typically very high in these patients. In addition, circulating erythrocytes may contain Howell-Jolly bodies or, if anemia is profound, Cabot rings (see **i6.4**). Of importance, occasional patients with severe megaloblastic anemia will have a normal MCV, often the consequence of a combined anemia (eg, megaloblastic anemia and concurrent iron deficiency, thalassemia, or anemia of chronic disease) **i6.32** [Chan 2007].

In patients with megaloblastic anemia, the bone marrow is characteristically hypercellular, with an increase in all hematopoietic lineages **i6.33**. However, erythroid hyperplasia frequently predominates with a reverse in the myeloid-to-erythroid ratio. For all proliferating hematopoietic lineages, nuclear-cytoplasmic dissociation is evident, but this is most prominent for the erythroid lineage. These cells exhibit large nuclei with fine,

sieve-like, stippled chromatin, despite a relatively more mature cytoplasm **i6.34**, **i6.35**. Although the granulocytic maturation pyramid can be left-shifted, myeloblasts are not typically increased in the bone marrow of patients with megaloblastic anemia. The most prominent morphologic abnormalities in the granulocytic lineage reflecting nuclear-cytoplasmic dissociation include giant metamyelocytes, large "horseshoe" band neutrophils, and hypersegmented neutrophils **i6.36**, **i6.37**, **i6.38**. In addition, mild dyspoietic changes may be evident, especially in the erythroid lineage. These abnormalities include nuclear lobulation, minimal multinucleation, and increased sideroblastic iron **i6.39**. The bone marrow core biopsy is typically markedly hypercellular. Increased erythroblasts with oblong nucleoli may be prominent **i6.40**. Increased karyorrhexis may be evident, reflecting intramedullary cell death. However, because cytoplasmic maturation is unimpeded, hemoglobin production

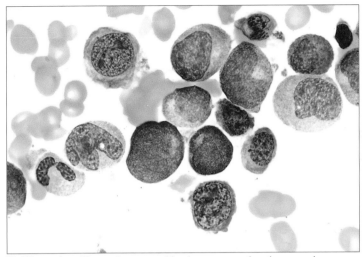

i6.35 *Erythroid hyperplasia, sieve-like chromatin, and nuclear-cytoplasmic dysynchrony are shown on this bone marrow aspirate smear from a patient with megaloblastic anemia. (Wright)*

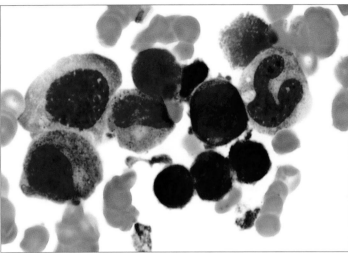

i6.36 *Bone marrow aspirate smear from patient with combined vitamin B₁₂ and iron deficiency. Note megaloblastic changes of granulocytic cells, while erythoid cells are less remarkable. (Wright)*

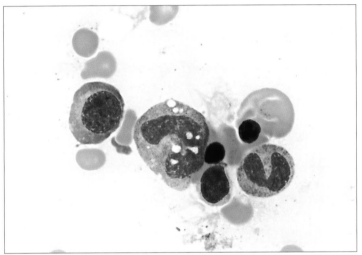

i6.37 *Giant band in bone marrow aspirate from patient with megaloblastic anemia. (Wright)*

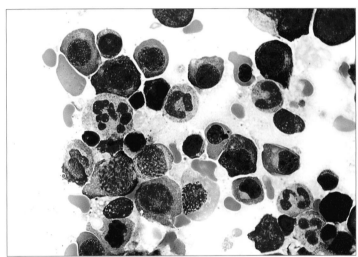

i6.38 *Bone marrow aspirate smear showing marked hypersegmentation of mature neutrophils as well as other megaloblastic changes in patient with megaloblastic anemia. (Wright)*

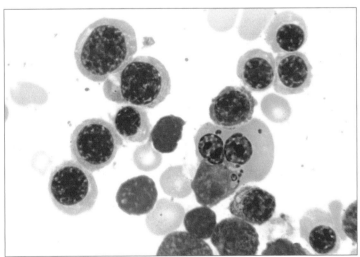

i6.39 *Mild dyserythropoiesis is evident on this bone marrow aspirate smear in a case of pernicious anemia. Note the multinucleation and Howell-Jolly bodies. (Wright)*

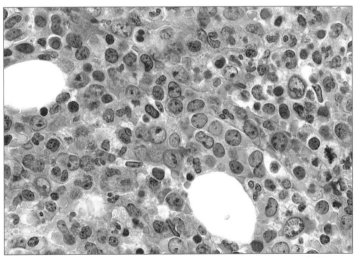

i6.40 *Increased, clustered erythroblasts with dispersed chromatin and oblong nucleoli are illustrated on a bone marrow biopsy section from a patient with megaloblastic anemia. (H&E)*

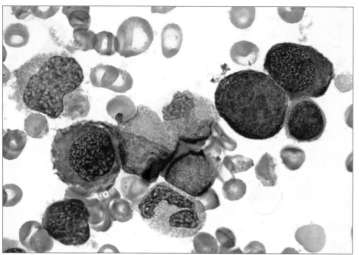

i6.41 *Bone marrow aspirate smear showing neonatal megaloblastic anemia secondary to vitamin B$_{12}$ deficiency in vegan mother. (Wright) (courtesy C Kjeldsberg, MD)*

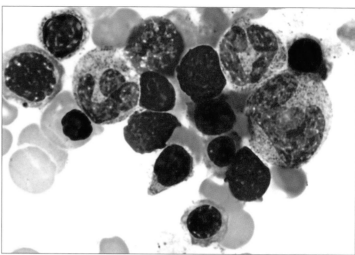

i6.42 *Partially treated megaloblastic anemia in bone marrow aspirate smear obtained from a patient 5 days after beginning vitamin B$_{12}$ therapy. Note persistence of marked granulocytic megaloblastic changes. (Wright)*

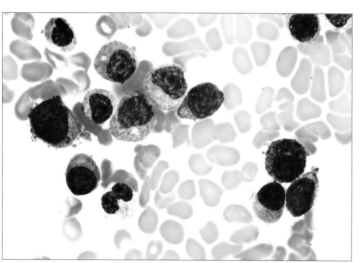

i6.43 *Bone marrow aspirate smear from patient with myelodysplasia mimicking megaloblastic anemia. Macrocytosis was present in the blood. Note megaloblastic changes in conjunction with increased myeloblasts. (Wright)*

in erythrocytes and granule production in neutrophils are both normal. Storage iron is frequently increased.

Patients with megaloblastic anemia may develop concurrent iron deficiency anemia, which will mask many of the classic RBC changes [Chan 2007]. Although the RDW is increased, the MCV in these cases of combined deficiency may either fall within normal range or reflect the more severe deficiency. However, the megaloblastic changes of the granulocyte lineage in bone marrow and peripheral blood are not masked by concurrent iron deficiency **i6.36**.

Megaloblastic anemia in infants and young children is also a diagnostic challenge because many of these children present with "failure to thrive." Although some cases of infantile megaloblastic anemia result from rare mutations in cobalamin or folate receptor or transporter genes, more commonly megaloblastic anemia in infants is

the consequence of extreme maternal dietary restrictions **i6.41** [Fyfe 2004, Katar 2006, Weiss 2004, Whitehead 2006, Zhao 2007]. A high clinical suspicion and rapid diagnosis and treatment are essential to avert progression of neurologic defects.

Rapid changes in peripheral blood and bone marrow occur in patients effectively treated for megaloblastic anemia. Erythroid precursors demonstrate normal morphologic characteristics within 2 to 3 days, while granulocyte hypersegmentation resolves in approximately 1 week. Because of the high proliferation rate in megaloblastic anemia, a rapid reticulocytosis is seen in response to appropriate therapy and may reach a peak of 50% to 70% within 4 to 10 days after the onset of therapy. The hemogram reverts to normal approximately 1 to 2 months after initiation of treatment for megaloblastic anemia. Erythroid abnormalities may resolve sooner than granulocytic abnormalities as noted in patients undergoing bone marrow examination after initiation of cobalamin therapy **i6.42**.

The differential diagnosis of megaloblastic anemia includes myelodysplasia, and sometimes this distinction may be challenging **i6.43**. Other causes of megaloblastic features in bone marrow are listed in **t6.8** and include constitutional disorders, drug and toxins, and primary hematopoietic neoplasms [Aminoff 1999, Carmel 2009, Diaz 1999, Fleming 1999, Foucar 2008, 2009a, Labay 1999, Ward 2002, Wickramasinghe 2006].

Iron Deficiency Anemia

Iron deficiency is, by far, the most common type of acquired cytoplasmic RBC maturation defect with an estimated 3 billion affected people worldwide [Andrews 2008, Moy 2006]. Iron deficiency anemia is almost always an acquired disorder secondary to blood loss, inadequate intake, or both [Andrews 2008, Hershko 2009]. Autoimmune gastritis with underlying *Helicobacter pylori* infection is a more recently identified

t6.8 Causes of Bone Marrow Megaloblastosis

Rare Constitutional Genetic Disorders

Orotic aciduria

Lesch-Nyhan syndrome

Transcobalamin II deficiency

Congenital megaloblastic anemia*

Congenital dyserythropoietic anemia

Congenital sideroblastic anemia

Methionine synthetase deficiency

Homocystinosis

Acquired Megaloblastic Disorders

Megaloblastic anemia (vitamin B$_{12}$ or folate deficiency)

Myelodysplastic syndromes

Acute myelogenous leukemia, especially erythroleukemias

Chemotherapeutic agents that primarily interfere with purine or pyrimidine synthesis

Zidovudine[†] (inhibits reverse transcriptase)

Drugs associated with impaired absorption or other causes of decreased availability of vitamin B$_{12}$ or folate (anticonvulsants, antibiotics, antimalarial agents, oral contraceptives, alcohol)

Toxins (benzene, arsenic)[‡]

*Multiple genetic types described including mutations in thiamine transporter gene and cubulin (intrinsic factor receptor) gene
[†]Treatment used to suppress retroviral replication in human immunodeficiency virus 1-positive patients
[‡]Marked karyorrhexis is also present

References: [Aminoff 1999, Carmel 2009, Diaz 1999, Fleming 1999, Foucar 2008, 2009b, Labay 1999, Ward 2002, Wickramasinghe 2006]

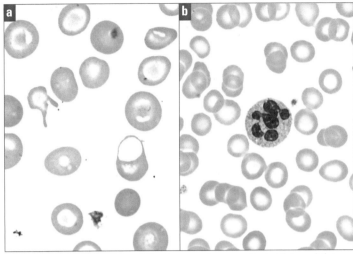

i6.44 *Composite of peripheral blood smears from a patient with iron deficiency showing hypochromia with prekaratocytes* **a** *and prominent hypersegmentation* **b** *mimicking megaloblastic anemia. (Wright)*

(transferrin) [Angeles Vazquez Lopez 2006, Baillie 2003, Danise 2008, Harrington 2008, Moy 2006, Umbreit 2005].

The differential diagnosis of iron deficiency anemia includes β-thalassemia minor, anemia of chronic disease, and other microcytic anemias. The distinction of these disorders is usually based on CBC, other laboratory tests, and family history i6.44 [Harrington 2008, Holme 2007, Sirdah 2008, Urrechaga 2009]. Recent reports suggest that the identification of prekaratocytes and pencil cells is helpful in distinguishing iron deficiency (increased) from β-thalassemia minor and anemia of chronic disease i6.44 [Harrington 2008]. Although the reduction in RBC count usually parallels the severity of iron deficiency anemia, relatively higher RBC counts may be evident in iron-deficient infants and young children [Aslan 2003]. Markedly elevated RBC count is present in patients with severe hypoxia, often secondary to cardiac defects, in whom therapy consists of chronic phlebotomy to induce iron deficiency (see Chapter 9). A similar picture can be seen in patients undergoing regular phlebotomy for polycythemia vera.

Erythroid hyperplasia, although variable, is a predictable bone marrow finding in patients with acquired cytoplasmic maturation defects. The absence of both erythrocyte and storage iron distinguishes iron deficiency anemia from other cytoplasmic maturation defects.

Sideroblastic Anemias

Other disorders characterized by cytoplasmic maturation defects include sideroblastic anemias and other disorders that result from porphyrin ring defects t6.9 [Camaschella 2008, Finsterer 2007, Foucar 2008, Natelson 2007, Nearman 2007, Perkins 2004, Willis 2005]. Both markedly increased storage and erythroid iron characterize the porphyrin ring abnormalities that cause sideroblastic anemias. Because the excessive sideroblastic iron becomes deposited in mitochondria, ring sideroblasts (ie, a ring of iron granules

cause of iron deficiency [Andrews 2008, Hershko 2009]. Rare genetic defects cause iron deficiency, secondary to mutations in genes encoding iron transport proteins (transferrin) as well as other genes, *DMTI* and *GLRX5*. All of these constitutional disorders are extremely uncommon and rarely encountered in clinical practice [Andrews 2008, Beaumont 2006, Iolascon 2006].

The blood smear and CBC parameters are often diagnostic of iron deficiency anemia. This constellation includes reduced RBC count, low MCV, low MCHC, elevated RDW in conjunction with pale erythrocytes, prekaratocytes, and pencil cells (elliptocytes) on the blood smear. Platelets are often increased and hypersegmented neutrophils may be present i6.44 [Westerman 1999].

Because of the prevalence of iron deficiency anemia in both children and adults, the initial evaluation of a patient with an acquired microcytic hypochromic anemia should always include an evaluation of serum iron and ferritin levels [Andrews 2008]. Additional laboratory tests include protoporphyrin, soluble transferrin receptor, and total iron-binding capacity

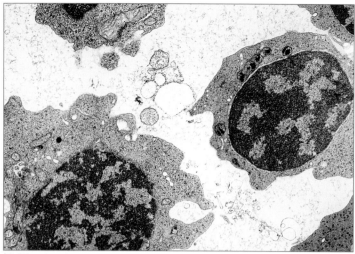

i6.45 *Abundant iron within perinuclear mitochondria of 2 normoblasts is evident by electron micrography in a patient with acquired sideroblastic anemia.*

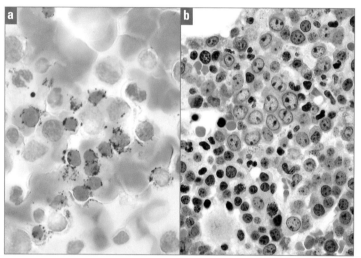

i6.46 *Composite of iron stain **a** and bone marrow core biopsy section **b** in patient with acquired sideroblastic anemia showing numerous ring sideroblasts and marked erythroid hyperplasia including numerous erythroblasts with oblong nuclei. (Prussian blue, H&E)*

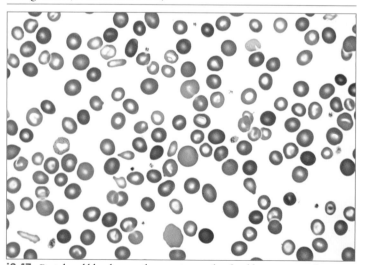

i6.47 *Peripheral blood smear from patient with sideroblastic anemia showing striking dimorphic erythrocyte picture. (Wright)*

t6.9 Causes of Ring Sideroblastosis in Bone Marrow

Bone Marrow Neoplasms

Myelodysplasia (multiple subtypes)*

Therapy-induced myelodysplasia and T-AML

Acute myelogenous leukemia (AML), especially erythroleukemias

Toxins

Alcohol abuse

Arsenic

Benzene

Lead poisoning

Zinc abuse (leading to copper deficiency)

Medications/Homeopathic Remedies

Isoniazid

Azathioprine

Pyrazinamide

Chloramphenicol

Cycloserine

Zinc therapy/denture adhesive (leading to copper deficiency)

Genetic Disorders

Congenital sideroblastic anemias (very rare)[†]

Congenital dyserythropoietic anemia (very rare)

Pearson marrow-pancreas syndrome (very rare)

Thiamine-responsive anemia with diabetes and deafness (TRMA)

Wolfram syndrome (very rare)

---

*Mutations in hemochromatosis-associated genes noted at higher frequency than controls [Nearman 2007]
[†]Both X-linked and autosomal recessive types described

References: [Camaschella 2008, Finsterer 2007, Foucar 2008, Lewis 2007, Natelson 2007, Nearman 2007, Perkins 2004, Sibley 2009, Willis 2005]

adjacent to the nuclear membrane) are prominent **i6.45**, **i6.46**. Despite the iron excess, hemoglobin synthesis is impaired. Although these cells are often slightly macrocytic, they are also hypochromic. Frequently, a dimorphic RBC picture is evident in blood **i6.47**. Some cases of acquired sideroblastic anemia occur in patients with hematologic neoplasms, either myelodysplasia (MDS) or acute myeloid leukemias (AML), while other cases of acquired sideroblastic anemia are nonclonal and result from metabolic abnormalities of mitochondria or porphyrin ring constituents (see Chapters 16 and 18). In patients with MDS/AML, the ring sideroblasts are generally accompanied by other multilineage dysplastic abnormalities reflecting the stem cell nature of these clonal neoplasms. Cytogenetic abnormalities may be identified in these neoplastic disorders, especially in the higher-grade processes. Mutations in hemochromatosis-related genes have also been noted with increased frequency in patients with myeloid

t6.10 Erythrocyte Survival Defects

Constitutional (intrinsic RBC defect)		Pathophysiology
Membrane	Hereditary sphyerocytosis, hereditary elliptocytosis, hereditary pyropoikilocytosis	Mutations in various ankyrin, spectrin genes result in loss of RBC deformability
Enzyme	G6PD deficiency, pyruvate kinase deficiency, phosphoglycerate kinase deficiency	Numerous mutations described, resulting in decreased enzyme stability and increased susceptibility to acute hemolysis secondary to toxins, infections, medications
Hemoglobinopathy	Sickle cell anemia, hemoglobin C	Mutant hemoglobin results in polymerization of hemobglobin leading to premature RBC destruction and many systemic vasculopathies
Constitutional (extrinsic RBC defect)		
Membrane	Congenital TTP	Mutations in *ADAMTS13* gene family
Acquired (intrinsic RBC defect)		
	Paroxysmal noctural hemoglobinuria	Acquired somatic mutation at the hematopoietic stem cell level of *PIGA* gene resulting in defective anchoring proteins on RBC membrane causing increased susceptibility to complement-mediated hemolysis
Acquired (extrinsic defect)		
	Immune-mediated hemolytic anemia	Allo- or autoantibody production induced by numerous mechanisms; idiopathic autoantibodies also common. Antibody binding to RBC results in membrane loss in spleen with formation of spherocytes with shortened survival time
	Microangiopathic hemolytic anemia	Endothelial damage or formation of platelet microthrombi are primary causes of erythrocyte fragmentation; genetic predisposition to some MAHAs, notably hemolytic uremic syndrome (mutations in complement regulatory protein genes); autoimmune mechanisms also described

G6PD = glucose-6-phosphate dehydrogenase; MAHA = microangiopathic hemolytic anemia; *PIGA* = phosphatidylinositol glycan complementation class A gene; RBC = red blood cell

References: [An 2008, Arndt 2005, Ayi 2008, Beutler 2007, 2008, Brodsky 2009, Caprioli 2006, Cataland 2007, Costa 2005, Davenport 2005, Delaunay 2007, Gaetani 2008, Hill 2007, Kato 2007, Levy 2001, Mason 2007, Mohandas 2008, Packman 2008, Parker 2005, Petz 2008, Platt 2008, Ramos 2007, Rock 2005, Semple 2005, Zanella 2007]

neoplasms exhibiting ring sideroblasts [Nearman 2007]. Many non-neoplastic conditions are also linked to increased bone marrow ring sideroblasts **t6.9** [Foucar 2008, Holme 2007, Natelson 2007, Perkins 2004, Sassa 2006, Willis 2005]. Drugs and toxic exposures probably induce ring sideroblasts via inhibition of porphyrin ring enzymes. Occasionally erythroblasts and myeloid precursors are prominently vacuolated in patients with acquired sideroblastic anemia, especially cases associated with copper deficiency, which may be secondary to excess dietary zinc [Willis 2005].

[6.4.5]   **Erythrocyte Survival Defects**

Both intrinsic and extrinsic RBC defects can result in decreased erythrocyte survival time **t6.4** p 95, **t6.10**. If this decreased erythrocyte survival time exceeds the compensatory capacity of the bone marrow, a hemolytic anemia results. As opposed to proliferation and maturation defects, both an erythroid hyperplasia in the bone marrow and a brisk reticulocytosis in blood characterize these RBC survival defects. Except for PNH, the intrinsic RBC defects are constitutional; the erythrocytes that are produced cannot survive normal physiologic challenges. In contrast, extrinsic RBC

defects result from an environmental abnormality; normal erythrocytes are produced but released into an environment that adversely affects survival time.

Constitutional Erythrocyte Survival Defects

The constitutional erythrocyte survival defects can be categorized into membrane defects, enzyme deficiencies, and hemoglobinopathies that all result in the production of RBCs that fail to survive normally in blood **t6.4** p 95, **t6.10**. In general, these constitutional RBC defects were preserved in populations because of increased resistance to severe forms of malaria **sidebar 6.4** [Mohandas 2008]. The most common intrinsic RBC membrane defect is hereditary spherocytosis, while glucose-6-phosphate dehydrogenase deficiency and sickle cell anemia represent prototypic intrinsic enzyme and hemoglobin defects, respectively [An 2008, Arndt 2005, Ayi 2008, Beutler 2007, 2008, Brodsky 2008, Costa 2005, Davenport 2005, Delaunay 2007, Gaetani 2008, Hill 2007, Kato 2007, Mason 2007, Packman 2008, Parker 2005, Petz 2008, Platt 2008, Ramos 2007, Semple 2005, Zanella 2007]. Although much is known about the specific genetic defects responsible for these constitutional erythrocyte survival defects, discussion in this chapter will be primarily focused on standard features

[sidebar 6.4] Red Blood Cell Disorders and the Malaria Hypothesis

In 1948, JBS Haldane proposed that the geographic overlap between areas of endemic thalassemia and malaria infection suggested a protective effect of the former against the latter, thus formulating the so-called "malaria hypothesis" for red blood cell disorders. Substantial epidemiologic and laboratory evidence has since been gathered to support the hypothesis, and thalassemias and some hemoglobinopathies are generally regarded as conferring some protection against *Plasmodium* infection. Although this association has become a commonplace, it nevertheless constitutes one of the most remarkable explanations for a constellation of mutations yet encountered in human genetics. Thus, it is worth examining the evidence for these associations in more detail, and also questioning what other red blood cell disorders might be attributable to the malaria hypothesis.

Absent de novo mutation, alleles that confer disadvantage (as in the case of homozygosity for HgbS) should be eliminated from a given population, unless they also give significant benefit in some settings, in which case a carrier rate will be achieved that balances the advantages and disadvantages in the face of the selective pressure. The fact that hemoglobinopathy and thalassemia alleles achieve polymorphic frequency in some African and Asian populations is strong evidence for their partly advantageous nature. Moreover, haplotype analysis has shown that many of these mutations arose independently, again implicating selective pressure [Flint 1993].

While such observations indeed suggest these alleles may be protective, numerous epidemiologic and in vitro studies have been necessary to specifically demonstrate the association of these phenotypes with malarial resistance. These case-control studies and experimental data for HgbS, HgbC, HgbE, the thalassemias, and glucose-6-phosphate dehydrogenase (G6PD) deficiency are summarized in **tS6.4**. In general, these alleles are thought to confer malaria resistance via 2 potential mechanisms. First, in some cases they are associated with in vitro resistance to parasitic invasion or growth, perhaps due to structural changes or altered expression of membrane proteins. HgbC cells show decreased expression of the *Plasmodium falciparum* erythroid membrane protein 1 (PfEMP-1), a virulence factor that mediates endothelial adhesion and severe complications [Fairhurst 2005]. α-thalassemia cells have decreased expression of CR1, a complement receptor critical for RBC rosetting, an event associated with the development of severe malaria [Cockburn 2004]. Second, in many of these disorders, red blood cells are more susceptible to phagocytosis at the early ring stage of infection, a critical advantage because at later stages the presence of hemozoin pigment inhibits many functions of the macrophage [Min-Oo 2005, Schwarzer 2008]. The same mechanisms that cause hemolytic anemia may compromise the red blood cell sufficiently that even early, low-level parasitic infections are unsustainable and rapidly cleared.

Links between parasite protection and other RBC abnormalities have also been proposed. Hereditary elliptocytosis occurs in a worldwide distribution, but the prevalence of mutations is particularly high (2%) in western Africa. In vitro studies suggest some protective effeczt from this mutation [Dhermy 2007]. Southeast Asian ovalocytosis, due to a band 3 mutation, is apparently lethal in the homozygous state but confers protection to cerebral malaria in the heterozygous form, perhaps by increasing the affinity of infected cells for endothelial receptors expressed only outside of the brain [Cortes 2005]. Two groups have recently documented protective effects in vitro for homozygous pyruvate kinase deficiency, though epidemiologic support for this connection remains to be collected [Ayi 2008, Durand 2008]. Protection by blood-group-based polymorphisms without morphologic effects (eg, the Duffy and Gerbich systems) has also been documented [Chitnis 2008, Maier 2003].

Worldwide, malaria continues to exact a staggering price in morbidity and mortality. Up to 500 million people each year sustain acute infections, leading to 1 to 2 million deaths; in Africa, it is estimated that a child dies of malaria every 30 seconds [Min-Oo 2005]. The incidence of red blood cell abnormalities is similarly impressive, estimated at 1 in 6 humans worldwide [Mohandas 2008]. These observations, in combination with the experimental and epidemiologic evidence presented herein, suggest that malaria is the unseen force behind many of the anemia-causing mutations described in this chapter.

tS6.4 Epidemiologic & Experimental Evidence Implicating Malarial Pressure in the Evolution of RBC Disorders

Defect	Epidemiologic Studies	Experimental Studies
HgbS	RR = 0.45 for HgbAS vs HgbAA, all causes mortality, ages 2-26 months [Aidoo 2002] RR = 0.29 for HgbAS vs HgbAA, *P falciparum* infection [Willcox 1983b]	↑ susceptibility to phagocytosis at ring stage of RBC infection [Ayi 2004] ↓ expression of PfEMP-1, ↓ cytoadherance of infected RBCs [Cholera 2008]
HgbC	OR = 0.22 (severe), 0.14 (cerebral) malaria, HgbAC vs HgbAA [Agarwal 2000] 29% risk reduction HgbAC vs HgbAA; 93% reduction HgbCC vs AbAA, clinical malaria [Modiano 2001]	Impaired parasite maturation and membrane knob formation [Fairhurst 2003] ↓ expression of PfEMP-1, ↓ cytoadherance of infected RBCs [Fairhurst 2005]
HgbE	6.9 × greater risk of severe malaria complication in normals vs HgbAE [Hutagalung 1999]	Reduced *P falciparum* invasion of HgbAE RBCs [Chotivanich 2002] ↑ phagocytosis of infected RBCs [Yuthavong 1990]
α-thalassemia	RR = 0.40 and 0.66 for α-thalassemia+ heterozygotes, homozygotes vs normals, severe malaria [Allen 1997] OR = 0.74 for α-thalassemia+ heterozygotes vs normals, severe malaria [Mockenhaupt 2004] α-thalassemia associated with ↑ incidence of asymptomatic *P vivax* infection at young age, potentially providing later immunity [Williams 1996]	↑ IgG binding to RBCs [Luzzi 1991] ↓ CR1 surface expression, leading to ↓ rosette formation [Cockburn 2004] ↑ phagocytosis of infected RBCs [Yuthavong 1990]
β-thalassemia	RR = 0.41 to 0.45 for β-thalassemia trait vs normal, ages 1-9 yrs; significant parasite density [Willcox 1983a] RR = 0.49 for β-thalassemia heterozygotes vs normal, *P falciparum* infection [Willcox 1983b]	↑ susceptibility to phagocytosis at ring stage of RBC infection [Ayi 2004] ↑ IgG binding to RBCs [Luzzi 1991]
G6PD deficiency	Risk reduction of 46%-58% for male hemizygotes and female heterozygotes, severe malaria [Ruwende 1995]	↑ susceptibility to phagocytosis at ring stage of RBC infection [Cappadoro 1998] ↑ killing of parasites by H_2O_2 [Yuthavong 1990]

G6PD = glucose-6-phosphate dehydrogenase; IgG = immunoglobulin; OR = odds ratio; RBC = red blood cell; RR = relative risk;

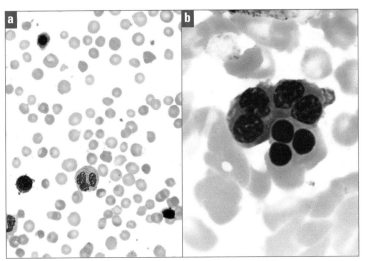

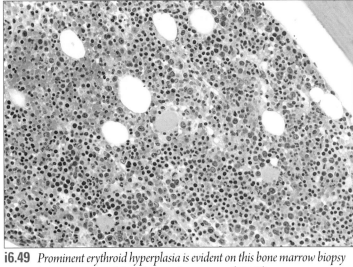

i6.48 *This composite illustrates the peripheral blood* **a** *and bone marrow aspirate smear* **b** *findings in a patient with hereditary spherocytosis. Note spherocytes in blood and frequent multinucleation of erythroid cells in the bone marrow, a consequence of the high proliferation rate. (Wright)*

i6.49 *Prominent erythroid hyperplasia is evident on this bone marrow biopsy section from a patient with hereditary spherocytosis. (H&E)*

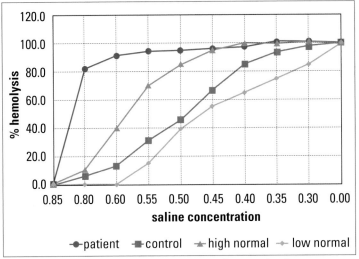

f6.1 *24-hour incubation graph showing increased osmotic fragility in patient compared with high normal and low normal control samples.*

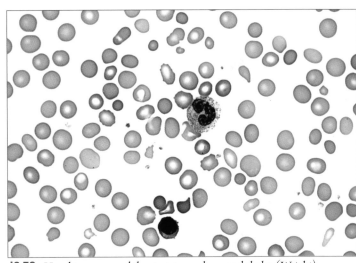

i6.50 *Hereditary pyropoikilocytosis in newborn male baby. (Wright)*

such as blood findings and laboratory test results [Mohandas 2008]. Morphologic review of peripheral blood smears for distinctive erythrocyte abnormalities and polychromasia, clinicopathologic correlations, and various laboratory tests are generally sufficient for the classification of constitutional (intrinsic) RBC membrane disorders. In addition to the identification of spherocytes on smears, tests for osmotic fragility or cryohemolysis also indicate spherocytosis **f6.1** [An 2008, Delaunay 2007]. Other less common membrane defects, such as hereditary elliptocytosis, can also be identified on blood smears. These constitutional membrane defects are apparent at birth and are characterized by bone marrow erythroid hyperplasia and sustained reticulocytosis **i6.48, i6.49**. Very rare neonates with hereditary elliptocytosis present with striking RBC fragmentation and extreme anisopoikilocytosis, termed hereditary pyropoikilocytosis **i6.50** [Costa 2005, Ramos 2007]. The extreme degree

of RBC fragmentation and microspherocytes interferes with accurate automated CBC testing [Ramos 2007]. In apparent de novo cases of hemolytic anemia, evaluation of parental blood may be useful to document a genetic disorder **i6.51**.

Assays of erythrocyte enzymes or oxidant stress tests for induction of Heinz bodies can be used to detect glucose-6-phosphate dehydrogenase deficiency, the most common type of hereditary RBC enzyme defect [Beutler 2008, Mason 2007]. Worldwide about 400 million people harbor X-linked mutations in the *G6PD* gene, which confer increased resistance to malarial infection (see **sidebar 6.4**) [Mason 2007]. The distinctive clinical picture of intermittent "fragmentation" type hemolysis associated with drug ingestion or other oxidant exposure can be useful in identifying these patients, though these patients are often otherwise asymptomatic [Mason 2007]. Other less common RBC enzyme defects, such as pyruvate kinase deficiency

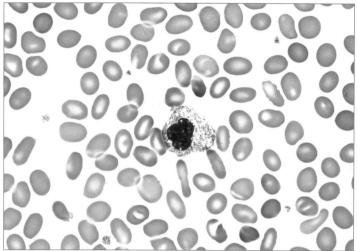

i6.51 *Blood smear from asymptomatic father of newborn baby with hereditary pyropoikilocytosis showing subclinical hereditary elliptocytosis in father (see i6.50). (Wright)*

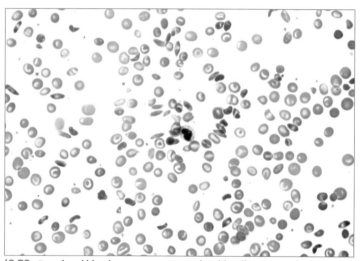

i6.52 *Peripheral blood smear in patient with sickle cell anemia in blast crisis showing numerous sickle cells and target cells. (Wright)*

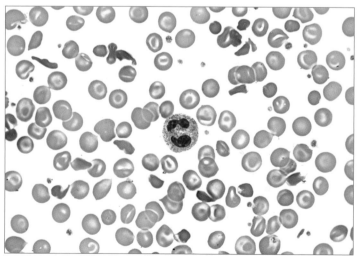

i6.53 *Peripheral blood smear from patient with sickle/thalassemia in crisis showing sickle cells and prominent erythrocyte targeting. (Wright)*

and phosphoglycerate kinase deficiency, are characterized by sustained survival defects with persistently elevated reticulocyte counts and bone marrow erythroid hyperplasia [Beutler 2007, Zanella 2007]. Erythrocyte morphology is generally unremarkable in these rarer types of RBC enzyme defects.

The prototypic hemoglobinopathy that causes lifelong hemolytic anemia is sickle cell anemia, an inherited disorder resulting from a point mutation in the β-globin chain gene (see **sidebar 6.3** p 105, **sidebar 6.4** p 116) [Kato 2007, Platt 2008]. Coinheritance of other hemoglobin mutations such as Hgb S/β⁺-thalassemia, SC disease, and Hgb SE may occur [Masiello 2007]. Homozygous hemoglobin S, sickle cell anemia, typically becomes clinically apparent after γ chain production is gradually replaced by β-chain production during the first few months of life, and is characterized by variably severe, lifelong sickling crises [Kato 2007, Platt 2008]. Even though hemoglobin electrophoresis is the most reliable way to detect hemoglobinopathies, the distinctive sickle cells in patients with sickle cell anemia, or hemoglobin crystals in patients with hemoglobin C can be useful findings on blood smears that prompt this testing. Other blood findings in sickle cell crises include neutrophilia and thrombocytosis. In addition to sickle cells, polychromasia and nucleated RBCs are present **i6.52**, **i6.53**.

Bone marrow examination is generally not necessary to establish the diagnosis of any of these intrinsic erythrocyte disorders. However, bone marrow studies may be useful in patients with a sudden reduction in erythrocyte production, as evidenced by a sharp decrease in the reticulocyte count in conjunction with an exacerbation of the anemia. Acute parvovirus infection, resulting in a transient red cell aplasia, is a relatively common cause of this type of abrupt decompensation in patients with chronic hemolytic anemias (see Chapters 8 and 33). Also, folate deficiency is postulated to cause a similar exacerbation of the underlying anemia. In addition, extensive bone marrow necrosis may occur in patients with sickle cell anemia; systemic embolization of this necrotic marrow, termed *acute chest syndrome*, is a major cause of morbidity and mortality in these patients **i6.54** [Dang 2005, Gladwin 2008, Medoff 2005].

Acquired Erythrocyte Survival Defects (Paroxysmal Nocturnal Hemoglobinuria)

The only recognized type of acquired clonal intrinsic erythrocyte survival disorder is PNH, a rare disorder characterized by complement-mediated RBC lysis [Brodsky 2008, Brodsky 2009, de Latour 2008, Hill 2007, Parker 2005]. Both RBC proliferation and survival defects occur in PNH; proliferation defects often eventually dominate, leading some authors to suggest that all cases of PNH are linked to underlying bone marrow failure **t6.4** p 95, **t6.10** p 115 [Hill 2007] (see Chapter 7 for a detailed discussion of PNH in bone marrow failure disorders). Although some

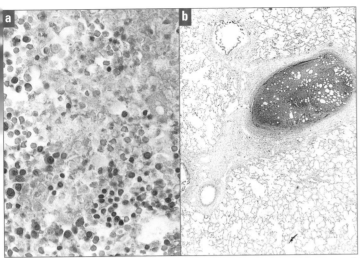

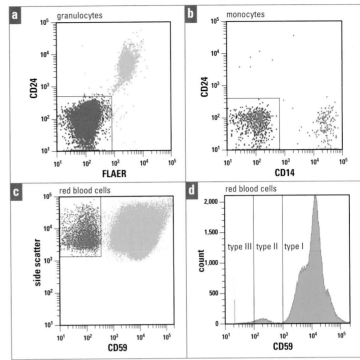

i6.54 *This composite illustrates extensive bone marrow necrosis* **a** *in a patient with sickle cell disease who developed fatal acute chest syndrome with extensive embolization of necrotic bone marrow in lungs* **b** *and multiple other organs. (H&E)*

f6.2 *Detection of paroxysmal nocturnal hemoglobinuria (PNH) using flow cytometry and fluorescently-labeled inactive aerolysin (FLAER). A major PNH clone is identified (red population) in the granulocytic* **a**, *monocytic* **b**, *and red blood cell (RBC) populations* **c**, **d**. *The PNH clone (red) shows typical loss of FLAER and CD24 compared to background monocytes (cyan) b. RBCs (red) show loss of CD59 c. A fraction of the PNH RBCs show reduced CD59 (type II RBCs, middle panel of* **d***) or absent CD59 (type III RBCs, left panel of* **d***).*

patients present with a de novo hemolytic picture of PNH, in other cases PNH occurs following profound bone marrow suppression or aplasia [de Latour 2008]. The susceptibility to complement-mediated lysis is secondary to multiple genetic abnormalities that result in defects in the biochemically complex protein anchor that holds many proteins onto cell membranes; all bone marrow lineages are affected [Brodsky 2008, 2009, Hill 2007, Parker 2005, Sutherland 2009]. In the absence of this functional anchoring protein, blood cells lack a variety of complement regulatory proteins; the consequence of this defect is increased susceptibility to complement-mediated destruction of mature cells, especially erythrocytes. PNH can be diagnosed by evaluating blood cells, for expression of the various glycosylphosphatidyl-inositol-linked complement regulatory proteins; most commonly assessed are CD55 and CD59 **f6.2** [Gupta 2007]. New PNH testing uses fluorescently-labeled inactive aerolysin (FLAER) to detect PNH clones in granulocytes and monocytes with increased sensitivity [Sutherland 2009].

Although the blood, bone marrow, and clinical findings are quite variable in patients with PNH, "classic" features include continuous low-grade hemolysis that is worse at night, secondary to physiologic mild nocturnal acidosis **i6.55**, **i6.56**. The bone marrow typically exhibits erythroid hyperplasia reflecting the dominant RBC survival defect in this subset of PNH patients, while the bone marrow may be markedly hypocellular in other patients **t6.11**, **i6.57**. Because patients developing this clonal hematopoietic disorder have an increased incidence of bone marrow failure and subsequent myelodysplasia or overt leukemia, some authors suggest that PNH is one manifestation of an aplasia/myelodysplasia spectrum (see Chapters 7 and 16) [Brodsky 2008, Hill 2007, Tiu 2007]. Humanized monoclonal antibody therapy directed against complement has resulted in reduction of hemolysis and improved RBC parameters in clinical trials [Brodsky 2009, Schubert 2008].

[6.4.6] **Other Extrinsic RBC Survival Defects**

All other types of acquired RBC survival defects are extrinsic, that is, they occur as a result of some abnormality of blood vessels or the environment within the blood that decreases erythrocyte survival time **t6.4** p 95, **t6.10**. Immune-mediated extrinsic erythrocyte defects may be autoimmune, alloimmune, isoimmune, or drug-related, and either cold or warm autoantibodies have been described [Arndt 2005, Davenport 2005, Packman 2008, Petz 2008, Semple 2005]. Autoimmune hemolytic anemias are classified as primary (idiopathic) or secondary, occurring in patients with various collagen vascular disorders, lymphoid neoplasms, mycoplasmal or viral infections, and solid tumors [Packman 2008]. Both autoimmune and alloimmune hemolytic anemia may occur in neonates. These 2 types of immune-mediated RBC destruction are secondary to maternal antibodies that are either directed exclusively toward fetal erythrocytes or attack both maternal and fetal erythrocytes **i6.58** [Glader 2005, Waldron 2005].

In patients with drug-mediated immune disorders, an antibody is produced that is directed to the drug or to the drug-RBC complex. Various categories of these drug-related immune hemolytic anemias have been delineated [Arndt 2005, Petz 2008]. In patients with all types of immune-mediated hemolysis, erythrocyte destruction is mediated by immunoglobulin and/or complement, and spherocytes may be

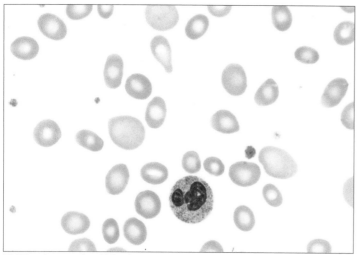

i6.55 *This peripheral blood smear is from a patient with paroxysmal nocturnal hemoglobinuria who had a 21-year history of dark urine in the morning. Note severe anemia, polychromasia, and abnormal erythrocytes. (Wright)*

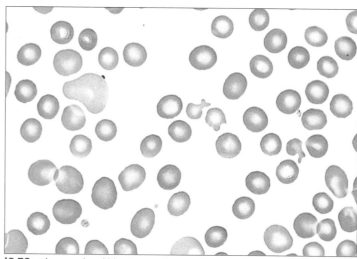

i6.56 *This peripheral blood smear from a patient with paroxysmal nocturnal hemoglobinuria illustrates an enlarged reticulocyte as well as unusually shaped erythrocyte fragments. (Wright) (courtesy C Leith, MD)*

t6.11 Paroxysmal Nocturnal Hemoglobinuria (PNH)

Mechanism of disease	Primary mechanism may be either production defect (most cases) or a survival defect (classic cases); intermediate forms common
Genetic defect	Acquired somatic mutation at stem cell level of *PIGA* gene that results in defective anchoring protein (GPI) in the membrane of blood cells
Hemolysis	Due to defect in GPI, complement regulating proteins are not appropriately bound to cell surface membranes, rendering erythrocytes susceptible to complement-mediated intravascular hemolysis
	Symptoms of intravascular hemolysis include hemoglobinuria (often in the morning), abdominal pain, dysphagia, thrombosis, and lethargy
Diagnosis	Flow cytometric immunophenotyping to assess for levels of GPI-associated proteins (CD55 and CD59) on the surface of neutrophils, monocytes, and erythrocytes
	CD59, complement inhibitory protein
	Recent flow cytometry techniques use FLAER to assess loss of PIGA proteins on neutrophils and monocytes **f6.2**
Disease associations	Acquired somatic mutation often follows aplastic episode
	Association with eventual development of myelodysplasia, acute myeloid leukemia, or overt aplastic anemia
	Increased incidence of thrombosis
Treatment	Terminal complement inhibitor therapy (humanized monoclonal antibody, Eculizumab) improves anemia by blocking complement-mediated hemolysis

FLAER = fluorescently-labeled inactive toxin **ae**rolysin; GPI = glycosylphosphatidyl-inositol; *PIGA* = phosphatidylinositol glycan complementation class A gene

References: [Brodsky 2008, 2009, de Latour 2008, Gupta 2007, Hill 2007, Olteanu 2006, Parker 2005, Schubert 2008, Sutherland 2009, Tiu 2007]

prominent. In cases of paroxysmal cold hemoglobinuria, the blood picture is unique in that, in addition to spherocytes and polychromasia, erythrophagocytosis by neutrophils and monocytes is often striking, the result of acute, severe intravascular hemolysis **i6.59** [Gertz 2007, Win 2005, 2008]. Agglutination is a prominent feature of cold agglutinin syndrome, but most patients with cold agglutinins do not experience significant hemolysis due to the low thermal range of the cold antibody [Petz 2008] **i6.60**. Bone marrow examination is generally required only if an unexpected complication occurs or if bone marrow examination is needed for the underlying disorder, such as a neoplasm.

One type of extrinsic RBC survival defect, termed *microangiopathic hemolytic anemia*, results from widespread endothelial damage or platelet/fibrin thrombi. Many conditions are linked to this type of erythrocyte fragmentation syndrome, including thrombotic thrombocytopenic purpura, hemolytic uremic syndrome, "march" hemoglobinuria, thermal injury, post-mitomycin C therapy, other drug treatments, toxin-producing infections, snake or spider venom, widespread dissemination of mucin-producing adenocarcinomas, human immunodeficiency virus (HIV)-1 infection, various obstetric complications, and turbulent blood flow (see Chapters 31 and 33) [Boyd 2009, Cataland 2007, Delvaeye 2009,

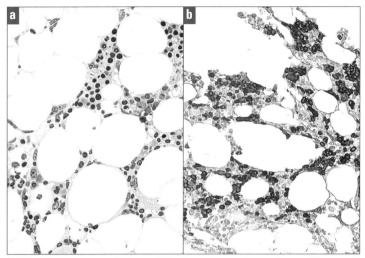

i6.57 *This composite of a hypocellular bone marrow biopsy from a 30-year-old woman with paroxysmal nocturnal hemoglobinuria reveals overall hypocellularity and relative erythroid hyperplasia* **a**, *which is highlighted by hemoglobin A staining* **b**. *(H&E, hemoglobin A) (courtesy C Leith, MD)*

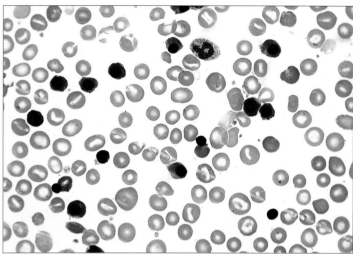

i6.58 *Peripheral blood smear from a newborn with hemolytic disease of the newborn with striking polychromasia and numerous nucleated red blood cells. (Wright)*

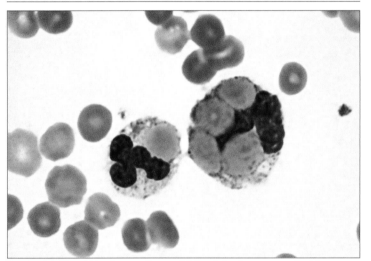

i6.59 *Peripheral blood smear from a child with fatal paroxysmal cold hemoglobinuria showing striking ingestion of red blood cells by monocytes and neutrophils. (Wright)*

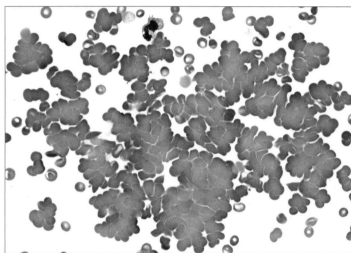

i6.60 *Peripheral blood smear showing striking red cell agglutination. (Wright)*

Eremina 2008, Fremeaux-Bacchi 2008, Mulliken 2004, Rock 2005]. Patients who develop some of these disorders, such as hemolytic uremic syndrome (HUS), may have underlying mutations in complement regulatory protein genes, rendering them more susceptible to developing HUS following infection or other inciting factors [Caprioli 2006]. Different mutations have been described in atypical HUS [Delvaeye 2009, Fang 2008, Fremeaux-Bacchi 2009]. Thrombotic thrombocytopenic purpura (TTP) is now recognized as an autoimmune disorder secondary to an acquired antibody inhibitor of ADAMTS13 (a disintegrin and metalloproteinase with thrombospondin type 1 motif, member 13) **sidebar 6.5** [Cataland 2007]. Congenital TTP has also been characterized by markedly reduced ADAMTS13 [Levy 2001].

In all of these microangiopathic disorders, the peripheral blood shows prominent fragmentation of erythrocytes and, depending on the duration of the anemia, reticulocytosis

may be present **i6.61**. Thrombocytopenia frequently accompanies these RBC abnormalities. Although bone marrow erythroid hyperplasia is an expected finding in all sustained fragmentation syndromes, bone marrow examination is not generally required in patients with microangiopathic hemolytic anemia. Even though earlier reports recommended bone marrow biopsy to assess for intravascular thrombi in patients with presumed TTP **i6.62**, bone marrow examination is not required to establish this diagnosis and should be restricted to those patients with other indications for this procedure.

Finally, blood loss is also considered a type of extrinsic survival defect. No distinctive erythrocyte findings occur in patients with acute blood loss unless microvascular abnormalities are also present; bone marrow examination is generally not necessary.

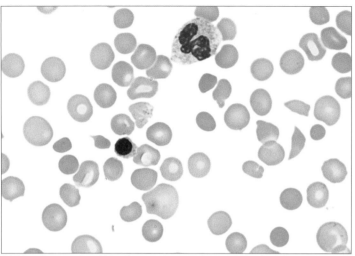

i6.61 *This peripheral blood smear shows striking red blood cell fragmentation, microspherocytes, and circulating normoblasts in a patient with thrombotic thrombocytopenic purpura. (Wright)*

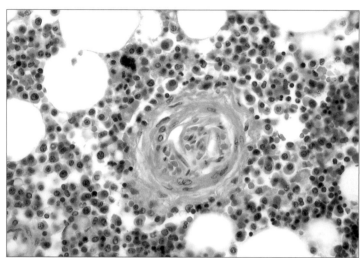

i6.62 *Bone marrow core biopsy showing intravascular thrombus in patient with thrombotic cytopenic purpura. (H&E)*

[6.5] Miscellaneous Causes of Anemia

Patients with copper deficiency, lead exposure, or arsenic exposure can develop anemias. Marked dyserythropoiesis with karyorrhexis and coarse basophilic stippling are seen in arsenic poisoning. Lead exposure is characterized by similar changes, but they may not be as dramatic [Eichner 1984].

In recent years, homeopathic zinc ingestion and excess denture adhesive use have resulted in an increased number of cases of zinc-induced copper deficiency [Rowin 2005, Sibley 2009, Willis 2005]. Copper deficiency, related either to zinc ingestion or other causes, produces a blood and bone marrow picture that mimics myelodysplasia [Gregg 2002, Harless 2006, Huff 2007, Kumar 2005]. A

[sidebar 6.5] Thrombotic Microangiopathies as Molecular Diseases

For many years following the initial descriptions of thrombotic thrombocytopenic purpura (TTP) (1924) and hemolytic uremic syndrome (HUS) (1955), the peripheral blood findings in cases of thrombotic microangiopathy were both dramatic and mysterious. It now appears that TTP and HUS, in fact following a pattern seen repeatedly in benign hematology, are common endpoints that may be reached through intrinsic constitutional mutations or secondary to extrinsic triggers.

TTP is diagnosed based on the pentad of thrombocytopenia, microangiopathic hemolytic anemia, neurologic symptoms and signs, renal compromise, and fever without other explanation; however, given the safety and efficacy of plasmapheresis, these criteria are more loosely applied in practice [Zheng 2008]. TTP is a disorder of the metalloproteinase ADAMTS13, which, under conditions of high shear, cleaves von Willebrand factor multimers into lower-molecular-weight components with relatively decreased thrombogenic potential. (A TTP-like picture may also arise independent of ADAMTS13 function, following direct endothelial damage). In most cases, TTP is caused by autoantibodies against ADAMTS13 [Studt 2003]. The autoantibodies are produced in various clinical settings, but genotype can influence

the process: the possession of HLA-DR53 is protective [Joseph 1994]. Approximately 50 different mutations have also been described in the *ADAMTS13* gene itself, producing the syndrome of familial TTP [Zheng 2008]. Importantly for diagnostic purposes, familial TTP manifests itself intermittently and, in approximately half of cases, only in adolescence or adulthood [Furlan 2001]. Affected individuals are usually compound heterozygotes for 2 separate mutations, and carriers show approximately 50% of normal ADAMTS13 levels without apparent physiologic consequence. The described mutations run the gamut from changes in critical cysteine residues to alterations in splice sites and frameshifts, affecting synthesis, secretion, or activity of the enzyme. Interestingly, a number of single nucleotide polymorphisms are also present which, on their own, have no direct impact of ADAMTS13 synthesis or function, but which, in the presence of certain mutations, modulate the severity of the defect [Plaimauer 2006].

Hemolytic uremic syndrome follows a similar acquired/constitutional dichotomy. Classical HUS arises in the setting of enteric infection by *E coli* O157:H7. Shiga toxins produced by this organism directly damage endothelial cells by inhibiting ribosomal RNA function, causing apoptosis, which exposes the thrombogenic

basement membrane [Tsai 2006, Zheng 2008]. However, approximately 5% to 10% of HUS cases were long-described as "atypical" HUS, in that no infection or diarrhea accompanied the onset of disease. It is now clear that many of these atypical HUS cases are directly attributable to inherited mutations affecting the function of complement. Mutations most frequently occur in genes encoding complement factor H and complement membrane cofactor protein (CD46), both of which inhibit C3b deposition on endothelial cells [Tsai 2006, Zheng 2008]. Mutations affecting these proteins therefore allow increased complement activity on endothelial surfaces, leading to damage and thrombotic microangiopathy.

Although the division of these entities into cases associated with mutations and those with extrinsic triggers is conceptually useful, this dichotomy fails to fully capture the complex interplay among genotype, environment, and phenotype. Although an individual may carry mutations associated with familial TTP, the disease may occur during childhood, adulthood, or not at all. Similarly, familial HUS mutations seem to confer only a variable predisposition to the disease. In both entities, second "hits" in the form of endothelial insult or generalized complement activation are likely required to produce clinical disease.

high index of suspicion is needed to recognize the distinctive blood and bone marrow profile of copper deficiency: anemia, neutropenia, vacuolated erythroblasts, vacuolated myeloblasts and promyelocytes, and variable numbers of ring sideroblasts **i6.63** [Willis 2005]. Diagnosis of copper deficiency is clinically important because of the significant myeloneuropathies that can occur in these patients [Kumar 2005, Rowin 2005].

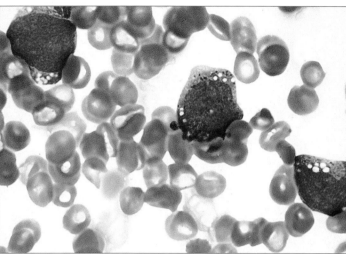

i6.63 *Bone marrow aspirate smear from patient with copper deficiency showing marked vacuolization of erythroid and granulocytic precursors. (Wright)*

[6.6] Age-Related Anemias

The incidences of these diverse types of constitutional and acquired anemias vary with patient age. For example, in neonates, hemorrhage and hemolysis (both survival defects) are the most likely causes of an anemia (see Chapters 30 and 31). Hemorrhage, sometimes inapparent, may be secondary to obstetric accidents, internal hemorrhage, fetomaternal hemorrhage, or twin-to-twin transfusion. Of the many possible causes of hemolysis in neonates, the most frequent include infections, disseminated intravascular coagulation, vascular lesions, and various maternal immune-mediated hemolytic processes. Although much less common, constitutional RBC enzyme defects and hereditary membrane defects also both produce a hemolytic anemia blood picture in neonates. In contrast, neonates with RBC proliferation defects such as Diamond-Blackfan anemia, congenital leukemia, or some congenital infections causing bone marrow suppression will demonstrate a reticulocytopenic anemia with normal erythrocyte morphologic characteristics [Downes 2006, Glader 2005, Lane 2005, Waldron 2005] (see Chapter 30 for more details).

In older children, iron deficiency is the most common cause of anemia. Other relatively common causes of anemia in children include anemia of chronic disease, bone marrow replacement disorders such as acute lymphoblastic leukemia, and hereditary RBC disorders such as thalassemias, sickle cell anemia, or hereditary spherocytosis.

In adults, iron deficiency is also the most common cause of anemia; anemia of chronic disease is also prevalent in this age group. In addition to bone marrow replacement by neoplasms or fibrosis, drug suppression of bone marrow or drug-mediated immune disorders are also fairly common causes of anemia in adults.

The assessment of an elderly patient for anemia is uniquely challenging because the definition of anemia versus normal age-related values is not clear cut. Based on the criterion of hemoglobin values of <13 g/dL (130 g/L) in men and <12 g/dL (120 g/L) in women, up to a quarter of elderly people are anemic (see Chapter 32) [Denny 2006, Eisenstaedt 2006, Guralnik 2004]. Anemia is more common in elderly blacks than whites [Denny 2006, Patel 2007]. In a significant proportion of these elderly patients a specific cause for the anemia cannot be determined [Ferrucci 2007, Guralnik 2004]. The most frequently determined causes of anemia in the elderly include nutritional deficiency (iron and folate), vitamin B_{12} deficiency, anemia of chronic disease, and anemia secondary to chronic renal failure [Artz 2004, Eisenstaedt 2006, Ferrucci 2007, Guralnik 2004]. Symptoms of vitamin B_{12} deficiency may be subtle in the elderly; causes of this deficiency vary, but malabsorption seems to be the predominant cause [Dharmarajan 2003].

[6.7] Diagnosis of Anemias

For straightforward, uncomplicated anemias, the diagnosis and assessment of dominant mechanism is often clear cut by blood smear review. For more complex anemias, bone marrow examination is necessary and the diagnostic interpretation is much more problematic, requiring that the pathologist provide substantially more information to clinicians to define the mechanism and possible etiology of the anemia **t6.12**.

[6.8] Clues and Caveats

1. In general, bone marrow examination is restricted to those patients whose anemia is "unexplained" after integration of clinical, hematologic, and laboratory findings, or to those patients in whom a bone marrow neoplasm (primary or secondary) is suspected.

2. Evaluation of bone marrow erythroid elements is necessary for the subclassification of CDAs, while bone marrow examination is not required for many other types of anemia.

3. Erythrocyte proliferation and maturation disorders are characterized by inappropriately low reticulocyte

t6.12 Components of Diagnostic Interpretation of Anemias*

Complete description of erythrocytes: eg, normocytic, macrocytic, hypochromic; uniformity, abnormal forms/inclusions

Peripheral blood evidence of erythrocyte production: eg, reticulocyte count, polychromasia, nucleated red blood cells

Other peripheral blood abnormalities; assess each lineage for qualitative and quantitative abnormalities

Bone marrow cellularity, bone, bone marrow stroma

Assessment of erythropoiesis: eg, relative or absolute erythroid hyperplasia

Assessment of erythroid maturation: intact or maturation failure, normal or dysplastic

Assessment of erythroid and storage iron

Assessment of morphologic features of all bone marrow lineages

By integration of clinical, laboratory, and hematologic parameters, provide judgment regarding:

the mechanism of the anemia (proliferation, maturation, or survival defect)
whether the anemia is constitutional vs acquired
exact etiology of the anemia, if apparent
recommendations for additional testing, if appropriate

*Interpretation much more abbreviated in straightforward cases

counts, while reticulocytosis is a feature of erythrocyte survival defects.

4. Erythroid or multilineage hypoplasia typifies the bone marrow picture in patients with congenital and most acquired erythrocyte proliferation disorders, while erythroid hyperplasia is characteristic of erythrocyte maturation and survival disorders.

5. Nutritional deficiencies (iron, vitamin B_{12}, and folate) all cause erythrocyte maturation defects. However, deficiencies of vitamin B_{12} and folate affect all proliferating cells, while the effects of iron deficiency are largely restricted to the erythroid lineage.

6. Concurrent iron deficiency can mask erythroid abnormalities in patients with megaloblastic anemia; granulocyte abnormalities persist.

7. Patients with megaloblastic anemia may have a normal MCV.

8. Florid megaloblastic anemia may mimic myelodysplasia with a paradoxical picture of blood cytopenias and hypercellular bone marrow; myeloblasts are not typically increased in megaloblastic anemia, and overall bone marrow architecture is intact (CD34 by immunoperoxidase may be useful in assessing blasts).

9. Numerous ring sideroblasts can be evident in the bone marrow in patients with clonal disorders (myelodysplasia and acute myeloid leukemia) as well as many

acquired nonclonal disorders primarily linked to drug/toxic exposures; rare constitutional sideroblastic anemias have also been described.

10. Secondary parvovirus infection can cause transient red cell aplasia in patients with chronic hemolytic anemias or constitutional maturation disorders such as severe thalassemias.

11. All intrinsic erythrocyte disorders are constitutional (evident at birth or shortly thereafter) except PNH, an *acquired* intrinsic RBC production/survival disorder resulting from an acquired somatic mutation at the hematopoietic stem cell level that results in defective anchoring proteins in the cell membrane.

12. PNH is a clonal hematopoietic disorder that is closely linked to aplastic episodes; evolution to either myelodysplasia or acute leukemia has been described in PNH.

13. PNH is most reliably diagnosed by flow cytometric analysis for decreased expression of a variety of GPI-associated complement regulatory surface membrane proteins such as CD55 and CD59.

14. Numerous disorders are linked to microangiopathic hemolytic anemia. Recent evidence suggests that TTP is an autoimmune disorder and that patients who develop HUS have mutations in several genes encoding complement regulatory protein.

15. Cytopenias, neurologic abnormalities, vacuoles in erythroid and granulocytic precursors, and ring sideroblasts are all features of copper deficiency which may be secondary to excess zinc intake.

16. Anemia is common in the elderly, more so in older black patients. The cause of anemia in the elderly is often indeterminate.

[6.9] References

Agarwal A, Guindo A, Cissoko Y, et al [2000] Hemoglobin C associated with protection from severe malaria in the Dogon of Mali, a West African population with a low prevalence of hemoglobin S. *Blood* 96:2358-2363.

Aidoo M, Terlouw DJ, Kolczak MS, et al [2002] Protective effects of the sickle cell gene against malaria morbidity and mortality. *Lancet* 359:1311-1312.

Allen SJ, O'Donnell A, Alexander ND, et al [1997] Alpha+-thalassemia protects children against disease caused by other infections as well as malaria. *Proc Natl Acad Sci USA* 94:14736-14741.

Aminoff M, Carter JE, Chadwick RB, et al [1999] Mutations in CUBN, encoding the intrinsic factor-vitamin B_{12} receptor, cubilin, cause hereditary megaloblastic anaemia 1. *Nat Genet* 21:309-313.

An X, Mohandas N [2008] Disorders of red cell membrane. *Br J Haematol* 141:367-375.

Andres E, Affenberger S, Zimmer J, et al [2006] Current hematological findings in cobalamin deficiency: a study of 201 consecutive patients with documented cobalamin deficiency. *Clin Lab Haematol* 28:50-56.

Andrews NC [2008] Forging a field: the golden age of iron biology. *Blood* 112:219-230.

Angeles Vazquez Lopez M, Molinos FL, Carmona ML, et al [2006] Serum transferrin receptor in children: usefulness for determining the nature of anemia in infection. *J Pediatr Hematol Oncol* 28:809-815.

Arndt PA, Garratty G [2005] The changing spectrum of drug-induced immune hemolytic anemia. *Semin Hematol* 42:137-144.

Artz AS, Fergusson D, Drinka PJ, et al [2004] Mechanisms of unexplained anemia in the nursing home. *J Am Geriatr Soc* 52:423-427.

Aslan D, Altay C [2003] Incidence of high erythrocyte count in infants and young children with iron deficiency anemia: re-evaluation of an old parameter. *J Pediatr Hematol Oncol* 25:303-306.

Ayi K, Min-Oo G, Serghides L, et al [2008] Pyruvate kinase deficiency and malaria. *N Engl J Med* 358:1805-1810.

Ayi K, Turrini F, Piga A, Arese P [2004] Enhanced phagocytosis of ring-parasitized mutant erythrocytes: a common mechanism that may explain protection against falciparum malaria in sickle trait and beta-thalassemia trait. *Blood* 104:3364-3371.

Baillie FJ, Morrison AE, Fergus I [2003] Soluble transferrin receptor: a discriminating assay for iron deficiency. *Clin Lab Haematol* 25:353-357.

Bain BJ [2005] Diagnosis from the blood smear. *N Engl J Med* 353:498-507.

Beaumont C, Delaunay J, Hetet G, et al [2006] Two new human DMT1 gene mutations in a patient with microcytic anemia, low ferritinemia, and liver iron overload. *Blood* 107:4168-4170.

Beutler E [2007] PGK deficiency. *Br J Haematol* 136:3-11.

Beutler E [2008] Glucose-6-phosphate dehydrogenase deficiency: a historical perspective. *Blood* 111:16-24.

Beutler E, Waalen J [2006] The definition of anemia: what is the lower limit of normal of the blood hemoglobin concentration? *Blood* 107:1747-1750.

Beutler E, West C [2005] Hematologic differences between African-Americans and whites: the roles of iron deficiency and alpha-thalassemia on hemoglobin levels and mean corpuscular volume. *Blood* 106:740-745.

Boyd SD, Mobley BC, Regula DP, Arber DA [2009] Features of hemolysis due to *Clostridium perfringens* infection. *Int J Lab Hematol* 31:364-367.

Brodsky RA [2008] Advances in the diagnosis and therapy of paroxysmal nocturnal hemoglobinuria. *Blood Rev* 22:65-74.

Brodsky RA [2009] How I treat paroxysmal nocturnal hemoglobinuria. *Blood* 113:6522-6527.

Buttarello M, Bulian P, Farina G, et al [2002] Five fully automated methods for performing immature reticulocyte fraction: comparison in diagnosis of bone marrow aplasia. *Am J Clin Pathol* 117:871-879.

Calis JC, Phiri KS, Faragher EB, et al [2008] Severe anemia in Malawian children. *N Engl J Med* 358:888-899.

Camaschella C [2008] Recent advances in the understanding of inherited sideroblastic anaemia. *Br J Haematol* 143:27-38.

Camaschella C [2009] Hereditary sideroblastic anemias: pathophysiology, diagnosis, and treatment. *Semin Hematol* 46:371-377.

Cappadoro M, Giribaldi G, O'Brien E, et al [1998] Early phagocytosis of glucose-6-phosphate dehydrogenase (G6PD)-deficient erythrocytes parasitized by *Plasmodium falciparum* may explain malaria protection in G6PD deficiency. *Blood* 92:2527-2534.

Caprioli J, Noris M, Brioschi S, et al [2006] Genetics of HUS: the impact of MCP, CFH, and IF mutations on clinical presentation, response to treatment, and outcome. *Blood* 108:1267-1279.

Carmel R [2008a] How I treat cobalamin (vitamin B_{12}) deficiency. *Blood* 112:2214-2221.

Carmel R [2008b] Nutritional anemias and the elderly. *Semin Hematol* 45:225-234.

Carmel R [2009] Megaloblastic anemias: disorders of impaired DNA synthesis. In: Greer JP, Foerster J, Rodgers G, et al, eds [2009] *Wintrobe's Clinical Hematology.* 12th ed: Lippincott Williams & Wilkins; 1143-1172.

Carpenter SL, Zimmerman SA, Ware RE [2004] Acute parvovirus B19 infection mimicking congenital dyserythropoietic anemia. *J Pediatr Hematol Oncol* 26:133-135.

Cataland SR, Jin M, Lin S, et al [2007] Cyclosporin and plasma exchange in thrombotic thrombocytopenic purpura: long-term follow-up with serial analysis of ADAMTS13 activity. *Br J Haematol* 139:486-493.

Chan CW, Liu SY, Kho CS, et al [2007] Diagnostic clues to megaloblastic anaemia without macrocytosis. *Int J Lab Hematol* 29:163-171.

Chasis JA, Mohandas N [2008] Erythroblastic islands: niches for erythropoiesis. *Blood* 112:470-478.

Chen JJ [2007] Regulation of protein synthesis by the heme-regulated eIF2alpha kinase: relevance to anemias. *Blood* 109:2693-2699.

Cheng CK, Chan J, Cembrowski GS, van Assendelft OW [2004] Complete blood count reference interval diagrams derived from NHANES III: stratification by age, sex, and race. *Lab Hematol* 10:42-53.

Chitnis CE, Sharma A [2008] Targeting the *Plasmodium vivax* Duffy-binding protein. *Trends Parasitol* 24:29-34.

Cholera R, Brittain NJ, Gillrie MR, et al [2008] Impaired cytoadherence of *Plasmodium falciparum*-infected erythrocytes containing sickle hemoglobin. *Proc Natl Acad Sci USA* 105:991-996.

Chotivanich K, Udomsangpetch R, Pattanapanyasat K, et al [2002] Hemoglobin E: a balanced polymorphism protective against high parasitemias and thus severe *P falciparum* malaria. *Blood* 100:1172-1176.

Cockburn IA, Mackinnon MJ, O'Donnell A, et al [2004] A human complement receptor 1 polymorphism that reduces *Plasmodium falciparum* rosetting confers protection against severe malaria. *Proc Natl Acad Sci USA* 101:272-277.

Cooke BM, Mohandas N, Coppel RL [2004] Malaria and the red blood cell membrane. *Semin Hematol* 41:173-188.

Cortes A, Mellombo M, Mgone CS, et al [2005] Adhesion of *Plasmodium falciparum*-infected red blood cells to CD36 under flow is enhanced by the cerebral malaria-protective trait southeast Asian ovalocytosis. *Mol Biochem Parasitol* 142:252-257.

Costa DB, Lozovatsky L, Gallagher PG, Forget BG [2005] A novel splicing mutation of the alpha-spectrin gene in the original hereditary pyropoikilocytosis kindred. *Blood* 106:4367-4369.

D'Souza E, Sawant PM, Nadkarni AH, et al [2008] Evaluation of the use of monoclonal antibodies and nested PCR for noninvasive prenatal diagnosis of hemoglobinopathies in India. *Am J Clin Pathol* 130:202-209.

Dallalio G, Law E, Means RT, Jr [2006] Hepcidin inhibits in vitro erythroid colony formation at reduced erythropoietin concentrations. *Blood* 107:2702-2704.

Dang NC, Johnson C, Eslami-Farsani M, Haywood LJ [2005] Bone marrow embolism in sickle cell disease: a review. *Am J Hematol* 79:61-67.

Danise P, Maconi M, Morelli G, et al [2008] Reference limits and behaviour of serum transferrin receptor in children 6-10 years of age. *Int J Lab Hematol* 30:306-311.

Davenport RD [2005] Pathophysiology of hemolytic transfusion reactions. *Semin Hematol* 42:165-168.

de Alarcon P, Werner E [2005] Normal values and laboratory methods. In: de Alarcon P, Werner E, eds. *Neonatal Hematology.* Cambridge: Cambridge University; 406-430.

de Latour RP, Mary JY, Salanoubat C, et al [2008] Paroxysmal nocturnal hemoglobinuria: natural history of disease subcategories. *Blood* 112:3099-3106.

Delaunay J [2007] The molecular basis of hereditary red cell membrane disorders. *Blood Rev* 21:1-20.

Delvaeye M, Noris M, De Vriese A, et al [2009] Thrombomodulin mutations in atypical hemolytic-uremic syndrome. *N Engl J Med* 361:345-357.

Denny SD, Kuchibhatla MN, Cohen HJ [2006] Impact of anemia on mortality, cognition, and function in community-dwelling elderly. *Am J Med* 119:327-334.

Dgany O, Avidan N, Delaunay J, et al [2002] Congenital dyserythropoietic anemia type I is caused by mutations in codanin-1. *Am J Hum Genet* 71:1467-1474.

Dharmarajan TS, Adiga GU, Norkus EP [2003] Vitamin B_{12} deficiency. Recognizing subtle symptoms in older adults. *Geriatrics* 58:30-34, 37-38.

Dhermy D, Schrevel J, Lecomte MC [2007] Spectrin-based skeleton in red blood cells and malaria. *Curr Opin Hematol* 14:198-202.

Diaz GA, Banikazemi M, Oishi K, et al [1999] Mutations in a new gene encoding a thiamine transporter cause thiamine-responsive megaloblastic anaemia syndrome. *Nat Genet* 22:309-312.

Dokal I, Vulliamy T [2008] Inherited aplastic anaemias/bone marrow failure syndromes. *Blood Rev* 22:141-153.

Downes K, Sarode R [2006] Hemolytic disease of the fetus and newborn caused by ABO, Rhesus, and other blood group alloantibodies. In: Bick R, Frenkel E, Baker W, Sarode R, eds. *Hematological Complications in Obstetrics, Pregnancy, and Gynecology* Cambridge: Cambridge University; 103-121.

Durand PM, Coetzer TL [2008] Pyruvate kinase deficiency protects against malaria in humans. *Haematologica* 93:939-940.

Eichner ER [1984] Erythroid karyorrhexis in the peripheral blood smear in severe arsenic poisoning: a comparison with lead poisoning. *Am J Clin Pathol* 81:533-537.

Eisenstaedt R, Penninx BW, Woodman RC [2006] Anemia in the elderly: current understanding and emerging concepts. *Blood Rev* 20:213-226.

Eremina V, Jefferson JA, Kowalewska J, et al [2008] VEGF inhibition and renal thrombotic microangiopathy. *N Engl J Med* 358:1129-1136.

Fairhurst RM, Baruch DI, Brittain NJ, et al [2005] Abnormal display of PfEMP-1 on erythrocytes carrying haemoglobin C may protect against malaria. *Nature* 435:1117-1121.

Fairhurst RM, Fujioka H, Hayton K, et al [2003] Aberrant development of *Plasmodium falciparum* in hemoglobin CC red cells: implications for the malaria protective effect of the homozygous state. *Blood* 101:3309-3315.

Fang CJ, Fremeaux-Bacchi V, Liszewski MK, et al [2008] Membrane cofactor protein mutations in atypical hemolytic uremic syndrome (aHUS), fatal Stx-HUS, C3 glomerulonephritis, and the HELLP syndrome. *Blood* 111:624-632.

Ferrucci L, Guralnik JM, Bandinelli S, et al [2007] Unexplained anaemia in older persons is characterised by low erythropoietin and low levels of pro-inflammatory markers. *Br J Haematol* 136:849-855.

Finsterer J [2007] Hematological manifestations of primary mitochondrial disorders. *Acta Haematol* 118:88-98.

Fleming JC, Tartaglini E, Steinkamp MP, et al [1999] The gene mutated in thiamine-responsive anaemia with diabetes and deafness (TRMA) encodes a functional thiamine transporter. *Nat Genet* 22:305-308.

Flint J, Harding RM, Clegg JB, Boyce AJ [1993] Why are some genetic diseases common? Distinguishing selection from other processes by molecular analysis of globin gene variants. *Hum Genet* 91:91-117.

Foucar K, Viswanatha D, Wilson C [2008] Non-neoplastic erythroid lineage disorders. In: King D, Gardner W, Sobin L, et al, eds [2008] *Non-Neoplastic Disorders of Bone Marrow (AFIP fascicle).* Washington, DC: American Registry of Pathology; 75-124.

Foucar K [2010a] Anemia of chronic disease and normochromic, normocytic non-hemolytic anemias In: Kjeldsberg C, ed. *Practical Diagnosis of Hematologic Disorders.* 5th ed. Chicago: ASCP.

Foucar K [2010b] Megaloblastic anemia In: Kjeldsberg C, ed. *Practical Diagnosis of Hematologic Disorders.* 5th ed. Chicago: ASCP.

Fremeaux-Bacchi V, Miller EC, Liszewski MK, et al [2008] Mutations in complement C3 predispose to development of atypical hemolytic uremic syndrome. *Blood* 112:4948-4952.

Furlan M, Lammle B [2001] Aetiology and pathogenesis of thrombotic thrombocytopenic purpura and haemolytic uraemic syndrome: the role of von Willebrand factor-cleaving protease. *Best Pract Res Clin Haematol* 14:437-454.

Fyfe J, Madsen M, Hojrup P, et al [2004] The functional cobalamin (vitamin B_{12})—intrinsic factor receptor is a novel complex of cubilin and amnionless. *Blood* 103:1573-1579.

Gaetani M, Mootien S, Harper S, et al [2008] Structural and functional effects of hereditary hemolytic anemia-associated point mutations in the alpha spectrin tetramer site. *Blood* 111:5712-5720.

Gasparini P, Miraglia del Giudice E, Delaunay J, et al [1997] Localization of the congenital dyserythropoietic anemia II locus to chromosome 20q11.2 by genomewide search. *Am J Hum Genet* 61:1112-1116.

Gazda HT, Sieff CA [2006] Recent insights into the pathogenesis of Diamond-Blackfan anaemia. *Br J Haematol* 135:149-157.

Gertz MA [2007] Management of cold haemolytic syndrome. *Br J Haematol* 138:422-429.

Glader B, Allen G [2005] Neonatal hemolysis. In: de Alarcon P, Werner E, eds. *Neonatal Hematology* Cambridge: Cambridge University Press; 132-162.

Gladwin MT, Vichinsky E [2008] Pulmonary complications of sickle cell disease. *N Engl J Med* 359:2254-2265.

Grasbeck R [2006] Imerslund-Grasbeck syndrome (selective vitamin B_{12} malabsorption with proteinuria). *Orphanet J Rare Dis* 1:17.

Green R [2005] Unreliability of current assays to detect cobalamin deficiency: "Nothing gold can stay." *Blood* 105:910.

Gregg XT, Reddy V, Prchal JT [2002] Copper deficiency masquerading as myelodysplastic syndrome. *Blood* 100:1493-1495.

Gupta R, Pandey P, Choudhry R, et al [2007] A prospective comparison of 4 techniques for diagnosis of paroxysmal nocturnal hemoglobinuria. *Int J Lab Hematol* 29:119-126.

Guralnik JM, Eisenstaedt RS, Ferrucci L, et al [2004] Prevalence of anemia in persons 65 years and older in the United States: Evidence for a high rate of unexplained anemia. *Blood* 104:2263-2268.

Harless W, Crowell E, Abraham J [2006] Anemia and neutropenia associated with copper deficiency of unclear etiology. *Am J Hematol* 81:546-549.

Harrington AM, Ward PC, Kroft SH [2008] Iron deficiency anemia, beta-thalassemia minor, and anemia of chronic disease: a morphologic reappraisal. *Am J Clin Pathol* 129:466-471.

Heimpel H, Anselstetter V, Chrobak L, et al [2003] Congenital dyserythropoietic anemia type II: Epidemiology, clinical appearance, and prognosis based on long-term observation. *Blood* 102:4576-4581.

Heimpel H, Schwarz K, Ebnother M, et al [2006] Congenital dyserythropoietic anemia type I (CDA I): Molecular genetics, clinical appearance, and prognosis based on long-term observation. *Blood* 107:334-340.

Hershko C, Ronson A, Souroujon M, et al [2006] Variable hematologic presentation of autoimmune gastritis: age-related progression from iron deficiency to cobalamin depletion. *Blood* 107:1673-1679.

Hershko C, Skikne B [2009] Pathogenesis and management of iron deficiency anemia: emerging role of celiac disease, *Helicobacter pylori*, and autoimmune gastritis. *Semin Hematol* 46:339-350.

Higgs DR, Garrick D, Anguita E, et al [2005] Understanding alpha-globin gene regulation: aiming to improve the management of thalassemia. *Ann N Y Acad Sci* 1054:92-102.

Higgs DR, Wood WG [2008] Long-range regulation of alpha globin gene expression during erythropoiesis. *Curr Opin Hematol* 15:176-183.

Hill A, Richards SJ, Hillmen P [2007] Recent developments in the understanding and management of paroxysmal nocturnal haemoglobinuria. *Br J Haematol* 137:181-192.

Holme SA, Worwood M, Anstey AV, et al [2007] Erythropoiesis and iron metabolism in dominant erythropoietic protoporphyria. *Blood* 110:4108-4110.

Huff JD, Keung YK, Thakuri M, et al [2007] Copper deficiency causes reversible myelodysplasia. *Am J Hematol* 82:625-630.

Hughes JR, Cheng JF, Ventress N, et al [2005] Annotation of cis-regulatory elements by identification, subclassification, and functional assessment of multispecies conserved sequences. *Proc Natl Acad Sci USA* 102:9830-9835.

Hutagalung R, Wilairatana P, Looareesuwan S, et al [1999] Influence of hemoglobin E trait on the severity of Falciparum malaria. *J Infect Dis* 179:283-286.

Iolascon A, d'Apolito M, Servedio V, et al [2006] Microcytic anemia and hepatic iron overload in a child with compound heterozygous mutations in DMT1 (SCL11A2). *Blood* 107:349-354.

Ivory K, Sarria B, Fairweather-Tait SJ, Hughes DA [2007] Reticulated platelets interfere with flow cytometric reticulocyte counts. *Int J Lab Hematol* 29:352-360.

Jebnoun S, Kacem S, Mokrani CH, et al [2001] A family study of congenital malabsorption of folate. *J Inherit Metab Dis* 24:749-750.

Joseph G, Smith KJ, Hadley TJ, et al [1994] HLA-DR53 protects against thrombotic thrombocytopenic purpura/adult hemolytic uremic syndrome. *Am J Hematol* 47:189-193.

Katar S, Nuri Ozbek M, Yaramis A, Ecer S [2006] Nutritional megaloblastic anemia in young Turkish children is associated with vitamin B-12 deficiency and psychomotor retardation. *J Pediatr Hematol Oncol* 28:559-562.

Kato GJ, Gladwin MT, Steinberg MH [2007] Deconstructing sickle cell disease: reappraisal of the role of hemolysis in the development of clinical subphenotypes. *Blood Rev* 21:37-47.

Kumar N, Elliott MA, Hoyer JD, et al [2005] "Myelodysplasia," myeloneuropathy, and copper deficiency. *Mayo Clin Proc* 80:943-946.

Labay V, Raz T, Baron D, et al [1999] Mutations in SLC19A2 cause thiamine-responsive megaloblastic anaemia associated with diabetes mellitus and deafness. *Nat Genet* 22:300-304.

Lane P [2005] Neonatal screening for hemoglobinopathies. In: de Alarcon P, Werner E, eds. *Neonatal Hematology* Cambridge: Cambridge University; 163-170.

Lanzara C, Ficarella R, Totaro A, et al [2003] Congenital dyserythropoietic anemia type II: Exclusion of 7 candidate genes. *Blood Cells Mol Dis* 30:22-29.

Latvala J, Parkkila S, Niemela O [2004] Excess alcohol consumption is common in patients with cytopenia: studies in blood and bone marrow cells. *Alcohol Clin Exp Res* 28:619-624.

Lavelle D, Vaitkus K, Hankewych M, et al [2006] Developmental changes in DNA methylation and covalent histone modifications of chromatin associated with the epsilon-, gamma-, and beta-globin gene promoters in Papio anubis. *Blood Cells Mol Dis* 36:269-278.

Levy GG, Nichols WC, Lian EC, et al [2001] Mutations in a member of the ADAMTS gene family cause thrombotic thrombocytopenic purpura. *Nature* 413:488-494.

Lew VL, Daw N, Etzion Z, et al [2007] Effects of age-dependent membrane transport changes on the homeostasis of senescent human red blood cells. *Blood* 110:1334-1342.

Lewis G, Wise MP, Poynton C, Godkin A [2007] A case of persistent anemia and alcohol abuse. *Nat Clin Pract Gastroenterol Hepatol* 4:521-526.

Libani IV, Guy EC, Melchiori L, et al [2008] Decreased differentiation of erythroid cells exacerbates ineffective erythropoiesis in beta-thalassemia. *Blood* 112:875-885.

Lind L, Sandstrom H, Wahlin A, et al [1995] Localization of the gene for congenital dyserythropoietic anemia type III, CDAN3, to chromosome 15q21-q25. *Hum Mol Genet* 4:109-112.

Lipton JM [2006] Diamond blackfan anemia: new paradigms for a "not so pure" inherited red cell aplasia. *Semin Hematol* 43:167-177.

Luzzi GA, Merry AH, Newbold CI, et al [1991] Surface antigen expression on *Plasmodium falciparum*-infected erythrocytes is modified in alpha- and beta-thalassemia. *J Exp Med* 173:785-791.

Means R, Glader B. Anemia: general considerations [2009] In: Greer J, Foerster J, Rodgers G, et al, eds [2009] *Wintrobe's Clinical Hematology.* 12th ed. Philadelphia: Lippincott Williams & Wilkins; 779-809.

Maier AG, Duraisingh MT, Reeder JC, et al [2003] *Plasmodium falciparum* erythrocyte invasion through glycophorin C and selection for Gerbich negativity in human populations. *Nat Med* 9:87-92.

Masiello D, Heeney MM, Adewoye AH, et al [2007] Hemoglobin SE disease: a concise review. *Am J Hematol* 82:643-649.

Mason PJ, Bautista JM, Gilsanz F [2007] G6PD deficiency: the genotype-phenotype association. *Blood Rev* 21:267-283.

Medoff BD, Shepard JA, Smith RN, Kratz A [2005] Case records of the Massachusetts General Hospital. Case 17-2005. A 22-year-old woman with back and leg pain and respiratory failure. *N Engl J Med* 352:2425-2434.

Menzel S, Garner C, Gut I, et al [2007] A QTL influencing F cell production maps to a gene encoding a zinc-finger protein on chromosome 2p15. *Nat Genet* 39:1197-1199.

Min SH, Oh SY, Karp GI, et al [2008] The clinical course and genetic defect in the PCFT gene in a 27-year-old woman with hereditary folate malabsorption. *J Pediatr* 153:435-437.

Min-Oo G, Gros P [2005] Erythrocyte variants and the nature of their malaria protective effect. *Cell Microbiol* 7:753-763.

Mockenhaupt FP, Ehrhardt S, Gellert S, et al [2004] Alpha(+)-thalassemia protects African children from severe malaria. *Blood* 104:2003-2006.

Modiano D, Luoni G, Sirima BS, et al [2001] Haemoglobin C protects against clinical *Plasmodium falciparum* malaria. *Nature* 414:305-308.

Mohandas N, Gallagher PG [2008] Red cell membrane: past, present, and future. *Blood* 112:3939-3948.

Moridani M, Ben-Poorat S [2006] Laboratory investigation of vitamin B_{12} deficiency. *Labmedicine* 37:166-174.

Moy RJ [2006] Prevalence, consequences and prevention of childhood nutritional iron deficiency: a child public health perspective. *Clin Lab Haematol* 28:291-298.

Mulliken JB, Anupindi S, Ezekowitz RA, Mihm MC, Jr [2004] Case records of the Massachusetts General Hospital. Weekly clinicopathological exercises. Case 13-2004. A newborn girl with a large cutaneous lesion, thrombocytopenia, and anemia. *N Engl J Med* 350:1764-1775.

Nakai Y, Inoue K, Abe N, et al [2007] Functional characterization of human proton-coupled folate transporter/heme carrier protein 1 heterologously expressed in mammalian cells as a folate transporter. *J Pharmacol Exp Ther* 322:469-476.

Natelson EA [2007] Benzene exposure and refractory sideroblastic erythropoiesis: is there an association? *Am J Med Sci* 334:356-360.

Nearman ZP, Szpurka H, Serio B, et al [2007] Hemochromatosis-associated gene mutations in patients with myelodysplastic syndromes with refractory anemia with ringed sideroblasts. *Am J Hematol* 82:1076-1079.

Neufeld EJ, Mandel H, Raz T, et al [1997] Localization of the gene for thiamine-responsive megaloblastic anemia syndrome, on the long arm of chromosome 1, by homozygosity mapping. *Am J Hum Genet* 61:1335-1341.

Obeid R, Morkbak AL, Munz W, et al [2006] The cobalamin-binding proteins transcobalamin and haptocorrin in maternal and cord blood sera at birth. *Clin Chem* 52:263-269.

Olteanu H, Karandikar NJ, McKenna RW, Xu Y [2006] Differential usefulness of various markers in the flow cytometric detection of paroxysmal nocturnal hemoglobinuria in blood and bone marrow. *Am J Clin Pathol* 126:781-788.

Packman CH [2008] Hemolytic anemia due to warm autoantibodies. *Blood Rev* 22:17-31.

Parker C, Omine M, Richards S, et al [2005] Diagnosis and management of paroxysmal nocturnal hemoglobinuria. *Blood* 106:3699-3709.

Patel KV, Harris TB, Faulhaber M, et al [2007] Racial variation in the relationship of anemia with mortality and mobility disability among older adults. *Blood* 109:4663-4670.

Pauling L, Itano HA, et al [1949] Sickle cell anemia, a molecular disease. *Science* 109:443.

Perkins SL [2004] Pediatric red cell disorders and pure red cell aplasia. *Am J Clin Pathol* 122 Suppl:S70-86.

Petz LD [2008] Cold antibody autoimmune hemolytic anemias. *Blood Rev* 22:1-15.

Phillips JD, Steensma DP, Pulsipher MA, et al [2007] Congenital erythropoietic porphyria due to a mutation in GATA1: The first trans-acting mutation causative for a human porphyria. *Blood* 109:2618-2621.

Plaimauer B, Fuhrmann J, Mohr G, et al [2006] Modulation of ADAMTS13 secretion and specific activity by a combination of common amino acid polymorphisms and a missense mutation. *Blood* 107:118-125.

Platt OS [2008] Hydroxyurea for the treatment of sickle cell anemia. *N Engl J Med* 358:1362-1369.

Quadros EV [2010] Advances in the understanding of cobalamin assimilation and metabolism. *Br J Haematol* 148:195-204.

Quek L, Thein SL [2007] Molecular therapies in beta-thalassaemia. *Br J Haematol* 136:353-365.

Ramos MC, Schafernak KT, Peterson LC [2007] Hereditary pyropoikilocytosis: a rare but potentially severe form of congenital hemolytic anemia. *J Pediatr Hematol Oncol* 29:128-129.

Raz T, Barrett T, Szargel R, et al [1998] Refined mapping of the gene for thiamine-responsive megaloblastic anemia syndrome and evidence for genetic homogeneity. *Hum Genet* 103:455-461.

Renella R, Wood WG [2009] The congenital dyserythropoietic anemias. *Hematol Oncol Clin North Am* 23:283-306.

Repapinou Z, Karababa P, Boussiou M, et al [2007] An improved method for the diagnostic approach of alpha+-thalassaemia. *Int J Lab Hematol* 29:45-51.

Rhodes MM, Kopsombut P, Bondurant MC, et al [2008] Adherence to macrophages in erythroblastic islands enhances erythroblast proliferation and increases erythrocyte production by a different mechanism than erythropoietin. *Blood* 111:1700-1708.

Robins EB, Blum S [2007] Hematologic reference values for African American children and adolescents. *Am J Hematol* 82:611-614.

Rock G, Clark W, Sternbach M, et al [2005] Haemolytic uraemic syndrome is an immune-mediated disease: role of anti-CD36 antibodies. *Br J Haematol* 131:247-252.

Rowin J, Lewis SL [2005] Copper deficiency myeloneuropathy and pancytopenia secondary to overuse of zinc supplementation. *J Neurol Neurosurg Psychiatry* 76:750-751.

Rund D, Rachmilewitz E [2005] Beta-thalassemia. *N Engl J Med* 353:1135-1146.

Ruwende C, Khoo SC, Snow RW, et al [1995] Natural selection of hemi- and heterozygotes for G6PD deficiency in Africa by resistance to severe malaria. *Nature* 376:246-249.

Sankaran VG, Menne TF, Xu J, et al [2008] Human fetal hemoglobin expression is regulated by the developmental stage-specific repressor BCL11A. *Science*.

Sassa S [2006] Modern diagnosis and management of the porphyrias. *Br J Haematol* 135:281-292.

Saunthararajah Y, Molokie R, Saraf S, et al [2008] Clinical effectiveness of decitabine in severe sickle cell disease. *Br J Haematol* 141:126-129.

Sawada K, Fujishima N, Hirokawa M [2008] Acquired pure red cell aplasia: updated review of treatment. *Br J Haematol* 142:505-514.

Schubert J, Hillmen P, Roth A, et al [2008] Eculizumab, a terminal complement inhibitor, improves anaemia in patients with paroxysmal nocturnal haemoglobinuria. *Br J Haematol* 142:263-272.

Schwarzer E, Skorokhod OA, Barrera V, Arese P [2008] Hemozoin and the human monocyte—a brief review of their interactions. *Parassitologia* 50:143-145.

Semple JW, Freedman J [2005] Autoimmune pathogenesis and autoimmune hemolytic anemia. *Semin Hematol* 42:122-130.

Shalev H, Kapelushnik J, Moser A, et al [2004] A comprehensive study of the neonatal manifestations of congenital dyserythropoietic anemia type I. *J Pediatr Hematol Oncol* 26:746-748.

Sibley A, Maddox AM [2009] Myelodysplasia and copper deficiency induces by denture paste. *Am J Hematol* 84:612.

Sirdah M, Tarazi I, Al Najjar E, Al Haddad R [2008] Evaluation of the diagnostic reliability of different RBC indices and formulas in the differentiation of the beta-thalassaemia minor from iron deficiency in Palestinian population. *Int J Lab Hematol* 30:324-330.

Skeppner G, Kreuger A, Elinder G [2002] Transient erythroblastopenia of childhood: prospective study of 10 patients with special reference to viral infections. *J Pediatr Hematol Oncol* 24:294-298.

So CC, Song YQ, Tsang ST, et al [2008] The HBS1L-MYB intergenic region on chromosome 6q23 is a quantitative trait locus controlling fetal haemoglobin level in carriers of beta-thalassaemia. *J Med Genet* 45:745-751.

Solomon LR [2005] Cobalamin-responsive disorders in the ambulatory care setting: unreliability of cobalamin, methylmalonic acid, and homocysteine testing. *Blood* 105:978-985.

Solomon LR [2007] Disorders of cobalamin (vitamin B$_{12}$) metabolism: emerging concepts in pathophysiology, diagnosis and treatment. *Blood Rev* 21:113-130.

Sripichai O, Makarasara W, Munkongdee T, et al [2008] A scoring system for the classification of beta-thalassemia/Hb E disease severity. *Am J Hematol* 83:482-484.

Studt JD, Kremer Hovinga JA, Alberio L, et al [2003] Von Willebrand factor-cleaving protease (ADAMTS-13) activity in thrombotic microangiopathies: diagnostic experience 2001/2002 of a single research laboratory. *Swiss Med Wkly* 133:325-332.

Suchi M, Mizuno H, Kawai Y, et al [1997] Molecular cloning of the human UMP synthase gene and characterization of point mutations in 2 hereditary orotic aciduria families. *Am J Hum Genet* 60:525-539.

Sutherland DR, Kuek N, Azcona-Olivera J, et al [2009] Use of a FLAER-based WBC assay in the primary screening of PNH clones. *Am J Clin Pathol* 132:564-572.

Tamary H, Dgany O, Proust A, et al [2005] Clinical and molecular variability in congenital dyserythropoietic anaemia type I. *Br J Haematol* 130:628-634.

Tamary H, Shalmon L, Shalev H, et al [1998] Localization of the gene for congenital dyserythropoietic anemia type I to a <1-cM interval on chromosome 15q15.1-15.3. *Am J Hum Genet* 62:1062-1069.

Thein SL [2008] Genetic modifiers of the beta-haemoglobinopathies. *Br J Haematol* 141:357-366.

Thein SL, Craig JE [1998] Genetics of Hb F/F cell variance in adults and hetero-cellular hereditary persistence of fetal hemoglobin. *Hemoglobin* 22:401-414.

Thein SL, Wainscoat JS, Sampietro M, et al [1987] Association of thalassaemia intermedia with a beta-globin gene haplotype. *Br J Haematol* 65:367-373.

Theurl I, Theurl M, Seifert M, et al [2008] Autocrine formation of hepcidin induces iron retention in human monocytes. *Blood* 111:2392-2399.

Thompson CA, Steensma DP [2006] Pure red cell aplasia associated with thymoma: clinical insights from a 50-year single-institution experience. *Br J Haematol* 135:405-407.

Tiu R, Gondek L, O'Keefe C, Maciejewski JP [2007] Clonality of the stem cell compartment during evolution of myelodysplastic syndromes and other bone marrow failure syndromes. *Leukemia* 21:1648-1657.

Tritipsombut J, Sanchaisuriya K, Fucharoen S, et al [2008] Hemoglobin profiles and hematologic features of thalassemic newborns: application to screening of alpha-thalassemia 1 and hemoglobin E. *Arch Pathol Lab Med* 132:1739-1745.

Tsai HM [2006] The molecular biology of thrombotic microangiopathy. *Kidney Int* 70:16-23.

Uda M, Galanello R, Sanna S, et al [2008] Genome-wide association study shows BCL11A associated with persistent fetal hemoglobin and amelioration of the phenotype of beta-thalassemia. *Proc Natl Acad Sci USA* 105:1620-1625.

Umbreit J [2005] Iron deficiency: a concise review. *Am J Hematol* 78:225-231.

Urrechaga E [2009] Red blood cell microcytosis and hypochromia in the differential diagnosis of iron deficiency and beta-thalassaemia trait. *Int J Lab Hematol* 31:528-534.

van der Zee SP, Schretlen ED, Monnens LA [1968] Megaloblastic anaemia in the Lesch-Nyhan syndrome. *Lancet* 1:1427.

Vernimmen D, De Gobbi M, Sloane-Stanley JA, et al [2007] Long-range chromosomal interactions regulate the timing of the transition between poised and active gene expression. *Embo J* 26:2041-2051.

Wakeman L, Al-Ismail S, Benton A, et al [2007] Robust, routine haematology reference ranges for healthy adults. *Int J Lab Hematol* 29:279-283.

Waldron P, Cashore W [2005] Hemolytic disease of the fetus and newborn. In: de Alarcon P, Werner E, eds. *Neonatal Hematology* Cambridge: Cambridge University; 91-131.

Ward PC [2002] Modern approaches to the investigation of vitamin B_{12} deficiency. *Clin Lab Med* 22:435-445.

Weiss G, Goodnough LT [2005] Anemia of chronic disease. *N Engl J Med* 352:1011-1023.

Weiss R, Fogelman Y, Bennett M [2004] Severe vitamin B_{12} deficiency in an infant associated with a maternal deficiency and a strict vegetarian diet. *J Pediatr Hematol Oncol* 26:270-271.

Westerman DA, Evans D, Metz J [1999] Neutrophil hypersegmentation in iron deficiency anaemia: a case-control study. *Br J Haematol* 107:512-515.

Whitehead VM [2006] Acquired and inherited disorders of cobalamin and folate in children. *Br J Haematol* 134:125-136.

Wickramasinghe SN [2006] Diagnosis of megaloblastic anaemias. *Blood Rev* 20:299-318.

Wickramasinghe SN, Wood WG [2005] Advances in the understanding of the congenital dyserythropoietic anaemias. *Br J Haematol* 131:431-446.

Willcox M, Bjorkman A, Brohult J [1983a] *Falciparum* malaria and beta-thalassaemia trait in northern Liberia. *Ann Trop Med Parasitol* 77:335-347.

Willcox M, Bjorkman A, Brohult J, et al [1983b] A case-control study in northern Liberia of *Plasmodium falciparum* malaria in haemoglobin S and beta-thalassaemia traits. *Ann Trop Med Parasitol* 77:239-246.

Williams TN, Maitland K, Bennett S, et al [1996] High incidence of malaria in alpha-thalassaemic children. *Nature* 383:522-525.

Willis M, Monaghan S, Miller M, et al [2005] Zinc-induced copper deficiency. *Am J Clin Pathol* 123:125-131.

Win N, Roberts DJ [2008] Management of paroxysmal cold haemoglobinuria: not only avoiding cold but also keeping warm. *Br J Haematol* 142:668.

Win N, Stamps R, Knight R [2005] Paroxysmal cold haemoglobinuria/Donath-Landsteiner test. *Transfus Med* 15:254.

Young NS, Brown KE [2004] Parvovirus B19. *N Engl J Med* 350:586-597.

Yuthavong Y, Bunyaratvej A, Kamchonwongpaisan S [1990] Increased susceptibility of malaria-infected variant erythrocytes to the mononuclear phagocyte system. *Blood Cells* 16:591-597.

Zanella A, Fermo E, Bianchi P, et al [2007] Pyruvate kinase deficiency: the genotype-phenotype association. *Blood Rev* 21:217-231.

Zhao R, Min SH, Qiu A, et al [2007] The spectrum of mutations in the PCFT gene, coding for an intestinal folate transporter, that are the basis for hereditary folate malabsorption. *Blood* 110:1147-1152.

Aplastic Anemia and Multilineage Bone Marrow Failure Disorders

David Czuchlewski, MD

Bone marrow failure is best regarded not as a single disease entity, but rather as the common pathologic endpoint to a number of adverse congenital, environmental and/or genetic influences. An excellent analogy may be made to heart failure, in which a vast array of inborn errors, congenital malformations, dietary and lifestyle factors, inherent genetic susceptibilities, and derangements of extrinsic organ systems all contribute, individually or in aggregate, to the eventual development of the single pathophysiologic entity of heart failure. Just as a diagnosis of "heart failure" is merely a starting point for further investigation into the underlying cause, so too is a diagnosis of aplastic anemia or bone marrow failure an occasion for in-depth collaboration between clinician and pathologist to identify, if possible, a primary etiology.

[7.1] Definition and Categorization of Aplastic Anemia and Bone Marrow Failure

The terms "aplastic anemia" and "bone marrow failure" have the potential to create substantial confusion, especially since "aplastic anemia" is sometimes used as shorthand for acquired idiopathic aplastic anemia. Here we will define aplastic anemia more broadly, as multiple cytopenias with trilineage bone marrow hypoplasia in the absence of neoplasia and reticulin fibrosis, indicating a basic failure to produce normal hematopoietic elements. The more quantitatively precise criteria listed in **t7.1** are often applied. Thus defined, aplastic anemia is a very rare disease, with an incidence of approximately 2 cases per million [Young 2008a].

Aplastic anemia may be either a constitutional/congenital or an acquired disorder, with acquired aplastic anemia being substantially more common **f7.1**. Fanconi anemia and dyskeratosis congenita are the paradigmatic causes of constitutional aplastic anemia. While, in general, age at presentation is an important aid in distinguishing acquired from constitutional cases, it is essential to recognize that some constitutional cases may not come to clinical attention until adolescence or even adulthood. This is characteristic of dyskeratosis congenita, although delayed presentations of other constitutional syndromes are being increasingly identified; in some cases, these events are associated with heterozygosity for the implicated alleles [Vulliamy 2002, Yamaguchi 2005].

Acquired aplastic anemia is typically characterized by immune-mediated destruction of progenitor cells [Bagby 2007]. However, direct insults by drugs, toxins, or infectious agents may be initiating events in some cases. Therefore, acquired aplastic anemia is subdivided into secondary cases, in which the initiating insult can be identified, and truly idiopathic cases, in which no such etiology appears obvious.

In addition to categorization by cause, aplastic anemia may be subclassified as moderate, severe, and very severe based on the peripheral blood counts **t7.2**.

A further source of complexity in the categorization of aplastic anemia is its variable association with paroxysmal nocturnal hemoglobinuria (PNH). Hemolytic PNH and aplastic anemia may occur concurrently or sequentially, and granulocytes with PNH-type alterations have been detected (using highly sensitive techniques) in 50% - 90% of cases of idiopathic aplastic anemia [Marsh 2009, Wang 2001]. This association is considered in section "[7.5] Acquired Aplastic Anemia" on p 143.

A complete picture of a given case of aplastic anemia would incorporate *all* of these parameters, as they are not mutually exclusive **t7.3**. For example, one might consider a case of aplastic anemia to be acquired/idiopathic, not severe, and associated with a PNH clone, while another case might be constitutional, severe, and unrelated to a clonal process. Treatment and prognosis may differ substantially based upon such

t7.1 Proposed Criteria for Diagnosis of Aplastic Anemia

Both I and II must be fulfilled, in the absence of neoplasia

I. The patient must have at least 2 of the following CBC findings:

granulocytes <500/μL (<0.5 × 10⁹/L)
platelets <20,000/μL (<20 × 10⁹/L)
corrected reticulocyte count <20 × 10⁹/L

II. In addition the bone marrow must be either:

markedly hypoplastic (<25% of normal age-appropriate cellularity)
or
moderately hypoplastic (25%-50% of normal age-appropriate cellularity, with <30% of the cells being hematopoietic)

CBC = complete blood count

References: Modified from [Camitta 1976, D'Andrea 2002, Marsh 2009]

t7.2 Severity of Aplastic Anemia by Absolute Neutrophil Count (ANC)

ANC	Classification
>500/μL (>0.5 × 10⁹/L)	Non-severe
200–500/μL (0.2–0.5 × 10⁹/L)	Severe
<200/μL (<0.2 × 10⁹/L)	Very severe

Reference: Modified from [Bacigalupo 2007, Marsh 2009]

t7.3 Multiparametric Assessment of BM Failure

Choose 1 element from each column for assessment

Etiology	Severity	Association
Constitutional	Non-severe	PNH clone present
Acquired, secondary	Severe	PNH clone absent
Acquired, idiopathic	Very severe	

BM = bone marrow, PNH = paroxysmal nocturnal hemoglobinuria

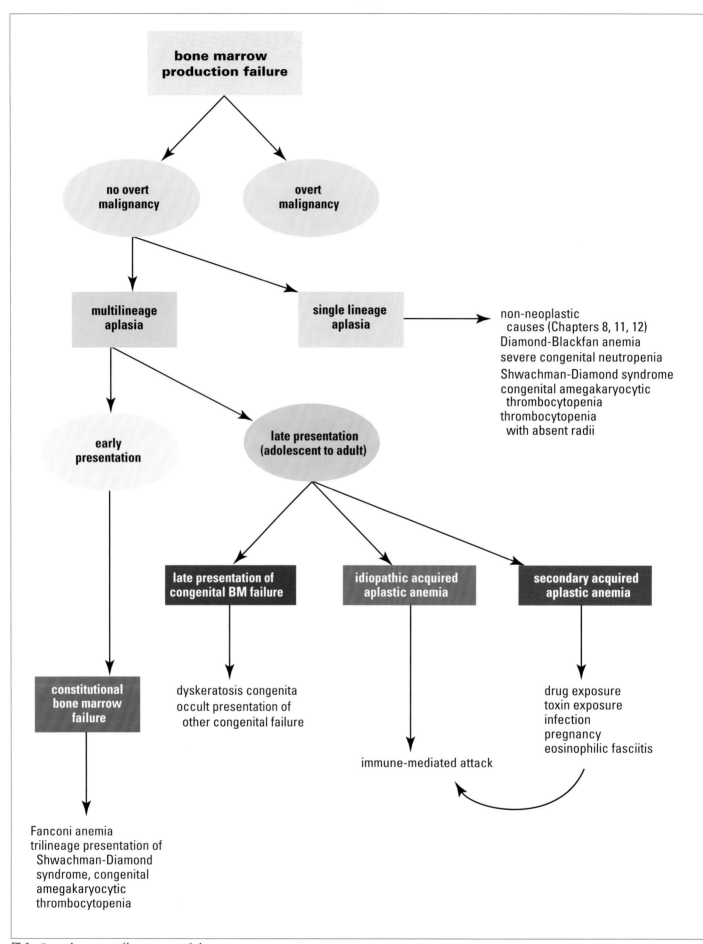

f7.1 *General overview of bone marrow failure.*

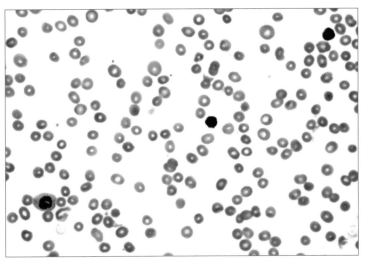

i7.1 *This peripheral blood smear is from an 86-year-old female with profound pancytopenia. (Wright)*

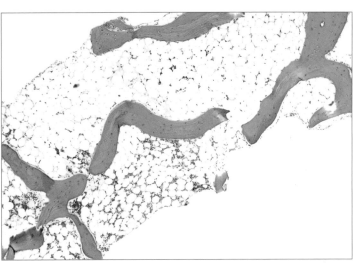

i7.2 *This bone marrow biopsy shows variable overall cellularity ranging from <5% to 20% cellularity. (H&E)*

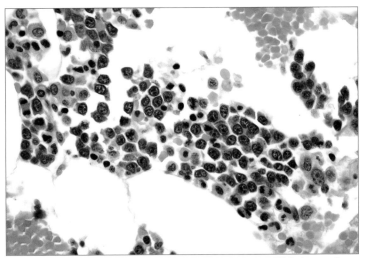

i7.3 *This bone marrow clot section from the same patient as i7.2 shows a focus of hematopoiesis, while all other particles were essentially acellular. (H&E)*

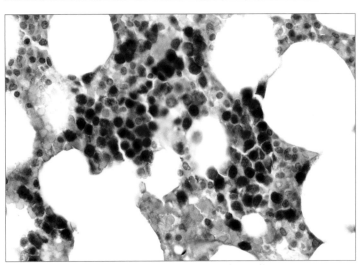

i7.4 *Immunoperoxidase for hemoglobin A shows focus of hematopoiesis consisting primarily of erythroid cells on bone marrow clot section. (immunoperoxidase for HgbA)*

considerations, underscoring the need for a multiparametric and collaborative approach to diagnosis.

If aplastic anemia represents *total* bone marrow failure, aplasias affecting single lineages are nevertheless instances of "bone marrow failure." While recent advances in molecular understanding have revealed intriguing biologic overlap between single lineage and multilineage heritable bone marrow failure, for ease of reference and conceptual integrity we discuss the predominantly single lineage aplasias in the chapters on neutropenia (Chapter 11), erythroblastopenia (Chapter 8), and megakaryocytic disorders (Chapter 12). However, certain of these primarily single lineage failure syndromes may also present in a multilineage fashion, and therefore enter the differential diagnosis of aplastic anemia. Indeed, multiple lineages are affected in some 40% of cases of Shwachman-Diamond syndrome (although true aplastic anemia is rare), and 91% of patients with congenital amegakaryocytic thrombocytopenia will progress to aplastic anemia by 5 years to 13 years of age

[Foucar 2008]. These entities are discussed in more detail in Chapters 11 and 12, respectively.

Finally, some would consider myelodysplastic syndrome (MDS) to be, technically, a form of bone marrow failure; again, for ease of reference, we limit the discussion of MDS here to the relationship between aplastic anemia and hypoplastic MDS, and refer the reader to Chapter 16 for a complete discussion of MDS.

[7.2] **Bone Marrow Morphology in Aplastic Anemia**

By definition **t7.1**, patients with aplastic anemia must exhibit both cytopenias in blood and a bone marrow cellularity no more than 1/4 of the age-related normal range *or* with significantly reduced hematopoiesis (<30% combined myeloid, erythroid, and megakaryocytic lineages) in the setting of hypocellularity (<50% age-related normal range) **i7.1, i7.2, i7.3, i7.4**. In practice, most cases demonstrate profound blood cytopenias, profound

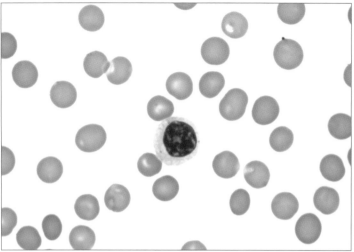

i7.5 *This peripheral blood smear is from a 25-year-old female with an absolute neutrophil count of <200/μL (0.2 × 10⁹/L). Patient presented with sepsis; complete blood count showed profound panycytopenia. (Wright)*

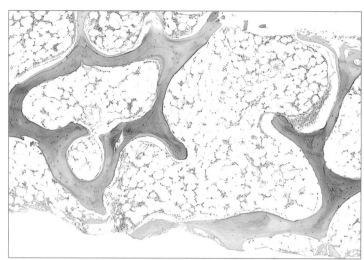

i7.6 *Low-power view of bone marrow biopsy sections demonstrating profound hypocellularity in a patient with acquired aplastic anemia. (H&E)*

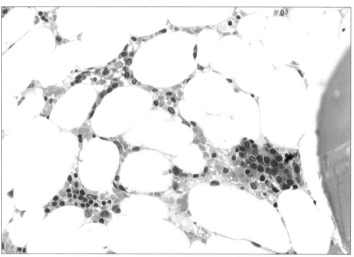

i7.7 *A rare residual island of monotypic immature cells is present on this bone marrow biopsy section from a patient with severe acquired aplastic anemia. (H&E)*

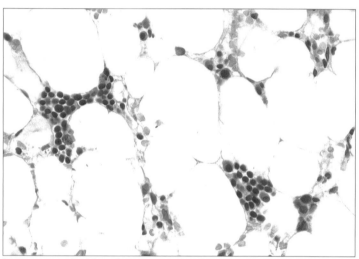

i7.8 *Rare residual foci of maturing erythroid cells are evident on this bone marrow biopsy section from a child who developed acquired aplastic anemia following hepatitis. (H&E)*

hypoplasia, and overall cellularity ranging between 5% and 10% **i7.5**, **i7.6**, **i7.7**, **i7.8**. Fat cells predominate and are diffusely distributed throughout the hematopoietic cavity. In most patients, neither the bony trabeculae nor the bone marrow stroma is abnormal, although occasional patients exhibit fibrillary stromal abnormalities **i7.9**. It is critical that the bone marrow biopsy be large enough and deep enough to accurately represent the cellularity of the marrow cavity, as subcortical marrow is often hypocellular even in normal individuals. Therefore, when aplastic anemia enters the differential diagnosis, the pathologist is fully justified in raising his or her threshold for what constitutes an adequate specimen. A good quality 2 cm biopsy has been specifically required by some to permit the diagnosis of aplastic anemia [Marsh 2009].

All hematopoietic lineages are markedly decreased on aspirate, clot section, and core biopsy preparations **i7.10**, **i7.11**,

i7.12, **i7.13**. However, either agranulocytosis or red cell aplasia can precede aplastic anemia **i7.14**. Some dyspoiesis may be identified, likely reflecting the effects of attempted hematopoietic production under stress [Marsh 2009, Shimamura 2006]. While it is impossible to definitively diagnose a given constitutional bone marrow failure syndrome based on morphologic findings alone, there may be some morphologic clues to specific constitutional disorders. For example, congenital amegakaryocytic thrombocytopenia (as a predominantly single lineage aplasia that often *evolves* into multilineage failure) may retain a predominantly megakaryocytic hypoplasia. In addition, residual megakaryocytes in congenital amegakaryocytic thrombocytopenia are often small and hypolobated, although this is a nonspecific finding (see Chapter 12) [D'Andrea 2002].

Much of the residual nonhematopoietic cellularity in cases of aplastic anemia consists of macrophages,

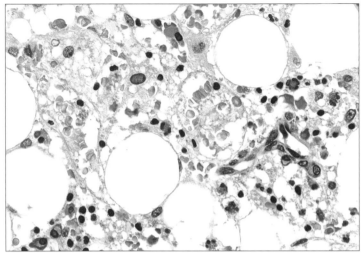

i7.9 *This bone marrow biopsy section illustrates eosinophilic fibrillary bone marrow stroma in a patient with chronic renal failure who developed abrupt aplastic anemia. (H&E)*

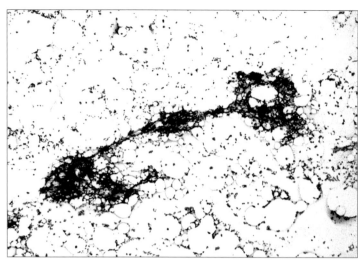

i7.10 *Low magnification of a bone marrow aspirate smear shows a virtually acellular bone marrow particle. (Wright)*

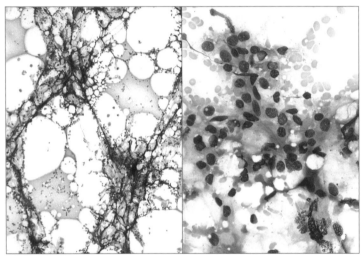

i7.11 *Bone marrow aspirate smears demonstrate profound loss of hematopoietic elements within bone marrow particles. Note abundance of bone marrow stromal cells, macrophages, and plasma cells. (Wright)*

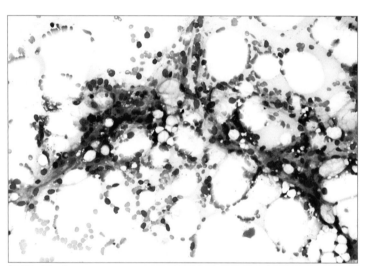

i7.12 *This bone marrow aspirate smear from a patient with aplastic anemia shows that the bone marrow particle contains only residual macrophages and lymphocytes without hematopoietic cells. (Wright)*

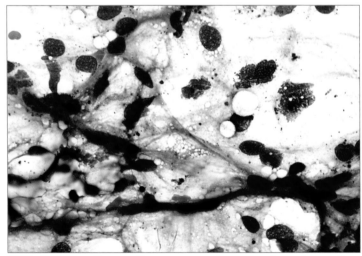

i7.13 *High magnification of bone marrow aspirate smear shows absence of hematopoiesis and fibrillar stromal damage. (Wright)*

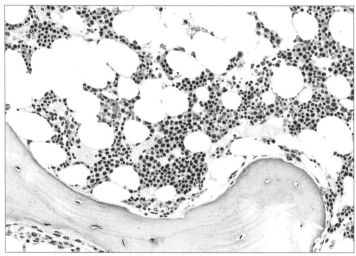

i7.14 *In this bone marrow biopsy section from a child, agranulocytosis preceded overt aplastic anemia. Note the preservation of the erythroid lineage. (H&E)*

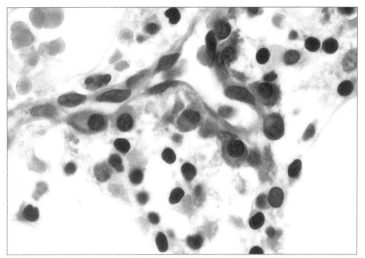

i7.15 *Prominent perivascular plasma cells are evident on this bone marrow biopsy section from a patient with acquired aplastic anemia. (H&E)*

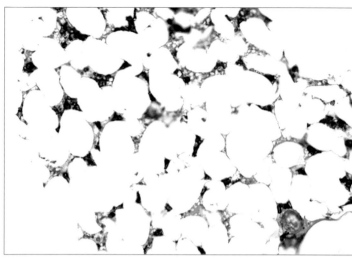

i7.16 *CD138+ plasma cells account for most of the cellularity in the bone marrow core biopsy specimen from a patient with aplastic anemia. (immunoperoxidase for CD138)*

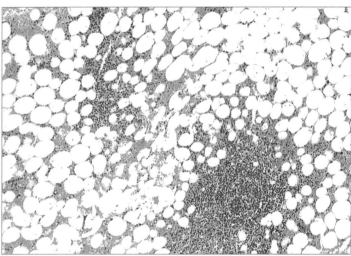

i7.17 *Low-power view of a clot section illustrates profound hematopoietic hypocellularity as well as a single lymphoid aggregate. (H&E)*

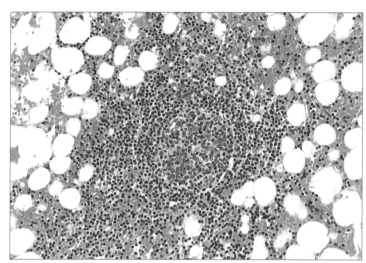

i7.18 *Higher magnification of* **i7.17** *shows a well-formed germinal center in this lymphoid aggregate in this clot section from a patient with aplastic anemia. (H&E)*

lymphocytes, and plasma cells **i7.15, i7.16**. These lymphocytes and plasma cells are often perivascular in distribution. Occasionally, patients with aplastic anemia may have such prominent lymphoid aggregates or lymphoplasmacytic and immunoblastic infiltrates that a diagnosis of lymphoblastic leukemia, multiple myeloma, or lymphoma must be excluded by immunophenotypic studies **i7.17, i7.18, i7.19, i7.20, i7.21**. Caution should be exercised in diagnosing these patients, because these florid polyclonal lymphoid infiltrates that efface the bone marrow may sometimes mask occult underlying neoplasms **i7.20, i7.21**.

In addition to hypocellularity, various other morphologic abnormalities have been identified in some patients with aplastic anemia, and studies have been performed that attempt to correlate these abnormalities

with disease outcome. These abnormalities include increased mast cells, various lymphoid infiltrates, increased eosinophils, fat necrosis, fibrosis, and stromal edema **i7.17, i7.18** [Krech 1985]. Fibrosis may rarely be evident at presentation in patients with aplastic anemia. Although unpredictable, some reports generally suggest resolution of this fibrosis following successful treatment [Soll 1995, Yan 1996]. Although the extent of lymphoid infiltration may correlate with response to immunosuppressive therapy, there is no clear-cut association between disease outcome and any of these morphologic abnormalities. However, increased mast cells, fat necrosis, necrobiotic cells, proteinaceous edema, and stromal damage all suggest a toxic insult to the bone marrow as a possible cause of the aplasia [Krech 1985].

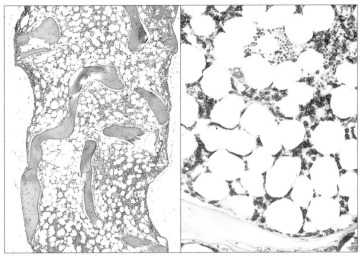

i7.19 *This composite of a bone marrow biopsy section from a patient with hypocellular hairy cell leukemia illustrates the value of CD20 immunoperoxidase staining in highlighting the extensive, yet subtle, infiltrates of hairy cells. (H&E and immunoperoxidase for CD20)*

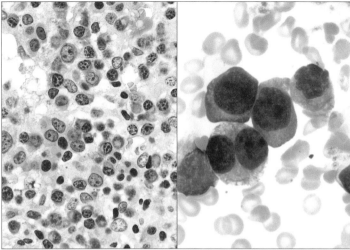

i7.20 *Bone marrow biopsy section and aspirate smear depict a florid plasma-cellular and immunoblastic reaction associated with profound hematopoietic (especially granulocytic) suppression that preceded the development of acute lymphoblastic leukemia by 4 months in this child* **i7.21**. *(H&E; Wright)*

[7.3] Differential Diagnostic Approach in Suspected Aplastic Anemia

A 4-step diagnostic algorithm is presented in **f7.2** for cases of suspected aplastic anemia. The first step is relatively straightforward: the quantitative targets for cytopenias and marrow cellularity as detailed in **t7.1** must be fulfilled. Vitamin B$_{12}$ levels, folate levels and an autoantibody screen should be obtained to exclude nutritional and autoimmune etiologies.

Once this is accomplished, the second step involves excluding the presence of a neoplastic process, in particular, hairy cell leukemia, myelodysplastic syndrome, acute myeloid leukemia (AML), and acute lymphoblastic leukemia, all of which may atypically present in a hypoplastic fashion. While any number of reasonable approaches may be taken to this end, the pathologist may wish to consider immuno-histochemistry and/or flow cytometric analysis for CD20+ B cells to assist in the identification of potentially subtle hairy cell leukemia infiltrates **i7.19**. Similarly, immunophenotypic evidence of aberrant early lymphoid maturation should be sought to exclude the rare case of occult acute lymphoblastic leukemia with a hypocellular presentation **i7.20, i7.21**.

Careful evaluation of blood and bone marrow for evidence of leukemic infiltrates or myelodysplastic features must be performed in all cases of presumed acquired aplastic anemia **i7.22, i7.23, i7.24, i7.25, i7.26** [Elghetany 1997, Guinan 1997]. The presence of *significant* morphologic dysplasia or increased blasts would support a diagnosis of hypocellular MDS **i7.27**. However, it is essential to recognize that cases of both acquired and constitutional aplastic anemia may show dyserythropoietic features consistent with "stress" hemato-poiesis. Therefore, a particularly high threshold should be used for establishing the presence of myelodysplasia in a

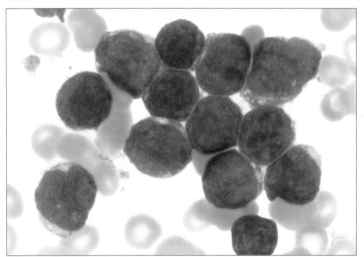

i7.21 *On this bone marrow aspirate smear, acute lymphoblastic leukemia replaces bone marrow in a child with antecedent florid immunoblastic reaction and hematopoietic hypoplasia* **i7.20**. *(Wright)*

hypocellular setting, and greater weight should be placed on more robust evidence such as the presence of increased ring sideroblasts. In contrast, significant granulocytic or megakaryocytic dysplasia is seen in MDS but not in acquired aplastic anemia [Marsh 2009]. Immunoperoxidase staining for CD34 and myeloperoxidase may be particularly useful in identifying increased blasts in cases of suspected hypocellular myelodysplasia or hypocellular AML, thus excluding aplastic anemia **i7.27, i7.28, i7.29** [Maciejewski 2004, Marsh 2009]. In certain cases, the differential diagnosis between hypocellular MDS and aplastic anemia may be impossible to completely resolve; the clinical and pathologic significance of this distinction is discussed further in section "[7.5] Acquired Aplastic Anemia" on p 143.

The third step illustrated in **f7.2** involves identifying an initiating etiology of aplastic anemia, if possible. Inherited

step 1: establish cellular parameters *(see* t7.1*)*

step 2: exclude malignancy

hairy cell leukemia	flow cytometry or IPOX for B cells
myelodysplastic syndrome **acute myeloid leukemia**	examination for significant dysplasia increased numbers of CD34+ blasts Auer rods clonal cytogenic abnormalities
acute lymphoblastic leukemia	flow cytometry or IPOX for CD34, TdT, etc

step 3: investigate etiology

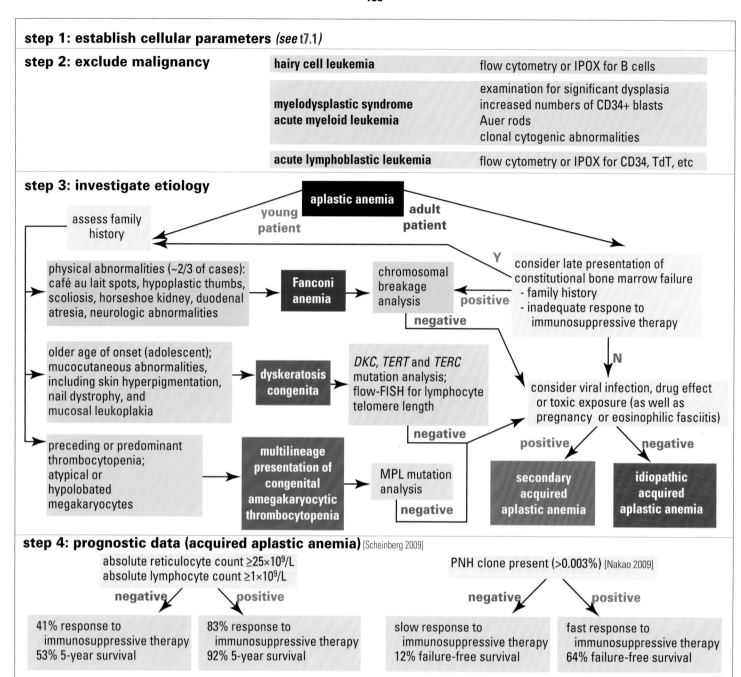

step 4: prognostic data (acquired aplastic anemia) [Scheinberg 2009]

absolute reticulocyte count ≥25×10⁹/L
absolute lymphocyte count ≥1×10⁹/L

negative / **positive**

41% response to immunosuppressive therapy
53% 5-year survival

83% response to immunosuppressive therapy
92% 5-year survival

PNH clone present (>0.003%) [Nakao 2009]

negative / **positive**

slow response to immunosuppressive therapy
12% failure-free survival

fast response to immunosuppressive therapy
64% failure-free survival

f7.2 *Diagnostic algorithm for suspected bone marrow failure. High-sensitivity flow cytometic analysis via FLAER is increasingly available with sensitivity of 0.01%. This test should be performed on peripheral blood rather than bone marrow. Nakao cites sensitivity of 0.003%.*
References: [Nakao 2006, Scheinberg 2009, Shimamura 2009]

causes are more likely to be diagnosed in younger patients, although cryptic presentations of such syndromes may be seen in adolescents and adults, and dyskeratosis congenita in particular is typically diagnosed in this slightly older age group. Family history should be closely analyzed in cases of potential inherited bone marrow failure. Since most of these syndromes show a propensity to evolve into AML, a family history of AML should also be sought. In addition, **f7.2** lists important parameters that may assist in narrowing the differential diagnosis among these entities. If the patient is an adult with no apparent stigmata of a constitutional syndrome, clinical correlation should be

undertaken to identify exposure to drugs, toxins, or recent viral illnesses that may represent initiating causes of acquired aplastic anemia. If a case of apparently acquired aplastic anemia does not respond to immunosuppression, or if there is a family history of bone marrow failure or myeloid malignancy, then genetic testing for mutations associated with dyskeratosis congenita should be considered to more fully investigate the possibility of an occult presentation of constitutional bone marrow failure [Calado 2008].

Finally, in cases of acquired aplastic anemia, it is possible for the pathologist to gather and present important prognostic information at the time of diagnosis. The presence of a PNH

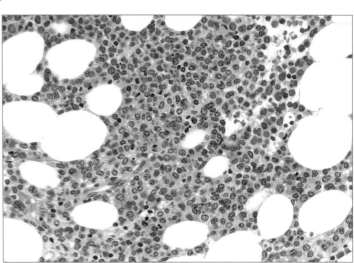

i7.22 *This bone marrow biopsy section is from a child with moderate to markedly decreased hematopoietic elements. Note prominent lymphoid aggregate. (H&E)*

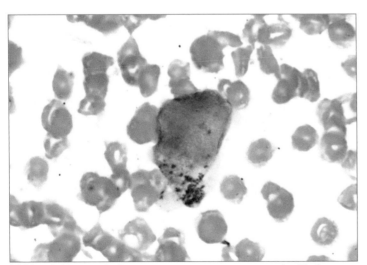

i7.23 *In other areas of the same biopsy section depicted in i7.22, large, nonparatrabecular foci of immature cells are evident. (H&E)*

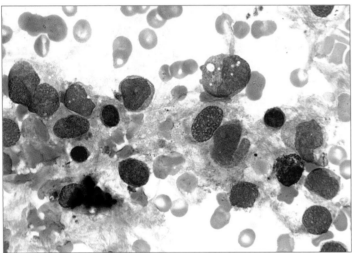

i7.24 *Although infrequent, distinct foci of increased blasts are present in occasional particles on this bone marrow aspirate particle crush smear from same case illustrated in i7.22, i7.23. (Wright)*

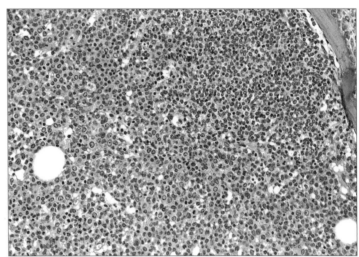

i7.25 *Within 6 months, the patient illustrated in i7.22, i7.23, i7.24 developed overt bone marrow replacement by blasts, as evidenced on this bone marrow biopsy section. (H&E)*

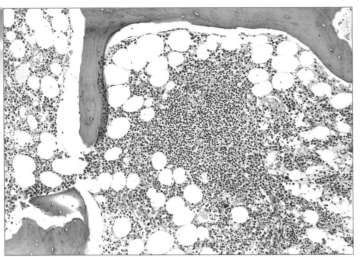

i7.26 *The blasts on this bone marrow aspirate smear were Sudan black B positive, confirming the morphologic impression of acute myeloid leukemia evolving from hypocellular myelodysplasia (see i7.22–i7.25). (Sudan black B)*

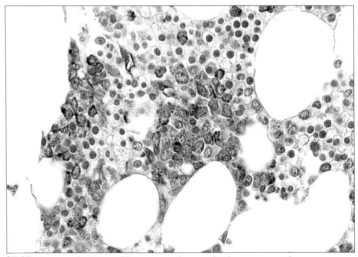

i7.27 *Increased CD34+ blasts are evident on this bone marrow biopsy section from a patient with hypocellular myelodysplasia. (immunoperoxidase)*

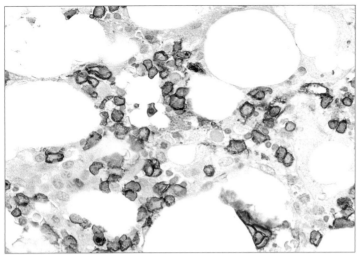

i7.28 *Blasts are highlighted by immunoperoxidase staining for CD34 in this bone marrow biopsy section from a patient with hypocellular acute myeloid leukemia. (immunoperoxidase for CD34)*

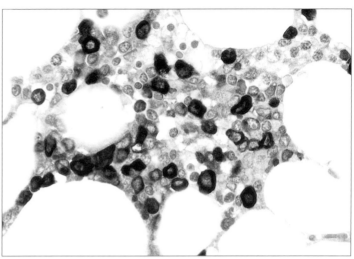

i7.29 *The myeloid lineage of the blasts illustrated in* **i7.28** *is confirmed by immunoperoxidase staining for myeloperoxidase on this bone marrow biopsy section from a patient with hypocellular acute myeloid leukemia. (immunoperoxidase for MPO)*

clone by flow cytometric analysis is predictive of a good response to immunosuppressive therapy, as are relatively preserved absolute reticulocyte and lymphocyte counts [Nakao 2006, Young 2008b].

[7.4] Specific Inherited Multilineage Bone Marrow Failure Disorders

Given our increased understanding of the constitutional bone marrow failure disorders and the biologic defects that some hold in common, one can consider these disorders according to their impaired molecular functions (including DNA repair pathways, telomere maintenance, and ribosomal biogenesis), or by the specific genes that have been implicated **t7.4, t7.5**.

Possible screening and confirmatory laboratory tests are summarized in **t7.2**. In these entities, bone marrow transplant may be attempted for cure, but inherent susceptibility to genetic damage often complicates the choice of conditioning regimen.

[7.4.1] Fanconi Anemia

Fanconi anemia is a genotypically and phenotypically heterogeneous disorder characterized by progressive trilineage bone marrow failure, generally presenting within the first decade of life **i7.30**. Most patients with Fanconi anemia demonstrate somatic congenital anomalies, including café au lait spots, hypoplastic thumbs, scoliosis, horseshoe kidney, duodenal atresia, or neurologic abnormalities; however, up to one-third of Fanconi anemia patients will lack such findings [Dokal 2008]. There is also substantially increased risk for secondary malignancies, including myelodysplasia, AML, and solid tumors. The detection of a clonal abnormality in the bone marrow of a Fanconi anemia patient strongly correlates with progression to MDS [Cioc 2010].

While Fanconi anemia usually behaves in an autosomal recessive fashion, X-linked recessive forms of the disease are also known. Mutations in any of 13 separate genes can give rise to the Fanconi phenotype, a situation readily explicable by the fact that the affected genes code for proteins involved in the same DNA damage detection and repair pathway [Dokal 2008]. Most of the known mutations involve members of the "Fanconi anemia core complex," which assists in the recognition of DNA damage and interacts with DNA repair proteins such as BRCA1 and BRCA2 [Levitus 2006]. Some Fanconi mutations more directly involve this secondary repair step by disabling partner proteins of BRCA1 or BRCA2 [Reid 2007]. Biallelic *BRCA2* mutations also give rise to Fanconi anemia [De Nicolo 2008, Howlett 2002]. Ineffective hematopoiesis may be due to abnormal interaction between the Fanconi anemia core complex and mediators of the Notch developmental pathway [Tremblay 2008]. The inability to conduct DNA surveillance and repair is thought to underlie the susceptibility to malignancies.

Cells with such mutations are exquisitely susceptible to DNA cross-linking, a feature that is exploited in a diagnostic test for Fanconi anemia. When patient cells and control cells are incubated with cross-linking agents such as diepoxybutane or mitomycin-C, the Fanconi mutations give rise to increased chromosomal breakage relative to the controls **f7.3**. This test is

t7.4 Molecular Pathogenesis of Constitutional Bone Marrow Failure Disorders

Defect	Disease
DNA repair pathways	Fanconi anemia
Telomere maintenance	Dyskeratosis congenita
Growth factor receptor mutation	Congenital amegakaryocytic thrombocytopenia

References: [Alter 2007a, Dokal 2008]

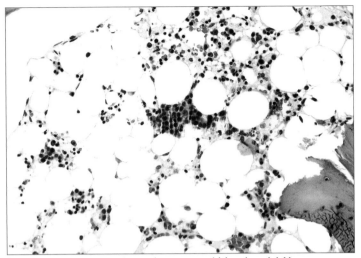

f7.30 *Bone marrow core biopsy from 5-year-old female with lifelong anemia and progressive cytopenias characteristic of Fanconi anemia. (H&E)*

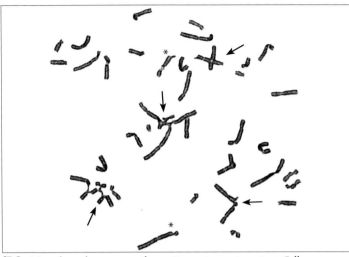

f7.3 *Metaphase chromosomes from a Fanconi anemia patient. Cells were grown in 40 ng/mL mitomycin C, harvested, and slides prepared according to standard protocol. Chromosomes were stained with Wright stain and 50 metaphases scored for breaks (asterisks) and radial formations (arrows).*

t7.5 Recognized Genetic Mutations in Inherited Bone Marrow Failure Syndromes*

Disease	Gene	Locus	Inheritance	% of Patients
Fanconi anemia	FANCA	16q24.3	AR	65%-70%
	FANCB	Xp22	XLR	<1%
	FANCC	9q22.3	AR	~10%
	FANCD1 (BRCA2)	13q12.3	AR	<1%
	FANCD2	3p25.3	AR	<1%
	FANCE	6p21.3	AR	4%-10%
	FANCF	11p15	AR	~4%
	FANCG	9p13	AR	10%-14%
	FANCI	15q26.1	AR	<1%
	FANCJ (BRIP1)†	17q22.3	AR	<5%
	FANCL	2p16.1	AR	<1%
	FANCM	14q21.3	AR	<1%
	FANCN (PALB2)†	16p12.1	AR	<1%
Dyskeratosis congenita	DKC1 (dyskerin)	Xq28	XLR	30%-36%
	TERC	3q26	AD	~5%
	TERT	5p15	AD, AR	<5%
	NOP10	15q14	AR	<1%
	TINF2	14q11.2	AD, often de novo	~11%
	NHP2	12q24.3	AR	<5%
Congenital amegakaryocytic thrombocytopenia	MPL	1p34	AR	~100%

*Genetic defects in some subpopulations of these syndromes remain uncharacterized
†*FANCJ/BRIP1* and *FANCN/PALB2* associate with *BRCA1* and *BRCA2*, respectively
AR = autosomal recessive; XLR = X-linked recessive; AD = autosomal dominant

References: [Alter 2007a, Dokal 2008]. See also [Vulliamy 2008, Walne 2008, 2009]

a critical element in the workup of all suspected bone marrow failure disorders, as Fanconi anemia is unique among these diseases in showing excessive chromosomal breakage and radial formation. Given the large number of affected genes and the variety of mutations described, genetic testing for Fanconi anemia, even by direct sequencing, is currently impractical for clinical purposes [Ameziane 2008].

[7.4.2] **Dyskeratosis Congenita**

Like Fanconi anemia, dyskeratosis congenita consistently results in trilineage hematopoietic failure and increased incidence of hematologic malignancy and solid tumors [Alter 2009]. However, dyskeratosis congenita is distinguished by a comparatively late onset, with bone marrow failure typically presenting in adolescence or young adulthood. Dyskeratosis congenita is also characterized by a distinct set of mucocutaneous abnormalities, including skin hyperpigmentation, nail dystrophy, and mucosal leukoplakia, though these manifestations demonstrate significant interindividual variability. When the integumentary changes are prominent, dyskeratosis congenita may be a relatively obvious diagnostic consideration. In contrast, given an adolescent or adult patient with bone marrow failure and minimal or absent skin changes, a constitutional bone marrow failure syndrome may not top the list of differential diagnoses. Even more confoundingly, as pancytopenia develops, the bone marrow may show an initial compensatory hypercellular response before hematopoiesis flags and the hypocellular state supervenes.

Dyskeratosis congenita is, like Fanconi anemia, a genotypically heterogeneous syndrome caused by mutations of a number of distinct genes that cluster in a single biochemical pathway. Inheritance may be X-linked recessive, autosomal dominant, or autosomal recessive, depending on the genetic lesion [Kirwan 2008]. Although the genetic abnormalities in most cases remain uncharacterized, all described mutations affect genes (including *DKC1*, *TERC*, *TERT*, *NOP10*, *NHP2*, *TINF2*) coding for either proteins or untranslated RNA molecules that associate with the telomerase complex [Savage 2008, Vulliamy 2008, Walne 2008]. This complex maintains the telomeres by using a reverse transcriptase (TERT) to add bases according to an untranslated RNA template (TERC). The abnormalities in these and associated genes, in addition to the consistent finding of abnormally short telomeres in cases of dyskeratosis congenita, indicates that dyskeratosis congenita is fundamentally a disorder of telomere maintenance [Calado 2008]. The effects of shortened telomeres would be expected to be most severe in tissue undergoing rapid and continual cellular division, likely accounting for the phenotypic prominence of skin and bone marrow changes [Blasco 2007]. Although current consensus focuses on the role of telomere maintenance in the disease, there is evidence that ribosomal biogenesis is also aberrant in some forms of the disease [Ganapathi 2008, Kirwan 2008]. See **sidebar 7.1** for further discussion of the relationship between telomere length, bone marrow failure and myeloid malignancy.

While family history and dermatologic changes may be crucial clues to the diagnosis of dyskeratosis congenita, several avenues of laboratory investigation are available. Cytogenetic analysis may reveal a propensity towards unbalanced in vitro chromosomal translocations [Dokal 2008].

[sidebar 7.1] **Telomeres and Bone Marrow Failure**

The ends of the chromosome present a special challenge to the cell. First, cellular machinery cannot readily distinguish naked chromosomal ends from double-stranded DNA breaks, a mistake that would lead to genetic chaos and apoptosis. Second, DNA replication on the lagging strand is discontinuous; in the middle of the chromosome, Okazaki fragments are joined by DNA ligase to complete replication, but at the end of the chromosome, the lagging strand has no terminal Okazaki fragment, leading to the continual loss of genetic material from these ends during replication. The ingenious solution to both of these problems is the telomere, a sequence of thousands of tandem repeats that caps and protects the chromosomal end. The telomerase complex is dedicated to the reverse transcription of this region from an untranslated RNA template, thus preserving the telomere in the face of repeated replication cycles.

Telomeres are abnormally short in many forms of bone marrow failure, including both constitutional and acquired aplastic anemia. Initially, this was thought to be a secondary effect of the rapid cellular division by stem cells attempting to preserve hematopoietic production. However, the realization that several components of the telomerase complex, including TERT, TERC, and dyskerin, are characteristically affected by mutations in dyskeratosis congenita has given rise to the theory that short telomeres may play a causative role in bone marrow failure syndromes. Short telomeres are found in up to one-third of cases of apparently acquired aplastic anemia, and in 8% of such patients constitutional mutations in *TERT* or *TERC* are present [Calado 2008]. *TERT* and *TERC* mutations are also present in some cases of familial aplastic anemia, MDS, and AML [Fogarty 2003, Kirwan 2008]. A significant number of apparently sporadic AML cases occur in individuals carrying these mutations. Cases with these mutations could thus be considered cryptic presentations or forma frusta of dyskeratosis

congenita with progression to clonal malignancies. The presence of shortened telomeres in the unmutated cases, as well as in Fanconi anemia and Shwachman-Diamond syndrome, also suggests a biologic continuum that implicates abnormalities of telomere maintenance in hematopoietic failure.

Interestingly, short telomeres also predispose to improper joining of chromosomal ends, either to one another or to more centromeric regions. Short telomeres in the bone marrow failure syndromes may thus account for some proportion of the risk of aneuploidy and malignant progression in the bone marrow failure syndromes [Calado 2008, Marrone 2004].

Telomere length may be increasingly utilized in the diagnosis of dyskeratosis congenita. Since other bone marrow failure syndromes share with dyskeratosis congenita a propensity for telomere shortening, examination of telomere length in granulocytes is not specific for this disorder. In contrast, the finding of abnormally short telomeres in *lymphocytes* has a sensitivity and specificity of 91% for the diagnosis of dyskeratosis congenita [Alter 2007b].

The *DKC1, TERT,* and *TERC* genes are amenable to direct sequencing for the identification of mutations [Bagby 2004], although these genes have been implicated in only about 1/2 of dyskeratosis congenita cases [Dokal 2008]. Finally, a combined flow cytometric/fluorescence in situ hybridization technique has been described to identify the very short telomeres characteristic of the disease (see **sidebar 7.1**) [Alter 2007b].

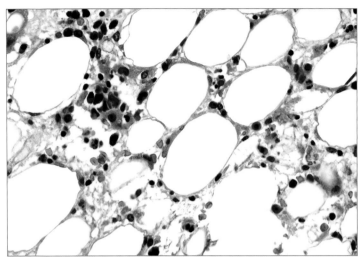

i7.31 *Bone marrow core biopsy from patient with aplastic anemia showing stromal damage and fibrillar necrosis following initiation of a new medication. (H&E) (courtesy C Sever, MD)*

[7.4.3]   **Familial Aplastic Anemia**

Rare cases of familial aplastic anemia do not fulfill diagnostic criteria of other constitutional bone marrow failure syndromes. Such cases are highly variable in phenotype, with diverse ages of presentation and associated physical findings. The responsible genetic lesions in these cases are not well-characterized. However, recently a number of patients diagnosed with familial aplastic anemia were discovered to harbor mutations affecting the telomerase complex, suggesting that their disease process was, in fact, a variant of dyskeratosis congenita lacking the full phenotypic expression of that syndrome [Fogarty 2003]. As rare cohorts of "familial aplastic anemia" are identified and scrutinized, it is likely that many will be found to represent such variants of specific heritable bone marrow failure disorders.

[7.5]   **Acquired Aplastic Anemia**

[7.5.1]   **Overview of Acquired Aplastic Anemia**

When Paul Ehrlich provided the first description of aplastic anemia in 1888, the etiology of the condition was entirely obscure. The intervening years have provided more insight into the pathogenesis of this process, but many aspects remain to be fully elucidated. In general, acquired aplastic anemia arises when bone marrow progenitor cells come under immune-mediated attack. In a subset of cases, there appears to be an inciting event that leads to this immune attack, most commonly exposure to a toxin, drug, or virus, though aplastic anemia may also develop in the setting of pregnancy or eosinophilic fasciitis through obscure mechanism. In idiopathic cases, although immune attack occurs, the inciting event (if any) is not apparent. In most instances the aplastic state is persistent, underscoring that lasting damage is occurring at the level of the progenitor cell [Young 2008b]. Indeed, the natural history of untreated aplastic anemia is almost universal mortality within 1-2 years, a prognosis that has thankfully been improved upon with immunosuppressive therapy and bone marrow transplantation.

[7.5.2]   **Pathogenesis of Aplastic Anemia**

There is a well-documented association between certain viral infections and the development of aplastic anemia. Aplastic anemia may complicate viral hepatitis, including infection with hepatitis A, B, and G viruses [Cengiz 2007]. In addition, up to 10% of cases of aplastic anemia develop following an episode of seronegative, cryptogenic hepatitis [Honkaniemi 2007]. In these cases findings on serologic studies are negative for the major recognized hepatitis viruses, leading some to propose a novel infectious agent. In one unusual case, mutations in an antigenic determining region of hepatitis B virus were documented, accounting for the seronegative status [Cariani 2007].

Epstein-Barr virus and HIV typically cause relatively mild suppression of hematopoiesis, but in rare cases they are associated with sustained aplasia [Grishaber 1988, Lau 1994, Shah 2005]. Similarly, although classic parvovirus infection is linked to suppression of erythropoiesis, in some cases severe aplastic anemia may develop. This is most frequently observed in chronically immunosuppressed patients, though cases of parvovirus-associated aplastic anemia in immunocompetent patients are reported [Yetgin 2004]. Interestingly, parvoviral DNA is detectable in a substantial number of cases of aplastic anemia of otherwise unknown etiology [Mishra 2005].

Aplastic anemia may also follow exposure to chemicals and therapeutic drugs. Some 27% of cases of aplastic anemia in the West may be attributable to medical drugs [Young 2008b]; the implicated substances range from those like chloramphenicol, which is strongly associated with the development of aplastic anemia, to drugs for which aplasia is a rare, idiosyncratic reaction **i7.31**. Benzene is the most common toxin associated with the development of aplastic anemia; however, recent epidemiologic data have suggested that benzene exposure accounts for a very minor proportion of cases of aplastic

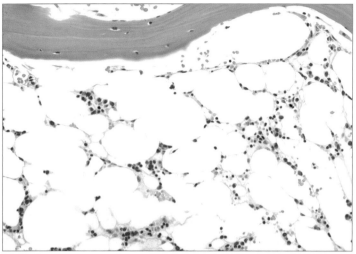

i7.32 *Bone marrow core biopsy from a 25-year-old female with aplastic anemia showing profound hypocellularity. (H&E)*

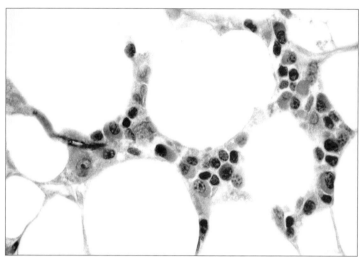

i7.33 *Immunoperoxidase staining for CD34 on bone marrow core biopsy from a 25-year-old female with aplastic anemia (see **i7.32**) shows virtually no CD34+ cells. (immunoperoxidase for CD34)*

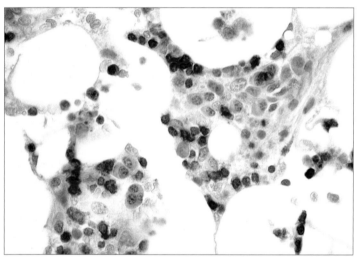

i7.34 *Immunoperoxidase staining of bone marrow core biopsy for CD3 shows increased T cells in a 25-year-old female with aplastic anemia (see **i7.32**, **i7.33**, **i7.35**.) (immunoperoxidase for CD3)*

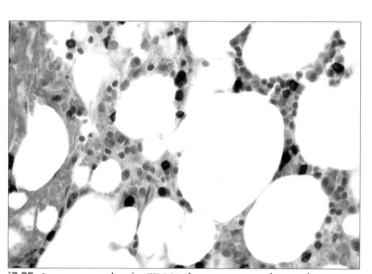

i7.35 *Immunoperoxidase for CD20 in bone marrow core biopsy of a 25-year-old patient with aplastic anemia showing scattered, dispersed B cells (see **i7.32**, **i7.33**, **i7.34**). (immunoperoxidase for CD20)*

anemia [Issaragrisil 2006, Young 2008b]. Other toxins, such as insecticides and solvents, have also been implicated. While it is difficult in such cases to prove direct causation, genetic polymorphisms that reduce the efficiency of enzymes involved in metabolizing toxins, including benzene derivatives, are associated with a significantly increased risk of aplastic anemia in some populations [Dirksen 2004, Dufour 2005, Lee 2001, Sutton 2004].

In the majority of aplastic anemia cases, no potential etiologic cause can be identified. These idiopathic cases likely represent a heterogeneous collection of processes. In some instances, the cause may be an unidentified viral infection or toxic exposure that, if recognized, would place the case squarely within the category of secondary aplastic anemia. In other cases, idiopathic aplastic anemia may represent a late or cryptic presentation of one of the constitutional bone marrow failure syndromes described herein [Alter 2005, Marrone 2007].

In most cases of idiopathic acquired aplastic anemia, stem cells are thought to come under immune-mediated attack, limiting their ability to maintain hematopoiesis **i7.32**, **i7.33**, **i7.34**, **i7.35**. The precise target of the immune response is unclear, and indeed may vary from patient to patient. Oligoclonal T cells are present in many cases [de Vries 2008, Piao 2005], suggesting that the immune response may have some degree of specificity. Certain HLA alleles are associated with acquired aplastic anemia, and autoantibodies have been demonstrated in some cases against cell surface proteins [Fuhrer 2007, Hirano 2003, 2005, Usman 2004]. Regardless of the exact target of the immune response, regulatory T cells are both numerically decreased and dysfunctional in patients with aplastic anemia at presentation, leading to uninhibited production of large amounts of interferon γ and tumor necrosis factor α, cytokines with the ability to suppress hematopoiesis and induce apoptosis in the stem cell and progenitor cell populations [Dubey 2005]. The centrality

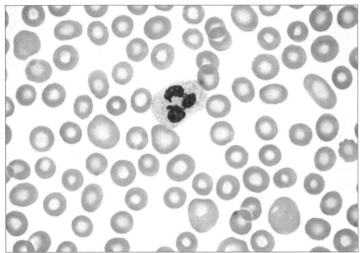

i7.36 *Peripheral blood smear from a patient with paroxysmal nocturnal hemoglobinuria who experienced progressive anemia and thrombocytopenia. (Wright)*

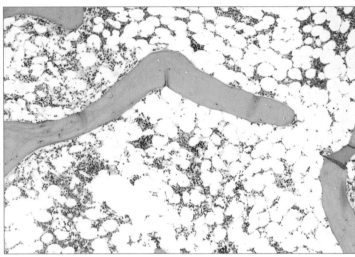

i7.37 *Bone marrow core biopsy from a 30-year-old female with paroxysmal nocturnal hemoglobinuria showing variable, but overall hypocellular picture (see **i7.36**). (H&E)*

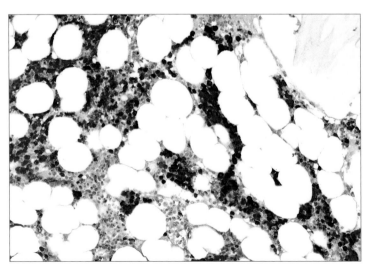

i7.38 *Immunoperoxidase staining for hemoglobin A on bone marrow core biopsy from a 30-year-old female with paroxysmal nocturnal hemoglobinuria shows a relative predominance of erythroid precursors (see **i7.36**). (immunoperoxidase for HgbA)*

[sidebar 7.2]   **Paroxysmal Nocturnal Hemoglobinuria and Ockham's Razor**

The medieval philosopher William of Ockham (1295-1349) formulated the principle of ontological parsimony that came to be known as Ockham's razor: namely, that in attributing a cause to a given effect the simplest explanation is usually the correct one; or, as famously summarized, *Entia non sunt multiplicanda praeter necessitatem* ("entities should not be multiplied unnecessarily"). Modern science often has recourse to Ockham's razor when constructing hypotheses or drawing conclusions regarding complex or poorly understood systems. Recently an elegant mathematic model of stem cell dynamics has led to the invocation of Ockham's razor in describing the pathogenesis of paroxysmal nocturnal hemoglobinuria (PNH).

As discussed in the accompanying text and in Chapter 6, PNH is a disease defined by the emergence of hematopoietic clones with mutations of *PIGA*, leading to loss of the glycosylphosphatidylinositol (GPI) membrane anchor and susceptibility of the resulting blood cells to complement-mediated lysis. A longstanding controversy surrounds the ontogeny of these cells. The leading hypothesis to explain the emergence of PNH cells is process of "natural selection," in which stem cells under immune-mediated attack face selective pressure, leading to a growth advantage for those few cells that randomly produce protective mutations [Brodsky 2008, Sugimori 2009]. This theory dovetails with the known immune-mediated etiology of acquired aplastic anemia, thus potentially explaining the association between these entities.

Among the findings offered in support of this theory are the observations that both the acquisition of clonal abnormalities and the loss of GPI-linked surface proteins confer increased resistance to natural killer cell–mediated apoptosis, potentially providing the type of advantage necessary to survive in the adverse environment of an aplastic marrow [Hanaoka 2006, 2009, Nagakura 2002]. However, the "clonal escape" theory remains controversial, with some evidence contradicting the putative survival advantage for GPI-negative cells [Araten 2002, Karadimitris 2000b].

It is in this context that a recent collaboration was undertaken between hematologists and computational biologists. Using data relating to the size of the stem cell pool according to age, the rate of stem cell replication and differentiation, and the documented rate of spontaneous *PIGA* mutation, Dingli et al constructed a model of stem cell dynamics [Dingli 2008]. They then ran their model with an important and unusual assumption: that the *PIGA* mutation confers *no* selective advantage to the cell in which it occurs. Thus, their model is essentially a thought experiment testing the null hypothesis regarding GPI's supposedly causative role in clonal hematopoiesis.

After modeling the stem cell dynamics of 10^9 virtual people, each of whom lived 100 years, Dingli et al calculated the number of individuals in whom clinical PNH would have occurred (based on the assumption that mutations must occupy at least 20% of the active stem cell pool to produce clinical PNH). The calculated incidence of disease was ~8 cases/million, with an average age of onset of 58 years. These values correspond quite closely to the characteristics of PNH observed in actual practice. Moreover, since the model assumes no selective advantage to *PIGA*-mutated cells and stem cell differentiation is a random, stochastic process, in approximately 12% of the virtual cases, the PNH clone disappeared after presentation. Again, this agrees with clinical observations regarding the natural history of PNH, in which the disease spontaneously remits in around 15% of patients [Hillmen 1995]. Finally, the Dingli model recapitulates the indisputable association between bone marrow failure and PNH. By varying the model to reflect known data regarding the stem cell pool and replication rate in bone marrow failure (ie, fewer stem cells replicating more rapidly to preserve hematopoiesis), the model predicts a 10-fold increase in the incidence of PNH, with a younger age at onset and larger clonal populations—all features consistent with the clinical behavior of PNH clones in bone marrow failure syndromes.

If computational biology suggests an answer that would have greatly pleased William of Ockham, the finding is nevertheless difficult to reconcile with other data suggesting the presence of immune-mediated selective pressure in the development of PNH (eg, the increased response to immunosuppressive therapy in aplastic anemia patients with significant PNH clones) [Wang 2001]. Very recent data suggests that the behavior of the PNH clone differs depending on whether it arises in a hematopoietic stem cell or a hematopoietic progenitor cell [Sugimori 2009]. Thus, the matter of selective advantage and GPI-linked proteins remains an open experimental question.

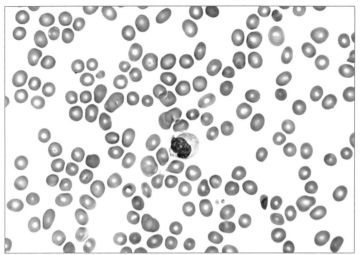

i7.39 *Peripheral blood smear from a 74-year-old female with paroxysmal nocturnal hemoglobinuria and pancytopenia. (Wright) (courtesy P Armell, MD)*

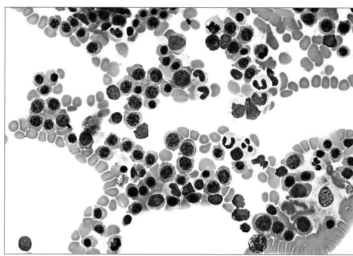

i7.40 *Bone marrow aspirate from a 74-year-old female with paroxysmal nocturnal hemoglobinuria shows erythroid hyperplasia. (Wright) (courtesy P Armell, MD)*

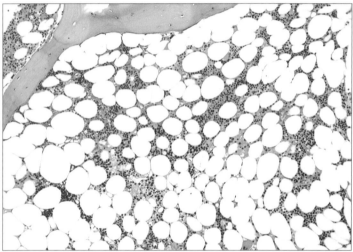

i7.41 *Bone marrow core biopsy showing variable but overall hypocellularity in a 74-year-old female with paroxysmal nocturnal hemoglobinuria. (H&E) (courtesy P Armell, MD)*

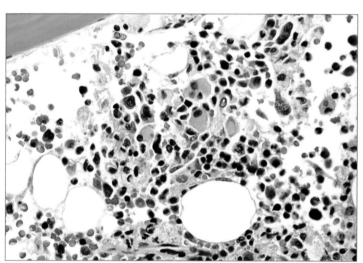

i7.42 *Bone marrow core biopsy from a 51-year-old male with longstanding aplastic anemia who developed acquired monosomy 7. Note abnormal megakaryocytes. (H&E) (courtesy C Sever, MD)*

of these T-cell-produced cytokines to the pathogenesis of acquired aplastic anemia is underscored by the success of immunosuppressive therapy, the clinical efficacy of which correlates with the degree of T-cell suppression [Bagby 2007]. Polymorphisms in genes that heighten or dampen the efficiency of the cytokine-driven immune response have also been shown to increase the risk of acquired aplastic anemia [Gidvani 2007]. In short, the central event in acquired aplastic anemia is said to be a T-cell driven "microenvironmental cytokine storm" in the bone marrow [Bagby 2007].

[7.5.3]   **Association of Acquired Aplastic Anemia with Clonal Disorders of Hematopoiesis**

Several lines of evidence suggest an association between aplastic anemia and PNH. Low level, subclinical circulating PNH cells are detectable in up to 90% of patients with

acquired aplastic anemia using highly-sensitive flow techniques [Wang 2001]. Clinically apparent hemolytic PNH will supervene in 5% - 10% of cases of aplastic anemia **i7.36, i7.37, i7.38** [Marsh 2003]. Abnormal hematopoiesis is a consistent feature of PNH, and some cases of PNH evolve to outright bone marrow failure [Young 2008b]. Recent studies document an abnormal T-cell repertoire in PNH, analogous to T-cell defects that are linked to progenitor cell destruction in aplastic anemia [Karadimitris 2000a]. Patients with hemolytic PNH and overt PNH in the setting of bone marrow failure have similar prognoses [de Latour 2008]. These overlapping clinical features and presentations have led some to propose that aplastic anemia and PNH may in fact represent a spectrum of a single disease. See **sidebar 7.2** for a further discussion of the theories advanced to account for the relationship between PNH and aplastic anemia.

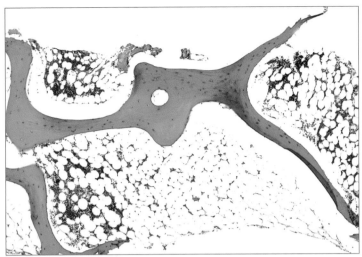

i7.43 *Bone marrow core biopsy from a 38-year-old male with cytogenetics showing del(13q) and aplastic anemia picture. (H&E) (courtesy C Sever, MD)*

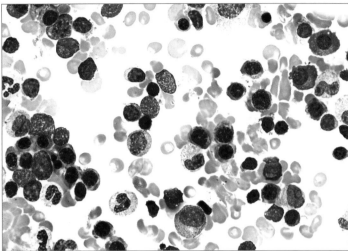

i7.44 *Bone marrow aspirate smear from a 38-year-old male showing focus of hematopoiesis consisting primarily of erythroid precursors in patient with aplastic anemia picture and del(13q) (see **i7.43**). (Wright) (courtesy C Sever, MD)*

Similarly, some cases of aplastic anemia show significant overlap with hypocellular MDS. Indeed, as described in section "[7.2] Bone Marrow Morphology in Aplastic Anemia" on p 133, it may be quite difficult in some cases to reliably distinguish between these entities **i7.39, i7.40, i7.41**. Historically, the identification of clonal cytogenetic abnormalities has been thought to support a diagnosis of hypocellular MDS over aplastic anemia [Maciejewski 2004], but some cases nevertheless fall into a "gray zone" between these entities, with abnormal cytogenetic clones detectable in up to 12% of cases of aplastic anemia [Marsh 2009]. The term "aplastic anemia with cytogenetic abnormalities" has been used by some to describe such cases. It is currently believed that the presence or absence of increased CD34+ blasts better discriminates aplastic anemia from hypocellular MDS than does the detection of cytogenetic abnormalities [Xu 2009].

Further complicating this relationship, cases of uncomplicated aplastic anemia also have a propensity to evolve into MDS and AML **i7.42, i7.43, i7.44**. The presence of monosomy 7 indicates a poor prognosis with a high likelihood of progression to AML and refractoriness to immunosuppressive therapy [Maciejewski 2002, Marsh 2009, Young 2008b]; in contrast, patients with trisomy 8 and other cytogenetic abnormalities will generally respond to immunosuppressive therapy [Maciejewski 2002, Marsh 2009].

[7.6] Clues and Caveats

1. **t7.6** lists several helpful questions the pathologist may wish to consider, and perhaps explicitly address, in rendering a diagnosis of aplastic anemia or bone marrow failure.
2. Acquired aplastic anemia is much more common than its constitutional counterpart.

t7.6 Components for Diagnostic Interpretation in Aplastic Anemia

1. Is the bone marrow truly hypocellular and not simply a subcortical sample?

2. What is the severity of the aplastic anemia (determined by peripheral counts, degree of hypocellularity)?

3. Is there evidence to suggest a constitutional bone marrow failure syndrome?

    Family history (including family history of MDS/AML)

    Congenital abnormalities

    Age of presentation

    Preceding single-lineage aplasia

4. Have hypocellular presentations of hematopoietic malignancies been ruled out via IHC and/or cytogenetics?

    Hairy cell leukemia

    Acute lymphoblastic leukemia

    MDS

    AML

5. Is there evidence of concomitant PNH, either clinically or by flow cytometric analysis?

6. Is there clinical history of drug/toxin exposure or viral infection to support diagnosis of secondary acquired aplastic anemia?

7. In cases of previously diagnosed acquired aplastic anemia:

    Has the current material been compared to prior specimens to assess for progressive dysplasia?

    Has cytogenetic analysis been ordered?

AML = acute myeloid leukemia; IHC = immunohistochemistry; MDS = myelodysplastic syndrome; PNH = paroxysmal nocturnal hemoglobinuria

3. Most patients with constitutional bone marrow failure syndromes demonstrate hematologic abnormalities in infancy and early childhood, and often have associated bone, skin, renal, and central nervous system abnormalities; however, initial presentation sometimes occurs in older children and adults.

4. Fanconi anemia may be diagnosed with cytogenetic studies for increased sensitivity to cross-linking agents. Other inherited bone marrow failure syndromes may show characteristic genetic abnormalities, but do *not* share with Fanconi anemia the sensitivity to chromosomal breakage.

5. In adults, especially older patients, true hematopoietic hypoplasia/aplasia must be distinguished from technical artifacts such as small core biopsy specimens that consist largely of the physiologically hypocellular subcortical zone.

6. Hypoplastic MDS, AML, and hairy cell leukemia should be excluded from consideration before making a diagnosis of acquired aplastic anemia. In addition, rare hypocellular presentations of acute lymphoblastic leukemia may be obscured by florid immunoblastic proliferations.

7. Neither increased bone marrow myeloblasts nor significant dysplasia of hematopoietic elements in blood or bone marrow are features of typical acquired aplastic anemia and instead suggest a diagnosis of hypocellular MDS or AML.

8. Assessment of CD34 and myeloperoxidase by immunoperoxidase techniques is useful in highlighting immature cells in cases of hypoplastic MDS/AML.

9. Standard cytogenetic analysis is useful in identifying clonal abnormalities in cases of aplastic anemia and hypocellular MDS/AML, but hypocellular specimens may limit meta analysis, and FISH panels may therefore be useful.

10. CD20 staining by immunoperoxidase techniques is very valuable in identifying subtle infiltrates of B-cells in cases of hypocellular hairy cell leukemia.

11. In addition to hypocellularity, a wide variety of lymphoid, bone marrow stromal, and other types of abnormalities are occasionally found in the bone marrow of patients with acquired aplastic anemia.

12. Although rare, some patients with aplastic anemia have prominent bone marrow lymphoid and even immunoblastic infiltrates that may require immunophenotypic or molecular assessment for clonality.

13. Pure red cell, granulocytic, and, rarely, megakaryocytic aplasia may occasionally precede overt trilineage aplasia in acquired and constitutional aplastic anemias.

14. Patients with aplastic anemia who are treated with immune-modulating agents (often in conjunction with colony-stimulating factor therapy) have an increased risk of developing MDS/AML that exhibits morphologic and genetic features of a therapy-related neoplasm.

15. Assessment for PNH clones is important in aplastic anemia; sensitivity of the flow cytometry assay is a critical variable in this determination.

[7.7] References

Alter BP [2005] Bone marrow failure: a child is not just a small adult (but an adult can have a childhood disease). *Hematology (Am Soc Hematol Educ Program)* 2005:96-103.

Alter BP [2007a] Diagnosis, genetics, and management of inherited bone marrow failure syndromes. *Hematology (Am Soc Hematol Educ Program)* 2007:29-39.

Alter BP, Baerlocher GM, Savage SA, et al [2007b] Very short telomere length by flow fluorescence in situ hybridization identifies patients with dyskeratosis congenita. *Blood* 110:1439-1447.

Alter BP, Giri N, Savage SA, Rosenberg PS [2009] Cancer in dyskeratosis congenita. *Blood* 113:6549-6557.

Ameziane N, Errami A, Leveille F, et al [2008] Genetic subtyping of Fanconi anemia by comprehensive mutation screening. *Hum Mutat* 29:159-166.

Araten DJ, Bessler M, McKenzie S, et al [2002] Dynamics of hematopoiesis in paroxysmal nocturnal hemoglobinuria (PNH): No evidence for intrinsic growth advantage of PNH clones. *Leukemia* 16:2243-2248.

Bacigalupo A [2007] Aplastic anemia: pathogenesis and treatment. *Hematology (Am Soc Hematol Educ Program)* 2007:23-28.

Bagby G, Lipton J, Sloand E, Schiffer C [2004] Marrow failure. *Hematology (Am Soc Hematol Educ Program)* 2004:318-336.

Bagby GC, Meyers G [2007] Bone marrow failure as a risk factor for clonal evolution: prospects for leukemia prevention. *Hematology (Am Soc Hematol Educ Program)* 2007:40-46.

Blasco MA [2007] Telomere length, stem cells and aging. *Nat Chem Biol* 3:640-649.

Brodsky RA [2008] Advances in the diagnosis and therapy of paroxysmal nocturnal hemoglobinuria. *Blood Rev* 22:65-74.

Calado RT, Young NS [2008] Telomere maintenance and human bone marrow failure. *Blood* 111:4446-4455.

Calado RT, Regal JH, Hills M, et al [2009] Constitutional hypomorphic telomerase mutations in patients with acute myeloid leukemia. *Proc Natl Acad Sci USA* 106:1187-1192.

Camitta BM, Thomas ED, Nathan DG, et al [1976] Severe aplastic anemia: a prospective study of the effect of early marrow transplantation on acute mortality. *Blood* 48:63-70.

Cariani E, Pelizzari AM, Rodella A, et al [2007] Immune-mediated hepatitis-associated aplastic anemia caused by the emergence of a mutant hepatitis B virus undetectable by standard assays. *J Hepatol* 46:743-747.

Cengiz C, Turhan N, Yolcu OF, Yilmaz S [2007] Hepatitis associated with aplastic anemia: do CD8(+) kupffer cells have a role in the pathogenesis? *Dig Dis Sci* 52:2438-2443.

Cioc AM, Wagner JE, MacMillan M, et al [2010] Diagnosis of myelodysplastic syndrome among a cohort of 119 patients with Fanconi anemia. *Am J Clin Pathol* 133(1):92-100.

D'Andrea AD, Dahl N, Guinan EC, Shimamura A [2002] Marrow failure. *Hematology (Am Soc Hematol Educ Program)* 2002:58-72.

de Latour RP, Mary JY, Salanoubat C, et al [2008] Paroxysmal nocturnal hemoglobinuria: natural history of disease subcategories. *Blood* 112:3099-3106.

De Nicolo A, Tancredi M, Lombardi G, et al [2008a] A novel breast cancer-associated BRIP1 (FANCJ/BACH1) germ-line mutation impairs protein stability and function. *Clin Cancer Res* 14:4672-4680.

de Vries AC, Langerak AW, Verhaaf B, et al [2008b] T-cell receptor Vbeta CDR3 oligoclonality frequently occurs in childhood refractory cytopenia (MDS-RC) and severe aplastic anemia. *Leukemia* 22:1170-1174.

Dingli D, Luzzatto L, Pacheco JM [2008] Neutral evolution in paroxysmal nocturnal hemoglobinuria. *Proc Natl Acad Sci USA* 105:18496-18500.

Dirksen U, Moghadam KA, Mambetova C, et al [2004] Glutathione S transferase theta 1 gene (GSTT1) null genotype is associated with an increased risk for acquired aplastic anemia in children. *Pediatr Res* 55:466-471.

Dokal I, Vulliamy T [2008] Inherited aplastic anaemias/bone marrow failure syndromes. *Blood Rev* 22:141-153.

Dubey S, Shukla P, Nityanand S [2005] Expression of interferon gamma and tumor necrosis factor alpha in bone marrow T cells and their levels in bone marrow plasma in patients with aplastic anemia. *Ann Hematol* 84:572-577.

Dufour C, Svahn J, Bacigalupo A, et al [2005] Genetic polymorphisms of CYP3A4, GSTT1, GSTM1, GSTP1 and NQO1 and the risk of acquired idiopathic aplastic anemia in Caucasian patients. *Haematologica* 90:1027-1031.

Elghetany MT, Hudnall SD, Gardner FH [1997] Peripheral blood picture in primary hypocellular refractory anemia and idiopathic acquired aplastic anemia: an additional tool for differential diagnosis. *Haematologica* 82:21-24.

Fogarty PF, Yamaguchi H, Wiestner A, et al [2003] Late presentation of dyskeratosis congenita as apparently acquired aplastic anaemia due to mutations in telomerase RNA. *Lancet* 362:1628-1630.

Foucar K, Viswanatha D, Wilson C [2008] Bone marrow failure disorders. In: King D, Gardner W, Sobin L, et al, eds. *Non-Neoplastic Disorders of Bone Marrow (AFIP fascicle)*. Washington, DC: American Registry of Pathology; 221-248.

Fuhrer M, Durner J, Brunnler G, et al [2007] HLA association is different in children and adults with severe acquired aplastic anemia. *Pediatr Blood Cancer* 48:186-191.

Ganapathi KA, Shimamura A [2008] Ribosomal dysfunction and inherited marrow failure. *Br J Haematol* 141:376-387.

Gidvani V, Ramkissoon S, Sloand EM, Young NS [2007] Cytokine gene polymorphisms in acquired bone marrow failure. *Am J Hematol* 82:721-724.

Grishaber JE, McClain KL, Mahoney DH, Jr [1988] Fernbach DJ. Successful outcome of severe aplastic anemia following Epstein-Barr virus infection. *Am J Hematol* 28:273-275.

Guinan EC [1997] Clinical aspects of aplastic anemia. *Hematol Oncol Clin North Am* 11:1025-1044.

Hanaoka N, Kawaguchi T, Horikawa K, et al [2006] Immunoselection by natural killer cells of PIGA mutant cells missing stress-inducible ULBP. *Blood* 107:1184-1191.

Hanaoka N, Nakakuma H, Horikawa K, et al [2009] NKG2D-mediated immunity underlying paroxysmal nocturnal haemoglobinuria and related bone marrow failure syndromes. *Br J Haematol* 146:538-545.

Hillmen P, Lewis SM, Bessler M, et al [1995] Natural history of paroxysmal nocturnal hemoglobinuria. *N Engl J Med* 333:1253-1258.

Hirano N, Butler MO, Guinan EC, et al [2005] Presence of anti-kinectin and anti-PMS1 antibodies in Japanese aplastic anaemia patients. *Br J Haematol* 128:221-223.

Hirano N, Butler MO, Von Bergwelt-Baildon MS, et al [2003] Autoantibodies frequently detected in patients with aplastic anemia. *Blood* 102:4567-4575.

Honkaniemi E, Gustafsson B, Fischler B, et al [2007] Acquired aplastic anaemia in 7 children with severe hepatitis with or without liver failure. *Acta Paediatr* 96:1660-1664.

Howlett NG, Taniguchi T, Olson S, et al [2002] Biallelic inactivation of BRCA2 in Fanconi anemia. *Science* 297:606-609.

Issaragrisil S, Kaufman DW, Anderson T, et al [2006] The epidemiology of aplastic anemia in Thailand. *Blood* 107:1299-1307.

Karadimitris A, Manavalan JS, Thaler HT, et al [2000a] Abnormal T-cell repertoire is consistent with immune process underlying the pathogenesis of paroxysmal nocturnal hemoglobinuria. *Blood* 96:2613-2620.

Karadimitris A, Notaro R, Koehne G, et al [2000b] PNH cells are as sensitive to T-cell-mediated lysis as their normal counterparts: implications for the pathogenesis of paroxysmal nocturnal haemoglobinuria. *Br J Haematol* 111:1158-1163.

Kirwan M, Dokal I [2008] Dyskeratosis congenita: a genetic disorder of many faces. *Clin Genet* 73:103-112.

Krech R, Thiele J [1985] Histopathology of the bone marrow in toxic myelopathy. A study of drug induced lesions in 57 patients. *Virchows Arch A Pathol Anat Histopathol* 405:225-235.

Lau YL, Srivastava G, Lee CW, et al [1994] Epstein-Barr virus associated aplastic anaemia and hepatitis. *J Paediatr Child Health* 30:74-76.

Lee KA, Kim SH, Woo HY, et al [2001] Increased frequencies of glutathione S-transferase (GSTM1 and GSTT1) gene deletions in Korean patients with acquired aplastic anemia. *Blood* 98:3483-3485.

Levitus M, Joenje H, de Winter JP [2006] The Fanconi anemia pathway of genomic maintenance. *Cell Oncol* 28:3-29.

Maciejewski JP, Risitano A, Sloand EM, et al [2002] Distinct clinical outcomes for cytogenetic abnormalities evolving from aplastic anemia. *Blood* 99:3129-3135.

Maciejewski JP, Selleri C [2004] Evolution of clonal cytogenetic abnormalities in aplastic anemia. *Leuk Lymphoma* 45:433-440.

Marrone A, Dokal I [2004] Dyskeratosis congenita: molecular insights into telomerase function, aging and cancer. *Expert Rev Mol Med* 6:1-23.

Marrone A, Sokhal P, Walne A, et al [2007] Functional characterization of novel telomerase RNA (TERC) mutations in patients with diverse clinical and pathological presentations. *Haematologica* 92:1013-1020.

Marsh JC, Elebute MO [2003] Stem cells in paroxysmal nocturnal haemoglobinuria and aplastic anaemia: increasing evidence for overlap of haemopoietic defect. *Transfus Med* 13:377-386.

Marsh JC, Ball SE, Cavenagh J, et al [2009] Guidelines for the diagnosis and management of aplastic anaemia. *Br J Haematol* 147:43-70.

Mishra B, Malhotra P, Ratho RK, et al [2005] Human parvovirus B19 in patients with aplastic anemia. *Am J Hematol* 79:166-167.

Nagakura S, Ishihara S, Dunn DE, et al [2002] Decreased susceptibility of leukemic cells with PIGA mutation to natural killer cells in vitro. *Blood* 100:1031-1037.

Nakao S, Sugimori C, Yamazaki H [2006] Clinical significance of a small population of paroxysmal nocturnal hemoglobinuria-type cells in the management of bone marrow failure. *Int J Hematol* 84:118-122.

Piao W, Grosse J, Czwalinna A, et al [2005] Antigen-recognition sites of micromanipulated T cells in patients with acquired aplastic anemia. *Exp Hematol* 33:804-810.

Reid S, Schindler D, Hanenberg H, et al [2007] Biallelic mutations in PALB2 cause Fanconi anemia subtype FA-N and predispose to childhood cancer. *Nat Genet* 39:162-164.

Savage SA, Giri N, Baerlocher GM, et al [2008] TINF2, a component of the shelterin telomere protection complex, is mutated in dyskeratosis congenita. *Am J Hum Genet* 82:501-509.

Scheinberg P, Wu CO, Nunez O, Young NS [2009] Predicting response to immunosuppressive therapy and survival in severe aplastic anaemia. *Br J Haematol* 144:206-216.

Shah I, Murthy AK [2005] Aplastic anemia in an HIV infected child. *Indian J Pediatr* 72:359-361.

Shimamura A [2006] Shwachman-Diamond syndrome. *Semin Hematol* 43:178-188.

Shimamura A [2009] Clinical approach to marrow failure. *Hematology (Am Soc Hematol Edu Program)* 2009:329-337.

Soll E, Massumoto C, Clift RA, et al [1995] Relevance of marrow fibrosis in bone marrow transplantation: a retrospective analysis of engraftment. *Blood* 86:4667-4673.

Sugimori C, Mochizuki K, Qi Z, et al [2009] Origin and fate of blood cells deficient in glycosylphosphatidylinositol-anchored protein among patients with bone marrow failure. *Br J Haematol* 147:102-112.

Sutton JF, Stacey M, Kearns WG, et al [2004] Increased risk for aplastic anemia and myelodysplastic syndrome in individuals lacking glutathione S-transferase genes. *Pediatr Blood Cancer* 42:122-126.

Tremblay CS, Huang FF, Habi O, et al [2008] HES1 is a novel interactor of the Fanconi anemia core complex. *Blood* 112:2062-2070.

Usman M, Adil SN, Moatter T, et al [2004] Increased expression of HLA DR2 in acquired aplastic anemia and its impact on response to immunosuppressive therapy. *J Pak Med Assoc* 54:251-254.

Vulliamy T, Beswick R, Kirwan M, et al [2008] Mutations in the telomerase component NHP2 cause the premature ageing syndrome dyskeratosis congenita. *Proc Natl Acad Sci USA* 105:8073-8078.

Vulliamy T, Marrone A, Dokal I, Mason PJ [2002] Association between aplastic anaemia and mutations in telomerase RNA. *Lancet* 359:2168-2170.

Walne AJ, Vulliamy TJ, Beswick R, et al [2008] TINF2 mutations result in very short telomeres: analysis of a large cohort of patients with dyskeratosis congenita and related bone marrow failure syndromes. *Blood* 145:164-172.

Walne AJ, Dokal I [2009] Advances in the understanding of dyskeratosis congenita. *Br J Haematol* 145:164-172.

Wang H, Chuhjo T, Yamazaki H, et al [2001] Relative increase of granulocytes with a paroxysmal nocturnal haemoglobinuria phenotype in aplastic anaemia patients: the high prevalence at diagnosis. *Eur J Haematol* 66:200-205.

Xu H, Li A, Yu Y, et al [2009] Comparative analysis of G-CSFR and GM-CSFR expressions on CD34+ cells in patients with aplastic aneia and myelodysplastic syndrome. *Int J Lab Hematol* 31:591-602.

Yamaguchi H, Calado RT, Ly H, et al [2005] Mutations in TERT, the gene for telomerase reverse transcriptase, in aplastic anemia. *N Engl J Med* 352:1413-1424.

Yan XQ, Lacey D, Hill D, et al [1996] A model of myelofibrosis and osteosclerosis in mice induced by overexpressing thrombopoietin (mpl ligand): Reversal of disease by bone marrow transplantation. *Blood* 88:402-409.

Yetgin S, Cetin M, Ozyurek E, et al [2004] Parvovirus B19 infection associated with severe aplastic anemia in an immunocompetent patient. *Pediatr Hematol Oncol* 21:223-226.

Young NS, Kaufman DW [2008a] The epidemiology of acquired aplastic anemia. *Haematologica* 93:489-492.

Young NS, Scheinberg P, Calado RT [2008b] Aplastic anemia. *Curr Opin Hematol* 15:162-168.

CHAPTER

Erythroblastopenia

Kathryn Foucar, MD

ffective erythropoiesis requires hematopoietic stem cells, erythroid progenitor cells, an adequate bone marrow microenvironment, and appropriate regulatory factors. Any defect in this complex system may result in failure of the bone marrow to produce adequate erythroid cells, termed either *erythroblastopenia* or *red cell aplasia*. In this disorder the bone marrow typically demonstrates few maturing erythroid cells, often only widely scattered erythroblasts. These erythroblastopenic disorders can be classified into 3 groups: congenital red cell aplasia, acquired transient erythroblastopenic disorders, and acquired sustained red cell aplasias (so-called pure red cell aplasia) **t8.1**. Depending on both the duration of the red cell aplasia and the basal lifespan of the individual patient's erythrocytes, these patients display a variable degree of anemia; patients in whom erythroblastopenia is sustained will develop severe normocytic normochromic anemia with a markedly reduced reticulocyte count. Furthermore, even transient erythroblastopenia may result in severe exacerbation of anemia in patients with underlying constitutional red blood cell (RBC) disorders. These constitutional RBC disorders include RBC survival defects (eg, hereditary spherocytosis) as well as familial disorders in which the cause of anemia is multifactorial but sustained high levels of erythropoiesis are required for compensation (eg, thalassemias). A hallmark of any erythroblastopenic disorder is an inappropriately low reticulocyte count indicating decreased RBC production.

[8.1] Incidence and Epidemiology of Red Cell Aplasia

The incidence of red cell aplasia varies by specific subtype, the rarest being the constitutional disorder Diamond-Blackfan anemia (DBA), with an incidence of 5 per million births [Dokal 2008]. This disorder equally affects males and females and is more common in patients of European descent. Transient erythroblastopenia of childhood (TEC) usually affects children 6 months to 3 years of age, with an annual incidence rate of 4 per 100,000 in isolated countries in which these data are available [Skeppner 2002]. The true incidence of TEC is probably higher due to the likelihood of underdiagnosis in spontaneously resolving, clinically occult cases [Prassouli 2005]. Similarly, parvovirus is a common childhood viral infection, and it is likely that there are substantial numbers of clinically occult, transient cases of viral-induced red cell aplasia. The incidence of sustained red cell aplasia from chronic parvoviral infection is significant in immunosuppressed populations [Mylonakis 1999]. Other causes of acquired, sustained red cell aplasia are uncommon, occurring in only a minority of patients with leukemias, thymomas, lymphomas, and other neoplasms.

t8.1 Erythroblastopenic Disorders (Red Cell Aplasia)

Constitutional*

Diamond-Blackfan anemia

Acquired Red Cell Aplasia

Transient

    Transient erythroblastopenia of childhood

    Parvovirus infection (usually transient)[†]

Sustained red cell aplasia (pure red cell aplasia)

    Primary (idiopathic)

    Secondary to various immune aberrations, drug therapy, underlying neoplasms, or infections

*Fanconi anemia can occasionally initially manifest with red cell aplasia, although subsequent multilineage aplasia develops
[†]Parvoviral infections may be sustained/chronic in immunocompromised patients and in very rare, apparently immunocompetent patients

References: [Dokal 2008, Fujishima 2008, Perkins 2004, Sawada 2008, Skeppner 2002, Vlachos 2008]

[8.2] Congenital Red Cell Aplasia

Although red cell aplasia can occasionally be the initial manifestation of Fanconi anemia (a congenital cause of aplastic anemia), the only congenital disorder characterized initially by isolated and sustained red cell aplasia is DBA, a rare disorder commonly associated with short stature, various craniofacial and thumb skeletal abnormalities, as well as other malformations **t8.2, t8.3** [Dokal 2008, Flygare 2007a, 2007b, Gazda 2006, Lipton 2006, Ohene-Abuakwa 2005]. With rare exception, anemia is present either at birth or develops within the first year of life. Several erythrocyte abnormalities characterize DBA, including a significant macrocytosis with mean corpuscular volumes ranging from 110-140 fL. In addition to size abnormalities, these erythrocytes retain increased amounts of hemoglobin F, express i antigen on their surface, and have increased levels of RBC adenosine deaminase [Dokal 2008, Flygare 2007b, Gazda 2006, Lipton 2009]. As a consequence of the red cell aplasia, the reticulocyte count is profoundly decreased, and severe anemia develops despite markedly increased erythropoietin levels.

[8.2.1] Pathogenesis

Several familial types of DBA have been described, but many cases are sporadic **t8.2**. Although genetically heterogeneous, several specific mutations have been identified in family kindred studies [Dokal 2008, Farrar 2008, Lipton 2009]. The primary molecular/genetic defect in DBA appears to be faulty ribosomal biogenesis resulting in defective ribosomal function [Farrar 2008, Shimamura 2008]. How this defect produces red cell aplasia is not clear, and intrinsic progenitor cell defects have also been proposed [Dokal 2008, Flygare 2007b, Gazda 2006, Lipton 2009, Ohene-Abuakwa 2005].

t8.2 Diamond-Blackfan Anemia

Incidence	5 per million births; equal sex ratio
Presentation	Most cases diagnosed in early infancy (95% diagnosed by 1 year); very rare cases present in adulthood
Inheritance	45% familial (autosomal dominant); ~55% de novo mutations Usually autosomal dominant inheritance pattern
Anomalies	Common; 50% have skeletal defects, especially thumb and craniofacial; cardiac and urogenital malformations also common 30% short stature
Blood	Moderate to severe macrocytic anemia Reticulocytopenia (profound) WBC (absolute neutrophil count) usually normal to slightly decreased Platelet count normal to slightly increased
Bone marrow	Red cell aplasia with only rare erythroblasts (usually < 5% erythroid cells) Other hematopoietic elements unremarkable (overall cellularity normal/near normal) Infants may have increased benign lymphoid precursors termed hematogones* Eventual development of global hypoplasia, especially in steroid-refractory cases
Molecular defect(s)	Genetically heterogeneous; faulty ribosome biogenesis hypothesized as underlying defect resulting in defective ribosomal function due to mutations in structural ribosomal proteins Evidence suggests a number of intrinsic progenitor cell defects in proliferation, differentiation, apoptosis, and cytokine response Genetic defects: 9 genes, all associated with ribosomal biogenesis, have been found to be mutated in a total of ~53% of cases *RPS19* (~25%), *RPL5* (~6.6%), *RPS10* (~6.4%), *RPL11* (~4.8%), *RPL35A* (~3.5%), *RPS26* (~2.6%), *RPS24* (~2%), *RPS17* (~1%), *RPS7* (~1%)
Disease course	Frontline corticosteroid therapy and transfusions (majority of patients respond); other therapies include chronic transfusions and bone marrow/stem cell transplantation Increased lifetime risk of acute myeloid leukemia/myelodysplasia

*See Chapter 21 for discussion on hematogones

References: [Doherty 2010, Dokal 2008, Farrar 2008, Flygare 2007a, 2007b, Gazda 2006, Lipton 2006, 2009, Ohene-Abuakwa 2005, Vlachos 2008]

[8.2.2] **Morphology**

Patients with DBA manifest with profound anemia without polychromasia i8.1; other lineages are generally preserved. Bone marrow examination in DBA reveals either complete loss of the erythroid lineage or scattered, isolated, morphologically unremarkable erythroblasts i8.2, i8.3. Increased numbers of B-lymphocyte precursor cells, termed *hematogones,* are often present in the bone marrow, especially in infants and young children i8.2. These cells exhibit a high nuclear-cytoplasmic ratio and can diffusely infiltrate the bone marrow, potentially mimicking an acute leukemia (see Chapter 21). In contrast to this worrisome finding, granulocytic and megakaryocytic lineages are preserved in the bone marrow, and levels of neutrophils and platelets in the blood are often normal. Acute leukemia manifesting with isolated erythroblastopenia is very unusual; if necessary, flow cytometric immunophenotyping can be used to distinguish hematogones from lymphoblasts (see Chapter 21). Although isolated red cell aplasia may persist for many years, long-term follow-up of patients with DBA reveals that progressive multilineage bone marrow hypoplasia with associated neutropenia and/or thrombocytopenia may develop in a substantial number, especially in those who do not respond to therapy. Thus, DBA may actually be another type of multilineage bone marrow failure disorder [Dokal 2008, Lipton 2006] (see Chapter 7). The risk of developing acute myeloid leukemia/myelodysplasia in long-term survivors exceeds expected rates t8.2 [Dokal 2008, Lipton 2009].

t8.3 Comparison of Erythroblastopenic Disorders

Disorder	Onset	Erythrocytes	Reticulocyte Count	Additional Features
Congenital				
Diamond-Blackfan anemia	At birth through infancy	↑ mean corpuscular volume ↑ hemoglobin F i antigen present ↑ RBC adenosine deaminase	↓	Either complete loss of erythroid lineage or only earliest forms present Other hematopoietic lineages unremarkable; mild thrombocytosis common Increased bone marrow hematogones; may mimic ALL (B lymphoblastic leukemia) Corticosteroid therapy successful in 2/3 of patients; others may require allogeneic bone marrow or cord blood transplantation Progressive global hypoplasia in non-responders
Acquired				
Transient erythroblastopenia of childhood	Usually >1 yr of age (occasionally occurs <1 year)	Normal morphology Normal mean corpuscular volume (may be ↑ during recovery)	↓ (↑ during recovery)	Either complete loss of erythroid lineage or only earliest forms present Other hematopoietic lineages unremarkable; mild neutropenia common Increased bone marrow hematogones; may mimic ALL (B lymphoblastic leukemia) No associated abnormalities Frequent history of presumed viral infection Association with human herpesvirus-6, parvovirus, Kawasaki disease described
Parvovirus-induced red cell aplasia (usually transient, but may be sustained) (see t8.5)	Any age, predominates in children Patient typically has underlying chronic anemia or immunodeficiency disorder	Variable, depending on underlying disorder	↓ (↑ during recovery)	Most frequently recognized in patients with chronic red blood cell disorders associated with a shortened life span; infection self-limited Also occurs as subclinical infection of erythroblasts in normal patients; infection self-limited In immunocompromised patients, infections are sustained and cause prolonged red cell aplasia or aplasia of other lineages (agranulocytosis) Parvovirus infects erythroblasts and other mitotically active erythroid cells; intranuclear inclusions visible in rare residual erythroblasts; rest of lineage usually absent Other hematopoietic lineages generally unremarkable Spontaneous recovery occurs, except in immunosuppressed patients who cannot mount neutralizing antibody response
Acquired sustained red cell aplasia (see t8.6)	Adolescence through adulthood	Normal morphology Normal mean corpuscular volume	↓	Both primary (one half) and secondary types (one half) Erythroid lineage absent or only earliest forms present Other hematopoietic lineages unremarkable Secondary cases linked to T-cell large granular lymphocytic leukemia, other B- and T-cell lymphoproliferative neoplasms, thymoma, viral infections, autoimmune disorders, drug toxicities, medications Immune pathophysiologic mechanisms likely; autoantibody directed against erythroid progenitors in some patients, while T-cell mediated suppression of erythropoiesis occurs in others; antibodies to rh erythropoietin in patients on long-term therapy Clonal T-cell defects detected in some cases Therapy: discontinue all antecedent drug therapy; immune-modulating agents may be required; assess for occult T-cell clones

ALL = acute lymphoblastic leukemia; rh = recombinant human

References: [Bennett 2005, Casadevall 2002, Cherrick 1994, Dokal 2008, Lipton 2009, Masuda 2005, Mori 2003, Prassouli 2005, Sawada 2009, Skeppner 2002, Thompson 2006, Vlachos 2008, Wang 2007]

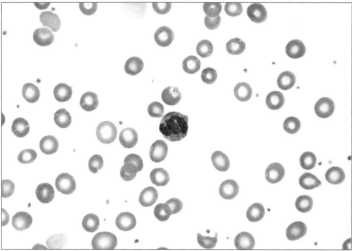

i8.1 *Profound anemia without polychromasia is evident in the peripheral blood in patient with Diamond-Blackfan anemia. Neutrophils and platelets were normal. (Wright)*

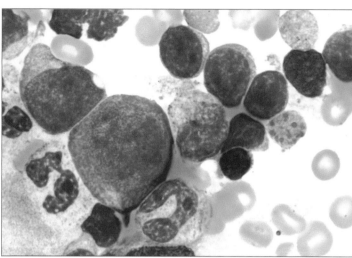

i8.2 *Only rare erythroblasts are evident on this bone marrow aspirate smear from a child with Diamond-Blackfan anemia. Note abundant lymphoid cells with uniformly condensed chromatin characteristic of hematogones. (Wright)*

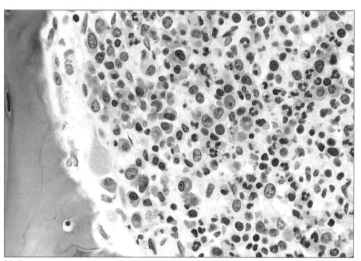

i8.3 *This bone marrow biopsy section from a child with long-standing Diamond-Blackfan anemia shows intact granulopoiesis with an absence of identifiable erythroid islands. (H&E)*

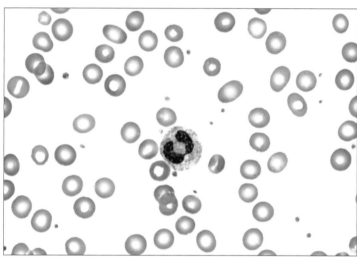

i8.4 *Blood smear from a child with transient erythroblastopenia of childhood shows marked normocytic, normochromic anemia without polychromasia. Other cell counts preserved. (Wright)*

[8.3] ## Acquired Transient Erythroblastopenic Disorders

Acquired erythroblastopenia may be either transient or sustained **t8.1, t8.3**. The 2 well-described types of transient erythroblastopenia are so-called TEC and parvovirus-related erythroblastopenia. Despite proposed differences between these 2 disorders, overlap is likely, especially now that highly sensitive and specific genetic techniques are available to document acute parvovirus infection (see **sidebar 8.1**) [Prassouli 2005].

[8.3.1] ### Transient Erythroblastopenia of Childhood

The term *TEC* has been applied to an idiopathic, self-limited disorder characterized by normocytic, normochromic anemia, profound reticulocytopenia, and decreased erythroid cells in the bone marrow [Cherrick 1994, Prassouli 2005]. Although most patients are older than 1 year of age, TEC has been described in infants, including newborns, causing differential diagnostic difficulties with DBA [Farhi 1998, Miller 1994, Tugal 1994]. A substantial portion of children with TEC are also neutropenic [Cherrick 1994].

Pathogenesis

A viral cause for TEC has been postulated for years; associations of TEC with human herpesvirus 6 infection (PCR assessment of bone marrow DNA), parvovirus, and Kawasaki disease have been published [Frank 1994, Penchansky 1997, Prassouli 2005, Skeppner 2002]. Rare reports describe familial TEC [Gustavson 2002].

Morphology

Like patients with DBA, those with TEC may manifest significant anemia, typically normocytic/normochromic, without polychromasia **i8.4**. Similarly, there is either complete

[sidebar 8.1] Beyond Koch's Postulates: Molecular Diagnosis and Parvovirus

When considering the surprisingly complex relationship between parvovirus and the human host, one may long for the elegant simplicity of Koch's postulates, the classic criteria for proving that a particular infectious agent causes a particular disease. In his 1882 article, *Die Aetiologie der Tuberculose*, Koch proposed that to prove causation, it is necessary to isolate a microorganism from the host, grow the organism in pure culture, and produce the disease in a second host upon inoculation with the pure organism [Koch 1942]. The strength of Koch's approach is that it focuses on the physiologic response of the organism as a whole to the infection: if the test subject becomes prostrate and febrile, then there is excellent evidence for a pathogenic process. In the case of parvovirus, however, as with many other microorganisms, Koch's approach fails to capture the considerable variability in disease, the inconsistency in host interactions, and the multiplicity of genotypes. Most importantly, the exquisite sensitivity of molecular techniques for parvovirus detection (and for infectious agents in general) complicates our understanding of the very relationship between the presence of the infectious agent and disease. Here we consider, in the context of parvovirus, the investigational and diagnostic challenges created by these factors.

As detailed in the accompanying chapter, parvovirus is responsible for a wide array of pathologies, the variability of which depends to some degree on host characteristics: in those with underlying red blood cell disorders, transient aplasia may occur, while in those incapable of robust immune response, sustained aplasia may be the result. In addition, parvovirus has been implicated in spontaneous abortion and congenital anemia in the setting of prenatal infection. Parvovirus more routinely causes the uncomplicated viral exanthem erythema infectiosum, or fifth disease. The parvovirus receptor is known to be, at least in part, the P antigen expressed on the surface of the red blood cell [Brown 1993]; however, as this receptor is also expressed on other cell types, including endothelial cells [Cooling 1995], parvovirus has been hypothesized to play a pathologic role in organ systems and locations further afield from the hematopoietic. Parvovirus has also been linked (with varying degrees of certainty) to juvenile idiopathic arthritis syndrome, autoimmune diseases, and cardiomyopathy [Bock 2005, Gonzalez 2007, Tsay 2006]. Much of the evidence implicating parvovirus in these latter syndromes comes from molecular analysis, which, as we will see, highlights the challenges of demonstrating pathogenic causation in a molecular world.

The most obvious prerequisite for designing a molecular test for a microorganism is to have a clear and accurate rendering of target genetic sequences. However, particularly in the case of some viruses, this is a more difficult challenge than might initially be apparent. The nucleic acid replication of such microorganisms may be purposefully imprecise, compared with the mammalian and human processes, such that random mutations are frequently inserted during nucleic acid replication [Duffy 2008]. This variability allows the pathogen to "hit upon" beneficial mutations that bolster infectivity or evade host responses. It also means that in some cases, from the perspective of laboratory investigation, the genomic sequence is a moving or elusive target. The *Parvoviridae*, for example, (despite being DNA viruses) show a rate of mutation more in keeping with the highly changeable RNA viruses [Lopez-Bueno 2006, Norja 2008]. Partly because of this inherent variability, several different genotypic strains of parvovirus B19 have been described. While the most common strain is considered "genotype 1," strains A6 and K71 are classified as "genotype 2" and V9 as "genotype 3," each diverging from the reference sequence on the order of 10% [Corcoran 2004, Ekman 2007]. In the 1970s, genotype 1 appears to have almost completely replaced genotype 2 as the dominant circulating strain in most of the world, for unknown reasons [Norja 2008]. Commonly used commercial polymerase chain reaction (PCR)–based assays for parvovirus are not equally sensitive to these variant strains, and in some cases may entirely fail to detect their presence [Hokynar 2004], a limitation somewhat mitigated by the fact that the full biologic function and pathogenic potential of the alternate strains are yet unknown [Ekman 2007].

A second major problem with sequence-based detection of microorganisms arises from the exquisite sensitivity of the PCR assay. Whereas serologic testing for anti-parvovirus antibodies may, in cases of subpar immune response, show false-negative results [Kurtzman 1988], we encounter the opposite problem in the molecular realm: it is possible using such techniques as representational difference analysis to detect as few as a single copy of a viral DNA in a host tissue or blood sample [Lisitsyn 1993]. Given that some microorganisms may show low background colonization associated with subclinical infection or an asymptomatic carrier state, a key requirement for such molecular testing is to establish quantitative cutoffs for the number of microorganisms consistent with a symptomatic infection. Indeed, a detailed study of parvovirus viremia in a convalescent, immunocompetent individual found that a PCR assay could detect residual parvovirus sequence up to 3 full years after primary infection [Cassinotti 2000].

While such a result is not a false positive, in that the virus is presumably indeed still present, it could be clinically misinterpreted if a prior parvovirus infection were to be detected and assigned responsibility for an unrelated cause of anemia or erythroblastopenia. This situation led the World Health Organization (WHO) to develop a publicly available parvovirus standard (NIBSC 99/800), to be used in quantitative PCR reactions, such that measures of viremia could be accurate and reproducible. Nevertheless, it is important to understand the diagnostic difference between detecting 10^{14} DNA genome equivalents, as is typical of active infection, and lower levels that might indicate residual viremia.

The sensitivity of sequence-based detection significantly complicates not only clinical diagnosis of parvovirus infection, but also the assignment of specific pathology to the presence of the virus. For instance, as noted above, parvovirus has been detected by PCR analysis in cardiac tissue samples in patients with otherwise unexplained cardiomyopathy and heart failure. Since heart muscle expresses the P glycoprotein, it seems reasonable to infer that parvovirus is a cause of heart failure. However, parvovirus has *also* been detected in tissue samples from completely asymptomatic individuals [Soderlund-Venermo 2002], raising the possibility that the parvovirus detected in patients with heart failure may be latent and entirely unrelated to the pathology in question [Modrow 2006]. Similarly, a recent case-control study analyzing a purported role for parvovirus infection in juvenile dermatomyositis found no evidence of increased parvovirus infection in such patients, and cautioned against anecdotal associations between parvovirus and autoimmune syndromes in general [Mamyrova 2005]. An analogous study failed to confirm a role for parvovirus in juvenile idiopathic arthritis [Weissbrich 2007]. Controversy also surrounds transient erythroblastopenia of childhood (TEC), which has been associated inconclusively (as noted in the accompanying chapter) with both parvovirus and human herpesvirus 6 infection.

Thus, at this level of sensitivity, Koch's original postulates are rendered at least problematic, if not largely inoperable. Some have proposed a new set of "guidelines" for establishing microbial disease causation using molecular techniques [Fredericks 1996]. It is a fascinating paradox that such a rigorously empirical laboratory technique demands a corresponding philosophical analysis, but as illustrated by the diseases examined in this chapter, such considerations will be important as sequence-based investigation of microbial pathogenesis becomes even more widely applied.

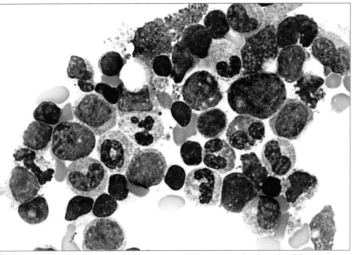

i8.5 *Bone marrow aspirate smear shows only rare residual erythroblasts in patient with transient erythroblastopenia of childhood. (Wright)*

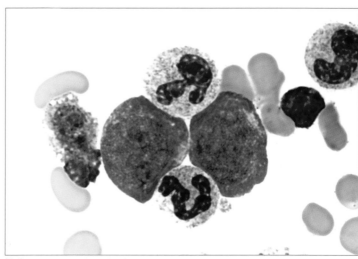

i8.6 *Two normal residual erythroblasts evident in bone marrow aspirate smear from patient with transient erythroblastopenia of childhood. (Wright)*

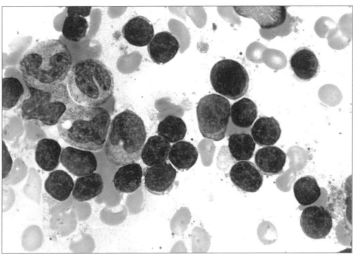

i8.7 *In addition to marked lymphocytosis, only rare erythroblasts are evident on this bone marrow aspirate smear from a child with transient erythroblastopenia who experienced a spontaneous recovery. Lymphocytes exhibit nuclear features of hematogones. (Wright)*

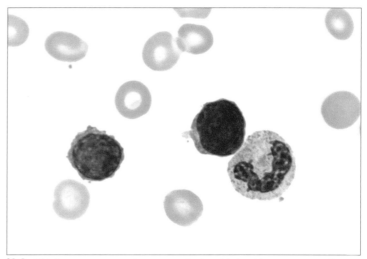

i8.8 *This bone marrow aspirate smear depicts side-by-side comparison of a normal lymphocyte (left) with a hematogone (right) in a child with transient erythroblastopenia of childhood. (Wright)*

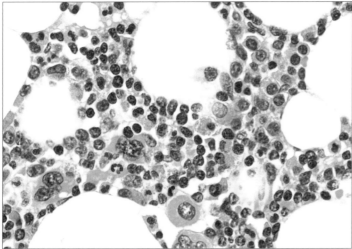

i8.9 *Normal granulocytic and megakaryocytic cells are present on this bone marrow biopsy section from a patient with transient profound erythroblastopenia. Note diffuse increase in lymphoid cells. (H&E)*

absence of the erythroid lineage or only scattered, morphologically unremarkable erythroblasts in the bone marrow **i8.5**, **i8.6**. Both the granulocytic and megakaryocytic lineages are usually preserved and exhibit normal morphologic characteristics. Also, as with DBA, a marked increase in bone marrow hematogones (lymphocyte precursors) may be present in patients with TEC, and these cells must be distinguished from those of acute lymphoblastic leukemia **i8.7**, **i8.8**, **i8.9** (see Chapter 21). The proportion of bone marrow hematogones present is often more impressive in patients with acquired TEC than in similar-age patients with DBA [Penchansky 1997].

Differential Diagnosis and Outcome

Because the cytopathic effects of parvovirus infection can be subtle and variable, this infection should be excluded by serum PCR studies before a diagnosis of TEC is established.

The differential diagnosis of TEC also includes DBA; various phenotypic and hematologic parameters can be used to help distinguish DBA from TEC at presentation, while the differences in clinical course generally allow definitive distinction **t8.2**, **t8.3**. Spontaneous recovery of TEC generally occurs within 1-2 months and is associated with an increased mean corpuscular volume, a marked reticulocytosis, and recovery of absolute neutrophil counts.

[8.3.2] **Parvovirus-Related Erythroblastopenia**

Incidence and Epidemiology

The features and hematologic manifestations of parvovirus B19 infection in humans are detailed in **t8.3**, **t8.4**, **t8.5**. Although parvovirus-induced red cell aplasia is a well-characterized disorder, both the spectrum of abnormalities induced by this virus and the types of patients developing significant parvovirus-induced disease have expanded in recent years. The disease manifestations of acute parvovirus infection vary widely based on the patient age and the underlying immune and hematologic status of the patient **t8.5** [Florea 2007, Young 2004]. Parvovirus B19 infection was initially recognized as a cause of transient red cell aplasia in patients with underlying erythrocyte disorders, such as

t8.4 Features of Parvovirus B19

Features	Comments
Infection in humans	Only human pathogenic parvovirus
	Common worldwide infection; most adults seropositve
Infection of erythroid lineage/ other lineages	Cellular receptor for B19 is blood group P antigen (globoside); erythroid cells expressing P are susceptible to parvovirus B19 infection; erythroid progenitor cells only known natural host of parvovirus B19
	Parvovirus can also rarely infect other hematopoietic lineage progenitor cells (eg, megakaryocyte progenitors) and endothelial cells
Viral replication (single-stranded DNA virus)	B19 requires mitotically active cells for replication; as virus replicates drives infected erythroid cells to premature death via apoptosis
Disease manifestations	Vary widely based on age of patient and underlying immune and hematologic status of patient
	Includes erythema infectiosum, transient aplastic crisis, sustained pure red cell aplasia, hydrops fetalis/congenital anemia, and polyarthropathy syndrome

References: [Florea 2007, Weigel-Kelley 2003, Young 2004]

t8.5 Hematologic Manifestations of Parvovirus B19 Infection

Immune Status	Hematologic Status	Comments
In utero		
Under development	High RBC production	Intrauterine demise may occur (hydrops fetalis) due to impaired RBC production or surviving neonate may be severely anemic; spontaneous recovery *in utero* has been described
Children/adults		
Intact	Normal RBC production	Typical disease picture is erythema infectiosum in children while polyarthropathy syndrome predominates in adults; although RBC production ceases briefly (transient aplastic crisis), there are no clinical/hematologic manifestations
Intact	Basal accelerated erythrocyte production (hemolytic anemias, thalassemia, rare iron deficiency anemia)	Transient aplastic crisis, even though self-limited, leads to precipitous drop in hemoglobin, hematocrit
		Bone marrow notable for striking paucity of maturing erythroid cells; rare viral inclusions in erythroblasts; variable lymphocytosis (especially prominent in young children)
		Extensive bone marrow necrosis with systemic embolization (acute chest syndrome) may occur in sickle cell anemia patients who develop secondary parvovirus B19 infection
Immunocompromised/ immunodeficient (unable to mount neutralizing antibody to eradicate B19 virus)	Usually no constitutional disorders associated with accelerated erythropoiesis, although patient may have baseline anemia of chronic disease or bone marrow suppression from underlying disease/therapy and following bone marrow transplantation	Sustained red cell aplasia with anemia and reticulocytopenia
		Variable bone marrow picture; usually paucity of erythroid lineage; rare giant erythroblasts with viral inclusions may be found
		In rare instances, erythroid lineage intact and numerous viral inclusions evident (some AIDS patients)
		Some patients with chronic parvovirus B19 infection will develop infection associated hemophagocytic syndrome

References: [Fattet 2004, Florea 2007, Hayes-Lattin 2004, Young 2004]

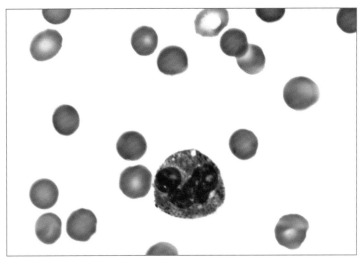

i8.10 *Profound anemia is evident in this patient with hereditary spherocytosis who developed acute parvovirus infection. Note absence of polychromasia. (Wright)*

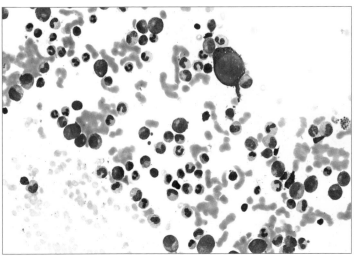

i8.11 *Rare giant erythroblasts evident on low magnification scanning of bone marrow aspirate smear in patient with acute parvovirus infection. (Wright)*

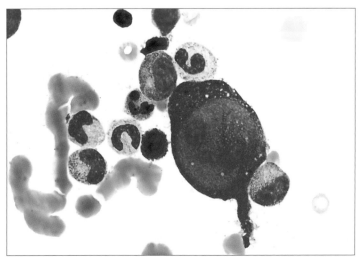

i8.12 *High magnification of rare giant erythroblast shows sparse cytoplasmic vacuoles and prominent nucleoli/inclusions. (Wright)*

hereditary spherocytosis, sickle cell anemia, and severe thalassemia, which are characterized by both a shortened RBC lifespan (less dramatic in thalassemia) and accelerated production of erythrocytes in the bone marrow with marked erythroid hyperplasia [Young 2004]. In this clinical situation, a patient with a known chronic anemia presents with an abrupt onset of severe symptoms associated with a profound decrease in reticulocyte count and marked exacerbation of the underlying anemia. This phenomenon of red cell aplasia superimposed on chronic hemolytic anemia has been termed *transient aplastic crisis.*

Parvovirus B19 is also linked to hydrops fetalis/congenital anemia in pregnant women who become infected, secondary to the profound suppression of fetal erythropoiesis during a time of physiologically high erythrocyte production **t8.5** [Young 2004]. Although red cell aplasia also occurs in normal children and adults infected with parvovirus B19, there are typically no clinical or hematologic manifestations of this transient, self-limited interruption in RBC production.

Because of the inability to mount a neutralizing antibody response, parvovirus B19 infection in immunodeficient/immunocompromised patients may result in prolonged infection, leading to sustained erythroblastopenia [Florea 2007, Young 2004]. As expected, these patients develop severe reticulocytopenic anemia.

Pathogenesis

Since the parvovirus cell surface receptor is the P antigen (with possible co-receptor), the specific tropism of parvovirus B19 for erythroid progenitor cells is well understood **t8.4 sidebar 8.1**. Replication of this single-stranded DNA virus in erythroblast nuclei drives these cells to premature death by apoptosis [Weigel-Kelley 2003, Young 2004]. However, nonproductive infection of either megakaryocytic or granulocytic precursors has also been described, explaining the occasional suppression of these lineages in chronically infected patients, especially immunosuppressed patients [Young 2004].

Morphology, Differential Diagnosis, and Outcome

In patients with underlying hemolytic anemia, even a transient cessation of erythropoiesis can result in a profound reticulocytopenic anemia **i8.10**. Parvovirus B19 infection produces very distinctive erythroid abnormalities in the bone marrow in conjunction with less conspicuous dyspoietic features in occasional patients **i8.11, i8.12, i8.13, i8.14, t8.5**. In addition to profound erythroid hypoplasia, the rare residual immature erythroid precursor cells may demonstrate enlarged overall size, cytoplasmic vacuolization, and intranuclear viral inclusions with peripheral chromatin

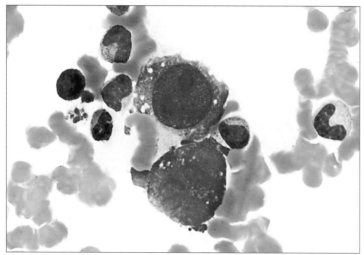

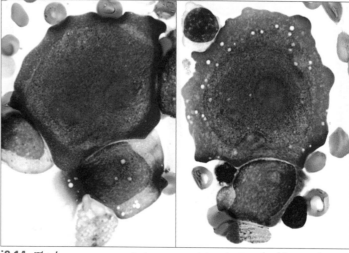

i8.13 *Two degenerating, giant erythroblasts with probable viral inclusions on bone marrow aspirate smear in patient with red cell aplasia secondary to acute parvovirus infection.*

i8.14 *This bone marrow aspirate smear contains giant erythroblasts with poorly demarcated possible intranuclear inclusions in a patient with hereditary spherocytosis who developed acute red cell aplasia. Note vacuolization of erythroblast and normal sized erythroblast adjacent to giant erythroblast (Wright) (courtesy P Ward, MD)*

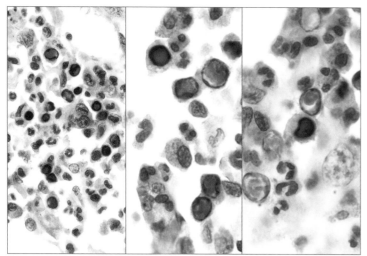

i8.15 *Erythroid precursor cells with distinctive, eosinophilic, parvoviral intranuclear inclusions (lantern cells) are evident on these bone marrow biopsy sections from an immunosuppressed transplant patient who developed acute red cell aplasia. (H&E) (courtesy C Sever, MD)*

condensation, so-called lantern cells **i8.14** [Brown 1995, 1997, Krause 1992, Liu 1997]. These viral inclusions are generally more readily apparent on bone marrow core biopsy or clot sections **i8.15, i8.16, i8.17**. On aspirate smears, the viral inclusions may more resemble a large nucleolus than an actual inclusion **i8.12, i8.13**. Giant erythroblasts show evidence of cell dissolution in association with acute parvovirus infection **i8.17** [Koduri 1998]. Because erythroid precursors are usually decreased, the identification of these suspicious/diagnostic cells may require careful review of several slides **i8.11, i8.16**. Immunoperoxidase stains for hemoglobin A/glycophorin A can be very useful in highlighting the rare residual erythroid cells on clot and biopsy sections, facilitating the search for viral inclusions or viral cytopathic effect such as dissolution

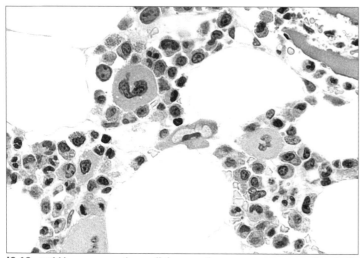

i8.16 *Mild bone marrow hypocellularity and rare inconspicuous erythroid cells are evident on this bone marrow biopsy section from a 21-year-old male with acute parvovirus infection. Center cell represents erythroblast with possible viral inclusion. (H&E) (courtesy C Sever, MD)*

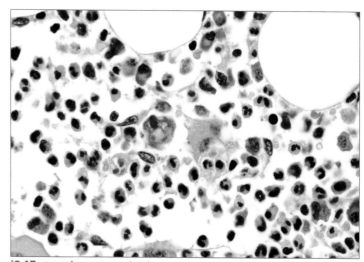

i8.17 *Rare degenerating-dissolving erythroid precursors evident on bone marrow core biopsy section in patient with acute parvovirus infection. (H&E)*

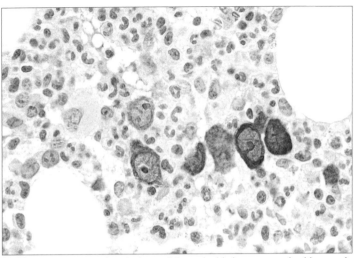

i8.18 *Immunoperoxidase for hemoglobin A highlights giant erythroblasts with possible viral inclusions in this case of acute parvovirus infection. (immunoperoxidase) (courtesy C Sever, MD)*

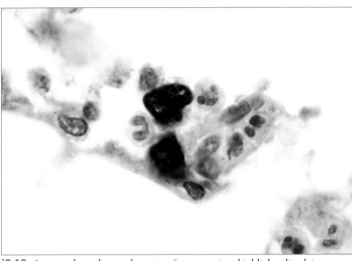

i8.19 *Immunohistochemical staining for parvovirus highlights dissolving erythroid precursors in bone marrow biopsy section from patient with acute parvovirus infection. (immunoperoxidase)*

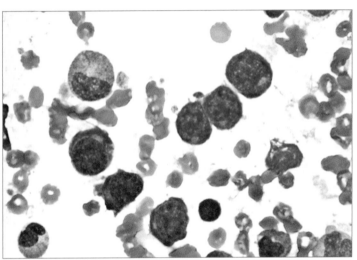

i8.20 *A wave of erythroblasts characterizes this bone marrow aspirate smear from a patient with early recovery from acute parvovirus infection. (Wright)*

of the nuclear membrane **i8.18**. In addition, both immunostaining with monoclonal antibodies directed against parvovirus B19 proteins and in situ hybridization techniques using parvovirus B19 DNA probes have been described **i8.19**. These techniques can be used to readily document parvovirus B19 infection in bone marrow from patients with suspected parvovirus-induced red cell aplasia **i8.19**. With B19 DNA in situ hybridization techniques, underlying parvovirus B19 infection can also be identified in approximately 10% of randomly selected bone marrow specimens from AIDS patients in whom parvovirus infection was not the primary consideration [Liu 1997]. Although rare, both agranulocytosis and amegakaryocytosis have been noted in patients with sustained parvovirus infection [Nagai 1992, Pont 1992]. Associated dysplasia of rare residual granulocytic and megakaryocytic cells may be evident in these cases, although, in general, these other

hematopoietic lineages are morphologically unremarkable with intact maturation. During the early recovery phase from acute parvovirus infection, a wave of regenerating erythroblasts may be evident on bone marrow specimens **i8.20**.

A unique bone marrow profile has been identified in rare immunodeficient/immunocompromised patients with concurrent parvovirus infection. In this small group, the erythroid lineage is intact with maturation despite chronic parvovirus B19 infection [Crook 2000]. Numerous viral inclusions in various stages of erythroid cells have been identified in this small cohort of patients **i8.21, i8.22**. Parvovirus B19 infection has also been linked to several additional bone marrow abnormalities. For example, evidence suggests an association between parvovirus B19 infection and acute chest syndrome in patients with sickle cell anemia [Goldstein 1995, Lowenthal 1996]. In these patients, parvovirus is thought to cause extensive bone marrow necrosis. Systemic embolization of this necrotic bone marrow results in the severe respiratory symptoms that define acute chest syndrome (see Chapter 6). In immunocompromised/immunodeficient patients, sustained parvovirus B19 infection may trigger systemic histiocytic hyperplasia with hemophagocytosis, so-called infection-associated hemophagocytic syndrome, in addition to sustained red cell aplasia. In these patients, the bone marrow will exhibit increased cytologically bland histiocytes containing ingested hematopoietic elements (see Chapter 27) [Tsuda 1994, Yufu 1997]. There have also been rare reports of parvovirus infection associated with recurrent agranulocytosis and immune thrombocytopenia [Carper 1996, Murray 1994]. Finally, chronic parvovirus infection has been rarely reported to produce a bone marrow and blood picture that mimics myelodysplasia [Hasle 1994]. In these patients, the bone marrow is hypercellular with dysplastic granulocytic cells, in conjunction with erythroblastopenia. The peripheral blood is characterized

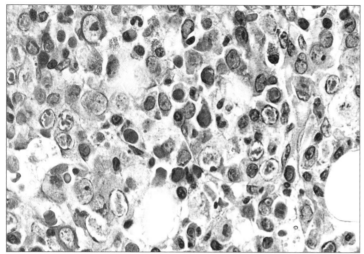

i8.21 *Bone marrow biopsy section from an AIDS patient with chronic parvovirus infection reveals abundant erythroid cells with evidence of maturation; note prominent viral inclusions in erythroblasts and more mature forms. (H&E) (courtesy R McKenna, MD)*

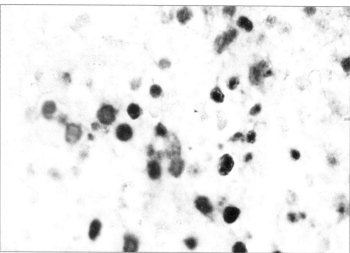

i8.22 *The parvovirus inclusions are highlighted on this in situ hybridization preparation on the bone marrow biopsy section illustrated in **i8.21**. (in situ hybridization using parvovirus B19 probe) (courtesy R McKenna, MD)*

by pancytopenia with multilineage dysplasia. In these rare cases, these abnormalities have been reported to resolve after treatment for the parvovirus.

The differential diagnosis of parvovirus logically includes the other types of red cell aplasia, especially TEC. Indeed, some cases diagnosed as TEC may actually be parvovirus induced [Prassouli 2005]. Neonatal parvovirus infection can mimic DBA [Tugal 1994]. Other more unique differential diagnostic considerations involve cases in which the patient has a clinically occult/unknown underlying hematologic disorder. Chronic parvovirus infection in patients with clinically occult glucose-6-phosphate dehydrogenase deficiency can masquerade as DBA, while acute parvovirus infection in a patient with unsuspected hereditary spherocytosis was associated with bone marrow morphologic findings that suggested congenital dyserythropoietic anemia [Carpenter 2004, Parekh 2005]. Consequently, a high index of suspicion for acute or chronic parvovirus infection is warranted in any case of erythroblastopenia and also in cases in which a wave of recovery erythroblasts is noted. Similarly, even cases in which the erythroid lineage is intact with maturation, parvovirus infection may still be present, especially if there is underlying severe immunodeficiency [Crook 2000]. Cases of acute parvovirus associated with increased bone marrow hematogones (benign lymphoid precursors) may be misinterpreted as acute lymphoblastic leukemia [Yetgin 2004].

Except for immunosuppressed patients, spontaneous recovery is the rule and generally occurs within 1-2 weeks after disease onset. Patients who have underlying immuno-deficiency disorders or who are immunocompromised from prior therapy may require high-dose intravenous immuno-globulin therapy or other immunomodulatory agents to eradicate parvovirus infection [Fattet 2004, Florea 2007, Hayes-Lattin 2004, Young 2004].

Acquired Sustained Red Cell Aplasia (Pure Red Cell Aplasia)

[8.4.1]   ### Incidence and Epidemiology

Acquired sustained red cell aplasia, also called pure red cell aplasia, predominates in adolescents and adults, but can affect patients of all ages [Praditpornsilpa 2009, Sawada 2008, Sawada 2009]. A severe normochromic, normocytic to slightly macrocytic anemia results, with morphologically normal erythrocytes and a markedly decreased reticulocyte count. General features of patients with acquired sustained pure red cell aplasia, including both primary and secondary types, are detailed in **t8.1**, **t8.3**, and **t8.6**.

Primary red cell aplasia is idiopathic, while secondary red cell aplasias are associated with a wide variety of neoplastic and nonneoplastic disorders **t8.3**, **t8.6** [Lipton 2009, Sawada 2008, 2009 Vlachos 2008]. Although phenytoin (Dilantin) is the most frequent drug associated with acquired red cell aplasia, at least 40 other drugs have been linked to this disorder [Erslev 1996]. In addition, secondary red cell aplasia is associated with thymoma, various hematolymphoid neoplasms, carcinomas, infections, and immune disorders [Fujishima 2008, Lipton 2009, Praditpornsilpa 2008, Sawada 2008, Vlachos 2008]. The most common neoplastic disorder associated with pure red cell aplasia in recent studies is T-cell large granular lymphocytic leukemia, a clonal disorder of cytotoxic T cells (see Chapter 22) [Fujishima 2008, Sawada 2008]. Clonal T-cell defects have also been identified in cases of pure red cell aplasia associated with B-cell chronic lymphocytic leukemia, thymoma, and rare patients without an established underlying overt hematologic neoplasm [Masuda 2005, Sawada 2009, Thompson 2006]. In addition to parvovirus B19, other viruses linked to secondary acquired red cell aplasia include mumps, hepatitis, Epstein-Barr virus, and rarely HIV-1 **t8.6** [Vlachos 2008].

t8.6 Classification of Acquired Sustained Red Cell Aplasia (Pure Red Cell Aplasia)

Primary (1/2 of cases)

Idiopathic

Secondary (1/2 of cases)

Large granular lymphocytic leukemia-T cell type*

Other B- and T-cell lymphoproliferative neoplasms: B-cell chronic lymphocytic leukemia, non-Hodgkin lymphoma, Hodgkin lymphoma

Drug treatments, many agents—diphenylhydantoin most common

Thymoma

Autoimmune disorders[†]

Pregnancy

Solid tumors (usually carcinomas)

Viral infections (parvovirus B19, mumps, hepatitis, Epstein-Barr virus)

Posttransplantation of ABO-incompatible bone marrow

Antibodies to recombinant erythropoietin[‡]

*Most common disorder associated with pure red cell aplasia; T-cell clone detected in many patients with red cell aplasia, even cases without overt T-cell large granular lymphocyte disorders [Masuda 2005, Mori 2003]
[†]Rare cases of systemic lupus erythematosus with combined red cell aplasia and autoimmune hemolytic anemia due to anti-erythropoietin antibodies
[‡]Occurs in patients requiring long-term recombinant erythropoietin therapy, eg, chronic renal failure patients [Hara 2008]

References: [Attar 2007, Bennett 2004, 2005, Casadevall 2002, Fujishima 2008, Hara 2008, Hirokawa 2009, Kako 2008, Lipton 2009, Masuda 2005, Mori 2003, Praditpornsilpa 2009, Sawada 2008, 2009, Thompson 2006, Vlachos 2008]

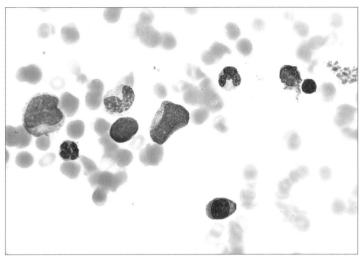

i8.23 *Dilute bone marrow aspirate smear from a patient with systemic lupus erythematosus who developed pure red cell aplasia; note intact granulocytic cells but paucity of erythroid precursors. (Wright)*

[8.4.2] Pathogenesis

Because of the diverse underlying disorders in patients with secondary pure red cell aplasia, many different pathologic mechanisms are probably responsible for the loss of this lineage. However, various immune mechanisms, including both humoral and cell-mediated factors, are likely to be responsible in most of these patients [Charles 1996, Erslev 1996, Lacy 1996, Sawada 2009]. Antierythroid antibodies may be detected in some patients, while the variety of clonal and nonclonal T-cell defects in patients with acquired pure red cell aplasia suggests a dominant role for cell-mediated immune defects in the genesis of this disease.

A unique type of acquired red cell aplasia occurs in patients who undergo allogeneic bone marrow transplantation from an ABO-incompatible donor. In these patients, the residual recipient antibodies directed against RBC antigens attack the donor erythroid lineage in the bone marrow [Erslev 1996]. Aggressive plasmapheresis is usually successful in removing this antibody, after which the erythroid lineage completely recovers.

Another unique type of acquired red cell aplasia results from the development of antibodies to recombinant erythropoietin [Bennett 2004, 2005, Casadevall 2002, McKoy 2008]. This acquired red cell aplasia is seen in patients receiving prolonged recombinant

erythropoietin, especially patients with chronic renal failure [Bennett 2004, 2005, Casadevall 2002]. Finally, the rare viruses (other than parvovirus) that have been linked to acquired red cell aplasia likely produce erythroblastopenia via regulatory defects rather than direct erythroblast destruction as seen in parvovirus infection.

[8.4.3] Morphology and Differential Diagnosis

Patients with acquired pure red cell aplasia have a profound normocytic, normochromic anemia without polychromasia. Other blood parameters are generally unremarkable. Bone marrow examination usually reveals either complete loss of the erythroid lineage or only scattered, morphologically unremarkable erythroblasts, which can be confirmed on immunohistochemical assessment **i8.23, i8.24, i8.25**. Other hematopoietic lineages are morphologically normal and show intact maturation. Depending on the cause of the secondary pure red cell aplasia, other blood and bone marrow features may be present.

Occult parvovirus infection must be excluded by PCR testing in all cases of secondary red cell aplasia (see **sidebar 8.1**). In addition, evaluation for any underlying condition such as T-cell large granular lymphocytic leukemia, thymoma, drug therapy, or immune disorder is important. Of note, T-cell large granular lymhocytic leukemia is the most common neoplasm linked to acquired pure red cell aplasia **i8.26, i8.27, i8.28**. Immune-modulating therapies, including antilymphocyte globulin, corticosteroid, or cyclosporine therapy may be successful, especially in patients with underlying lymphoproliferative or other immune disorders [Fujishima 2008, Sawada 2008, Sawada 2009]. Myelodysplasia must also be excluded because rare cases of myelodysplasia can present with red cell aplasia [Wang 2007]. In addition, patients with myelodysplasia may develop concurrent/subsequent red

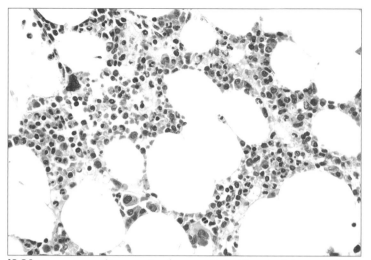

i8.24 Bone marrow biopsy section from a patient with systemic lupus erythematosus who developed pure red cell aplasia shows overall hypocellularity with intact granulocytic and megakaryocytic cells. Erythroid colonies are virtually absent (see i8.23). (H&E)

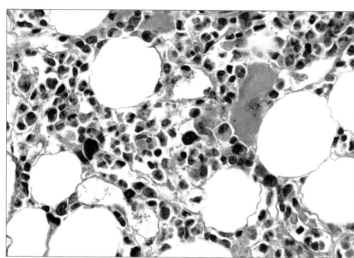

i8.25 Immunoperoxidase for hemoglobin A highlights rare erythroid cells in bone marrow core biopsy section from patient with red cell aplasia. (immunoperoxidase)

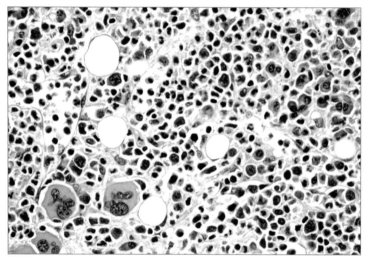

i8.26 Bone marrow core biopsy section in patient with T-cell large granular lymphocytic leukemia-associated red cell aplasia. Note subtle infiltrate of lymphoid cells and absence of erythroid colonies. (H&E)

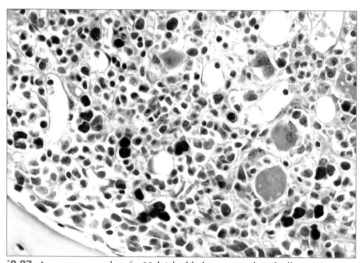

i8.27 Immunoperoxidase for HgbA highlights rare erythroid cell in patient with T-cell large granular lymphocytic leukemia-associated red cell aplasia. (immunoperoxidase)

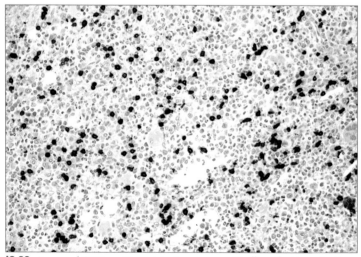

i8.28 Increased CD8 positive cytotoxic suppressor T cells evident in patient with T-cell large granular lymphocytic leukemia-associated red cell aplasia. (immunoperoxidase)

cell aplasia, often ultimately determined to be secondary to parvovirus infection i8.29, i8.30, i8.31.

[8.5] Differential Diagnosis of Erythroblastopenia

The differential diagnosis of congenital red cell aplasia is fairly limited. In neonates and infants with this disorder, a distinction between DBA and Fanconi anemia is important. Because of the different phenotypic abnormalities associated with these 2 disorders and the different underlying genetic defects, this differential diagnosis is generally not difficult (see Chapter 7). DBA also must be distinguished from congenital parvovirus infection; documentation of maternal infection and molecular testing are useful in making this distinction.

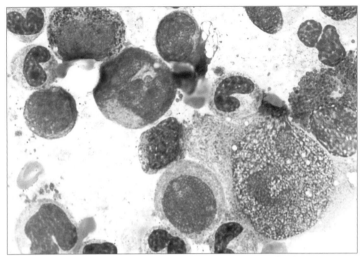

i8.29 *Bone marrow aspirate smear from patient with myelodysplasia who developed secondary acute parvovirus-induced red cell aplasia. Note degenerating giant erythroblast. (Wright)*

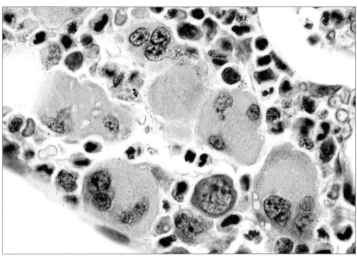

i8.30 *Bone marrow core biopsy section shows clustered, atypical megakaryocytes in conjunction with large degenerating erythroblasts (lower center) in a patient with myelodysplasia who developed secondary acute parvovirus infection. (H&E)*

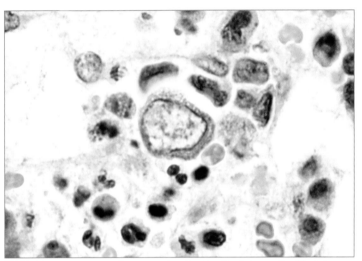

i8.31 *Bone marrow core biopsy section showing dissolving erythroblasts in patient with myelodysplasia and secondary acute parvovirus infection. (H&E)*

Similarly, rare cases of TEC are reported to occur in the neonatal period.

In older children and adults, the differential diagnosis of anemia with reticulocytopenia is broader and includes neoplasms such as myelodysplasia, dietary deficiency disorders such as megaloblastic anemia, as well as aplastic anemia. Although rare, patients with myelodysplasia may initially exhibit red cell hypoplasia [Wang 2007]. Therefore, careful review of both peripheral blood and bone marrow smears for evidence of multilineage dysplasia is important in patients with a presumptive diagnosis of acquired pure red cell aplasia. A substantially increased mean corpuscular volume, a reticulocyte count exceeding 1%, and dysplasia of either granulocytes or platelets all strongly suggest a diagnosis of myelodysplasia. Cytogenetic studies may be useful in distinguishing acquired pure red cell aplasia (normal karyotype)

from myelodysplasia (potential abnormal karyotype). Immunoperoxidase staining for CD34 may also be useful in highlighting increased or abnormally localized blast populations in cases of myelodysplasia. However, rare patients with overt myelodysplasia may develop secondary prolonged parvovirus infections yielding a complex morphologic picture of myelodysplasia with concurrent parvovirus-induced changes i8.29, i8.30, i8.31. Finally, very rarely, red cell aplasia may precede the development of overt aplastic anemia in the non-neonatal setting. This diagnosis of evolving aplastic anemia can be made by monitoring successive bone marrow and peripheral blood smears.

Either serologic or serum PCR tests for parvovirus-related antibodies or parvovirus DNA are indicated in any patient with acquired red cell aplasia, but it must be recognized that antibody results may be negative in immunosuppressed patients unable to mount an antibody response (see **sidebar 8.1**). Thus PCR for parvovirus testing is the most sensitive and specific test available to confirm acute parvovirus infection. Because this test is inexpensive and widely available, this is the optimal test for patients of all ages with red cell aplasia. In children with a transient disorder, the diagnosis of TEC is applied when no evidence for parvovirus can be established. In addition to serologic studies, identification of viral inclusions in erythroid precursors substantiates a diagnosis of parvovirus infection, although either molecular or in situ hybridization techniques are more sensitive methods to assess for parvovirus infection. These findings help to distinguish parvovirus-induced red cell aplasia from other types of red cell aplasia. Finally, in pediatric patients with either constitutional or acquired red cell aplasia, the bone marrow may contain abundant benign lymphocyte precursors, so-called hematogones, which must be distinguished from acute lymphoblastic anemia (see Chapter 21).

[8.6] Components of the Diagnostic Interpretation in Red Cell Aplasia

The goal of the diagnostic process is to identify both the morphologic abnormality and the pathophysiologic mechanism for erythroblastopenia t8.7. Some disorders, such as acquired idiopathic pure red cell aplasia and transient erythroblastopenia of childhood, are essentially diagnoses of exclusion. Parvovirus infection should always be considered in cases of acquired erythroblastopenia; this diagnosis should be confirmed or refuted by molecular studies on serum. Although erythroblast morphologic characteristics may be useful in prompting these studies, morphology may be noncontributory in some cases. In AIDS patients chronically infected with parvovirus, several unique morphologic variants have been described.

[8.7] Clues and Caveats

1. The red cell aplasias are separated into constitutional and acquired types; both idiopathic and secondary types of acquired red cell aplasia are described.
2. DBA is the only defined type of constitutional red cell aplasia; mutations in ribosome synthesis genes have been detected.

t8.7 Components of Diagnostic Interpretation in Red Cell Aplasia

Correlate blood and bone marrow morphology including erythrocyte morphology as well as other lineages

Once erythroblastopenia is documented by bone marrow review, must determine if process is constitutional, acquired transient, or acquired sustained red cell aplasia*

Determination of transient vs sustained red cell aplasia may require clinical follow-up

Comment on erythroblast morphology: parvovirus infection should always be considered in cases of acquired red cell aplasia; diagnostic molecular tests can be performed on blood or parvoviral immunoglobulins can be assessed (note: parvovirus infection is often sustained in immunosuppressed patients)

In cases of parvovirus infection assess for evidence of an underlying hematologic disorder such as hereditary spherocytosis, which may have been clinically occult

Recommend clinical and laboratory evaluation to determine if acquired, sustained erythroblastopenia (so-called pure red cell aplasia) is idiopathic or secondary

Evaluate blood and bone marrow for possible T-large granular lymphocytic leukemia (flow cytometry or immunohistochemistry)

Perform T-cell clonality studies in acquired pure red cell aplasia to detect occult clones

Recommend additional tests, as appropriate

*Clinical evaluation, age at onset, family history, patient follow-up, and additional laboratory tests including genetic analyses are all useful in identifying constitutional disorders

3. Increased numbers of hematogones are often present in the bone marrow of infants and children with red cell aplasia; these cells closely mimic acute lymphoblastic leukemia on morphology and immunophenotype assessment.
4. TEC is a self-limited, presumed viral disorder, which must be distinguished from DBA and parvovirus B19–induced red cell aplasia; parvovirus infection should be excluded.
5. Clinically classic cases of TEC have been linked to parvovirus infection.
6. Serologic tests, viral B19 DNA assays in serum, and in situ hybridization of bone marrow samples are sensitive methods for detecting parvovirus B19 infection; antibody response may not occur in immunosuppressed patients.
7. When bone marrow erythroid cells are decreased, parvoviral intranuclear inclusions in giant erythroblasts must be sought on aspirate smears and biopsy sections; inclusions are usually more apparent on fixed specimens such as clot and biopsy sections.
8. Immunoperoxidase staining for hemoglobin A or glycophorin A can be useful in highlighting rare residual erythroid cells, facilitating assessment for parvovirus inclusions; immunohistochemistry/in situ hybridization for parvovirus is recommended for definitive histologic diagnosis.
9. Clinically significant parvovirus infection is not limited to patients with underlying RBC survival defects; parvovirus infection can result in sustained red cell aplasia in immunosuppressed patients.
10. Granulocytic and/or megakaryocytic lineages may also be suppressed in patients with parvovirus infection.
11. Acute parvovirus infection may be linked to the bone marrow necrosis that, when embolized, precipitates acute chest syndrome in sickle cell anemia patients.
12. Chronic parvovirus infection should be considered in AIDS patients with unexplained anemia and reticulocytopenia; results of conventional serologic studies for parvovirus antibodies may be negative.
13. In patients with acquired sustained red cell aplasia, evaluation for underlying neoplasms, especially T-cell lymphoproliferative neoplasms and thymoma, is warranted, along with assessment for immune disorders; occult T-cell clones can also be detected in patients with apparent idiopathic pure red cell aplasia.
14. Antibodies to recombinant erythropoietin can result in acquired, sustained pure red cell aplasia in patients with chronic renal failure.
15. Careful morphologic review for evidence of multilineage dysplasia is necessary to identify those rare patients with myelodysplasia who initially present with erythroid

hypoplasia; immunoperoxidase stains for CD34 and cytogenetic studies may be helpful.

[8.8] Acknowledgments

The author acknowledges the photographic contributions of R McKenna, MD, C Sever, MD, and P Ward, MD.

[8.9] References

Attar EC, Aquino SL, Hasserjian RP [2007] Case records of the Massachusetts General Hospital. Case 33-2007. A 49-year-old HIV-positive male with anemia. *N Engl J Med* 357:1745-1754.

Bennett CL, Cournoyer D, Carson KR, et al [2005] Long-term outcome of individuals with pure red cell aplasia and antierythropoietin antibodies in patients treated with recombinant epoetin: a follow-up report from the Research on Adverse Drug Events and Reports (RADAR) Project. *Blood* 106:3343-3347.

Bennett CL, Luminari S, Nissenson AR, et al [2004] Pure red-cell aplasia and epoetin therapy. *N Engl J Med* 351:1403-1408.

Bock CT, Klingel K, Aberle S, et al [2005] Human parvovirus B19: A new emerging pathogen of inflammatory cardiomyopathy. *J Vet Med B Infect Dis Vet Public Health* 52:340-343.

Brown KE, Anderson SM, Young NS [1993] Erythrocyte P antigen: cellular receptor for B19 parvovirus. *Science* 262:114-117.

Brown KE, Young NS [1995] Parvovirus B19 infection and hematopoiesis. *Blood Rev* 9:176-182.

Brown KE, Young NS [1997] Parvovirus B19 in human disease. *Annu Rev Med* 48:59-67.

Carpenter SL, Zimmerman SA, Ware RE [2004] Acute parvovirus B19 infection mimicking congenital dyserythropoietic anemia. *J Pediatr Hematol Oncol* 26:133-135.

Carper E, Kurtzman GJ [1996] Human parvovirus B19 infection. *Curr Opin Hematol* 3:111-117.

Casadevall N, Nataf J, Viron B, et al [2002] Pure red-cell aplasia and antierythro-poietin antibodies in patients treated with recombinant erythropoietin. *N Engl J Med* 346:469-475.

Cassinotti P, Siegl G [2000] Quantitative evidence for persistence of human parvovirus B19 DNA in an immunocompetent individual. *Eur J Clin Microbiol Infect Dis* 19:886-887.

Charles RJ, Sabo KM, Kidd PG, Abkowitz JL [1996] The pathophysiology of pure red cell aplasia: implications for therapy. *Blood* 87:4831-4838.

Cherrick I, Karayalcin G, Lanzkowsky P [1994] Transient erythroblastopenia of childhood. Prospective study of fifty patients. *Am J Pediatr Hematol Oncol* 16:320-324.

Cooling LL, Koerner TA, Naides SJ [1995] Multiple glycosphingolipids determine the tissue tropism of parvovirus B19. *J Infect Dis* 172:1198-1205.

Corcoran A, Doyle S [2004] Advances in the biology, diagnosis and host-pathogen interactions of parvovirus B19. *J Med Microbiol* 53:459-475.

Crook T, Barton Rogers B, McFarland R, et al [2000] Unusual bone marrow manifestations of parvovirus B19 infection in immunocompromised patients. *Hum Pathol* 31:161-168.

Doherty L, Sheen MR, Vlachos A, et al [2010] Ribosomal protein genes *RPS10* and *RPS26* are commonly mutated in Diamond-Blackfan anemia. *Am J Hum Genet* 86(2):222-228.

Dokal I, Vulliamy T [2008] Inherited aplastic anaemias/bone marrow failure syndromes. *Blood Rev* 22:141-153.

Duffy S, Shackelton LA, Holmes EC [2008] Rates of evolutionary change in viruses: patterns and determinants. *Nat Rev Genet* 9:267-276.

Ekman A, Hokynar K, Kakkola L, et al [2007] Biological and immuno-logical relations among human parvovirus B19 genotypes 1-3. *J Virol* 81:6927-6935.

Erslev AJ, Soltan A [1996] Pure red-cell aplasia: a review. *Blood Rev* 10:20-28.

Farhi DC, Luebbers EL, Rosenthal NS [1998] Bone marrow biopsy findings in childhood anemia: prevalence of transient erythroblastopenia of childhood. *Arch Pathol Lab Med* 122:638-641.

Farrar JE, Nater M, Caywood E, et al [2008] Abnormalities of the large ribosomal subunit protein, Rpl35a, in Diamond-Blackfan anemia. *Blood* 112:1582-1592.

Fattet S, Cassinotti P, Popovic MB [2004] Persistent human parvovirus B19 infection in children under maintenance chemotherapy for acute lymphocytic leukemia. *J Pediatr Hematol Oncol* 26:497-503.

Florea AV, Ionescu DN, Melhem MF [2007] Parvovirus B19 infection in the immunocompromised host. *Arch Pathol Lab Med* 131:799-804.

Flygare J, Aspesi A, Bailey JC, et al [2007a] Human RPS19, the gene mutated in Diamond-Blackfan anemia, encodes a ribosomal protein required for the maturation of 40S ribosomal subunits. *Blood* 109:980-986.

Flygare J, Karlsson S [2007b] Diamond-Blackfan anemia: erythropoiesis lost in translation. *Blood* 109:3152-3154.

Frank GR, Cherrick I, Karayalcin G, et al [1994] Transient erythroblastopenia in a child with Kawasaki syndrome: a case report. *Am J Pediatr Hematol Oncol* 16:271-274.

Fredericks DN, Relman DA [1996] Sequence-based identification of microbial pathogens: a reconsideration of Koch's postulates. *Clin Microbiol Rev* 9:18-33.

Fujishima N, Sawada K, Hirokawa M, et al [2008] Long-term responses and outcomes following immunosuppressive therapy in large granular lymphocyte leukemia-associated pure red cell aplasia: a Nationwide Cohort Study in Japan for the PRCA Collaborative Study Group. *Haematologica* 93:1555-1559.

Gazda HT, Sieff CA [2006] Recent insights into the pathogenesis of Diamond-Blackfan anaemia. *Br J Haematol* 135:149-157.

Goldstein LJ, Strenger R, King TC, et al [1995] Retrospective diagnosis of sickle cell-hemoglobin C disease and parvovirus infection by molecular DNA analysis of postmortem tissue. *Hum Pathol* 26:1375-1378.

Gonzalez B, Larranaga C, Leon O, et al [2007] Parvovirus B19 may have a role in the pathogenesis of juvenile idiopathic arthritis. *J Rheumatol* 34:1336-1340.

Gustavson P, Klar J, Matsson H, et al [2002] Familial transient erythroblastopenia of childhood is associated with the chromosome 19q13.2 region but not caused by mutations in coding sequences of the ribosomal protein S19 (RPS19) gene. *Br J Haematol* 119:261-264.

Hara A, Wada T, Kitajima S, et al [2008] Combined pure red cell aplasia and autoimmune hemolytic anemia in systemic lupus erythematosus with anti-erythropoietin autoantibodies. *Am J Hematol* 83:750-752.

Hasle H, Kerndrup G, Jacobsen BB, et al [1994] Chronic parvovirus infection mimicking myelodysplastic syndrome in a child with subclinical immunode-ficiency. *Am J Pediatr Hematol Oncol* 16:329-333.

Hayes-Lattin B, Seipel TJ, Gatter K, et al [2004] Pure red cell aplasia associated with parvovirus B19 infection occurring late after allogeneic bone marrow transplantation. *Am J Hematol* 75:142-145.

Hirokawa M, Sawada K, Fujishima N, et al [2009] Acquired pure red cell aplasia associated with malignant lymphomas: a nationwide cohort study in Japan for the PRCA Collaborative Study Group. *Am J Hematol* 84:144-148.

Hokynar K, Norja P, Laitinen H, et al [2004] Detection and differentiation of human parvovirus variants by commercial quantitative real-time PCR tests. *J Clin Microbiol* 42:2013-2019.

Kako S, Kanda Y, Oshima K, et al [2008] Late onset of autoimmune hemolytic anemia and pure red cell aplasia after allogeneic hematopoietic stem cell transplantation using in vivo alemtuzumab. *Am J Hematol* 83:247-249.

Koch J [1942] Die aetiologie der tuberculose, translated as "The aetiology of tuberculosis" (1882). In: Clark D, ed. *Source Book of Medical History*. New York: Dover.

Koduri PR [1998] Novel cytomorphology of the giant proerythroblasts of parvovirus B19 infection. *Am J Hematol* 58:95-99.

Krause JR, Penchansky L, Knisely AS [1992] Morphological diagnosis of parvovirus B19 infection. A cytopathic effect easily recognized in air-dried, formalin-fixed bone marrow smears stained with hematoxylin-eosin or Wright-Giemsa. *Arch Pathol Lab Med* 116:178-180.

Kurtzman GJ, Cohen B, Meyers P, et al [1988] Persistent B19 parvovirus infection as a cause of severe chronic anaemia in children with acute lymphocytic leukaemia. *Lancet* 2:1159-1162.

Lacy MQ, Kurtin PJ, Tefferi A [1996] Pure red cell aplasia: association with large granular lymphocyte leukemia and the prognostic value of cytogenetic abnormalities. *Blood* 87:3000-3006.

Lipton JM [2006] Diamond blackfan anemia: new paradigms for a "not so pure" inherited red cell aplasia. *Semin Hematol* 43:167-177.

Lipton JM, Ellis SR [2009] Diamond-Blackfan anemia: diagnosis, treatment, and molecular pathogenesis. *Hematol Oncol Clin North Am* 23:261-282.

Lisitsyn N, Lisitsyn N, Wigler M [1993] Cloning the differences between 2 complex genomes. *Science* 259:946-951.

Liu W, Ittmann M, Liu J, et al [1997] Human parvovirus B19 in bone marrows from adults with acquired immunodeficiency syndrome: a comparative study using in situ hybridization and immunohistochemistry. *Hum Pathol* 28:760-766.

Lopez-Bueno A, Villarreal LP, Almendral JM [2006] Parvovirus variation for disease: a difference with RNA viruses? *Curr Top Microbiol Immunol* 299:349-370.

Lowenthal EA, Wells A, Emanuel PD, et al [1996] Sickle cell acute chest syndrome associated with parvovirus B19 infection: case series and review. *Am J Hematol* 51:207-213.

Mamyrova G, Rider LG, Haagenson L, et al [2005] Parvovirus B19 and onset of juvenile dermatomyositis. *JAMA* 294:2170-2171.

Masuda M, Teramura M, Matsuda A, et al [2005] Clonal T cells of pure red-cell aplasia. *Am J Hematol* 79:332-333.

McKoy JM, Stonecash RE, Cournoyer D, et al [2008] Epoetin-associated pure red cell aplasia: past, present, and future considerations. *Transfusion* 48:1754-1762.

Miller R, Berman B [1994] Transient erythroblastopenia of childhood in infants < 6 months of age. *Am J Pediatr Hematol Oncol* 16:246-248.

Modrow S [2006] Parvovirus B19: The causative agent of dilated cardiomyopathy or a harmless passenger of the human myocard? *Ernst Schering Res Found Workshop* 2006:63-82.

Mori KL, Furukawa H, Hayashi K, et al [2003] Pure red cell aplasia associated with expansion of CD3+ CD8+ granular lymphocytes expressing cytotoxicity against HLA-E+ cells. *Br J Haematol* 123:147-153.

Murray JC, Kelley PK, Hogrefe WR, McClain KL [1994] Childhood idiopathic thrombocytopenic purpura: association with human parvovirus B19 infection. *Am J Pediatr Hematol Oncol* 16:314-319.

Mylonakis E, Dickinson BP, Mileno MD, et al [1999] Persistent parvovirus B19 related anemia of 7 years' duration in an HIV-infected patient: complete remission associated with highly active antiretroviral therapy. *Am J Hematol* 60:164-166.

Nagai K, Morohoshi T, Kudoh T, et al [1992] Transient erythroblastopenia of childhood with megakaryocytopenia associated with human parvovirus B19 infection. *Br J Haematol* 80:131-132.

Norja P, Eis-Hubinger AM, Soderlund-Venermo M, et al [2008] Rapid sequence change and geographical spread of human parvovirus B19: Comparison of B19 virus evolution in acute and persistent infections. *J Virol* 82:6427-6433.

Ohene-Abuakwa Y, Orfali KA, Marius C, Ball SE [2005] Two-phase culture in Diamond-Blackfan anemia: localization of erythroid defect. *Blood* 105:838-846.

Parekh S, Perez A, Yang XY, Billett H [2005] Chronic parvovirus infection and G6PD deficiency masquerading as Diamond-Blackfan anemia. *Am J Hematol* 79:54-57.

Penchansky L, Jordan JA [1997] Transient erythroblastopenia of childhood associated with human herpesvirus type 6, variant B. *Am J Clin Pathol* 108:127-132.

Perkins SL [2004] Pediatric red cell disorders and pure red cell aplasia. *Am J Clin Pathol* 122Suppl:S70-86.

Pont J, Puchhammer-Stockl E, Chott A, et al [1992] Recurrent granulocytic aplasia as clinical presentation of a persistent parvovirus B19 infection. *Br J Haematol* 80:160-165.

Praditpornsilpa K, Kupatawintu P, Mongkonsritagoon W, et al [2009] The association of anti-r-HuEpo-associated pure red cell aplasia with HLA-DRB1*09-DQB1*0309. *Nephrol Dial Transplant* 24:1545-1549.

Prassouli A, Papadakis V, Tsakris A, et al [2005] Classic transient erythroblastopenia of childhood with human parvovirus B19 genome detection in the blood and bone marrow. *J Pediatr Hematol Oncol* 27:333-336.

Sawada K, Fujishima N, Hirokawa M [2008] Acquired pure red cell aplasia: updated review of treatment. *Br J Haematol* 142:505-514.

Sawada K, Hirokawa M, Fujishima N [2009] Diagnosis and management of acquired pure red cell aplasia. *Hematol Oncol Clin North Am* 23:249-259.

Shimamura A [2008] Diamond-Blackfan anemia: a new facet. *Blood* 112:1552-1553.

Skeppner G, Kreuger A, Elinder G [2002] Transient erythroblastopenia of childhood: prospective study of 10 patients with special reference to viral infections. *J Pediatr Hematol Oncol* 24:294-298.

Soderlund-Venermo M, Hokynar K, Nieminen J, et al [2002] Persistence of human parvovirus B19 in human tissues. *Pathol Biol* (Paris) 50:307-316.

Thompson CA, Steensma DP [2006] Pure red cell aplasia associated with thymoma: clinical insights from a 50-year single-institution experience. *Br J Haematol* 135:405-407.

Tsay GJ, Zouali M [2006] Unscrambling the role of human parvovirus B19 signaling in systemic autoimmunity. *Biochem Pharmacol* 72:1453-1459.

Tsuda H, Maeda Y, Nakagawa K, et al [1994] Parvovirus B19-associated haemophagocytic syndrome with prominent neutrophilia. *Br J Haematol* 86:413-414.

Tugal O, Pallant B, Shebarek N, Jayabose S [1994] Transient erythroblastopenia of the newborn caused by human parvovirus. *Am J Pediatr Hematol Oncol* 16:352-355.

Vlachos A, Ball S, Dahl N, et al [2008] Diagnosing and treating Diamond Blackfan anaemia: results of an international clinical consensus conference. *Br J Haematol* 142:859-876.

Wang SA, Yue G, Hutchinson L, et al [2007] Myelodysplastic syndrome with pure red cell aplasia shows characteristic Clinicopathological features and clonal T-cell expansion. *Br J Haematol* 138:271-275.

Weigel-Kelley KA, Yoder MC, Srivastava A [2003] Alpha5beta1 integrin as a cellular coreceptor for human parvovirus B19: requirement of functional activation of beta1 integrin for viral entry. *Blood* 102:3927-3933.

Weissbrich B, Suss-Frohlich Y, Girschick HJ [2007] Seroprevalence of parvovirus B19 IgG in children affected by juvenile idiopathic arthritis. *Arthritis Res Ther* 9:R82.

Yetgin S, Cetin M, Aslan D, et al [2004] Parvovirus B19 infection presenting as pre-B-cell acute lymphoblastic leukemia: a transient and progressive course in 2 children. *J Pediatr Hematol Oncol* 26:689-692.

Young NS, Brown KE [2004] Parvovirus B19. *N Engl J Med* 350:586-597.

Yufu Y, Matsumoto M, Miyamura T, et al [1997] Parvovirus B19-associated haemophagocytic syndrome with lymphadenopathy resembling histiocytic necrotizing lymphadenitis (Kikuchi's disease). *Br J Haematol* 96:868-871.

Erythrocytosis

Kathryn Foucar, MD

Depending upon the clinical practice patient population, elevated red blood cell (RBC) parameters may require astute differential diagnosis decision-making or the cause may be straightforward. Patient age is a significant factor. For example, the approach to polycythemia (erythrocytosis) in neonates is entirely different from that used in older children and adults **t9.1**. Often the cause of erythrocytosis can be discerned by evaluation for any disorder associated with either decreased plasma volume producing a *relative* erythrocytosis (dehydration, emesis) or common causes of hypoxia-driven secondary erythrocytosis (smoking, obesity, sleep apnea, cardiopulmonary disease). Once these relatively straightforward causes of erythrocytosis have been excluded, more elaborate evaluation may be required **t9.1**. The role of bone marrow examination in the workup of erythrocytosis is generally restricted to patients with possible clonal myeloid disorders, typically polycythemia vera (see Chapter 14 for a comprehensive discussion of all chronic myeloproliferative neoplasms).

[9.1] Definitions and Terminology

Erythrocytosis is defined as hemoglobin, hematocrit, and RBC count above age/sex-related normal ranges [McMullin 2008, O'Malley 2005, Spivak 2008, Tefferi 2006a]. In the neonate, polycythemia is generally defined as a hematocrit of 65% or more, but other criteria are sometimes used such as standard deviations above normal [Rosenkrantz 2005]. The role of red cell mass (volume) in establishing a diagnosis of absolute erythrocytosis is controversial. Red cell mass is claimed to be an essential test in the classification of erythrocytoses by some authors, whereas other reports claim that this radionucleic test is too problematic to be of clinical value in light of more recently developed tests [Means 2009, Spivak 2008, Tefferi 2006a].

Nomenclature is also controversial. Some authors use erythrocytosis and polycythemia interchangeably, while others restrict the term *polycythemia* to those cases in which elevated red cell mass has been documented, while erythrocytosis is noted when RBC count is elevated [Means 2009, Van Maerken 2004]. In this chapter, erythrocytosis and polycythemia will be used interchangeably as is conventionally done.

---

t9.1 General Approach to Erythrocytosis

Apply standard criteria to define erythrocytosis/polycythemia

　Hgb, Hct, RBC count above age/sex-related normal ranges
　Elevated red cell mass (termed polycythemia)—measurement problematic

Consider relative erythrocytosis

　Any plasma volume depletion disorder (many causes, common)

Consider constitutional vs acquired likelihood

　Assess age at onset, family history, other CBC abnormalities, spleen size, hematologic assessment of family members
　Neonatal erythrocytosis requires assessment for possible placental, maternal, and fetal factors
　Assess for chronic hypoxia—many conditions
　Consider medications, illicit rh EPO, androgens
　Consider esoteric causes: high O_2 affinity hemoglobin (rare), increased carboxyhemoglobin (smokers, otherwise rare), EPO-producing tumors/conditions (occasional), 2, 3-BPG mutase deficiency (rare), renal artery stenosis (occasional)

Consider categorization based on EPO level

　Consistently decreased EPO level in polycythemia vera due to constitutive JAK2 activation and congenital erythrocytosis due to *EPOR* gene mutation
　Elevated EPO level in secondary erythrocytosis
　Normal EPO level in relative erythrocytosis

Apply genetic testing in appropriate circumstances

　JAK2 mutation and *BCR-ABL1* fusion gene analysis in cases of possible polycythemia vera
　EPOR, VHL, HIF1A, EPAS1 (*H1F2A*), *BPGM* (2,3 mutase) gene mutation analyses in *rare* cases of suspected familial (congenital) erythrocytosis

BCR-ABL = breakpoint cluster region-Ableson oncogene; BPG = biphosphoglycerate; CBC = complete blood count; EPO = erythropoietin; EPOR = erythropoietin receptor; Hct = hematocrit; Hgb = hemoglobin; HIF = hypoxia-inducible factor; JAK = Janus kinase; RBC = red blood cell; rh = recombinant human; VHL = von Hippel-Lindau

t9.2 General Definitions and Categories of Erythrocytoses

Category	Definition
Absolute erythrocytosis (true polycythemia)	Increased red blood cell mass (volume)
Primary	
Polycythemia vera	Acquired clonal stem cell neoplasm with autonomous overproduction of erythroid and other lineages
Familial polycythemia	Hypersensitivity to erythropoietin secondary to various mutations in erythropoietin receptor gene
Secondary	
Physiologically appropriate (hypoxia-mediated)	Secondary to residence at high altitude, many chronic hypoxic disorders (including neonatal polycythemia), many renal abnormalities including renal artery stenosis,* or gene mutations causing hemoglobinopathies/ erythrocyte enzyme defects that are associated with decreased oxygen delivery to tissues
Physiologically inappropriate (abnormal erythropoietin production)	Secondary to dysregulated erythropoietin production or production of other erythropoietic substances by neoplasms of the kidney, liver, adrenal, central nervous system, breast, thymus, lung, ovary, uterus, and testes
	Familial cases linked to mutations in genes encoding components of oxygen sensing regulatory pathway
Drug-associated	Androgen therapy, illicit rh EPO or androgen ingestion
Relative erythrocytosis	Normal red blood cell mass; decreased plasma volume from fluid loss, ie, dehydration (eg, gastrointestinal or renal disorders, heavy smoking,† hantavirus pulmonary syndrome), and Gaisbock syndrome

*Conditions associated with local renal hypoxia
†Polycythemia in heavy smokers linked to both secondary and relative erythrocytosis [Leifert 2008]

References: [Delanghe 2008, Foucar 2008, Gordeuk 2004, Hoyer 2004, Koster 2001, Kralovics 2005b, Leifert 2008, McMullin 2008, Means 2009, O'Malley 2005, Pastore 2003b, Percy 2008a, 2008b, 2009, Rad 2008, Rosenkrantz 2005, Tefferi 2006b, Van Maerken 2004]

t9.3 2008 World Health Organization Diagnostic Criteria for Polycythemia Vera*

Major criteria

Elevated hemoglobin, other evidence of increased red cell volume†

Presence of *JAK2* V617F or functionally similar mutation such as *JAK2* exon 12 mutation

Minor criteria

Bone marrow trilineage myeloproliferation

Subnormal erythropoietin level

Endogenous erythroid colony formation in vitro

*See Chapter 14 for a detailed discussion of polycythemia vera
†See Chapter 14 for specific male, female hemoglobin, hematocrit levels

References: [Tefferi 2008b, Thiele 2008]

with autonomous overproduction of erythrocytes [Kralovics 2005b, Spivak 2008, Tefferi 2006a]. Secondary absolute erythrocytosis results from either physiologically appropriate (hypoxia-driven) or inappropriate excess production of erythropoietin or erythropoietin-like compounds. In both primary and secondary types of absolute erythrocytosis, the RBC mass is increased. Because of the sustained increased erythrocyte production, erythroid hyperplasia is a predicted bone marrow finding, but bone marrow examination is not required in most cases. Both storage and erythroid iron may be diminished in the bone marrow, especially in patients undergoing therapeutic phlebotomy. In contrast, relative (apparent) erythrocytosis results when plasma volume is decreased, while RBC mass is normal, and no specific bone marrow abnormalities would be expected.

[9.2.1] **Primary Acquired Erythrocytosis (Polycythemia Vera)**

Polycythemia vera occurs almost exclusively in adults and requires the integration of clinical, laboratory, and peripheral blood findings to establish the diagnosis. The diagnosis of polycythemia vera is based on major and minor criteria, and distinction from other acquired erythrocytotic disorders is necessary (see Chapter 14) t9.3, t9.4.

Pathogenesis

A major advance in the understanding of the pathogenetic mechanisms of polycythemia vera occurred in 2005 when 4 research laboratories nearly simultaneously identified gain of function *JAK2* V617F mutations in patients with polycythemia vera and other chronic myeloproliferative neoplasms [Baxter 2005, James 2005, Kralovics 2005a, Levine 2005]. This gain of function mutation resulted in constitutive *JAK2* activation in the absence of erythropoietin binding to the erythropoietin receptor (EPOR). Subsequent studies have confirmed that *JAK2* V617F or a similar mutation is present in virtually

[9.2] **Classification of Erythrocytotic Disorders**

Erythrocytotic disorders can be divided into absolute and relative categories. The absolute erythrocytoses are further subclassified into primary and secondary types t9.2. Although rare families with primary familial/congenital erythrocytosis due to mutations in the erythropoietin receptor gene are well-described, by far the more common type of primary erythrocytosis is polycythemia vera, an acquired clonal stem cell bone marrow disorder associated

t9.4 Comparison of Laboratory Tests Useful in Classifying Acquired Polycythemic (Erythrocytotic) Disorders

Test	Polycythemia Vera	Acquired Secondary Erythrocytosis	Acquired Secondary Erythrocytosis (Inappropriate)	Relative Erythrocytosis
Red blood cell volume (mass)*	↑	↑	↑	Normal
Erythropoietin levels	↓	↑	↑	Normal
Arterial oxygen saturation	Normal	Often ↓	Normal	Normal
White blood cell count	↑	Usually normal	Usually normal	Variable
Absolute basophilia	Present	Absent	Absent	Absent
Uric acid	↑	Normal	Usually normal	Normal
Histamine	↑	Normal	Normal	Normal
Serum iron	↑	Normal†	Normal	Normal
Storage iron	↓	Normal†	Normal	Normal
Hemoglobinopathy (high O$_2$ affinity)	Absent	Present in some cases	Absent	Absent
Carboxyhemoglobin (↓ O$_2$ carrying capacity)	Normal	May be increased	Usually normal	Usually normal
Clonal cytogenetic abnormalities	10%-20%	Absent	Absent	Absent
JAK2 mutation	100%	Absent	Absent	Absent
Spontaneous erythroid colony formation‡	Present	Absent	Absent	Absent
Bone marrow	Panhyperplasia	Erythroid hyperplasia	Erythroid hyperplasia	Normal

*Many problems in accurate measurement of red cell mass; often *not* used currently
†May be decreased in patients undergoing therapeutic phlebotomy
‡Cell culture studies that assess growth of erythroid colonies in the absence of exogenous erythropoietin
↑ = increased; ↓ = decreased

References: [Kralovics 2005b, Spivak 2008, Tefferi 2006a, 2008b]

100% of cases of polycythemia vera [Tefferi 2008a] (see Chapter 14 for a comprehensive discussion of polycythemia vera).

Morphology

The typical blood and bone marrow findings in polycythemia vera are listed in t9.5 (see Chapter 14). Compared with secondary erythrocytosis, the unique features of the blood picture in patients with polycythemia vera include variable circulating normoblasts and immature granulocytic cells, basophilia, and thrombocytosis i9.1. Patients with polycythemia vera often undergo chronic phlebotomies to reduce iron and red blood cells. Consequently, features of iron deficiency are often present; the complete blood count (CBC) may demonstrate erythrocytosis and hypochromic/ microcytic RBCs, in conjunction with white blood cell (WBC) and platelet abnormalities i9.2.

Bone marrow evaluation offers important diagnostic and prognostic information in polycythemia vera. Early in the disease course, the bone marrow is characteristically hypercellular with trilineage myeloproliferation, though erythroid cells generally predominate i9.3. Morphologic abnormalities, especially of megakaryocytes, are common in the bone marrow of patients with this stem cell disease

t9.5 Peripheral Blood and Bone Marrow Findings in Polycythemia Vera*

Blood

Increased hemoglobin, hematocrit†

Elevated RBC count†

Variable erythrocyte morphology

Normoblasts may be present

Mild to moderate leukocytosis; mild basophilia, neutrophilia

Thrombocytosis; rare cases with striking increase in platelets‡

Bone marrow

Moderate to marked hypercellularity

Increased erythropoiesis, granulopoiesis, and megakaryopoiesis; intact maturation

Abundant enlarged, hyperlobulated megakaryocytes in clusters

Decreased, often absent, storage iron

Dilated sinusoids with intravascular hematopoietic colonies

*See Chapter 14
†Concurrent iron deficiency is very common and will have an impact on levels
‡Thrombocytosis may be exacerbated by concurrent iron deficiency

References: [Campbell 2006, Tefferi 2008b, Thiele 2006]

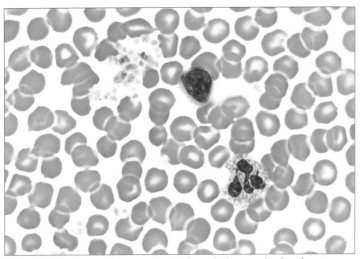

i9.1 *This blood smear from a patient with newly diagnosed polycythemia vera illustrates the elevated erythrocyte, granulocyte, and platelet levels that characterize this clonal stem cell disorder. (Wright)*

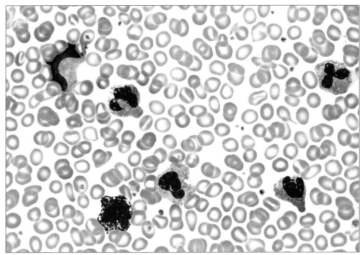

i9.2 *Peripheral blood smear from patient with iron-deficient polycythemia vera with prominent erythrocytosis (red blood cells, $7.6 \times 10^6/\mu L$ [$7.6 \times 10^{12}/L$]) and microcytosis (mean corpuscular volume, 65 fL). Other features of a myeloproliferative disorder including leukocytosis, basophilia, and thrombocytosis are present. (Wright)*

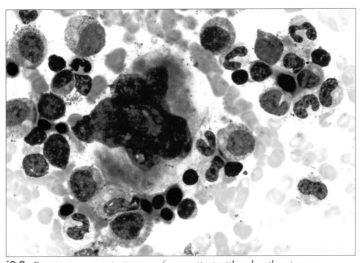

i9.3 *Bone marrow aspirate smear from patient with polycythemia vera showing hypercellularity as well as a markedly enlarged, hyperlobulated megakaryocyte (Wright)*

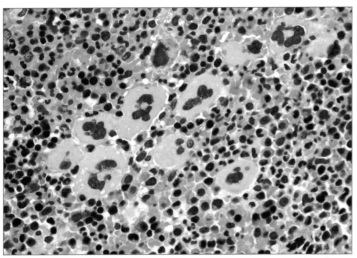

i9.4 *Bone marrow core biopsy showing markedly increased, clustered, and hyperlobulated megakaryocytes in patient with polycythemia vera. (H&E)*

and include clustering and hyperlobation of nuclei **t9.5, i9.4**. Because of prolonged erythrocyte overproduction, storage iron is often absent. Increased intramedullary cell death and high rates of cell turnover may result in hyperuricemia. Progressive fibrosis with decline in cellularity characteristically may occur after prolonged disease. Details of bone marrow morphology throughout the disease course of patients with polycythemia vera are presented in Chapter 14.

[9.2.2] **Familial/Congenital Primary Erythrocytosis**

Pathogenesis

At least 9 gain-of-function mutations of the erythropoietin receptor (*EPOR*) gene associated with familial and de novo primary erythrocytosis have been identified [Kralovics 2005b]. As with polycythemia vera, erythropoietin levels are low, since erythrocyte production is driven by the conformationally altered EPOR, which does not require erythropoietin binding for activation of downstream events, leading to autonomous erythrocyte production.

Morphology

Unlike polycythemia vera, other hematopoietic lineages are unremarkable—the CBC values and bone marrow morphology reflect isolated erythrocytosis in the blood and isolated erythroid hyperplasia in the bone marrow. Other parameters useful in the subclassification of primary erythrocytosis include age at presentation, family history, and genetic findings.

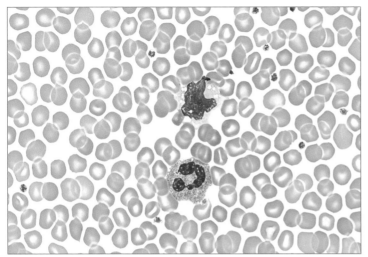

i9.5 *Marked erythrocytosis and polychromasia in patient with chronic hypoxia. (Wright)*

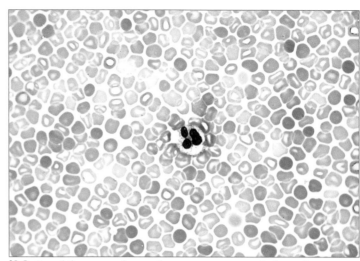

i9.6 *Iron-deficient secondary erythrocytosis in patient with chronic hypoxia undergoing phlebotomy therapy. (Wright)*

[9.2.3] **Secondary Erythrocytosis (Congenital and Acquired)**

Definition

The increased RBC mass in patients with the various secondary erythrocytotic disorders is the consequence of sustained increased levels of erythropoietin or erythropoietin-like substances.

Pathophysiology and Morphology

There are many causes of secondary erythrocytosis; these may be categorized as either physiologically appropriate or physiologically inappropriate **t9.2, t9.4**. Physiologically appropriate secondary erythrocytosis can result when chronic tissue hypoxia leads to sustained elevations in erythropoietin levels in blood **i9.5**. The cause of this hypoxia is often clinically apparent and includes various cardiac and pulmonary disorders. These patients often require chronic phlebotomy to reduce iron stores and blood viscosity, producing a blood picture of marked erythrocytosis with concurrent microcytic/hypochromic erythrocytes **i9.6**. Sophisticated laboratory tests may be required to document other types of physiologically appropriate secondary erythrocytosis, especially those caused by rare hemoglobinopathies or types of RBC enzyme mutations associated with decreased oxygen delivery to tissues. Careful evaluation for renal disease linked to local renal hypoxia is warranted [McMullin 2008].

Although isolated erythroid hyperplasia is a predictable finding, bone marrow examination is generally not required to establish a diagnosis of physiologically appropriate secondary erythrocytosis; storage iron is often depleted in the bone marrow due to chronic phlebotomy.

Patients with physiologically inappropriate erythrocytosis also have sustained overproduction of either erythropoietin or substances that secondarily induce erythropoietin production. However, the underlying disorder responsible for physiologically inappropriate secondary erythrocytosis is not hypoxia and is often clinically occult **t9.2**. Careful evaluation for occult neoplastic conditions is necessary. Many different erythropoietin-producing tumors have been identified, including neoplasms in liver, kidney, adrenal, central nervous system, uterus, lung, thymus, and breast [Foucar 2008, O'Malley 2005]. Tumors may also indirectly cause polycythemia via production of various erythropoietin-inducing hormones.

Dysregulated/sustained erythropoietin production also occurs in rare familial kindreds with mutations in genes encoding the oxygen sensing apparatus regulatory factors. These include mutations in genes that encode various hypoxia-inducible factor-α (HIF-α) and inactivators/regulators of HIF-α [Gordeuk 2004, Ladroue 2008, Lee 2008, Pastore 2003b, Percy 2008a, 2008b, 2009, Semenza 2009]. Because erythropoietin production is regulated by HIF, mutations in either *HIF* genes or *HIF* inactivator genes result in sustained, dysregulated erythropoietin production (so-called Chuvash polycythemia) [Gale 2008, Lee 2008, Percy 2009] (see **sidebar 9.1** for more details).

Although erythroid hyperplasia is a predicted bone marrow finding in patients with physiologically inappropriate erythrocytosis, bone marrow examination is generally not required to establish this diagnosis, but it may be necessary for other reasons such as tumor staging.

Oxygen Sensing and Erythrocytosis

Oxygen, which was originally present on earth only in trace quantities, was toxic to the earliest anaerobic forms of life on earth. Following the sudden and rapid accumulation of oxygen in the atmosphere (the "Great Oxidation Event"), organisms quickly adapted to the newly aerobic environment [Buick 2008]. Ironically, what had before been toxic was now vital, and a new problem presented itself: what to do when there is not enough? Cells evolved complex responses to hypoxia, including the reduction of energy-intensive processes like DNA transcription and replication, the switch to alternative pathways of metabolism and, in more complex organisms, the production of extracellular signals intended to provide more oxygen.

Critical to all of these steps is the initial recognition that insufficient oxygen is available. *Escherichia coli*, for example, accomplishes this mainly by incorporating iron molecules into a critical regulator of transcription. In the presence of oxygen, the redox state of the iron molecule causes a conformational change that alters the binding properties of the protein [Bailey-Serres 2005].

Evolution has conserved this general approach, and in humans the oxygen-sensing pathway is largely dependent on 2 separate components: hypoxia inducible factor (HIF), the transcription factor responsible for orchestrating the cellular response, and prolyl hydroxylases (PHDs), molecules that contain nonheme iron. In the presence of oxygen, PHDs hydroxylate HIF at specific amino acid residues, allowing the von Hippel-Lindau tumor suppressor protein (VHL) to ubiquitinate HIF; thus targeted for degradation, HIF cannot promote transcription of hypoxia-inducible genes [Percy 2009, Rocha 2007]. However,

similar to the strategy employed by *E coli*, the absence of oxygen renders the iron-bearing PHD enzyme nonfunctional; in this state, HIF is not targeted for destruction, and increased transcription of its target genes commences [Kaelin 2008]. A separate oxygen-dependent enzyme, FIH (factor-inhibiting HIF), retains its ability to modify HIF at different domains and at lower oxygen concentrations, potentially permitting the cell to calibrate cellular activity to the specific level of hypoxia [Koivunen 2004, Percy 2009]. HIF targets a wide variety of genes relating to oxygen supply, cellular metabolism, growth and apoptosis [Rocha 2007]. Recently, a number of microRNAs have also been shown to be HIF-inducible, raising the possibility that signaling through HIF may not only *promote* the expression of certain genes, but actively *prevent* translation of other proteins, thus more globally altering the state of the cell [Ivan 2008].

Familial erythrocytosis-associated mutations have been described in the several components of the oxygen-sensing pathway. Various mutations affecting the active site of PHD2, for example, diminish the hydroxylation and, therefore the degradation, of HIF [Al-Sheikh 2008, Percy 2007, 2009]. Gain-of-function mutations in an isoform of HIF have also recently been described [Gale 2008, Percy 2008b]. The common end result of these defects is the increased expression of genes under transcriptional control by HIF, including erythropoietin, which in turn leads to increased erythropoiesis.

However, mutation of another key component of the oxygen sensing pathway, *VHL*, may be the most commonly identified defect in idiopathic erythrocytosis [Lee 2006, Percy 2009]. A specific mutation, R200W (C598T), is characteristic of so-called Chuvash polycythemia (named for the Chuvashia

region of Russia, where familial erythrocytosis is endemic). An identical mutation is present in an endemic cluster of familial erythrocytosis identified on the island of Ischia, in the Bay of Naples [Perrotta 2006]. The maintenance of a relatively high allelic frequency (0.07 in Ischia), despite significant thrombosis-related mortality, has led some to hypothesize that the allele may be advantageous in some settings, similar to the protective role ascribed to hemoglobin S [Perrotta 2006]. Other rare erythrocytosis-associated mutations of *VHL* have been identified, often affecting the same region of the VHL protein as the Chuvash mutation [Bento 2005, Cario 2005, Lee 2006, Pastore 2003a, 2003b, Randi 2005], and these have recently been comprehensively reviewed [Lee 2008]. Interestingly, patients with Chuvash polycythemia or similar mutations do *not* show evidence of von Hippel-Lindau disease, the cancer susceptibility syndrome defined by mutations in *VHL* [Lee 2006]. The converse is also true: although patients with von Hippel-Lindau disease develop highly vascularized tumors, consistent with VHL's role in the oxygen sensing pathway, these patients do not generally show erythrocytosis in the absence of an erythropoietin-producing tumor [Roberts 2008]. As VHL sits at the crossroads of numerous regulatory pathways within the cell, it is possible that the *VHL* mutations impact discrete pathways and thereby generate different phenotypes [Kapitsinou 2008, Roberts 2008]. Alternatively, the mutations may result in differing degrees of functional impairment of the protein [Lee 2006]. Indeed, the susceptibility to different types of tumors in different genetic subclasses of von Hippel-Lindau disease underscores the phenotypic variability conferred by different mutations of this fascinating gene [Shehata 2008].

Relative Erythrocytosis

Pathogenesis

Relative erythrocytosis is not the consequence of any RBC or bone marrow abnormality, but is instead secondary to reduced plasma volume. Often the cause of reduced plasma volume is readily clinically apparent and is related to disorders, such as gastrointestinal or renal diseases, which are associated with excess fluid loss. One relatively newly recognized disorder, hantavirus pulmonary syndrome, is characterized by a marked relative erythrocytosis secondary to florid pulmonary capillary plasma leak i9.7 [Koster 2001]. Other blood findings in hantavirus pulmonary syndrome are presented in Chapters 10, 21, and 33. Relative erythrocytosis can also develop in heavy smokers [Leifert 2008].

Morphology

Complete blood count data reflect hemoconcentration, and morphologic abnormalities would not be expected in erythroid or other cell lineages unless these abnormalities were caused

by the underlying disease. Bone marrow examination is usually not necessary for the management of patients with relative erythrocytosis, unless polycythemia vera is a strong diagnostic consideration.

One challenging diagnostic type of relative erythrocytosis is Gaisbock syndrome, characterized by sustained erythrocytosis, hypertension, obesity, and smoking [Means 2009, Stefanini 1978]. Blood and bone marrow examination may be performed in these patients to rule out a myeloproliferative neoplasm, especially if there is both erythrocytosis and leukocytosis in the blood i9.8. The bone marrow aspirate smear shows erythroid hyperplasia with intact maturation, while overall cellularity, bony trabeculae, and megakaryocytes are all normal on the bone marrow core biopsy i9.9, i9.10.

Neonatal Polycythemia

Polycythemia can occur in neonates; this disorder is more common in either infants with Down syndrome or offspring of diabetic mothers [Rosenkrantz 2005, Werner 1995]. When the venous

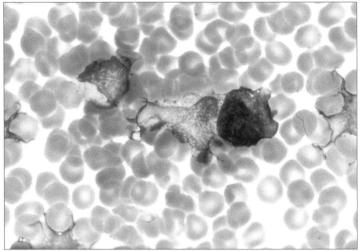

i9.7 *This blood smear from a patient with fatal florid hantavirus pulmonary syndrome illustrates striking relative erythrocytosis (hematocrit, >65% [0.65]) that occurs in this disease. Note neutrophilia with left shift presumably secondary to acute, profound respiratory distress. (Wright)*

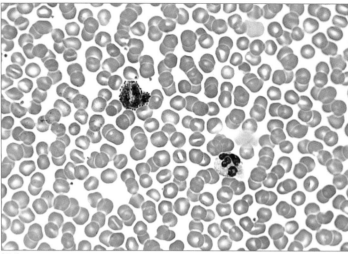

i9.8 *Peripheral blood showing relative erythrocytosis but unremarkable white blood cell and platelets in patient with Gaisbock syndrome. (Wright)*

hematocrit value exceeds 65% (0.65) in these neonates, aggressive management is required. Polycythemic infants may develop plethora, lethargy, cyanosis, or respiratory distress from hyperviscosity. Many of these infants also have associated hypoglycemia and hyperbilirubinemia, and rapid reduction in the hematocrit level is necessary to ameliorate these potentially life-threatening complications. The etiology of neonatal polycythemia includes placental, maternal, and fetal factors **t9.6**. One

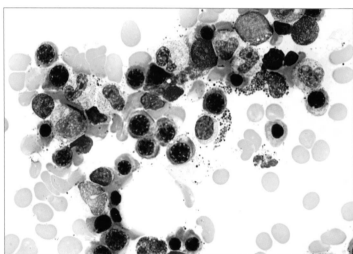

i9.9 *Bone marrow aspirate smear from patient with Gaisbock syndrome showing erythroid hyperplasia but unremarkable granulocytic lineage. (Wright)*

t9.6 Causes of Neonatal Polycythemia*

Placental factors

Delayed clamping umbilical cord

Twin-twin transfusion

Maternal-fetal transfusion

Perinatal asphyxia (acute hypoxia)

Intrauterine hypoxia (chronic hypoxia)

Diabetic mother

Maternal hypertension

Maternal smoking

Maternal cyanotic heart disease

Fetal factors

Trisomy 13, 18, 21

Hypothyroidism

Neonatal thyrotoxicosis

Congenital adrenal hyperplasia

Beckwith-Weidermann syndrome

High altitude

*See Chapter 30

References: [Rosenkrantz 2005, Werner 1995]

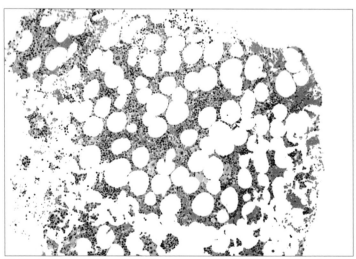

i9.10 *Bone marrow clot section from patient with Gaisbock syndrome showing overall normal cellularity without features of a chronic myeloproliferative neoplasm. (H&E)*

Neonatal Polycythemia and Down Syndrome

The occurrence of polycythemia in neonates with Down syndrome presents an intriguing etiologic puzzle. On the one hand, the neonatal period in infants with Down syndrome is characterized by abnormal hematopoiesis, with frequent CBC abnormalities in multiple lineages [Henry 2007] and, most dramatically, the Down syndrome-associated transient myeloproliferative disorder (see Chapter 30 for further details). On the other hand, polycythemia in the general neonatal population is a well-reported phenomenon often linked to chronic hypoxia during fetal development **t9.6**. The question then arises: Does polycythemia seen in the setting of Down syndrome represent a variant of the neonatal polycythemia seen in non-Down syndrome cases, or does it truly reflect a disease-specific transient dysregulation of erythropoiesis?

Epidemiologic data confirm that neonatal polycythemia is significantly more common in infants with Down syndrome than in unaffected neonates, suggesting that there is indeed a disease-specific association. Neonatal polycythemia is observed in 2% to 4% of the general newborn population and in 33% of those with Down syndrome [Foucar 2001, Henry 2007]. However, this finding alone does not rule out the possibility that the Down syndrome–associated cases might be secondary to some fetal or placental factor common to Down syndrome, eg, congenital abnormalities of the heart. In such a scenario, erythropoietin levels would be expected to be increased in response to hypoxia. In fact, the literature is contradictory on this point, with one study identifying significantly increased erythropoietin in cord blood samples of infants with Down syndrome, and another study showing no increase in erythropoietin levels in amniotic fluid samples of similar patients [Campbell 1994, Widness 1994].

The *GATA1* mutation is closely associated with the development of transient myeloproliferative disorder (transient abnormal myelopoiesis) of Down syndrome, being present in 97% of such cases. However, since only 4% of Down syndrome neonates harbor the *GATA1* mutation [Pine 2007], while some 33% develop neonatal polycythemia, it seems likely that factors independent of *GATA1* mutations must play a significant role in the development of neonatal polycythemia in the setting of Down syndrome. Increased dosage of genes in the duplicated region of chromosome 21 has itself been shown in mouse models to induce some of the CBC abnormalities seen in Down syndrome in the neonatal period [Kirsammer 2008].

At present, then, the specific mechanisms underlying the erythrocytosis seen in this patient population remain unclear. It is possible that neonatal polycythemia in this setting may comprise 2 distinct types. Some cases may represent variants of typical neonatal polycythemia exacerbated or facilitated by inherent abnormalities of hematopoiesis related to Down syndrome, while other cases may be variants of transient myeloproliferative disorder (transient abnormal myelopoiesis) showing marked normoblastosis instead of circulating immature blasts [Bozner 2002]. Further study is necessary to refine the classification and diagnostic criteria for these unusual cases.

---

common underlying mechanism is chronic hypoxia [Rosenkrantz 2005, Werner 1995] (see **sidebar 9.2** for more details).

In addition to neonatal polycythemia, rare cases of transient erythrocytosis with markedly increased circulating maturing normoblasts have been described in neonates with Down syndrome [Foucar 2001]. This spontaneously regressing disorder is likely a variant of the transient myeloproliferative disorders (transient abnormal myelopoiesis) in infants with Down syndrome that more commonly exhibit high numbers of circulating myeloblasts, erythroblasts, and megakaryoblasts. *GATA1* gene mutations are characteristic of neonatal Down syndrome–associated transient abnormal myelopoiesis. Recently *JAK3* mutations have also been described in these self-limited disorders in neonates [Tefferi 2008a] (see Chapter 30 for more details and illustrations).

[9.3] ### Differential Diagnosis, Laboratory Testing

Since acquired polycythemia is much more common than constitutional erythrocytosis, the differential diagnosis of acquired erythrocytosis will be discussed first.

The laboratory tests useful in distinguishing the various acquired polycythemic states are listed in **t9.4**. Some, such as the hematologic parameters and arterial oxygen saturation, should be routinely performed on virtually all patients with suspected primary or secondary polycythemia, while other tests are useful under more selected clinical circumstances. Laboratory testing for all patients with erythrocytosis should be directed by the unique clinical features of each patient.

With the assessment of complete blood count data and other laboratory test results, both secondary and relative erythrocytotic disorders can generally be distinguished from polycythemia vera. Erythropoietin levels are generally increased in patients with secondary erythrocytosis, normal in patients with relative erythrocytosis, and decreased in those with polycythemia vera and familial primary erythrocytosis [Delanghe 2008, Foucar 2008, Gordeuk 2004, Hoyer 2004, Koster 2001, Kralovics 2005b, Leifert 2008, O'Malley 2005, Pastore 2003b, Percy 2008a, 2008b, Rad 2008, Rosenkrantz 2005, Tefferi 2006b, Van Maerken 2004]. Polycythemia vera is further characterized by multilineage abnormalities in blood and bone marrow, *JAK2* mutations in virtually all cases, clonal cytogenetic abnormalities in 10% - 20%, and spontaneous erythrocyte colony formation in cell culture assays [Kralovics 2005b, Spivak 2008, Tefferi 2008b].

Although positive family history may be sufficient for clinical diagnosis, sophisticated gene mutation analysis may be necessary to confirm mutations in the erythropoietin receptor gene in cases of autosomal dominant primary familial erythrocytosis [Kralovics 2005b]. Other types of familial erythrocytosis are secondary, driven by sustained, physiologically inappropriate erythropoietin production. These rare, usually autosomal recessive disorders are due to mutations in genes encoding the oxygen-sensing apparatus regulatory factors, including genes encoding several isoforms of hypoxia-inducible factor-α (HIF-α), mutations in genes that encode hydroxylaters that inactivate HIF-α, and mutations in the von Hippel-Lindau gene responsible for degradation of hydroxylated HIF-α [Gordeuk 2004, Ladroue 2008, Lee 2008, Pastore 2003b, Percy 2008a, 2008b, 2009]. In these 3 types of mutations, the result is dysregulated, sustained erythropoietin production.

Finally, sophisticated testing to detect recombinant human erythropoietin in urine and serum is necessary for detecting illicit use by endurance athletes [Delanghe 2008]. Similarly, flow cytometry can be used to detect allogeneic blood transfusions (blood doping) used by athletes to increase RBC levels, increase oxygen concentration in arterial blood, and enhance performance [Arndt 2008].

[9.4]   Clues and Caveats

1. Polycythemia vera is a clonal stem cell disorder derived from *JAK2* V617F mutation and characterized by multilineage qualitative and quantitative abnormalities in blood and bone marrow, while isolated erythrocyte abnormalities in blood and bone marrow generally characterize secondary erythrocytoses.

2. Although generally mild in polycythemia vera, an increased absolute basophil count is characteristic of chronic myeloproliferative neoplasms. Other blood features include nucleated RBCs, variable neutrophilia with left shift and variable thrombocytosis; these features are not typically seen in secondary erythrocytoses.

3. Clonal cytogenetic defects and functional abnormalities of neutrophils and platelets are unique to polycythemia vera and are not characteristic of secondary or relative erythrocytotic disorders.

4. Rare families/individual patients have sustained primary erythrocytosis secondary to erythropoietin receptor gene mutations, conferring erythropoietin independence, while other familial erythrocytoses are secondary to constitutional mutations in oxygen-sensing regulatory factor genes, resulting in dysregulated erythropoietin production.

5. Erythropoietin levels are decreased in primary familial erythrocytosis and polycythemia vera, increased in secondary erythrocytosis, and normal in relative erythrocytosis.

6. Except for tumor-staging purposes, bone marrow examination is not generally required for patients with secondary and relative erythrocytosis. Instead, these diagnoses are based on the integration of clinical, laboratory, and sometimes radiographic data.

7. The secondary erythrocytoses, both physiologically appropriate and inappropriate, are mediated by erythropoietin or erythropoietin-like substances.

8. Polycythemia can occur in newborns and is linked to placental defects, maternal factors, including diabetes, and trisomy 13, 18, 21 in the fetus. In addition, neonates with Down syndrome may rarely have a pronounced normoblastemia that spontaneously regresses.

9. Hantavirus pulmonary syndrome is a cause of relative erythrocytosis via massive leakage of plasma into the lungs, producing rapid, dramatic hemoconcentration.

10. Consider Gaisbock syndrome as a possible cause of erythrocytosis in obese, hypertensive patients who smoke.

[9.5]   References

Al-Sheikh M, Moradkhani K, Lopez M, et al [2008] Disturbance in the HIF-1alpha pathway associated with erythrocytosis: further evidences brought by frameshift and nonsense mutations in the prolyl hydroxylase domain protein 2 (*PHD2*) gene. *Blood Cells Mol Dis* 40:160-165.

Anastasi J, Vardiman J [2010] Polycythemia vera. In: Kjeldsberg C, ed. *Practical Diagnosis of Hematologic Disorders*. Chicago: ASCP Press; 579-594.

Arndt PA, Kumpel BM [2008] Blood doping in athletes—detection of allogeneic blood transfusions by flow cytofluorometry. *Am J Hematol* 83:657-667.

Bailey-Serres J, Chang R [2005] Sensing and signalling in response to oxygen deprivation in plants and other organisms. *Ann Bot (Lond)* 96:507-518.

Baxter EJ, Scott LM, Campbell PJ, et al [2005] Acquired mutation of the tyrosine kinase JAK2 in human myeloproliferative disorders. *Lancet* 365:1054-1061.

Bento MC, Chang KT, Guan Y, et al [2005] Congenital polycythemia with homozygous and heterozygous mutations of von Hippel-Lindau gene: five new Caucasian patients. *Haematologica* 90:128-129.

Bozner P [2002] Transient myeloproliferative disorder with erythroid differentiation in Down syndrome. *Arch Pathol Lab Med* 126:474-477.

Buick R [2008] When did oxygenic photosynthesis evolve? *Philos Trans R Soc Lond B Biol Sci* 363:2731-2743.

Campbell J, Wathen N, Lewis M, et al [1994] Amniotic fluid erythropoietin levels in normal and Down's syndrome pregnancies. *Eur J Obstet Gynecol Reprod Biol* 56:191-194.

Campbell PJ, Green AR [2006] The myeloproliferative disorders. *N Engl J Med* 355:2452-2466.

Cario H, Schwarz K, Jorch N, et al [2005] Mutations in the von Hippel-Lindau (VHL) tumor suppressor gene and VHL-haplotype analysis in patients with presumable congenital erythrocytosis. *Haematologica* 90:19-24.

Delanghe JR, Bollen M, Beullens M [2008] Testing for recombinant erythropoietin. *Am J Hematol* 83:237-241.

Foucar K [2001] Neonatal hematopathology: special considerations. In: Collins R, Swerdlow S, eds. *Pediatric Hematopathology*. New York: Churchill Living; 173-184.

Foucar K [2008] Non-neoplastic erythroid lineage disorders. In: King D, Gardner W, Sobin L, et al, eds. *Non-Neoplastic Disorders of Bone Marrow (AFIP fascicle)*. Washington, DC: American Registry of Pathology; 75-124.

Gale DP, Harten SK, Reid CD, et al [2008] Autosomal dominant erythrocytosis and pulmonary arterial hypertension associated with an activating HIF2 alpha mutation. *Blood* 112:919-921.

Gordeuk VR, Sergueeva AI, Miasnikova GY, et al [2004] Congenital disorder of oxygen sensing: association of the homozygous Chuvash polycythemia VHL mutation with thrombosis and vascular abnormalities but not tumors. *Blood* 103:3924-3932.

Henry E, Walker D, Wiedmeier SE, Christensen RD [2007] Hematological abnormalities during the first week of life among neonates with Down syndrome: data from a multihospital healthcare system. *Am J Med Genet A* 143:42-50.

Hoyer JD, Allen SL, Beutler E, et al [2004] Erythrocytosis due to bisphospho-glycerate mutase deficiency with concurrent glucose-6-phosphate dehydro-genase (G-6-PD) deficiency. *Am J Hematol* 75:205-208.

Ivan M, Harris AL, Martelli F, Kulshreshtha R [2008] Hypoxia response and microRNAs: No longer 2 separate worlds. *J Cell Mol Med* 12:1426-1431.

James C, Ugo V, Le Couedic JP, et al [2005] A unique clonal *JAK2* mutation leading to constitutive signalling causes polycythaemia vera. *Nature* 434:1144-1148.

Kaelin WG, Jr [2008] Ratcliffe PJ. Oxygen sensing by metazoans: the central role of the HIF hydroxylase pathway. *Mol Cell* 30:393-402.

Kapitsinou PP, Haase VH [2008] The VHL tumor suppressor and HIF: Insights from genetic studies in mice. *Cell Death Differ* 15:650-659.

Kirsammer G, Jilani S, Liu H, et al [2008] Highly penetrant myeloprolif-erative disease in the Ts65Dn mouse model of Down syndrome. *Blood* 111:767-775.

Koivunen P, Hirsila M, Gunzler V, et al [2004] Catalytic properties of the asparaginyl hydroxylase (FIH) in the oxygen sensing pathway are distinct from those of its prolyl 4-hydroxylases. *J Biol Chem* 279:9899-9904.

Koster F, Foucar K, Hjelle B, et al [2001] Rapid presumptive diagnosis of Hantavirus Cardiopulmonary Syndrome by peripheral blood smear review. *Am J Clin Pathol* 116:665-672.

Kralovics R, Passamonti F, Buser AS, et al [2005a] A gain-of-function mutation of *JAK2* in myeloproliferative disorders. *N Engl J Med* 352:1779-1790.

Kralovics R, Skoda RC [2005b] Molecular pathogenesis of Philadelphia chromosome negative myeloproliferative disorders. *Blood Rev* 19:1-13.

Ladroue C, Carcenac R, Leporrier M, et al [2008] PHD2 mutation and congenital erythrocytosis with paraganglioma. *N Engl J Med* 359:2685-2692.

Lee FS [2008] Genetic causes of erythrocytosis and the oxygen-sensing pathway. *Blood Rev* 22:321-332.

Lee FS, Percy MJ, McMullin MF [2006] Oxygen sensing: Recent insights from idiopathic erythrocytosis. *Cell Cycle* 5:941-945.

Leifert JA [2008] Anaemia and cigarette smoking. *Int J Lab Hematol* 30:177-184.

Levine RL, Wadleigh M, Cools J, et al [2005] Activating mutation in the tyrosine kinase JAK2 in polycythemia vera, essential thrombocythemia, and myeloid metaplasia with myelofibrosis. *Cancer Cell* 7:387-397.

McMullin MF [2008] The classification and diagnosis of erythrocytosis. *Int J Lab Hematol* 30:447-459.

Means RT [2009] Erythrocytosis. In: Greer J, Foerster J, Rodgers G, et al, eds. *Wintrobe's Clinical Hematology.* 12th ed. Philadelphia: Lippincott Williams & Wilkins; 1261-1272.

O'Malley D, Vardiman J [2005] Polycythemia (erythrocytosis),including polycy-themia vera (PV). In: Kjeldsberg C, ed. *Practical Diagnosis of Hematologic Disorders.* Chicago: ASCP; 579-594.

Pastore Y, Jedlickova K, Guan Y, et al [2003a] Mutations of von Hippel-Lindau tumor-suppressor gene and congenital polycythemia. *Am J Hum Genet* 73:412-419.

Pastore YD, Jelinek J, Ang S, et al [2003b] Mutations in the VHL gene in sporadic apparently congenital polycythemia. *Blood* 101:1591-1595.

Percy MJ, Furlow PW, Beer PA, et al [2007] A novel erythrocytosis-associated PHD2 mutation suggests the location of a HIF binding groove. *Blood* 110:2193-2196.

Percy MJ, Beer PA, Campbell G, et al [2008a] Novel exon 12 mutations in the HIF2A gene associated with erythrocytosis. *Blood* 111:5400-5402.

Percy MJ, Furlow PW, Lucas GS, et al [2008b] A gain-of-function mutation in the HIF2A gene in familial erythrocytosis. *N Engl J Med* 358:162-168.

Percy MJ, Rumi E [2009] Genetic origins and clinical phenotype of familial and acquired erythrocytosis and thrombocytosis. *Am J Hematol* 84:46-54.

Perrotta S, Nobili B, Ferraro M, et al [2006] Von Hippel-Lindau-dependent polycythemia is endemic on the island of Ischia: Identification of a novel cluster. *Blood* 107:514-519.

Pine SR, Guo Q, Yin C, et al [2007] Incidence and clinical implications of GATA1 mutations in newborns with Down syndrome. *Blood* 110:2128-2131.

Rad FH, Ulusakarya A, Gad S, et al [2008] Novel somatic mutations of the VHL gene in an erythropoietin-producing renal carcinoma associated with secondary polycythemia and elevated circulating endothelial progenitor cells. *Am J Hematol* 83:155-158.

Randi ML, Murgia A, Putti MC, et al [2005] Low frequency of VHL gene mutations in young individuals with polycythemia and high serum erythro-poietin. *Haematologica* 90:689-691.

Roberts AM, Ohh M [2008] Beyond the hypoxia-inducible factor-centric tumour suppressor model of von Hippel-Lindau. *Curr Opin Oncol* 20:83-89.

Rocha S [2007] Gene regulation under low oxygen: holding your breath for transcription. *Trends Biochem Sci* 32:389-397.

Rosenkrantz T, Oh W [2005] Polycythemia and hyperviscosity in the newborn. In: de Alarcon P, Werner E, eds. *Neonatal Hematology* Cambridge: Cambridge University; 171-186.

Semenza GL [2009] Involvement of oxygen-sensing pathways in physiologic and pathologic erythropoiesis. *Blood* 114:2015-2019.

Shehata BM, Stockwell CA, Castellano-Sanchez AA, et al [2008] Von Hippel-Lindau (VHL) disease: an update on the clinico-pathologic and genetic aspects. *Adv Anat Pathol* 15:165-171.

Spivak JL, Silver RT [2008] The revised World Health Organization diagnostic criteria for polycythemia vera, essential thrombocytosis, and primary myelofibrosis: an alternative proposal. *Blood* 112:231-239.

Stefanini M, Urbas J, Urbs J [1978] Gaisbock's syndrome: Its hematologic, biochemical, and hormonal parameters. *Angiology* 29:520-533.

Tefferi A [2006a] The diagnosis of polycythemia vera: New tests and old dictums. *Best Pract Res Clin Haematol* 19:455-469.

Tefferi A [2008a] JAK and MPL mutations in myeloid malignancies. *Leuk Lymphoma* 49:388-397.

Tefferi A, Pardanani A [2006b] Mutation screening for *JAK2* V617F: When to order the test and how to interpret the results. *Leuk Res* 30:739-744.

Tefferi A [2008a] JAK and MPL mutations in myeloid malignancies. *Leuk Lymphoma* 49:388-397.

Tefferi A, Vardiman JW [2008b] Classification and diagnosis of myeloprolif-erative neoplasms: the 2008 World Health Organization criteria and point-of-care diagnostic algorithms. *Leukemia* 22:14-22.

Thiele J, Kvasnicka H, Orazi A, et al [2008] Polycythaemia vera. In: Jaffe E, Harris NL, Stein H, Vardiman JW, eds. *WHO Classification of Tumours: Pathology & Genetics: Tumours of Haematopoietic and Lymphoid Tissues.* Lyon, France: IARC Press; 2008:40-43.

Thiele J, Kvasnicka HM, Vardiman J [2006] Bone marrow histopathology in the diagnosis of chronic myeloproliferative disorders: a forgotten pearl. *Best Pract Res Clin Haematol* 19:413-437.

Van Maerken T, Hunninck K, Callewaert L, et al [2004] Familial and congenital polycythemias: a diagnostic approach. *J Pediatr Hematol Oncol* 26:407-416.

Werner EJ [1995] Neonatal polycythemia and hyperviscosity. *Clin Perinatol* 22:693-710.

Widness JA, Pueschel SM, Pezzullo JC, Clemons GK [1994] Elevated erythro-poietin levels in cord blood of newborns with Down's syndrome. *Biol Neonate* 66:50-55.

Non-Neoplastic Granulocytic and Monocytic Disorders, Excluding Neutropenia

Kaaren Reichard, MD

Knowledge of normal neutrophil, eosinophil, basophil, and monocyte morphology, and their respective counts in the peripheral blood and bone marrow is required in order to further investigate morphologic and numerical abnormalities of these cell types. Non-neoplastic etiologies underlying the numerical and morphologic abnormalities of these cells are the focus of this chapter. Non-neoplastic disorders of lymphoid cells are covered in Chapter 21, neutropenic conditions are covered in Chapter 11, and bone marrow histiocytic disorders are covered in Chapter 27. Although bone marrow pathology is the focus of this book, the majority of this chapter's discussion centers on peripheral blood findings, as most non-neoplastic disorders of these cell types seldom warrant bone marrow examination. However, peripheral blood abnormalities that would require further investigation by a bone marrow examination are addressed (morphologic and laboratory clues).

[10.1] Overview of Normal Cell Counts

As detailed in Chapter 1, myelopoiesis is a highly complicated and regulated process requiring stem cells, progenitor cells, an appropriate bone marrow milieu and coordinated regulatory factors. The end result of appropriate bone marrow maturation is circulating leukocytes, platelets, and red blood cells, which can be easily and routinely measured after venipuncture (see Chapters 6, 8, 9, and 12 for non-neoplastic red blood cell and platelet disorders). t10.1 shows age-related normal values in peripheral blood for white blood cell count, absolute neutrophil count, and the absolute cell counts above and below which a neutrophilic, eosinophilic, basophilic or monocytic disorder should be investigated [Foucar 2008]. Age-related variations should be recognized when a patient is evaluated for a constitutional or reactive myeloid disorder (see Chapter 2, **t2.1**, p 29).

[10.2] Neutrophils

[10.2.1] Neutrophilia

Neutrophil mobilization and maturation mechanisms underlie the various types of reactive neutrophilias discussed below [von Vietinghoff 2008]. For each of these mechanisms, the time course varies to achieve a detectable response. Demargination occurs largely through the action of epinephrine and is almost immediate (minutes). Approximately half of the neutrophils in circulation are attributable to the marginated pool. This generally results in

a transient increase in neutrophil count without significant toxic change. If there are sustained requirements for neutrophils (ie, prolonged/untreated infection or inflammation), an initial release of the storage compartment neutrophils is needed, which may take several hours, and ultimately increased neutrophil production by the marrow (days).

Neutrophilia is defined as an absolute increase in neutrophils above the established age-related normal range **t10.1**. The normal range is significantly different depending on age (eg, brisk neutrophilia at birth is expected, whereas beyond the neonatal period it is not). Non-neoplastic neutrophilias are typically the result of an acquired condition, although rare congenital disorders are known. Causes of non-neoplastic neutrophilias are listed in **t10.2**.

[10.2.2] Acquired Neutrophilia

Infectious and inflammatory disorders are the most frequent causes of non-neoplastic neutrophilia. Bacteria are the most common etiologic agent underlying infection-associated neutrophilia. The degree of white blood cell (WBC) elevation is generally proportional to the severity of the infection or inflammation, and neutrophils are rapidly mobilized [Burdon 2005, von Vietinghoff 2008]. The WBC count rarely exceeds 30×10^9/L, although in severe tissue damage/trauma the count may exceed 50×10^9/L. Any type of stressful situation (eg, phlebotomy, emotional

t10.1 Absolute Cell Counts by Patient Age*

	Newborn	<1 y	Child	Adult
WBC	15-30	11	8.5	7.5
ANC	10-25	3.5	3.5	3.5†
Neutrophilia	>28	>10	>8	>7
Neutropenia†	<7	<2.5	<1.5	<1.5
Eosinophilia	>0.5	>0.5	>0.5	>0.5
Eosinopenia	0	0	0	0
Basophilia	>0.1	>0.1	>0.1	>0.1
Basophilopenia	0	0	0	0
Monocytosis	>3.5	>0.8	>0.8	>0.8
Monocytopenia	<1	<0.2	<0.2	<0.2

*Units = cell count × 10³/µL (cell count × 10⁹/L)
†Absolute neutrophil counts may be physiologically lower in certain genetic groups, eg, African-American populations [Haddy 1999, Hsieh 2007, von Vietinghoff 2008]
ANC = absolute neutrophil count; WBC = white blood cell count

References: [Brugnara 2003, Foucar 2008a, 2010a, 2010b, Kjeldsberg 2010]

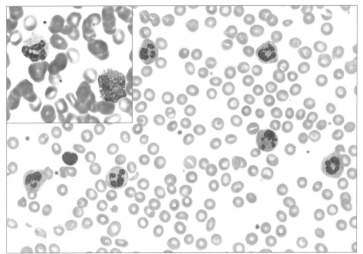

i10.1 *Peripheral blood smear illustrates a marked neutrophilia that consists primarily of mature neutrophils as well as occasional bands. Inset shows side-by-side comparison of normal neutrophil and eosinophil. (Wright)*

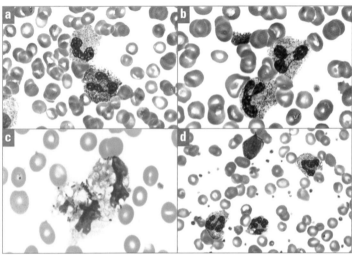

i10.2 *This composite shows a spectrum of toxic neutrophils in various infectious and noninfectious conditions. Note toxic granulation **a**, **b**, circulating neutrophil cytoplasmic fragment **b**, prominent vacuolization, a feature of sepsis—and note organisms **c** and toxic neutrophilia with left shift **d**. (Wright)*

stress, injury, surgery, exercise) may result in a mild transient absolute neutrophilia **t10.2**.

Nonactivated neutrophils are characterized by 4-5 nuclear lobes separated by a thin chromatin fiber, clumped chromatin, and an orange cytoplasmic hue (Wright stain) imparted by the numerous secondary granules **i10.1**. In contrast, activated neutrophils show toxic granulation, Döhle bodies and occasional vacuoles **t10.3**, **i10.2**. Toxic changes are typical of severe infections or recombinant colony-stimulating factor (CSF) therapy. Neutrophils with prominent cytoplasmic vacuoles in the presence of toxic granulation and Döhle bodies are suggestive of sepsis. Vacuolar change in neutrophils should be interpreted with caution, however, as aged and/or degenerated specimens often show vacuoles. Cytoplasmic vacuoles may also be seen in alcohol toxicity [Chetty-Raju 2004].

t10.2 Causes of Non-Neoplastic Neutrophilia

Acquired Conditions

Acute stress	Emotional stimuli
	Physical stress:
	Phlebotomy
	Trauma/injury
	Blood loss
	Seizures
	Postsurgery
	Exercise
	Pregnancy/delivery
	Tissue damage/necrosis:
	Burn
	Blunt injury
Infection	Bacterial, sepsis
	Viral:
	severe acute respiratory syndrome (SARS)
	hantavirus
Drugs/hormones	Epinephrine
	Lithium
	Colony-stimulating factors
	Beta-agonists
Chronic inflammatory conditions	Vasculitis
	Pancreatitis
	Hepatitis
	Colitis
	Autoimmune disorders
	Collagen vascular disease
	Sweet syndrome
Chronic noninfectious/ noninflammatory conditions	Chronic smoking
	Chronic blood loss
	Hypo/asplenism
Metabolic	Ketoacidosis
	Uremia
	Eclampsia
Malignancy	Carcinomas:
	bladder, hepatocellular, uterine, cervical
	Lymphomas
	Plasma cell myeloma
	Sarcomas

Constitutional Conditions

Leukocyte adhesion deficiency

Familial cold urticaria

Hereditary neutrophilia

References: [Ahn 2005, Araki 2007, Badolato 2004, Engsig 2007, Etzioni 2000, Focosi 2009, Ito 1993, Koster 2001, Lam 2004, Tsakonas 2007, Ward 1971]

t10.3 Granulocytic Morphologic Abnormalities

	Description	Non-Neoplastic Disease Etiologies
Nuclear		
Hyposegmentation **i10.16**	Nucleus with one or 2 nuclear lobes	Pelger-Huët anomaly **i10.17** Acquired pseudo Pelger-Huët (HIV-1, drugs, other infections) (Major differential diagnosis: myelodysplasia)
Hypersegmentation **i10.15**	Nucleus with >5 lobes	Vitamin B$_{12}$/folate deficiency HIV-1 Iron deficiency DNA inhibiting chemotherapeutic agent Myelokathexis (rare) **i10.24** (Differential diagnoses: primary myeloid neoplasm)
Pyknosis	Dark, round, homogeneous nucleus	Dying, apoptotic cell (Differential diagnosis: neoplastic cell of some sort)
Botryoid/grape-like	6 or more nuclear lobes, often with a pinwheel appearance	Hyperthermia (heat stroke) Hemorrhagic shock and encephalopathy syndrome (rare)
Cytoplasmic		
Toxic granulation **i10.2**	Enlarged, prominent, dark granules	Infection Acute severe stress CSF effect **i10.3**
Döhle bodies **i10.2**	Light blue inclusions Round to oval in shape Represent aggregated rough endoplasmic reticulum	Severe infection May-Hegglin (Döhle-body-like) CSF effect
Inclusions (excluding organisms)	Uniform, deep dark purple granules	Alder-Reilly anomaly **i10.19, i10.20, i10.21**
	Large azurophilic granules	Chédiak-Higashi **i10.23**
	Döhle-body-like	May-Hegglin **i10.22**
	Clear/lightly colored amorphous material	Cryoglobulinemia
	Howell-Jolly body-like	Immunosuppressive therapy Chemotherapy HIV-1
	Platelets	In vitro phenomenon Platelets may be ingested in cases of satellitism
Vacuoles		Bacteremia, artifact (aged specimen) **i10.2** Alcohol toxicity Medium chain AcylCoA dehydrogenase deficiency

AcylCoA = acyl-coenzyme A; CSF = colony-stimulating factor; HIV-1 = human immunodeficiency virus-1

Circulating cytoplasmic granulocyte fragments may rarely be present on blood smears; this finding is associated with sepsis or recombinant CSF therapy (see **i10.2b**) [Dalal 2002, Krauss 1989].

Accompanying the neutrophil toxic changes may be a shift to immaturity in the granulocytes (left shift), which, depending on the severity of infection, may include occasional circulating promyelocytes and blasts **i10.2d, i10.3**. A left shift is best recognized by circulating metamyelocytes and myelocytes, as neutrophilic band forms may be difficult to reliably distinguish from mature neutrophils [Buttarello 2008, Cornbleet 2002, van der Meer 2006].

t10.4 details morphologic features that may be seen in the peripheral blood and bone marrow in reactive neutrophilias. In the bone marrow, increased cellularity predominantly due to a granulocytic hyperplasia is seen, along with possible minimal/mild reticulin fibrosis (reversible), mild megakaryocytic hyperplasia with unremarkable morphology, mild polyclonal plasmacytosis, and reactive lymphoid

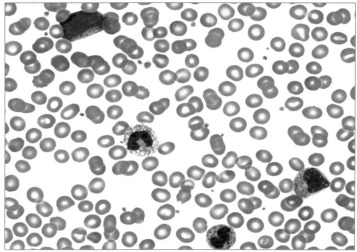

i10.3 *Left shift including circulating myelocytes and a circulating blast in conjunction with toxic neutrophils is evident on this peripheral blood smear from a patient receiving granulocyte colony-stimulating factor. (Wright)*

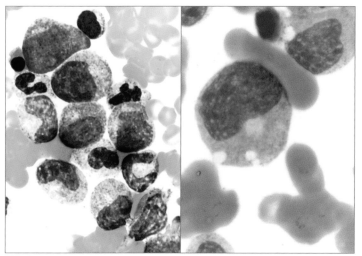

i10.4 *This bone marrow aspirate smear composite from a patient with adreno-cortical carcinoma shows marked granulocytic hyperplasia with prominent reactive features including paranuclear hofs. (Wright)*

aggregates **i10.4**. Granulomas may be seen in infectious and non-infectious states and are further discussed in Chapters 27 and 33. Autoimmune disorders/collagen vascular disease processes may show any or all of these findings **i10.5** (see Chapter 34) [Hunt 2009, Vlasoff 2006].

In patients receiving recombinant colony-stimulating factor (CSF therapy), the WBC count may be quite variable from 13×10^9/L to 100×10^9/L (rare) **i10.6** [Cummings 1999, Kerrigan 1989, Meyerson 1998, Orazi 1992]. The effects of recombinant granulocyte-CSF (G-CSF) or granulocyte-monocyte-CSF (GM-CSF) in the peripheral blood and bone marrow may extend from 3 days to 2 weeks post-administration, in our experience. The typical peripheral blood and bone marrow findings are presented in **t10.5**. The blood smear may show neutrophilic leukocytosis with left shift including blasts **i10.6**. Although blasts usually account for a minority of

t10.4 Morphologic Features of Reactive Neutrophilia in Blood and Bone Marrow

Blood	Comments
Leukocytosis	Usually <30 × 10⁹/L; higher WBC in young children
	Rarely >50 × 10⁹/L except in patients receiving cytokine therapy (or with cytokine-producing tumor)
Left shift	Bands* and metamyelocytes may be prominent
	In septic neonates may see circulating blasts and promyelocytes
Döhle bodies†	Retained portion of cytoplasm from more immature state of maturation
Toxic granulation	Etiology controversial, either retained primary granules or altered uptake of stain by secondary granules
Cytoplasmic vacuoles	Neutrophil vacuoles correlate with sepsis
Cytoplasmic fragments	Anuclear fragments of neutrophil cytoplasm found in patients with septic shock and in those receiving cytokine therapy
Other lineages	Thrombocytosis common; eosinophilia or monocytosis may accompany neutrophilia
	Basophilia not present
Bone Marrow	**Comments**
Cellularity	Usually mildly increased; greater cellularity in patients with increased endogenous or therapeutic cytokines
Granulocytic hyperplasia	Maturation intact, although may be left-shifted due to rapid release of more mature forms into blood
Reticulin fibrosis	Mild reticulin fibrosis noted in some reactive disorders
Increased megakaryocytes	Mild megakaryocytic hyperplasia (dysplasia absent to minimal)
Lymphoid aggregates	Found in some inflammatory processes, especially viral and autoimmune disorders
Granulomas	May be found in a variety of infectious diseases‡
Plasmacytosis	Increased polyclonal plasma cells common

*Morphologic identification of band neutrophils lacks reproducibility; recommend requirement of metamyelocytes for conclusive evidence of left shift
†In reactive neutrophilias, toxic granulation accompanies Döhle bodies; hypogranular cells with Döhle bodies are suggestive of myelodysplasia
‡Bone marrow granulomas discussed in detail in Chapters 27 and 33

References: [Foucar 2008, Hirokawa 1990, Hunt 2009, Kerrigan 1989, Seebach 1997, Strand 1991, Vlasoff 2006]

t10.5 Morphologic Features of Blood and Bone Marrow in Patients Receiving Recombinant Growth Factor Therapy*

Blood

Marked leukocytosis with increase in neutrophils (increase in monocytes, with variable increase in eosinophils, lymphocytes, and sometimes basophils in patients receiving GM-CSF)

Prominent toxic changes in mature and immature granulocytes

Leukoerythroblastic picture with circulating blasts (usually low percent)

Nuclear-cytoplasmic asynchrony[†]

Nuclear segmentation defects[†]

Transient increase in blasts prior to neutrophil recovery may mimic leukemia

Rare binucleate (tetraploid) neutrophils present (G-CSF)

Circulating myeloid cytoplasmic fragments

Bone Marrow[‡]

In patients with profound bone marrow suppression, early changes include interstitial foci of granulocyte precursors in hypocellular bone marrow

Increased cellularity with left shift in hematopoietic elements

Promyelocytic hyperplasia with reactive features during early phase of therapy

Rare reports of transient increase in blood and bone marrow blasts mimicking leukemia

Pronounced toxic changes of immature and mature granulocytic cells

Occasional binucleate promyelocytes and myelocytes

More mature granulocytes predominate after several weeks of therapy

Rare development of fibrosis with bony changes

Rare histiocytic proliferation (GM-CSF)

Rare development of acute bone marrow necrosis (G-CSF)

*Granulocyte monocyte colony-stimulating factor (GM-CSF) or granulocyte colony-stimulating factor (G-CSF)

[†]Bone marrow examination not routinely performed on most patients receiving recombinant cytokine therapy

[‡]Generally seen when growth factors used in conjunction with chemotherapeutic agents

Reference: [Foucar 2008]

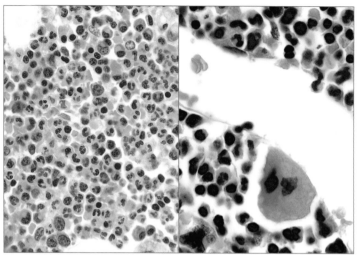

i10.5 *This bone marrow biopsy composite from an 8-year-old female with severe chronic inflammatory disease shows increased granulocytic precursors in conjunction with dilated sinuses. (H&E)*

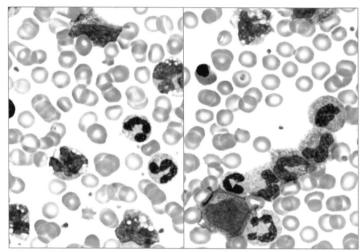

i10.6 *Prominent toxic neutrophilia in conjunction with numerous reactive-appearing monocytes and left shift is evident in this peripheral blood smear composite from a patient receiving granulocyte monocyte colony-stimulating factor. (Wright)*

WBCs, during the nadir in the WBC, blasts can account for a significant proportion of the sparse circulating cells. In the bone marrow, there is granulocytic hyperplasia with many cells showing a prominent paranuclear hof and binucleation i10.7, i10.8. Binucleation of neutrophils or precursors is often a major morphologic clue in the peripheral blood to CSF

administration. Another clue to recombinant CSF therapy is the intense and nearly universal enhanced toxic appearance of the granulocytes and monocytes. The cytoplasm bears a basophilic hue, vacuolization may be prominent, and toxic granules and Döhle bodies seem present in every granulocyte [Kerrigan 1989]. Blasts and promyelocytes may occasionally surpass 20% in the early phases of therapy and potentially mimic a myeloid malignancy [Meyerson 1998]. The increased blasts, although transient, should resemble typical myeloid blasts. Abnormal cytology (small size, minimal cytoplasm, Auer rods) should not be seen, nor should immunophenotypic aberrancy. Similarly, promyelocytes, in patients receiving CSF therapy, do not exhibit abnormal cytologic features (ie, prominent nuclear lobation rather than round nuclei, Auer

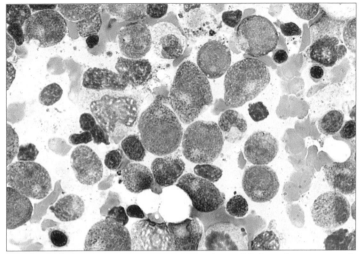

i10.7 *This bone marrow aspirate smear was obtained 3 days after initiation of granulocyte colony-stimulating factor therapy. Note wave of promyelocytes with prominent hof (Golgi region). (Wright)*

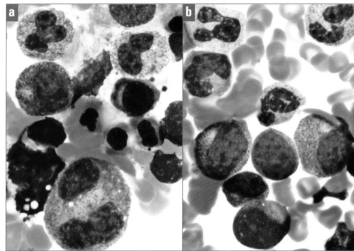

i10.8 *This bone marrow composite is from a patient with mantle cell lymphoma who was receiving granulocyte colony-stimulating factor after chemotherapy. Note the binucleate promyelocyte (**a** bottom), a typical feature. (Wright)*

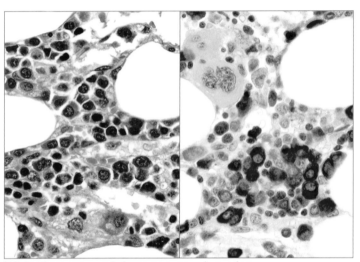

i10.9 *This composite of a bone marrow core biopsy from a patient receiving early treatment with granulocyte colony-stimulating factor shows markedly left-shifted granulopoiesis, which is highlighted by myeloperoxidase staining. (H&E and immunoperoxidase for myeloperoxidase)*

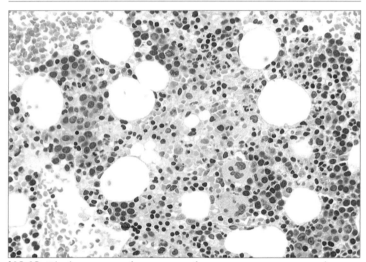

i10.10 *This bone marrow biopsy section from a patient receiving granulocyte monocyte colony-stimulating factor shows a focus of monocytic/histiocytic hyperplasia (center). (H&E)*

rods, lack of significant maturation), helping to exclude acute promyelocytic leukemia. The promyelocytes from patients receiving recombinant CSF therapy instead show prominent paranuclear hofs and prominent cytoplasmic granulation **i10.7**. In core biopsy sections, early CSF effect may be seen as clusters of immature, left-shifted granulocytes confirmed by myeloperoxidase immunohistochemistry **i10.9**. Occasionally, GM-CSF therapy may evoke a histiocytic response in the bone marrow, in addition to the expected granulocytic hyperplasia **i10.10** [Glasser 2007].

Overproduction of either endogenous colony-stimulating factor (CSF) or chemokines may be the result of an underlying malignancy. CSF-producing tumors often cause a marked toxic neutrophilic leukocytosis (40 - 80 × 10⁹/L) and thrombocytosis [Ahn 2005, Araki 2007, des Guetz 2004, Engsig 2007, Horio 1999, Ito 1993, Jardin 2005, Kimura 2005]. Excess endogenous chemokine production

by carcinoma cells (notably adrenocortical carcinoma) is linked to sustained toxic neutrophilia and granulocytic hyperplasia in the bone marrow (see **i10.4**).

Hantavirus pulmonary syndrome, when fatal, may demonstrate an absolute neutrophil count of >30 × 10⁹/L [Hallin 1996, Koster 2001, Nolte 1995, Zaki 1995]. This infection exhibits a distinctive set of peripheral blood hematologic and morphologic findings that are useful in the rapid diagnosis of this often fatal disease **t10.6** [Koster 2001]. The key findings, in the florid/symptomatic phase of the infection, include elevated hemoglobin, thrombocytopenia, circulating immunoblasts comprising >10% of lymphocytes, neutrophilia with left shift, and absence of toxic changes **i10.11**, **i10.12** [Koster 2001]. Prior to overt clinical symptomatology and pulmonary leak, the findings are much more subtle and may consist only of circulating immunoblasts, non-toxic left shift with normal

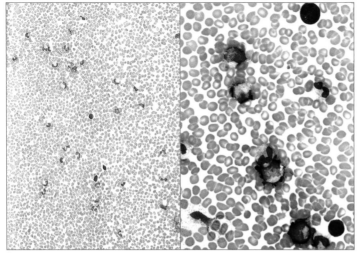

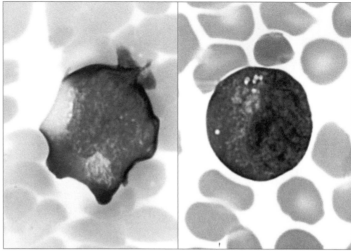

i10.11 *This low and high magnification of a blood smear from a patient with florid hantavirus pulmonary syndrome highlights all of the characteristic blood features, including hemoconcentration, thrombocytopenia, marked leukocytosis with left shift, lack of toxic changes of neutrophils, and circulating deeply basophilic immunoblasts. (Wright)*

i10.12 *Circulating immunoblasts characterize the blood picture in patients with hantavirus pulmonary syndrome. (Wright)*

absolute neutrophil count, and thrombocytopenia. In the appropriate clinical scenario, hantavirus infection should be suspected. Bone marrow examination in fatal cases of hantavirus pulmonary syndrome reveals a left shifted granulocytic lineage with abundant megakaryocytes i10.13. In suspected cases, repeat evaluation of the complete blood count and peripheral blood smear at least every 4 hours will aid in earlier detection. The ultimate confirmation of the diagnosis is identification of IgM antibodies in the patient's serum.

By integrating the clinical, hematologic, and morphologic findings, a reactive neutrophilia can generally be distinguished from a primary hematopoietic disorder in the peripheral blood such that a bone marrow examination need not be performed. Bone marrow examination may, however, be performed to obtain a specimen for culture, to evaluate

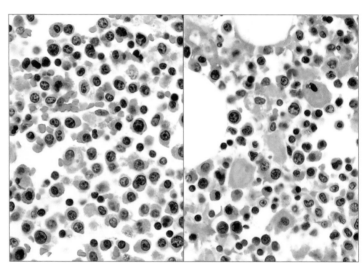

i10.13 *These composite bone marrow biopsy sections are from the autopsy specimen of a patient with fatal hantavirus pulmonary syndrome. Note abundance of megakaryocytes and paucity of mature granulocytes from antemortem release of maturation/storage compartment. (H&E)*

t10.6 Peripheral Blood Findings in Hantavirus Pulmonary Syndrome

Finding	Florid Phase (Capillary Leak)	Early Capillary Leak*
Hemoglobin/hematocrit	Markedly increased, especially in fatal cases	Normal, may be borderline increased
Neutrophils	Markedly increased with left shift to promyelocytes (toxic changes minimal or absent)	Normal number, minimal left shift may be evident on scanning; toxic changes absent
Platelet count	Substantially reduced, often $<50 \times 10^9$/L	Moderately reduced ($<100 \times 10^9$/L)
Immunoblasts	Account for >30% of lymphocytes, although absolute lymphocyte count usually normal	Account for >10% of lymphocytes; absolute lymphocyte count normal or decreased

*Repeat complete blood count and morphologic review within 4 hours often diagnostic

References: [Janic 2008, Koster 2001, Liu 2008, Malinge 2009]

t10.7 Peripheral Blood Clues in Neutrophilia to Suggest Bone Marrow Examination

Neutrophil dysplasia

Platelet dysplasia

Basophilia

Eosinophilia with abnormal basophilic granules

Auer rods

Circulating blasts without history of colony-stimulating factor therapy

Unexplained leukoerythroblastic blood picture

for granulomas, or to evaluate prolonged and unexplained neutrophilia. Peripheral blood findings that should suggest bone marrow examination are detailed in **t10.7**. Basophilia ($>0.5 \times 10^9/L$) and eosinophils with basophilic granules would be distinctly unusual in reactive neutrophilias and should prompt consideration of a primary myeloid neoplasm and bone marrow examination.

[10.2.3] **Constitutional Neutrophilia**

Congenital etiologies underlying neutrophilia are exceedingly rare and, as expected, frequently manifest in early childhood **t10.2** [Badolato 2004]. Patients with leukocyte adhesion deficiency-1 (LAD-1) have neutrophils that are unable to appropriately adhere to vascular endothelium and thus exhibit impaired/defective tissue diapedesis [Etzioni 2000]. This is an autosomal recessive disorder resulting in recurrent infections due to a deficiency of the β-2 integrin subunit (CD18) of the leukocyte cell adhesion molecule.

The neutrophil appearance is normal. Patients with LAD-III have been shown to have mutations in *FERMT3* affecting integrin activation [Moser 2009, Svensson 2009]. They have features of both LAD-I and Glanzmann thrombasthenia. Other very rare constitutional neutrophilias include familial cold urticaria, in which urticaria occurs after exposure to cold, and a poorly understood disorder termed hereditary neutrophilia [Galeazzi 2006, Neven 2008].

[10.2.4] **Neutrophilic Disorders Mimicking Neoplasia in Children**

Distinguishing reactive neutrophilia disorders from certain neoplastic processes in children can be quite challenging and requires clinical, laboratory, and morphologic correlation **t10.8**. Such disorders include transient abnormal myelopoiesis (TAM) (previously known as transient myeloproliferative disorder), juvenile rheumatoid arthritis, and chronic viral infections, particularly Epstein-Barr virus and (rarely) cytomegalovirus [Bloom 1998, Gupta 2009, Herrod 1983, Janic 2008, Kirby 1990, Webb 2007].

In 10% of newborns and infants with Down syndrome or trisomy 21 mosaicism, a unique, spontaneously remitting myeloproliferation occurs, termed TAM, and is a striking mimicker of overt acute myeloid leukemia (see Chapter 30) [Chou 2008, Malinge 2009]. The disorder typically presents within the first 6 months of life, remits spontaneously over a 4-8 week period, and is characterized by variable hepatosplenomegaly, a high WBC count, increased circulating blasts, and neutrophilia with left shift **i10.14**. The blasts are immunophenotypically heterogeneous, generally comprising a mixture of erythroid blasts, megakaryocytic blasts, and myeloblasts [Karandikar 2001]. Although

t10.8 Neutrophilic Disorders in Children That Mimic Overt Neoplastic Processes*

Disorder/Condition	Comments
Transient abnormal myelopoiesis (clonal)	Occurs in neonates/infants with Down syndrome; also documented in utero
	Transient leukocytosis with increased neutrophils and numerous blasts
	Blast morphology heterogeneous; megakaryoblasts often prominent; erythroblasts also numerous
	Spontaneous recovery within 4-6 weeks, although clonal by molecular studies
	GATA1 mutation
Juvenile rheumatoid arthritis (reactive)	Sustained leukocytosis with increased neutrophils and variable numbers of monocytes
	Hepatosplenomegaly common
	Lymphadenopathy common
Chronic Epstein-Barr virus infection[†] (reactive)	Patients usually have underlying immunodeficiency
	Sustained leukocytosis with neutrophilia and marked monocytosis
	Circulating immature forms may be evident
	Anemia, thrombocytopenia variable
	Bone marrow hypercellular and immature forms may be increased
	Lymphocytosis in bone marrow

*See Chapter 30 for illustrations and more discussion

[†]Rarely, chronic cytomegalovirus infection can cause a similar blood and bone marrow picture

References: [Foucar 2008, Gupta 2009, Janic 2008, Webb 2007]

there is a high rate of spontaneous remission, TAM is a clonal disorder, and a subset of these patients develops outright acute myeloid leukemia several years later.

Juvenile rheumatoid arthritis (JRA) may mimic chronic myelomonocytic leukemia or juvenile myelomonocytic leukemia (JMML) by exhibiting a granulocytic leukocytosis and monocytosis with clinical hepatosplenomegaly and lymphadenopathy mimicking [Janic 2008]. Leukopenia and thrombocytopenia are rare in JRA and, if present, may warrant bone marrow examination to exclude a malignancy [Bloom 1998, Koc 2000]. Occasionally a macrophage activation syndrome is seen, characterized by increased macrophages and hemophagocytosis in the bone marrow, which may be fatal [Zeng 2008].

Children with chronic Epstein-Barr virus (EBV) infection, generally seen in the setting of underlying immunodeficiency, may show a markedly abnormal peripheral blood picture with neutrophilic leukocytosis, left shift, and monocytosis [Liu 2008]. An increase in large granular lymphocytes is not uncommon. These findings, particularly when accompanied by hepatosplenomegaly or cytopenias, mimic a myeloproliferative neoplasm, and positive serologic EBV testing is required to establish the diagnosis [Herrod 1983]. The bone marrow is typically hypercellular with increased granulocytes and precursors, monocytes, and lymphocytes. Rarely, a hypocellular marrow may be seen [Liu 2008]. A similar abnormal blood and/or bone marrow picture has been reported in infants infected with cytomegalovirus [Kirby 1990], parvovirus [Gupta 2009, Yetgin 2000], and human herpesvirus 6 (HHV-6) infection [Lorenzana 2002]. Wiskott-Aldrich syndrome has been reported with JMML-like features [Watanabe 2007].

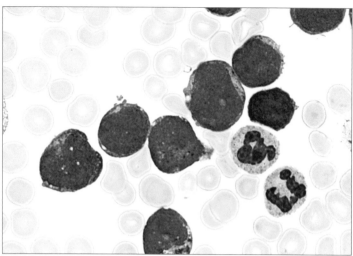

i10.14 *This peripheral blood smear is taken from an infant with Down syndrome at 32 weeks of gestation. The white blood cell count was $329 \times 10^3/\mu L$ ($329 \times 10^9/L$) with 80% blasts. The blasts are morphologically heterogeneous and include many megakaryoblasts based on immunophenotyping. (Wright) (courtesy R McKenna, MD)*

[10.2.5] **Abnormal Granulocyte Morphology**

Disorders with abnormal granulocyte morphology may be of constitutional or acquired origin. The disorder and the characteristic granulocyte morphologic abnormalities, hematologic parameters, and peripheral blood and bone marrow findings are listed in **t10.9** and **t10.10**. A concomitant neutropenia or neutrophilia may not be present (or other hematologic abnormalities).

Nuclear abnormalities of neutrophils most often involve the degree (over or under) of nuclear segmentation **i10.15**, **i10.16**. Cytoplasmic abnormalities include increased or decreased granulation, presence of primary granules,

t10.9 Non-Neoplastic Constitutional Disorders with Abnormal Granulocyte Morphology

Disorder	Hematologic Parameters	Neutrophil Abnormality	Peripheral Blood/Bone Marrow Findings	Molecular Defect
Chédiak-Higashi	Chronic neutropenia	Huge azurophilic cytoplasmic inclusions	May also see inclusions in lymphoid cells	*LYST* gene mutation
Alder-Reilly phenomenon (as component of mucopoly-saccaridosis)	Variable, may have cytopenias	Cytoplasmic, dark purple granules	May also see inclusions in lymphoid cells, monocytes Intense cytoplasmic granulation of all myeloid cells Eosinophils as "pseudobasophils"	Mucopolysaccaridosis: type VII (β-glucuronidase mutation) type VI (arylsulfatase β mutation)
May-Hegglin	Macrothrombocytopenia	Cytoplasmic, light blue, "Döhle-body"-like inclusions	May also see inclusions in eosinophils, basophils, and monocytes	*MYH9* mutations
Pelger-Huët anomaly	None	Unsegmented or bilobed neutrophils	Hyposegmentation of metamyelocytes, bands, neutrophils	Lamin β-receptor mutation
Myelokathexis	Chronic marked neutropenia	Neutrophils with thin interlobar strands	Granulocytic hyperplasia and hypersegmentation	WHIM syndrome: *CXCR4* mutation

References: [Aprikyan 2000, Cunningham 2009, Huizing 2008, Kawai 2009, Peterson 1982, Saito 2008, Stein 2003, Worman 2007]

t10.10 Non-Neoplastic Acquired Disorders with Abnormal Granulocyte Morphology

Disorder	Hematologic Parameters	Neutrophil Morphologic Abnormality	Peripheral Blood/Bone Marrow Findings
Infection			
Bacterial sepsis	Generally neutrophilia	Toxic granulation, vacuoles, Döhle-bodies	Granulocytic hyperplasia, toxic changes See **t10.4**, p 184
HIV-1	Generally neutrophilia	Detached nuclear fragments	See Chapter 33
	Variable lymphopenia	Pseudo-Pelger-Huët anomaly	
		Bizarrely shaped nuclei; high N:C ratio	
		Howell-Jolly body-like inclusions	
TB, mycoplasma	Monocytosis	Pseudo-Pelger-Huët	See Chapter 33
Nutritional deficiency			
Vitamin B$_{12}$/folate	Macrocytic anemia; occasionally pancytopenia	Hypersegmentation	Giant bands/metamyelocytes in BM Megaloblastosis of erythroid precursors with left shift (see Chapter 6)
Copper deficiency	Cytopenias	None	Vacuolization of granulocytic and erythroid precursors in BM (see Chapter 6)
Drugs			
CSF	Granulocytosis	Toxic granulation	Blasts 2%-50% (in hypocellular specimens) See **t10.5**, p 185
	Left shift, monocytosis	Bilobation of nuclei (more prominent in BM); blasts 2%-50%	
Chemotherapy (MTX)	Cytopenias	Nuclear segmentation abnormalities	Variable—ranges from hypo- to hypercellular
Ethanol	Cytopenias	Neutrophil vacuolization	Vacuolization of granulocytic precursors in BM, Mott cells
Sulfonamide, gancyclovir, valproic acid	Variable	Pseudo-Pelger-Huët	Marrow intact unless otherwise damaged from drug effect
Mycophenylate mofetil	Variable	Pseudo-Pelger-Huët	
Miscellaneous			
Hyperthermia	Variable	Abnormal nuclear budding/lobulation	

BM = bone marrow; CSF = colony-stimulating factor; HIV-1 = human immunodeficiency virus; MTX = methotrexate; N:C = nuclear-cytoplasmic ratio; TB = tuberculosis

References: [Akhtari 2009, Aprikyan 2000, Asmis 2003, Badolato 2004, Bain 1997, Best 2003, Chetty-Raju 2004, Cicchitto 1999, Dusse 2006, Etzell 2006, Maitra 2000, Saito 2008, Slagel 1994, Taegtmeyer 2005, Ward 2007]

inclusions (excluding organisms for this chapter), vacuoles, and aggregates of rough endoplasmic reticulum (Döhle bodies). **t10.3**, p 183 lists these various abnormalities and possible non-neoplastic situations in which they may be encountered.

[10.2.6] **Constitutional Conditions with Abnormal Granulocyte Morphology**

The Pelger-Huët anomaly (PHA) is characterized by unsegmented or bilobed mature neutrophil forms **i10.17** [Cunningham 2009, Worman 2007]. In this autosomal dominant inherited disorder, the majority/all of the neutrophils display the classic hyposegmented appearance both in

the blood and bone marrow **i10.18**. Neutrophil function is normal, and thus there is no clinical effect. PHA has been ascribed to lamin β-receptor mutations [Best 2003, Worman 2007].

The Alder-Reilly anomaly is characterized by uniform, distinctive, dark purple granules in the cytoplasm of neutrophils and bone marrow granulocyte precursors, and is often seen in association with the mucopolysaccharidoses **i10.19**, **i10.20** [Peterson 1982]. The morphology mimics toxic granulation, but other features that might suggest infection are absent (neutrophilia, left shift, and Döhle bodies). This intense cytoplasmic granulation may also be seen in monocytes and lymphoid cells. Eosinophils

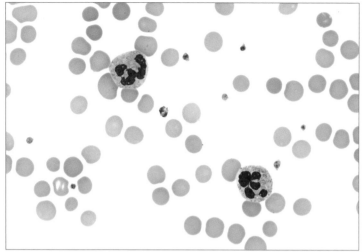

i10.15 *Hypersegmentation of neutrophil nuclei is evident in this peripheral blood smear from a patient who received aggressive chemotherapy followed by granulocyte colony-stimulating factor treatment. The hypersegmentation is a likely medication effect. (Wright)*

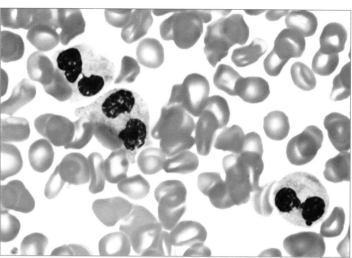

i10.16 *Striking neutrophil hypogranularity with Döhle bodies and nuclear hyposegmentation are evident in this peripheral blood smear from a patient with myelodysplasia. (Wright)*

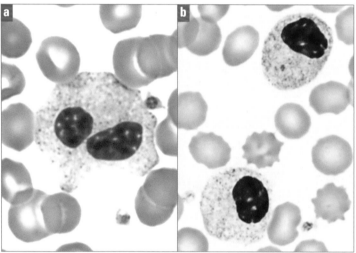

i10.17 *This composite smear shows the classic neutrophil morphology in familial Pelger-Huët anomaly in which most neutrophils exhibit either bilobation (pince-nez cell) **a**, or are nonlobated yet mature in terms of the degree of nuclear condensation (Stodmeister cells) **b**. (Wright)*

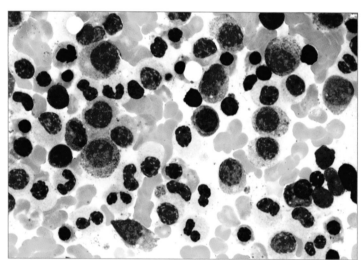

i10.18 *This bone marrow aspirate smear is from a patient with familial Pelger-Huët anomaly. Note the predominace of bilobed neutrophils with otherwise intact granulocytic maturation. (Wright) (courtesy S Kroft, MD)*

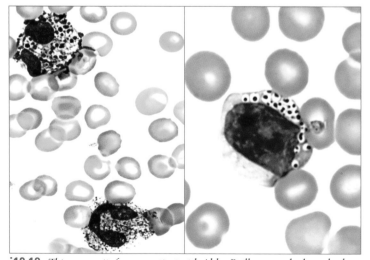

i10.19 *This composite from a patient with Alder-Reilly anomaly shows both the intensely hypergranular neutrophils and prominently vacuolated lymphoid cells that characterize this rare disorder that is often seen in association with a lysosomal enzyme deficiency. (Wright) (courtesy C Hanson, MD)*

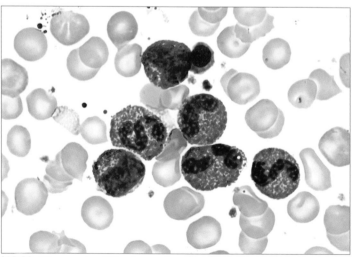

i10.20 *This peripheral blood smear from an infant with mucopolysaccharidosis shows striking eosinophilia of the neutrophil granules that characterizes Alder-Reilly anomaly. (Wright) (courtesy L Peterson, MD)*

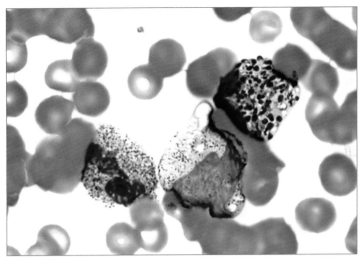

i10.21 *This peripheral blood smear shows a side-by-side comparison of a neutrophil (left), monocyte (center), and eosinophil with a distinctive "pseudo-basophil" appearance (right) in a patient with Alder-Reilly anomaly and Morteaux-Lamy syndrome. (Wright) (courtesy C Hanson, MD)*

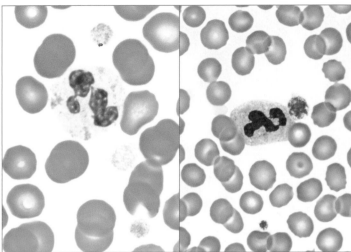

i10.22 *This peripheral blood composite is from 2 patients with May-Hegglin anomaly characterized by enlarged platelets and neutrophils that contain Döhle body-like inclusions. (Wright)*

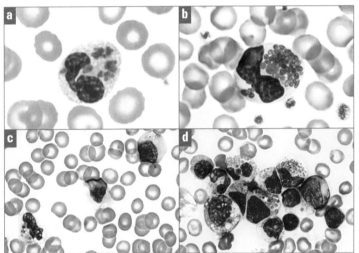

i10.23 *This composite of peripheral blood and bone marrow aspirate smears from 2 patients with Chédiak-Higashi syndrome illustrates the markedly enlarged and abnormal cytoplasmic granules in neutrophils **a**, eosinophils **b**, granulocytes and lymphoid cells **c**, and within maturing myeloid lineage cells of the bone marrow **d**. (Wright) (courtesy L Peterson, MD & R Brynes, MD)*

have a distinctive "pseudobasophil" appearance with large, basophilic/dark red cytoplasmic granules i10.21.

The May-Hegglin anomaly, an autosomal dominant disorder, is the result of mutations in the *MYH9* gene. Mutation of the myosin heavy chain type II-A results in *MYH9*-related hereditary macrothrombocytopenias, including 4 autosomal dominant platelet disorders: May-Hegglin anomaly, and Sebastian, Fechtner, and Epstein syndromes [Kunishima 2008, Nurden 2008]. This genetic aberration results in the accumulation and aggregation of myosin heavy chain II-A, which appears as the classic

"Döhle-body-like" inclusions in the cytoplasm of neutrophils, and occasionally monocytes, eosinophils and basophils i10.22 [Saito 2008]. These inclusions can be difficult to distinguish from true Döhle bodies; however toxic granulation is generally not present in an otherwise healthy individual with May-Hegglin anomaly. Other key features include thrombocytopenia, large platelets and occasional large platelets with diminished granulation/gray appearance i10.22.

Among the constitutional disorders, Chédiak-Higashi and myelokathexis (a component of WHIM syndrome) are generally classified as congenital neutropenic disorders and thus are described in detail in Chapter 11. In Chédiak-Higashi disorder, the hallmark peripheral blood finding is huge, azurophilic granules in the cytoplasm of granulocytes as well as monocytes and lymphocytes i10.23. In late stages of the disease (the accelerated phase), thought to be associated with Epstein-Barr virus infection, a systemic marked hemophagocytic lymphohistiocytic infiltration (which is often fatal) occurs, involving bone marrow, liver, spleen, and other organs [Certain 2000, Rubin 1985]. Rarely, pseudo-Chédiak-Higashi granules have been described in AML [Rao 2009].

Myelokathexis is a rare disorder characterized by chronic marked neutropenia with hypersegmentation of neutrophils, occasional cytoplasmic vacuoles, and degenerative (pyknotic) nuclei with excessively thin interlobar nuclear strands (see Chapter 11) i10.24 [Aprikyan 2000, Stein 2003]. The bone marrow is hypercellular with a marked granulocytic predominance and a full spectrum of maturation. The key morphologic feature

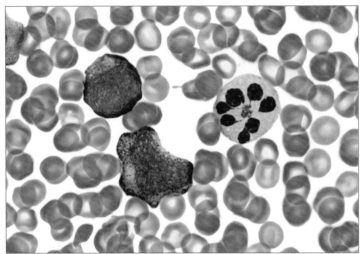

i10.24 *This bone marrow aspirate smear from a patient with myelokathexis shows a hypersegmented neutrophil with exceedingly thin connecting chromatin strands, while immature granulocytic cells are morphologically unremarkable. (Wright) (courtesy S Kroft, MD)*

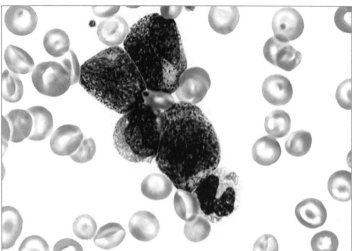

i10.25 *This peripheral blood smear from a patient who received colony-stimulating factor therapy following potent chemotherapy shows intensely hypergranular granulocytic cells at various stages of maturation in conjunction with a markedly hypogranular mature neutrophil showing a Döhle body (lower cell). This neutrophil with dysplastic features is the likely consequence of the multiagent chemotherapy, while the prominent left-shift with toxic granulation is likely the effect of granulocyte colony-stimulating factor therapy . (Wright)*

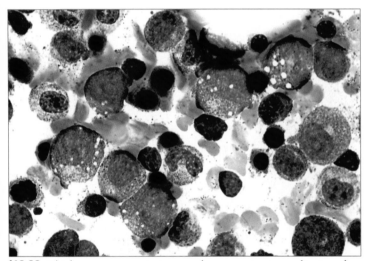

i10.26 *This bone marrow aspirate smear shows prominent vacuolization of granulocytic precursors in a patient with copper deficiency. (Wright)*

of myelokathexis is the long, thin filamentous strands connecting nuclear lobes of neutrophils. Since most of these morphologically abnormal neutrophils undergo apoptosis within the bone marrow, there is a striking neutropenia in the blood. Most of the rare neutrophils that do circulate are morphologically unremarkable.

[10.2.7] Acquired Conditions with Abnormal Granulocyte Morphology

A wide variety of acquired non-neoplastic consitions may exhibit abnormal granulocyte morphology **t10.10**. Infectious conditions and CSF therapy are the most common etiologies of toxic changes in the peripheral blood neutrophils and were previously discussed [10.2.2]. If recombinant CSF is given in conjunction with

chemotherapeutic agents for the treatment of neoplasms, one may see hybrid toxic and dysplastic features **i10.25**. Vacuolization of the neutrophil cytoplasm, if not ascribed to artifact, generally signifies severe infection/sepsis. In the bone marrow, vacuolization of granulocytic and erythroid progenitors is a hallmark feature of copper deficiency (see Chapter 6) **i10.26**.

Abnormal nuclear hypersegmentation of neutrophils is traditionally described in megaloblastic anemias as a result of vitamin B_{12} and/or folate deficiency (see Chapter 6) **t10.3**, p 183. However, such a change may also be seen in patients with human immunodeficiency virus (HIV)-1, iron deficiency, DNA-inhibiting chemotherapeutic agents, and corticosteroid therapy **i10.15**. Because many of these conditions may be associated with a cytopenia (eg, anemia), one must diligently assess the blood smears for additional clues to a primary myeloid neoplasm. Myelodysplastic syndromes (MDS) and some cases of chronic myelogenous leukemia (CML) may show neutrophil hypersegmentation. In such clonal diseases, various other morphologic abnormalities characteristic of those diseases may be evident. In CML, basophilia, left shift in the granulocytic lineage, and rare blasts are noted. In MDS, neutrophil hypo- and hypersegmentation may coexist, and may be associated with neutrophil/platelet hypogranularity.

Abnormal nuclear hyposegmentation of neutrophils is characterized as nonsegmented (monolobated) or bilobed mature forms and referred to as pseudo Pelger-Huët anomaly (PHA) if acquired **i10.27**. Generally it is

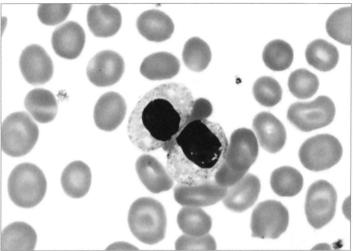

i10.27 *2 nonlobated, mature neutrophils are evident in this peripheral blood smear from a patient with pseudo-Pelger-Huët anomaly associated with myelodysplasia. (Wright)*

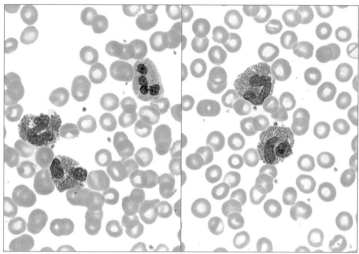

i10.28 *These peripheral blood smears are from 2 women who developed eosinophilia-myalgia syndrome following L-tryptophan ingestion. An absolute, mature eosinophilia was present in both patients. (Wright)*

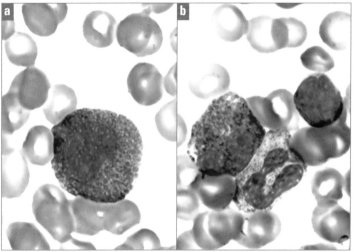

i10.29 *This composite of bone marrow aspirate smears shows 2 eosinophil precursors, a myelocyte **a** and a metamyelocyte **b**. Both eosinophil precursors show prominent secondary granules. (Wright)*

only a subset of the neutrophils that exhibit the pseudo Pelger-Huët appearance, as opposed to the inherited PHA, in which the majority of neutrophils are abnormal, providing the initial evidence for an acquired phenomenon. Causes of acquired non-neoplastic pseudo Pelger-Huët anomaly are myriad and include HIV-1, mycoplasma infection, certain medications (colchicines and sulfonamides), and chemotherapeutic agents **t10.3**, p 183 [Asmis 2003, Cunningham 2009, Dusse 2006, Etzell 2006, Taegtmeyer 2005]. Importantly, hyposegmented neutrophils are also a typical myelodysplastic finding. Therefore, careful evaluation for other clues to suggest a myeloid neoplasm is necessary (eg, blasts, abnormal platelets, and unexplained accompanying cytopenias).

[10.3] Eosinophils

Eosinophils normally comprise $<0.5 \times 10^9/L$ in the peripheral blood **t10.1**, p 181. They derive from the same granulocyte-monocyte progenitor cell as neutrophils (see Chapter 1), but are readily identified by their large, refractile, bright red/orange secondary granules present in the cytoplasm on a Wright-stained smear **i10.28** [Rothenberg 2006]. Given that eosinophils infiltrate tissues to combat an inciting organism or allergen, it follows that one of the gravest complications in tissue eosinophilia is the inappropriate release of eosinophil granules within blood or tissues, causing damage and fibrosis, particularly in the heart (due to degranulation in blood) and central nervous system [Klion 2005, Ogbogu 2007, Weller 1994].

The eosinophilic myelocyte is the first eosinophilic precursor to be recognized in the bone marrow and characteristically has a non-lobated, round nucleus, small nucleolus, and a variable admixture of brightly eosinophilic and purple (azurophilic) secondary granules in the cytoplasm **i10.29**. The mature eosinophil generally exhibits 2 nuclear lobes and minimal cytoplasmic azurophilic granules, though 3 or more nuclear lobes may be seen occasionally.

[10.3.1] Eosinophilia

Eosinophilia, defined as an absolute count of $>0.5 \times 10^3/\mu L$ ($>0.5 \times 10^9/L$) for all age groups, can be divided into 2 broad categories depending on whether the underlying etiology is a primary clonal disorder or a secondary reactive disorder [Gotlib 2006, Tefferi 2006, Sheikh 2009, Valent 2009b]. Eosinophilias are arbitrarily further classified as mild (0.5-$1.4 \times 10^3/\mu L$ [0.5-$1.4 \times 10^9/L$]), moderate (1.5-$5.0 \times 10^3/\mu L$ [1.5-$5.0 \times 10^9/L$]), or severe ($>5.0 \times 10^3/\mu L$ [$>5.0 \times 10^9/L$]) [Brito-Babapulle 2003]. Non-neoplastic causes of eosinophilia are generally regarded as cytokine-mediated, mainly through

t10.11 Causes of Secondary/Reactive Eosinophilia

Infection	Helminths
	Protozoa
	HIV-1
	Fungus
Allergic conditions	Allergic rhinitis
	Atopic dermatitis
	Allergic gastroenteritis
	Asthma
	Urticaria
	Allergic bronchopulmonary aspergillosis
Immunologic/autoimmune disorders	Rheumatoid arthritis
	Inflammatory bowel disease
	Polyarteritis nodosa
	Churg-Strauss
	Sarcoidosis
	Scleroderma
	Kimura disease
	Bullous pemphigoid
Drug hypersensitivity reactions	Antibacterial
	Anti-seizure
	Sulfonamides
	IL-2 therapy for renal carcinoma
	Numerous others
Hematopoietic neoplasms	Hodgkin and non-Hodgkin (T-and B-cell) lymphoma
	T-cell clonality of uncertain significance
	B-cell lymphoblastic leukemia with t(5;14)
Nonhematopoietic neoplasms	Lung carcinoma
	Gastric carcinoma
Other	Radiation

HIV-1 = human immunodeficiency virus

References: [Korenaga 1991, Ravoet 2009, Simon 2007, Vaklavas 2007, Wenzel 2009]

t10.12 Primary (Neoplastic) Eosinophilias

Disorder	Referenced in Chapter
Chronic myelogenous leukemia	14
Myeloid/lymphoid neoplasms with abnormalities of *PDGFRA*, *PDGFRB* and *FGFR1*	15
Systemic mastocytosis	14
Chronic eosinophilic leukemia	14
Chronic myeloproliferative neoplasms, subset	14
Myelodysplastic syndromes, subset	16
Acute myeloid leukemia with inv(16)(p13.1q22) or t(16;16)(p13.1;q22); *CBFB-MYH11*	18

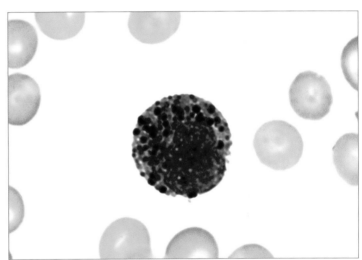

i10.30 *This bone marrow aspirate smear shows a single abnormal eosinophil with mixed eosinophil/basophil granules suggestive of acute myeloid leukemia with inv(16)(p13q22). (Wright)*

[10.3.2] **Abnormal Eosinophil Morphology**

Morphologic alterations of eosinophils may be seen in a spectrum of neoplastic and non-neoplastic eosinophilias [Fletcher 2007]. While in general they tend to predominate in neoplastic disorders, they are nonspecific and by themselves insufficient to distinguish a reactive from a clonal disorder. One major exception is finding basophil-like granules in addition to the typical eosinophil orange granules in mature eosinophils. This is distinctly unusual and, when prominent, should suggest an acute myeloid leukemia with a *CBFB-MYH11* fusion gene genetic abnormality i10.30. The remaining nonspecific changes include hypogranulation, nuclear segmentation abnormalities, abnormal localization/clustering of granules

the actions of interleukin IL-3 and IL-5 and are listed in **t10.11** [Korenaga 1991, Simon 2007, Wenzel 2009]. Patients with eosinophilia may harbor occult T-cell clones driving the eosinophilia. Furthermore, eosinophilia may be a feature of overt T-cell lymphoma [Ravoet 2009, Vaklavas 2007]. Clonal eosinophilias are listed in **t10.12** and are further discussed in other chapters of this book (see Chapters 14, 15, and 18). In the Western world, eosinophilia is primarily associated with allergic disorders, whereas in underdeveloped regions of the world, eosinophilia is most often attributed to a parasitic/helminthic infection. Other common causes of eosinophilia are drug reactions/hypersensitivity.

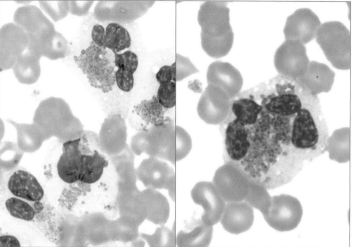

i10.31 *These peripheral blood smears illustrate dysplastic eosinophils from a patient with acute lymphoblastic leukemia with t(5;14)(q31;q32). Nuclear hypersegmentation, cytoplasmic degranulation, and cytoplasmic vacuolization are evident. (Wright)*

i10.32 *Increased, normal-appearing basophils are evident on a peripheral blood smear from a patient with mild reactive basophilia. (Wright)*

in cytoplasm, and cytoplasmic vacuolization **i10.31**. Rare cases showing dysplastic eosinophils are the result of neoplasm-induced cytokines rather than being part of the clone. When presented with such eosinophil morphologic abnormalities (often accompanied by eosinophilia), integration with the remainder of the CBC parameters, morphologic findings, and clinical and infectious history is necessary to determine if a bone marrow examination is needed. Peripheral blood clues to a possible clonal eosinophilic disorder are listed in **t10.13**.

[10.3.3]   **Eosinopenia**

An absolute decrease in the number of eosinophils is a relatively uncommon finding outside pancytopenic/leukopenic states. Certain conditions such as corticosteroid/dexamethasone therapy, acute stress (epinephrine), sepsis, and acute inflammatory states have all been associated

t10.13 Peripheral Blood Clues in Unexplained Eosinophilia to Suggest Bone Marrow Examination

Circulating blasts (myeloid or lymphoid)

Basophilia

Unexplained monocytosis

Eosinophils with basophilic granules (exclude rare Alder-Reilly anomaly)

Circulating mast cells

Unexplained anemia and/or thrombocytopenia

Dysplasia of granulocytes or platelets

Clinical workup has excluded common secondary causes (eg, drug, infection, allergy)

with eosinopenia [Abidi 2008]. Interestingly, isolated cases of eosinopenia in allergic patients are reported.

[10.4]   **Basophils**

In the normal situation, basophils comprise <1% of circulating leukocytes. The steady-state level of basophils remains low and constant despite diurnal, age, and gender variations [Arnalich 1987, Grattan 2003]. Basophils originate in the bone marrow from CD34+ pluripotent hematopoietic stem cells (see Chapter 1, **f1.3**, p 9) and are released into the peripheral blood as fully mature forms [Arock 2002, Iwasaki 2007]. The nature of stimuli promoting basophil development and maintenance of steady-state levels is not entirely clear. However, it has been suggested that the hematopoietic cytokine IL-3, mainly produced upon T-cell activation, plays a primary role in the differentiation of basophil precursors into mature basophils [Oh 2007, Ohmori 2009, Valent 2009a, Yoshimoto 1999].

Basophils are recognized in the peripheral blood and bone marrow by their distinctive, large, basophilic secondary granules, which tend to fill the cytoplasm and obscure the segmented nucleus **i10.32** [May 1984]. The granules are metachromatic (stain red or violet) with basic aniline dyes. These granules are rich in histamine, heparin, chondroitin sulfate, and other molecules. Basophils are myeloperoxidase negative, but a subset may be chloroacetate esterase positive.

[10.4.1]   **Basophilia**

Basophilia is generally defined as an absolute count of $>0.1 \times 10^3/\mu L$ ($>0.1 \times 10^9/L$) **t10.1**, p 181. Causes of non-neoplastic basophilia include allergic, inflammatory, endocrinopathic, and renal disorders, and also infrequently, carcinomas, radiotherapy, and certain drugs **t10.14** [Arnalich 1987,

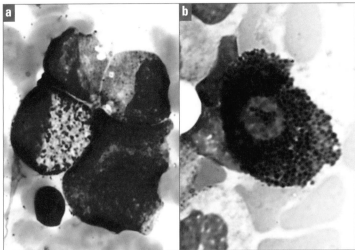

i10.33 *This bone marrow composite shows a comparison of mast cells (present in both **a** and **b**) with a basophil precursor adjacent to the mast cell in **a**. Note small, round nuclei of mast cells with abundant dark purple granular cytoplasm. (Wright)*

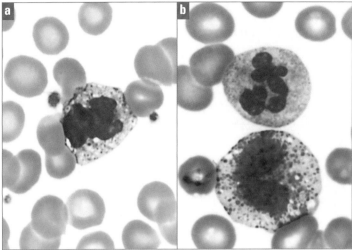

i10.34 *This composite of 2 peripheral blood smears from 2 patients with basophilia shows a partially degranulated basophil in a normal blood smear **a**, while **b** shows both a degranulated neutrophil and a degranulated basophil in a patient with a myeloproliferative neoplasm. (Wright)*

Mitre 2006, Tokuhira 2007]. In general, the degree of basophilia tends to be mild (<500/µL absolute count), and significant basophilia should prompt consideration of a neoplastic disorder **t10.15**. Such neoplastic disorders include myeloproliferative neoplasms and a subset of de novo and therapy-related acute myeloid leukemias and myelodysplastic syndromes [Chi 2008, Foucar 1979, Matsushima 2003, Tang 2009, Wimazal 2008].

t10.14 Causes of Reactive Basophilia in Blood and Bone Marrow

Allergic/hypersensitivity reactions	Allergic rhinitis
	Hypersensitivity to drugs, food
Chronic inflammatory conditions	Ulcerative colitis
	Rheumatoid arthritis
	Chronic renal insufficiency
	Autoimmune disease
Chronic infections	Chronic sinusitis
	Smallpox
	Varicella (chickenpox)
	Influenza
	Tuberculosis
	Helicobacter pylori
Other	Estrogen
	Hypothyroidism
	Iron deficiency anemia
	Secondary to pulmonary carcinoma (rare)
	Secondary to de novo large B-cell lymphoma (single reported case)

References: [Arnalich 1987, May 1984, Mitre 2006, Tokuhira 2007]

Despite the morphologic similarity between mast cells and basophils (and possible derivation from a common bone marrow precursor cell), mast cell disorders tend not to have increased basophils but may show increased eosinophils. Mast cells usually show a single round nucleus and cytoplasm packed with numerous purple, metachromatic granules **i10.33**. In difficult cases, immunophenotypic studies may help discriminate between mast cells and basophils, as mast cells are CD117+ and tryptase+ and basophils are CD123+, BB-1+, and 2D7+ [Agis 2006, Kepley 1995, McEuen 1999].

[10.4.2] **Abnormal Basophil Morphology**

In our experience, although basophils may show varying degrees of degranulation, this finding is of limited diagnostic usefulness in discriminating neoplastic from non-neoplastic basophil proliferations **i10.34**. If morphologically immature basophils are identified (fine chromatin, prominent nucleolus, diminished granules), and other clinical (splenomegaly) and/

t10.15 Neoplastic Differential Diagnostic Considerations of Basophilia

Chronic myelogenous leukemia, *BCR-ABL1*+

BCR-ABL1– myeloproliferative neoplasms

Myelodysplastic syndromes (<10%)

Acute myeloid leukemia (AML) with t(6;9)(p23;q34) (*DEK-NUP214*)

AML with basophil component

Acute lymphoblastic leukemia with basophil and/or eosinophil component

Therapy-related acute leukemias

Acute basophilic leukemia

References: [Chi 2008, Foucar 1979, Matsushima 2003, Tang 2009, Wimazal 2008]

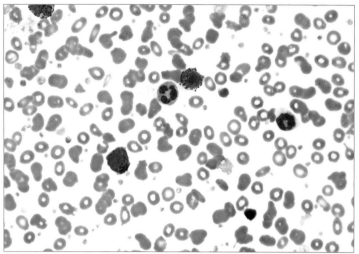

i10.35 *This peripheral blood smear is from a patient with chronic myelogenous leukemia in accelerated phase in which there are 10% circulating blasts and 20% circulating basophils with left-shifted basophils. (Wright)*

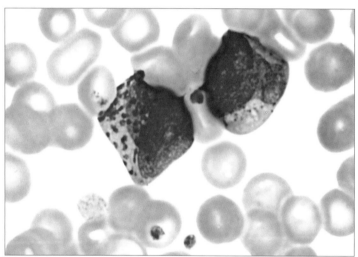

i10.36 *This bone marrow aspirate smear is from a patient with chronic myelogenous leukemia in basophilic blast phase. Note immature cell with prominent basophilic granules. (Wright)*

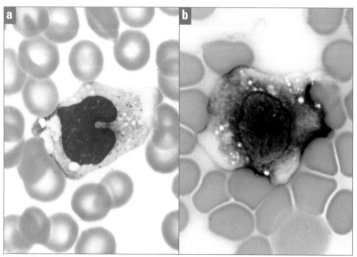

i10.37 *This composite of normal monocytes shows typical morphologic features by Wright stain **a**, while nonspecific esterase positivity is highlighted by cytochemical staining **b**. (Wright and nonspecific esterase cytochemical stain)*

t10.16 **Peripheral Blood Clues in Unexplained Basophilia to Suggest Bone Marrow Examination**

Circulating blasts

Non-toxic neutrophils with left shift and blasts

Majority of basophils with immature morphology

Unexplained eosinophilia

Unexplained abnormal platelet count

Neutrophil or platelet dysplasia

Teardrop red cells and/or circulating nucleated RBCs

or hematologic abnormalities are present to suggest a myeloid neoplasm, bone marrow examination is warranted for further investigation **t10.16**, **i10.35**, **i10.36**.

[10.4.3] **Basopenia**

A decreased number of circulating basophils, basophilopenia/basopenia, is difficult to define given the relatively low number of basophils in the normal state. However, basopenia has been reported in association with elevated corticosteroid levels (endogenous or exogenous), chronic urticaria, acute stress/acute inflammatory conditions, ovulation, and cigarette smoking [Dinauer 2003, Grattan 2003, Soni 1996, Walter 1980].

Also, except for 2 anecdotal reports of complex immunologic syndromes with a combined lack of eosinophils and basophils, there does not appear to be any genetic deficiency leading to the selective loss of basophils in humans [Falcone 2006, Juhlin 1977, Mitchell 1983].

[10.5] **Monocytes**

Monocytes normally comprise between 2% and 10% of the peripheral blood leukocytes with absolute monocyte counts of $<0.8 \times 10^3/\mu L$ ($<0.8 \times 10^9/L$). They are a component of the mononuclear phagocyte system and originate from the granulocyte-monocyte progenitor cell predominantly under the cytokine influence of GM-CSF and monocyte (M)-CSF (see Chapter 1 for more details) [Dale 2008, Hume 2006]. Differentiated blood monocytes circulate in the blood and then enter tissues to become resident tissue macrophages [Hume 2002]. In this chapter we focus on non-neoplastic disorders of monocytes in peripheral blood and bone marrow. Chapter 27 discusses histiocytic disorders of the bone marrow, while Chapters 17 and 18 cover malignant monocyte disorders.

Mature monocytes are readily identifiable in peripheral blood smears and are the direct result of sequential maturation of monoblasts to promonocytes to monocytes **i10.37**. In Wright-stained peripheral blood and bone marrow, monocytes average 12 µm-15 µm in diameter

t10.17 Causes of Non-Neoplastic Monocytosis

Infections	Tuberculosis*
	Viral:
	CMV*
	EBV
	Varicella
	Parvovirus
	Dengue hemorrhagic fever
	Malaria
	Brucellosis
	Leishmaniasis
	Fungal
	Bacterial endocarditis
Immunologic/ autoimmune disorders	SLE
	RA
	Autoimmune neutropenia
	Inflammatory bowel disease
	Myositis
	Sarcoidosis
Hematologic problems	Acute or chronic neutropenia
	Drug-induced neutropenia
	Hemolysis
	ITP
Drugs	GM-CSF
	Olanzapine
	Carbamazepine
	Phenytoin
	Phenobarbital
	Tetrachloroethane overdose
	Valproic acid
Neoplasms	Carcinoma
	Sarcoma
	Plasma cell myeloma
	Lymphoma
Stress	Severe trauma
	Myocardial infarction
	Splenectomy
Component of a congenital syndrome	Cyclic neutropenia
	Barth syndrome
	Wiskott-Aldrich syndrome
	Holoprosencephaly
Other	GM-CSF effect
	Intense exercise
	Subset of patients receiving IVIg for Kawaski disease

*May also show monocytopenia
CMV = cytomegalovirus; EBV = Epstein-Barr virus; SLE = systemic lupus erythematosus; RA = rheumatoid arthritis; ITP = immune-mediated thrombocytopenia; GM-CSF = granulocyte-monocyte colony-stimulating factor; IVIg = intravenous immunoglobulin

References: [Cooke 2006, Foucar 2008, Gulen 2005, Hong 2007, Jubinsky 2006, Kratz 2002, Lichtman 2006, Robinson 2003, Singh 2001, Tsolia 2002, Walsh 2005, William 2007, Wilson 2008]

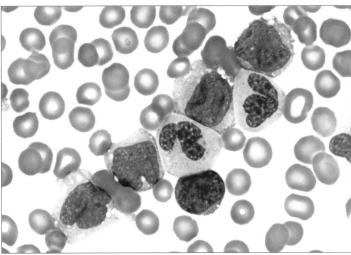

i10.38 *This peripheral blood smear shows numerous immature monocytic cells including monoblasts (upper right) and promonocytes (lower left) in a patient with acute myelomonocytic leukemia. (Wright)*

enzymes (eg, collagenase, esterases, elastase) that are vital for antimicrobial function. Mature monocyte nuclei show slight to moderate indentation, comprise one third to one half of the cell, lack nucleoli, and have a ropey pattern to the chromatin. The appearance of the chromatin and presence of nucleoli are crucial features in distinguishing mature monocytes from more immature forms i10.38. On occasion, the morphologic features of monocytes may be altered and their lineage confused with a granulocytic or lymphoid cell. In such a case, the morphology of the nucleus corresponding to each of those cell types aids in cell identification.

The enzymes within the monocyte granules are positive for a cytochemical nonspecific esterase stain (α-naphthyl butyrate esterase) and most often negative or very weakly positive for myeloperoxidase i10.37b. Such stains are useful in identifying monocytic lineage but are not useful in distinguishing mature monocytes from promonocytes. Distinguishing mature from immature monocytic cells may be a tricky morphologic endeavor, particularly when evaluating peripheral blood. Often, in cases of neoplastic monocytic disorders, the more readily identifiable immature monocytes (promonocytes and monoblasts) predominate in the bone marrow.

[10.5.1] Monocytosis

Monocytosis is defined as an absolute monocyte count of $>0.8 \times 10^3/\mu L$ ($>0.8 \times 10^9/L$) in adults and $>3.5 \times 10^3/\mu L$ ($>3.5 \times 10^9/L$) in neonates t10.1. Because of the key roles monocytes play in acute and chronic infections or inflammatory disorders, impaired immunologic conditions, hypersensitivity, and tissue repair, a monocytosis may result from a wide variety of non-neoplastic underlying disease

and demonstrate pale blue/gray cytoplasm. Fine, azurophilic (purple-red) granules and vacuoles may be seen in the cytoplasm in varying numbers i10.37a. These granules contain

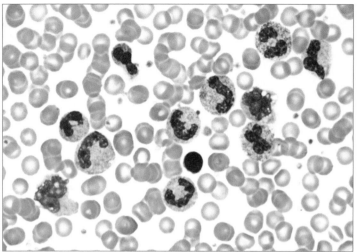

i10.39 *Both toxic neutrophils and monocytes are abundant in this peripheral blood smear from a patient treated with recombinant granulocyte monocyte colony-stimulating factor. (Wright)*

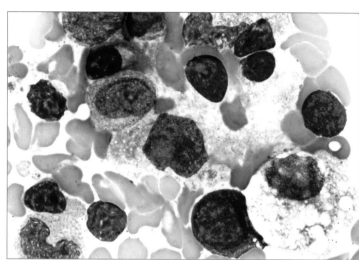

i10.40 *This bone marrow aspirate smear from an 11-month-old child with fever and pancytopenia shows increased monocytes and histiocytes. (Wright)*

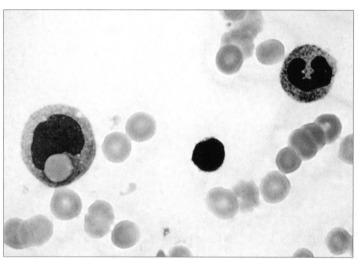

i10.41 *This peripheral blood smear from a patient with hemophagocytic syndrome shows ingestion of an erythrocyte by a mature monocyte. (Wright)*

t10.18 Peripheral Blood Clues in Unexplained/ Prolonged Monocytosis to Suggest Bone Marrow Examination

Circulating blasts

Conspicuous immature monocytic features (round nucleus, fine chromatin, nucleolus)

Unexplained leukoerythroblastic blood picture

Accompanying unexplained eosinophilia

states t10.17 [Cooke 2006, Hong 2007, Jubinsky 2006, Lichtman 2006, Liu 2004, Singh 2001, Tsolia 2002, Walsh 2005].

Monocytosis disorders, similar to the eosinophilias, can be classified based on primary (neoplastic/clonal) processes and secondary (non-neoplastic) conditions. Causes of non-neoplastic monocytosis include infections (mainly chronic), autoimmune disease, hematologic disorders, drug therapy, and acute stress among others t10.17. Rarely, monocytes may exhibit atypical features transiently after G-CSF treatment [Liu 2004]. Reactive vacuolization or toxic changes are not uncommon i10.39, i10.40. Peripheral monocytosis generally correlates with a similar increase in bone marrow. The monocytes may not, however, be as conspicuous in the bone marrow and are best visualized in cytologic preparations (eg, aspirate smear, touch preparation). In florid hemophagocytic syndrome, monocytes are increased

and ingest intact bone marrow cells i10.41. Increased monocytes and macrophages may also be seen in severe infection. In all cases, the monocyte morphology remains characteristically mature, though occasionally less mature chromatin or minimal indentation of the nucleus may be seen. In the latter scenario, the reactive nature of the monocytosis can be favored by a predominance of mature monocytes.

[10.5.2] **Abnormal Monocyte Morphology**

If there is prolonged monocytosis/cytopenias of uncertain etiology, dysplastic features in the granulocytes and blasts, or a predominance of immature-appearing monocytes, then additional workup, including bone marrow evaluation, to evaluate for a primary myeloid disorder is warranted t10.18. In these neoplastic disease entities, the monocyte count tends to be higher than in reactive conditions, and the monocytes exhibit more immature features (conspicuous nucleolus, finer [less ropey] dispersed chromatin, and a delicate nuclear membrane) i10.42, i10.43. In chronic myelomonocytic leukemia, hypercellularity, increased myelomonocytic cells, plasmacytoid dendritic cell nodules, and abnormal megakaryocytes may be seen (see Chapter 17) [Ngo 2008, Orazi 2006].

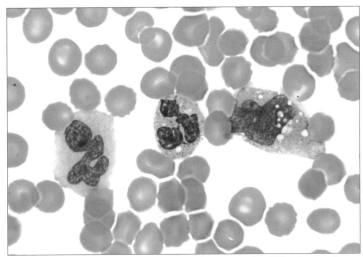

i10.42 *Dysplastic monocytes are illustrated on a peripheral blood smear from a child with myelodysplastic/myeloproliferative neoplasm. (Wright)*

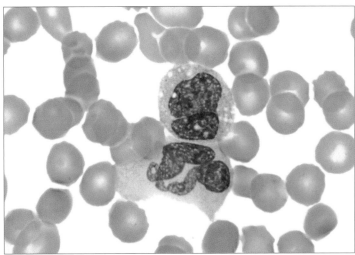

i10.43 *Dysplastic monocytes typically demonstrate nuclear immaturity, abnormal nuclear configuration, and hypogranular cytoplasm as shown on this blood smear (see **i10.42**). (Wright)*

With recombinant G-CSF, circulating blasts can be seen and dysplastic changes of granulocytes are not uncommon (occasional hypogranularity, abnormal nuclear segmentation) (see earlier discussion of G-CSF in this chapter).

[10.5.3] Monocytopenia

Monocytopenia, defined as an absolute monocyte count of $<0.2 \times 10^3/\mu L$ ($<0.2 \times 10^9/L$), is exceedingly rare in the absence of other hematologic abnormalities (eg, anemia and leukopenia). Non-neoplastic conditions associated with monocytopenia include aplastic anemia, glucocorticoid administration, hemodialysis, and sepsis [Nockher 2001]. Hairy cell leukemia is the most common neoplastic disorder associated with monocytopenia. Bone marrow examination is not required for non-neoplastic monocytopenias if the hematologic parameters improve upon resolution of the clinical incident. Clearly, non-transient cases of aplastic anemia or hairy cell leukemia will not show hematologic recovery, and bone marrow examination is usually warranted.

[10.6] Clues and Caveats

1. Acquired neutrophilias are much more common than their constitutional counterparts.
2. Toxic neutrophilias are typical of reactive conditions (eg, infection, colony-stimulating factor therapy) rather than myeloproliferative neoplasms.
3. Colony-stimulating factor therapy results in a striking granulocytic hyperplasia with toxic changes. Left shift and monocytosis in the bone marrow are most prominent for 3 to 10 days after drug administration. Blasts may be transiently increased but are cytologically and immunophenotypically normal.
4. Florid hantavirus pulmonary syndrome is characterized by marked nontoxic neutrophilia with left shift, hemoconcentration, thrombocytopenia, and circulating immunoblasts.
5. Rare causes of neutrophilia include underlying solid tumor malignancies.
6. In a subset of infants with Down syndrome, transient abnormal myelopoiesis (aka transient myeloproliferative disorder) occurs and mimics acute leukemia, particularly acute megakaryoblastic leukemia.
7. In children, chronic viral infection (eg, EBV and rarely cytomegalovirus) and juvenile rheumatoid arthritis may elicit a peripheral blood picture mimicking a myeloid neoplasm (chronic myelogenous leukemia, juvenile myelomonocytic leukemia).
8. In neutrophilic conditions with left shift, the presence of overt dysplasia, Auer rods, basophilia, or eosinophilia with basophilic granules should prompt consideration of a primary myeloid neoplasm.
9. Eosinophilias may be primary (clonal) or secondary (reactive). Distinctions require clinical, morphologic, and often genetic correlation.
10. Abnormal eosinophilic morphology may be seen in both reactive and clonal eosinophilic disorders. The presence of circulating blasts, mast cells, or basophilia should prompt consideration for bone marrow examination.
11. Non-neoplastic basophilia is uncommon and the absolute counts are not substantial. Distinction from a myeloproliferative neoplasm is necessary.
12. Reactive monocytosis is not accompanied by dysplasia of granulocytes or platelets, immature monocytic nuclear features, abnormal blasts, or abnormal eosinophils. Such features should suggest a primary myeloid neoplasm,

after exclusion of severe infection and colony-stimulating factor therapy.

[10.7] References

Abidi K, Khoudri I, Belayachi J, et al [2008] Eosinopenia is a reliable marker of sepsis on admission to medical intensive care units. *Crit Care* 12:R59.

Agis H, Krauth MT, Mosberger I, et al [2006] Enumeration and immunohistochemical characterisation of bone marrow basophils in myeloproliferative disorders using the basophil specific monoclonal antibody 2D7. *J Clin Pathol* 59:396-402.

Ahn HJ, Park YH, Chang YH, et al [2005] A case of uterine cervical cancer presenting with granulocytosis. *Korean J Intern Med* 20:247-250.

Akhtari M, Waller EK [2009] Howell-Jolly body-like inclusions in neutrophils. *Blood* 114(14):2860.

Aprikyan AA, Liles WC, Park JR, et al [2000] Myelokathexis, a congenital disorder of severe neutropenia characterized by accelerated apoptosis and defective expression of bcl-x in neutrophil precursors. *Blood* 95:320-327.

Araki K, Kishihara F, Takahashi K, et al [2007] Hepatocellular carcinoma producing a granulocyte colony-stimulating factor: Report of a resected case with a literature review. *Liver Int* 27:716-721.

Arnalich F, Lahoz C, Larrocha C, et al [1987] Incidence and clinical significance of peripheral and bone marrow basophilia. *J Med* 18:293-303.

Arock M, Schneider E, Boissan M, et al [2002] Differentiation of human basophils: an overview of recent advances and pending questions. *J Leukoc Biol* 71:557-564.

Asmis LM, Hadaya K, Majno P, et al [2003] Acquired and reversible Pelger-Huet anomaly of polymorphonuclear neutrophils in 3 transplant patients receiving mycophenolate mofetil therapy. *Am J Hematol* 73:244-248.

Badolato R, Fontana S, Notarangelo LD, Savoldi G [2004] Congenital neutropenia: Advances in diagnosis and treatment. *Curr Opin Allergy Clin Immunol* 4:513-521.

Bain BJ [1997] The haematological features of HIV infection. *Br J Haematol* 99:1-8.

Best S, Salvati F, Kallo J, et al [2003] Lamin B-receptor mutations in Pelger-Huet anomaly. *Br J Haematol* 123:542-544.

Bloom BJ, Smith P, Alario AJ [1998] Felty syndrome complicating juvenile rheumatoid arthritis. *J Pediatr Hematol Oncol* 20:511-513.

Brito-Babapulle F [2003] The eosinophilias, including the idiopathic hypereosinophilic syndrome. *Br J Haematol* 121:203-223.

Brugnara C [2003] Reference values in infancy and childhood. In: Nathan DG, Orkin SH, Ginsburg D, Look AT, eds. *Nathan and Oski's Hematology of Infancy and Childhood.* 6th ed. Philadelphia: WB Saunders; 1848-1851.

Burdon PC, Martin C, Rankin SM [2005] The CXC chemokine MIP-2 stimulates neutrophil mobilization from the rat bone marrow in a CD49d-dependent manner. *Blood* 105:2543-2548.

Buttarello M, Plebani M [2008] Automated blood cell counts: State of the art. *Am J Clin Pathol* 130:104-116.

Certain S, Barrat F, Pastural E, et al [2000] Protein truncation test of LYST reveals heterogenous mutations in patients with Chediak-Higashi syndrome. *Blood* 95:979-983.

Chetty-Raju N, Cook R, Erber WN [2004] Vacuolated neutrophils in ethanol toxicity. *Br J Haematol* 127:478.

Chi Y, Lindgren V, Quigley S, Gaitonde S [2008] Acute myelogenous leukemia with t(6;9)(p23;q34) and marrow basophilia: an overview. *Arch Pathol Lab Med* 132:1835-1837.

Chou ST, Opalinska JB, Yao Y, et al [2008] Trisomy 21 enhances human fetal erythro-megakaryocytic development. *Blood* 112:4503-4506.

Cicchitto G, Parravicini M, De Lorenzo S, et al [1999] Tuberculosis and Pelger-Huet anomaly. Case report. *Panminerva Med* 41:367-369.

Cooke ME, Potena L, Luikart H, Valantine HA [2006] Peripheral blood leukocyte counts in cytomegalovirus infected heart transplant patients: Impact of acute disease versus subclinical infection. *Transplantation* 82:1419-1424.

Cornbleet PJ [2002] Clinical utility of the band count. *Clin Lab Med* 22:101-136.

Cummings GH, Stevenson AJ [1999] The effect of growth factor therapy on blast percentages. *Am J Clin Pathol* 111:711-712.

Cunningham JM, Patnaik MM, Hammerschmidt DE, Vercellotti GM [2009] Historical perspective and clinical implications of the Pelger-Huet cell. *Am J Hematol* 84:116-119.

Dalal BI, Brigden ML [2002] Artifacts that may be present on a blood film. *Clin Lab Med* 22:81-100, vi.

Dale DC, Boxer L, Liles WC [2008] The phagocytes: Neutrophils and monocytes. *Blood* 112:935-945.

des Guetz G, Mariani P, Freneaux P, Pouillart P [2004] Paraneoplastic syndromes in cancer: case 2. Leucocytosis associated with liposarcoma recurrence: Original presentation of liposarcoma recurrence. *J Clin Oncol* 22:2242-2243.

Dinauer MC [2003] The phagocyte system and disorders of granulopoiesis and granulocyte function. In: Nathan DG, Orkin SH, eds. *Nathan and Oski's Hematology of Infancy and Childhood.* 6th ed. Philadelphia: WB Saunders; 923-1010.

Dusse LM, Morais ESRM, Freitas VM, et al [2006] Pseudo-Pelger-Huet in kidney-transplanted patients. *Acta Haematol* 116:272-274.

Engsig FN, Moller MB, Hasselbalch HK, et al [2007] Extreme neutrophil granulocytosis in a patient with anaplastic large cell lymphoma of T-cell lineage. *Apmis* 115:778-783.

Etzell JE, Wang E [2006] Acquired Pelger-Huet anomaly in association with concomitant tacrolimus and mycophenolate mofetil in a liver transplant patient: a case report and review of the literature. *Arch Pathol Lab Med* 130:93-96.

Etzioni A, Tonetti M [2000] Leukocyte adhesion deficiency II—from A to almost Z. *Immunol Rev* 178:138-147.

Falcone FH, Zillikens D, Gibbs BF [2006] The 21st century renaissance of the basophil? Current insights into its role in allergic responses and innate immunity. *Exp Dermatol* 15:855-864.

Fletcher S, Bain B [2007] Diagnosis and treatment of hypereosinophilic syndromes. *Curr Opin Hematol* 14:37-42.

Focosi D, Azzara A, Kast RE, et al [2009] Lithium and hematology: Established and proposed uses. *J Leukoc Biol* 85:20-28.

Foucar K, Viswanatha D, Wilson C [2008] Appendix. In: King D, Gardner W, Sobin L, et al, eds. *Non-Neoplastic Disorders of Bone Marrow (AFIP fascicle).* Washington, DC: American Registry of Pathology; 397-401.

Foucar K [2010a] Neutropenia. In: Kjeldsberg C, ed. *Practical Diagnosis of Hematologic Disorders.* 5th ed. Chicago: ASCP; 227-237.

Foucar K [2010b] Neutrophilia In: Kjeldsberg C, ed. *Practical Diagnosis of Hematologic Disorders.* 5th ed. Chicago: ASCP; 191-202.

Foucar K, McKenna RW, Bloomfield CD, et al [1979] Therapy-related leukemia: a panmyelosis. *Cancer* 43:1285-1296.

Galeazzi M, Gasbarrini G, Ghirardello A, et al [2006] Autoinflammatory syndromes. *Clin Exp Rheumatol* 24:S79-85.

Glasser L, Legolvan M, Horwitz HM [2007] Florid histiocytic hemophagocytosis following therapy with long acting G-CSF (pegfilgrastim). *Am J Hematol* 82:753-757.

Gotlib J, Cross NC, Gilliland DG [2006] Eosinophilic disorders: molecular pathogenesis, new classification, and modern therapy. *Best Pract Res Clin Haematol* 19:535-569.

Grattan CE, Dawn G, Gibbs S, Francis DM [2003] Blood basophil numbers in chronic ordinary urticaria and healthy controls: Diurnal variation, influence of loratadine and prednisolone and relationship to disease activity. *Clin Exp Allergy* 33:337-341.

Gulen H, Basarir F, Hakan N, et al [2005] Premature labor and leukoerythroblastosis in a newborn with parvovirus B19 infection. *Haematologica* 90 Suppl:ECR38.

Gupta N, Gupta R, Bakhshi S [2009] Transient myeloproliferation mimicking JMML associated with parvovirus infection of infancy. *Pediatr Blood Cancer* 52:411-413.

Haddy TB, Rana SR, Castro O [1999] Benign ethnic neutropenia: What is a normal absolute neutrophil count? *J Lab Clin Med* 133:15-22.

Hallin GW, Simpson SQ, Crowell RE, et al [1996] Cardiopulmonary manifestations of hantavirus pulmonary syndrome. *Crit Care Med* 24:252-258.

Herrod HG, Dow LW, Sullivan JL [1983] Persistent Epstein-Barr virus infection mimicking juvenile chronic myelogenous leukemia: Immunologic and hematologic studies. *Blood* 61:1098-1104.

Hirokawa M, Manabe T, Ishimatsu S, Yokotani Y [1990] Leukocytic fragments in blood smears. *Acta Pathol Jpn* 40:908-912.

Hong YJ, Jeong MH, Ahn Y, et al [2007] Relationship between peripheral monocytosis and nonrecovery of left ventricular function in patients with left ventricular dysfunction complicated with acute myocardial infarction. *Circ J* 71:1219-1224.

Horio H, Nomori H, Morinaga S, et al [1999] Granulocyte colony-stimulating factor-producing primary pericardial mesothelioma. *Hum Pathol* 30:718-720.

Hsieh MM, Everhart JE, Byrd-Holt DD, et al [2007] Prevalence of neutropenia in the U.S. population: Age, sex, smoking status, and ethnic differences. *Ann Intern Med* 146:486-492.

Huizing M, Helip-Wooley A, Westbroek W, et al [2008] Disorders of lysosome-related organelle biogenesis: clinical and molecular genetics. *Annu Rev Genomics Hum Genet* 9:359-386.

Hume DA [2006] The mononuclear phagocyte system. *Curr Opin Immunol* 18:49-53.

Hume DA, Ross IL, Himes SR, et al [2002] The mononuclear phagocyte system revisited. *J Leukoc Biol* 72:621-627.

Hunt K, Salama M, Sever C, Foucar K [2009] Characterization of collagen vascular disease-associated bone marrow changes by morphologic and immunohistochemical assessment. *Mod Pathol* 22(Suppl 1):268A Abstract [1218].

Ito T, Shimamura K, Shoji K, et al [1993] Urinary bladder carcinoma producing granulocyte colony-stimulating factor (G-CSF): A case report with immunohistochemistry. *Virchows Arch A Pathol Anat Histopathol* 422:487-490.

Iwasaki H, Akashi K [2007] Myeloid lineage commitment from the hematopoietic stem cell. *Immunity* 26:726-740.

Janic D, Loncarevic S, Krstovski N, et al [2008] Bone marrow findings in juvenile idiopathic arthritis. *Pediatr Hematol Oncol* 25:575-581.

Jardin F, Vasse M, Debled M, et al [2005] Intense paraneoplastic neutrophilic leukemoid reaction related to a G-CSF-secreting lung sarcoma. *Am J Hematol* 80:243-245.

Jubinsky PT, Shanske AL, Pixley FJ, et al [2006] A syndrome of holoprosencephaly, recurrent infections, and monocytosis. *Am J Med Genet A* 140:2742-2748.

Juhlin L, Michaelsson G [1977] A new syndrome characterised by absence of eosinophils and basophils. *Lancet* 1:1233-1235.

Karandikar NJ, Aquino DB, McKenna RW, Kroft SH [2001] Transient myeloproliferative disorder and acute myeloid leukemia in Down syndrome. An immunophenotypic analysis. *Am J Clin Pathol* 116:204-210.

Kawai T, Malech HL [2009] WHIM syndrome: Congenital immune deficiency disease. *Curr Opin Hematol* 16:20-26.

Kepley CL, Craig SS, Schwartz LB [1995] Identification and partial characterization of a unique marker for human basophils. *J Immunol* 154:6548-6555.

Kerrigan DP, Castillo A, Foucar K, et al [1989] Peripheral blood morphologic changes after high-dose antineoplastic chemotherapy and recombinant human granulocyte colony-stimulating factor administration. *Am J Clin Pathol* 92:280-285.

Kimura N, Ogasawara T, Asonuma S, et al [2005] Granulocyte-colony-stimulating factor- and interleukin 6-producing diffuse deciduoid peritoneal mesothelioma. *Mod Pathol* 18:446-450.

Kirby MA, Weitzman S, Freedman MH [1990] Juvenile chronic myelogenous leukemia: Differentiation from infantile cytomegalovirus infection. *Am J Pediatr Hematol Oncol* 12:292-296.

Kjeldsberg C [2010] Hematology reference values. In: *Practical Diagnosis of Hematologic Disorders.* 5th ed. Chicago: ASCP; 919-928.

Klion AD [2005] Recent advances in the diagnosis and treatment of hypereosinophilic syndromes. *Hematology Am Soc Hematol Educ Program* 209-214.

Koc A, Kosecik M, Tatli MM, et al [2000] Juvenile rheumatoid arthritis presented with thrombocytopenia. *Turk J Pediatr* 42:162-164.

Korenaga M, Hitoshi Y, Yamaguchi N, et al [1991] The role of interleukin-5 in protective immunity to *Strongyloides venezuelensis* infection in mice. *Immunology* 72:502-507.

Koster F, Foucar K, Hjelle B, et al [2001] Rapid presumptive diagnosis of Hantavirus cardiopulmonary syndrome by peripheral blood smear review. *Am J Clin Pathol* 116:665-672.

Kratz A, Lewandrowski KB, Siegel AJ, et al [2002] Effect of marathon running on hematologic and biochemical laboratory parameters, including cardiac markers. *Am J Clin Pathol* 118:856-863.

Krauss JS, Dover RK, Khankhanian NK, Tom GD [1989] Granulocytic fragments in sepsis. *Mod Pathol* 2:301-305.

Kunishima S, Hirano K, Hamaguchi M, Saito H [2008] Accumulation of MYH9 mRNA at leukocyte inclusion bodies in MYH9 disorders. *Eur J Haematol* 81:325-326.

Lam CW, Chan MH, Wong CK [2004] Severe acute respiratory syndrome: clinical and laboratory manifestations. *Clin Biochem Rev* 25:121-132.

Lichtman M [2006] Monocytosis and monocytopenia. In: *Williams Hematology.* 7th ed. New York, NY: McGraw Hill Medical; 983-987.

Liu CZ, Persad R, Inghirami G, et al [2004] Transient atypical monocytosis mimic acute myelomonocytic leukemia in post-chemotherapy patients receiving G-CSF: Report of 2 cases. *Clin Lab Haematol* 26:359-362.

Liu Y, Tang SQ, Liu LZ, et al [2008] [Characteristics of chronic active Epstein-Barr virus infection-associated hematological disorders in children]. *Zhongguo Shi Yan Xue Ye Xue Za Zhi* 16:574-578. Abstract only in English.

Lorenzana A, Lyons H, Sawaf H, et al [2002] Human herpesvirus 6 infection mimicking juvenile myelomonocytic leukemia in an infant. *J Pediatr Hematol Oncol* 24:136-141.

Maitra A, Ward PC, Kroft SH, et al [2000] Cytoplasmic inclusions in leukocytes. An unusual manifestation of cryoglobulinemia. *Am J Clin Pathol* 113:107-112.

Malinge S, Izraeli S, Crispino JD [2009] Insights into the manifestations, outcomes and mechanisms of leukemogenesis in Down syndrome. *Blood* 113:2619-2628.

Matsushima T, Handa H, Yokohama A, et al [2003] Prevalence and clinical characteristics of myelodysplastic syndrome with bone marrow eosinophilia or basophilia. *Blood* 101:3386-3390.

May ME, Waddell CC [1984] Basophils in peripheral blood and bone marrow. A retrospective review. *Am J Med* 76:509-511.

McEuen AR, Buckley MG, Compton SJ, Walls AF [1999] Development and characterization of a monoclonal antibody specific for human basophils and the identification of a unique secretory product of basophil activation. *Lab Invest* 79:27-38.

Meyerson HJ, Farhi DC, Rosenthal NS [1998] Transient increase in blasts mimicking acute leukemia and progressing myelodysplasia in patients receiving growth factor. *Am J Clin Pathol* 109:675-681.

Mitchell EB, Platts-Mills TA, Pereira RS, et al [1983] Acquired basophil and eosinophil deficiency in a patient with hypogammaglobulinaemia associated with thymoma. *Clin Lab Haematol* 5:253-257.

Mitre E, Nutman TB [2006] Basophils, basophilia and helminth infections. *Chem Immunol* Allergy 90:141-156.

Moser M, Bauer M, Schmid S, et al [2009] Kindlin-3 is required for beta2 integrin-mediated leukocyte adhesion to endothelial cells. *Nat Med* 15:300-305.

Neven B, Prieur AM, Quartier dit Maire P [2008] Cryopyrinopathies: Update on pathogenesis and treatment. *Nat Clin Pract Rheumatol* 4:481-489.

Ngo NT, Lampert IA, Naresh KN [2008] Bone marrow trephine morphology and immunohistochemical findings in chronic myelomonocytic leukaemia. *Br J Haematol* 141:771-781.

Nockher WA, Wiemer J, Scherberich JE [2001] Haemodialysis monocytopenia: Differential sequestration kinetics of CD14+CD16+ and CD14++ blood monocyte subsets. *Clin Exp Immunol* 123:49-55.

Nolte KB, Feddersen RM, Foucar K, et al [1995] Hantavirus pulmonary syndrome in the United States: a pathological description of a disease caused by a new agent. *Hum Pathol* 26:110-120.

Nurden P, Nurden AT [2008] Congenital disorders associated with platelet dysfunctions. *Thromb Haemost* 99:253-263.

Ogbogu PU, Rosing DR, Horne MK, 3rd [2007] Cardiovascular manifestations of hypereosinophilic syndromes. *Immunol Allergy Clin North Am* 27:457-475.

Oh K, Shen T, Le Gros G, Min B [2007] Induction of Th2 type immunity in a mouse system reveals a novel immunoregulatory role of basophils. *Blood* 109:2921-2927.

Ohmori K, Luo Y, Jia Y, et al [2009] IL-3 induces basophil expansion in vivo by directing granulocyte-monocyte progenitors to differentiate into basophil lineage-restricted progenitors in the bone marrow and by increasing the number of basophil/mast cell progenitors in the spleen. *J Immunol* 182:2835-2841.

Orazi A, Cattoretti G, Schiro R, et al [1992] Recombinant human interleukin-3 and recombinant human granulocyte-macrophage colony-stimulating factor administered in vivo after high-dose cyclophosphamide cancer chemotherapy: Effect on hematopoiesis and microenvironment in human bone marrow. *Blood* 79:2610-2619.

Orazi A, Chiu R, O'Malley DP, et al [2006] Chronic myelomonocytic leukemia: the role of bone marrow biopsy immunohistology. *Mod Pathol* 19:1536-1545.

Peterson L, Parkin J, Nelson A [1982] Mucopolysaccharidosis type VII. A morphologic, cytochemical, and ultrastructural study of the blood and bone marrow. *Am J Clin Pathol* 78:544-548.

Rao S, Kar R, Saxena R [2009] Pseudo-Chediak-Higashi anomaly in acute myelomonocytic leukemia. *Indian J Pathol Microbiol* 52:255-256.

Ravoet M, Sibille C, Gu C, et al [2009] Molecular profiling of CD3-CD4+ T cells from patients with the lymphocytic variant of hypereosinophilic syndrome reveals targeting of growth control pathways. *Blood* 114:2969-2983.

Robinson RL, Burk MS, Raman S [2003] Fever, delirium, autonomic instability, and monocytosis associated with olanzapine. *J Postgrad Med* 49:96.

Rothenberg ME, Hogan SP [2006] The eosinophil. *Annu Rev Immunol* 24:147-174.

Rubin CM, Burke BA, McKenna RW, et al [1985] The accelerated phase of Chediak-Higashi syndrome. An expression of the virus-associated hemophagocytic syndrome? *Cancer* 56:524-530.

Saito H, Kunishima S [2008] Historical hematology: May-Hegglin anomaly. *Am J Hematol* 83:304-306.

Seebach JD, Morant R, Ruegg R, et al [1997] The diagnostic value of the neutrophil left shift in predicting inflammatory and infectious disease. *Am J Clin Pathol* 107:582-591.

Sheikh J, Weller PF [2009] Advances in diagnosis and treatment of eosinophilia. *Curr Opin Hematol* 16:3-8.

Simon D, Simon HU [2007] Eosinophilic disorders. *J Allergy Clin Immunol* 119:1291-1300; quiz 1301-1292.

Singh KJ, Ahluwalia G, Sharma SK, et al [2001] Significance of haematological manifestations in patients with tuberculosis. *J Assoc Physicians India* 49:788, 790-784.

Slagel DD, Lager DJ, Dick FR [1994] Howell-Jolly body-like inclusions in the neutrophils of patients with acquired immunodeficiency syndrome. *Am J Clin Pathol* 101:429-431.

Soni R, Bose S, Gada D, Potnis V [1996] Basopenia as an indicator of ovulation (a short-term clinical study). *Indian J Physiol Pharmacol* 40:385-388.

Stein SM, Dale DC [2003] Molecular basis and therapy of disorders associated with chronic neutropenia. *Curr Allergy Asthma Rep* 3:385-388.

Strand CL, Goldstein D, Castella A [1991] Value of cytoplasmic vacuolization of neutrophils in the diagnosis of bloodstream infection. *Lab Med* 22:263-266.

Svensson L, Howarth K, McDowall A, et al [2009] Leukocyte adhesion deficiency-III is caused by mutations in KINDLIN3 affecting integrin activation. *Nat Med* 15:306-312.

Taegtmeyer AB, Halil O, Bell AD, et al [2005] Neutrophil dysplasia (acquired pseudo-Pelger anomaly) caused by ganciclovir. *Transplantation* 80:127-130.

Tang G, Woods LJ, Wang SA, et al [2009] Chronic basophilic leukemia: a rare form of chronic myeloproliferative neoplasm. *Hum Pathol* 40:1194-1199.

Tefferi A, Patnaik MM, Pardanani A [2006] Eosinophilia: Secondary, clonal and idiopathic. *Br J Haematol* 133:468-492.

Tokuhira M, Watanabe R, Iizuka A, et al [2007] De novo CD5+ diffuse large B cell lymphoma with basophilia in the peripheral blood: Successful treatment with autologous peripheral blood stem cell transplantation. *Am J Hematol* 82:162-167.

Tsakonas GP, Kallistratos MS, Balamoti EK, et al [2007] Rare and aggressive metastatic, axial multifocal local epithelioid sarcoma associated with paraneoplastic granulocytosis and hypoglycaemia. *Lancet Oncol* 8:82-84.

Tsolia M, Drakonaki S, Messaritaki A, et al [2002] Clinical features, complications and treatment outcome of childhood brucellosis in central Greece. *J Infect* 44:257-262.

Vaklavas C, Tefferi A, Butterfield J, et al [2007] "Idiopathic" eosinophilia with an occult T-cell clone: prevalence and clinical course. *Leuk Res* 31:691-694.

Valent P [2009a] Interleukin-33: A regulator of basophils. *Blood* 113:1396-1397.

Valent P [2009b] Pathogenesis, classification, and therapy of eosinophilia and eosinophil disorders. *Blood Rev* 23:157-165.

van der Meer W, van Gelder W, de Keijzer R, Willems H [2006] Does the band cell survive the 21st century? *Eur J Haematol* 76:251-254.

Vlasoff D, Morice W [2006] Non-neoplastic bone marrow pathology associated with autoimmune disorders. *Mod Pathol* 19(Suppl 1):250A Abstract [1162].

von Vietinghoff S, Ley K [2008] Homeostatic regulation of blood neutrophil counts. *J Immunol* 181:5183-5188.

Walsh DS, Thavichaigarn P, Pattanapanyasat K, et al [2005] Characterization of circulating monocytes expressing HLA-DR or CD71 and related soluble factors for 2 weeks after severe, non-thermal injury. *J Surg Res* 129:221-230.

Walter S, Nancy NR [1980] Basopenia following cigarette smoking. *Indian J Med Res* 72:422-425.

Ward HN, Reinhard EH [1971] Chronic idiopathic leukocytosis. *Ann Intern Med* 75:193-198.

Ward PC, McKenna RW, Kroft SH [2007] White blood cell changes in hyperthermia. *Br J Haematol* 138:130.

Watanabe N, Yoshimi A, Kamachi Y, et al [2007] Wiskott-Aldrich syndrome is an important differential diagnosis in male infants with juvenile myelomonocytic leukemia-like features. *J Pediatr Hematol Oncol* 29:836-838.

Webb D, Roberts I, Vyas P [2007] Haematology of Down syndrome. *Arch Dis Child Fetal Neonatal Ed* 92:F503-507.

Weller PF, Bubley GJ [1994] The idiopathic hypereosinophilic syndrome. *Blood* 83:2759-2779.

Wenzel SE [2009] Eosinophils in asthma: closing the loop or opening the door? *N Engl J Med* 360:1026-1028.

William BM, Corazza GR [2007] Hyposplenism: a comprehensive review. Part I: Basic concepts and causes. *Hematology* 12:1-13.

Wimazal F, Baumgartner C, Sonneck K, et al [2008] Mixed-lineage eosinophil/basophil crisis in MDS: A rare form of progression. *Eur J Clin Invest* 38:447-455.

Worman HJ, Bonne G [2007] "Laminopathies": A wide spectrum of human diseases. *Exp Cell Res* 313:2121-2133.

Yetgin S, Cetin M, Yenicesu I, et al [2000] Acute parvovirus B19 infection mimicking juvenile myelomonocytic leukemia. *Eur J Haematol* 65:276-278.

Yoshimoto T, Tsutsui H, Tominaga K, et al [1999] IL-18, although antiallergic when administered with IL-12, stimulates IL-4 and histamine release by basophils. *Proc Natl Acad Sci USA* 96:13962-13966.

Zaki SR, Greer PW, Coffield LM, et al [1995] Hantavirus pulmonary syndrome. Pathogenesis of an emerging infectious disease. *Am J Pathol* 146:552-579.

Zeng HS, Xiong XY, Wei YD, et al [2008] Macrophage activation syndrome in 13 children with systemic-onset juvenile idiopathic arthritis. *World J Pediatr* 4:97-101.

CHAPTER

Neutropenia and Agranulocytosis

David Czuchlewski, MD

While this chapter concerns quantitative abnormalities of granulocytes, a useful analogy may be made to anemia, which is often categorized as either "intrinsic," meaning that the anemia is secondary to some abnormality within the red blood cell itself, or "extrinsic," in which the anemia arises in the setting of factors unrelated to the internal environment of the cell, such as antibody-mediated attack or mechanical stress. Likewise, upon identifying a patient as neutropenic, one might ask: is the responsible abnormality *intrinsic* to the neutrophils, as in constitutional neutropenia? Or is the neutropenia instead a secondary phenomenon, a sign of pathology *extrinsic* to the neutrophil? Most frequently, extrinsic factors are indeed responsible; however, this realization hardly narrows the vast array of possible secondary causes of neutropenia—which include toxic effect, immune attack, peripheral destruction, and cytokine modulation—any of which may be operative, singly or in combination, in cases of drug-induced neutropenia, autoimmune syndromes, infection, systemic inflammation, and malignancies such as T-cell large granular lymphocytic leukemia. This chapter is devoted to the consideration and rational categorization of the diverse processes that result in neutropenia and agranulocytosis.

Although this chapter covers most aspects of isolated neutropenia, the differential diagnosis is significantly expanded when additional cytopenias accompany the neutropenia t11.1. In such cases, the reader is referred in particular to chapters describing myelodysplasia (Chapter 15), multilineage bone marrow failure (Chapter 7, p 140), nutritional deficiencies (Chapter 6), and hemophagocytic syndrome (Chapter 26). Importantly, rare cases of aplastic anemia, myelodysplastic syndrome, and acute lymphoblastic leukemia may present with initial *isolated* neutropenia.

t11.1 Selected Diagnostic Considerations When Neutropenia Occurs with Other Cytopenia(s)

Myelodysplastic syndrome

Aplastic anemia

Acute lymphoblastic leukemia

Infection

Medication/toxic exposure

Nutritional deficiency

Acute myeloid leukemia

General bone marrow infiltrative process

Constitutional bone marrow failure syndrome

Hemophagocytic syndrome

[11.1] Definition of Neutropenia and Agranulocytosis

Neutropenia is generally said to be present when neutrophils number $<1.5 \times 10^3/\mu L$ $(1.5 \times 10^9/L)$ in children and adults; however, normal ranges vary according to age, sex, and ethnicity (see next section and t11.2). Agranulocytosis is usually defined as an absolute neutrophil count (ANC) $<0.5 \times 10^3/\mu L$ $(0.5 \times 10^9/L)$. Agranulocytosis may be regarded as the most dramatic and consequential form of neutropenia, carrying with it a significant risk of secondary infection; however, it arises via some of the same causes and mechanisms as more moderate neutropenia, and thus differs from the latter quantitatively but not necessarily qualitatively. Therefore in this chapter we will speak in general of neutropenia, with the understanding that agranulocytosis is a condition subsumed by this larger category.

t11.2 Effects of Demographic Characteristics on Absolute Neutrophil Count (ANC)*

Age	ANC (Range) ($\times 10^9$/L)
Birth	11 (6.0-26.0)
12 hours	15.5 (6.0-28.0)
24 hours	11.5 (5.0-21.0)
1 week	5.5 (1.5-10.0)
2 weeks	4.5 (1.0-9.5)
1 month	3.8 (1.0-9.0)
6 months	3.8 (1.0-8.5)
1 year	3.5 (1.5-8.5)
2 years	3.5 (1.5-8.5)
4 years	3.8 (1.5-8.5)
6 years	4.3 (1.5-8.0)
8 years	4.4 (1.5-8.0)
10 years	4.4 (1.8-8.0)
16 years	4.4 (1.8-8.0)
21 years	4.4 (1.8-7.7)

Mean ANC by Sex and Race or Ethnicity

White male adult	4.3 (1.8-7.8)
White female adult	White male adult + 0.2
Black male adult	White male adult − 0.8
Black female adult	White male adult − 0.5
Mexican-American male adult	White male adult + 0.0
Mexican-American female adult	White male adult + 0.3

ANC by Tobacco Use

Smoker	Add 0.87 to nonsmoker reference range

*Reference ranges for individual laboratories will vary by analytic technique and patient population; laboratory-specific normal ranges should be measured and used for diagnostic purposes; these values in this table are provided solely to allow broad estimation of the impact of the listed features on ANC

References: [Geaghan 2008, Hsieh 2007, Lehmann 2007]

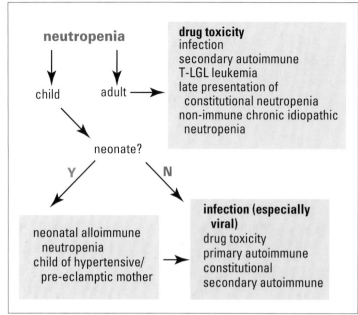

f11.1 *Key etiologies of isolated neutropenia, by age (bold indicates most common)*

t11.3 Mutations in Isolated Constitutional Neutropenia Syndromes

Syndrome	Gene	Inheritance Pattern
Shwachman-Diamond syndrome	*SBDS*	AR
Severe congenital neutropenia	*ELANE (ELA2)**	AD
	GFI1[†]	AD
	HAX1[†]	AR
	WAS[†]	XLR
	CSF3R[†]	AD
	G6PC3[†]	AR
Myelokathexis	*CXCR4*	AD
Chédiak-Higashi syndrome	*LYST*	AR

*ELANE mutations are seen in both severe congenital neutropenia and cyclic neutropenia (see **sidebar 11.2**, p 211)
[†]Mutations in these genes are rare causes of constitutional neutropenia
AR = autosomal recessive; AD = autosomal dominant; XLR = X-linked recessive

References: [Balabanian 2008, Berliner 2004, Dale 2009]

[11.2] Epidemiology of Neutropenia

Consideration of neutropenia from a population-based perspective is especially important, since the normal ranges quoted above may differ significantly by population. While some variation is seen by gender, of greater importance is the lower normal range seen in blacks. The mean ANC in black men is $3.5 \times 10^3/\mu L$ ($3.5 \times 10^9/L$), compared with $4.3 \times 10^3/\mu L$ ($4.3 \times 10^9/L$) for the white male US population [Hsieh 2007]. In addition, 5% of the black population shows an ANC $<1.5 \times 10^3/\mu L$ ($<1.5 \times 10^9/L$) without any apparent physiologic consequence [Hsieh 2007]. The specific genetic bases for these subtle differences are unknown but may relate to fundamental differences in myelopoietic capacity or the high prevalence in this population of a single nucleotide polymorphism (SNP) in the gene encoding the Duffy antigen [Grann 2008b, Mayr 2007, Rezvani 2001]. The phenomenon has been labeled *ethnic neutropenia*, but this term should be used with caution, because it implies the application of a population-wide normal range to a group with a distinctly lower, though still physiologic, normal distribution. Regardless, considering each patient in the context of the most appropriate reference range may avoid needless concern and unnecessary evaluation. Indeed, benign differences in neutrophil count have been implicated in treatment disparities by race [Grann 2008a, Hershman 2003, Kelly 2007].

In addition to gender and ethnic considerations, the environment may influence neutrophil count. Smoking, for example, is associated with higher mean neutrophil counts **t11.2** [Hsieh 2007]. More broadly, a longitudinal study documented a significant decrease in neutrophil count in a single US population between 1958 and 2002 which could not be attributed entirely to changes in smoking, obesity, or

physical activity over that time span [Ruggiero 2007], thus potentially implicating other undefined environmental factors.

While there is no age at which a given etiology of neutropenia is excluded, there is nevertheless a general pattern of incidence that may be useful in constructing differential diagnoses. Viral infection is a major cause of neutropenia in children, and it is also in this population that the constitutional neutropenia syndromes must be especially considered. In contrast, neutropenia in an adult patient is more likely to be secondary to drug administration, autoimmune processes or, as is often the case, multifactorial. Infection remains an important cause of neutropenia at all ages. These considerations are summarized in **f11.1**.

[11.3] Neutropenia of Intrinsic Etiology

In general, the intrinsic defects in neutrophils that produce isolated neutropenia are manifestations of heritable syndromes and mutations **t11.3**. These constitutional neutropenias are therefore most frequently diagnosed in children. However, it is essential to remember 2 caveats:

1. Even in children, neutropenia of extrinsic etiology is much more common.

2. Some of these syndromes may very rarely come to clinical attention for the first time in adolescence or adulthood, because of genetic heterogeneity [Bellane-Chantelot 2004].

If a constitutional neutropenia syndrome is suspected, **t11.4** and **t11.5** provide quick reference guides to diagnostic considerations and possible further workup.

t11.4 Syndromes Associated with Constitutional Neutropenia and Key Diagnostic Clues

Major constitutional neutropenia syndromes	Shwachman-Diamond syndrome	Pancreatic insufficiency
	Severe congenital neutropenia	Static neutropenia with granulocytic hypoplasia*
	Cyclic neutropenia	Periodicity of neutropenia (~ 21 day cycle)
Characteristically multilineage bone marrow failure (see Chapter 7, p 140)	Fanconi anemia	Increased chromosomal breakage with exposure to cross-linking agents
	Dyskeratosis congenita	Late onset of presentation
Immunodeficiency associated	Common variable immunodeficiency syndrome	Immunoglobulin subset irregularities and/or T/NK-cell dysfunction
	HyperIgM syndrome	
	X-linked agammaglobulinemia	
	Reticular dysgenesis	
Storage disorders	Glycogen storage disease, type Ib	Hypoglycemia
Trafficking disorders	Chédiak-Higashi syndrome	Large cytoplasmic granules in all lineages with granules; oculocutaneous albinism
	Griscelli syndrome, type 2	Neurologic impairment (usually); oculocutaneous albinism
	Hermansky-pudlak syndrome, type 2	Platelet function abnormalities; oculocutaneous albinism
Miscellaneous	Myelokathexis/WHIM syndrome	Granulocytic "right shift" with morphologic abnormalities, degenerative changes and apoptosis
		Warts
		Hypogammaglobulinemia
	Barth syndrome	Cardiomyopathy and skeletal myopathy
	Cohen syndrome	Psychomotor retardation
		Facial dysmorphism

*Severe congenital neutropenia must be differentiated from primary autoimmune neutropenia; molecular testing for *ELANE* mutations and serologic testing for antineutrophil antibodies may be indicated

WHIM = warts, hypogammaglobulinemia, infections, myelokathexis

References: [Balabanian 2005, Berliner 2004, Dokal 2008, James 2006]

t11.5 Morphologic Clues to Suspected Constitutional Neutropenia

Peripheral Blood

Chédiak-Higashi syndrome	Large neutrophilic granules
Myelokathexis	Morphologic abnormalities, degenerative changes

Bone Marrow

Granulocytic Hypoplasia or Aplasia; Left Shift		Granulocytic Hyperplasia	
Severe congenital neutropenia	Consider *ELANE* (*ELA2*) mutation analysis	Myelokathexis	Look for morphologic abnormalities, hypogammaglobulinemia
Neutropenic phase of cyclic neutropenia	Evaluate periodicity of neutropenia	Recovery phase of cyclic neutropenia	Evaluate periodicity of neutropenia
Shwachman-Diamond syndrome	Evaluate pancreatic function		

Also consider:

Fanconi anemia, dyskeratosis congenita (multilineage failure)

Infection (with direct damage to myeloid precursor)

Drug toxicity

Immune-mediated destruction

Also consider:

Infection (with peripheral consumption)

Altered distribution of neutrophils (total body neutrophil quantity normal)

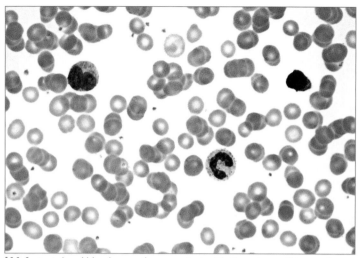

i11.1 *Peripheral blood smear from a patient with Shwachman-Diamond syndrome. Note rare neutrophil. (Wright) (courtesy P Izadi)*

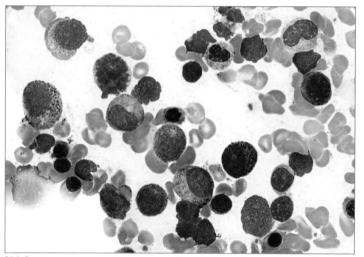

i11.2 *Bone marrow aspirate showing decreased granulocytic lineage cells in this patient with Shwachman-Diamond syndrome. (Wright) (courtesy P Izadi)*

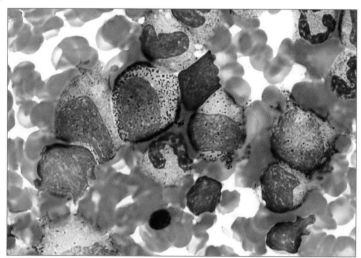

i11.3 *Bone marrow aspirate smear showing left-shifted granulopoiesis that is overall reduced in this patient with Shwachman-Diamond syndrome. (Wright) (courtesy P Izadi)*

[11.3.1]   **Shwachman-Diamond Syndrome**

Shwachman-Diamond syndrome, sometimes called Bodian-Shwachman syndrome, is an autosomal recessive disorder characterized most commonly by severe neutropenia, though multiple lineages are affected in some 40% of cases [Foucar 2008]. The neutropenia may be sustained or intermittent. Frequent coexisting abnormalities include insufficiency of the exocrine pancreas and metaphyseal chrondrodysplasia. In some patients, additional anomalies may include malformation of the thoracic rib cage, dental dysplasia, and icthyotic skin rash. Transformation to myelodysplasia and acute myeloid leukemia is a major cause of morbidity and mortality, occurring in approximately 1 in 4 cases, but the age at transformation is highly variable, ranging from 1-43 years [Dokal 2008].

Shwachman-Diamond patients typically present as infants with failure to thrive due to pancreatic insufficiency and gastrointestinal malabsorption, or infectious complications secondary to severe neutropenia [Burroughs 2009]. The blood shows profound neutropenia, while the bone marrow shows granulocytic hypoplasia with left-shifted maturation and variably preserved erythroid and megakaryocytic lineages **i11.1, i11.2, i11.3**. Cellularity is highly variable and does not necessarily correlate with the degree of cytopenia [Shimamura 2006].

[sidebar 11.1]   **Shwachman-Diamond Syndrome and Gene Conversion**

Mutations in the *SBDS* (Shwachman-Bodian-Diamond syndrome) gene at chromosome 7q11 have been detected in approximately 90% of Shwachman-Diamond patients [Boocock 2003]. An adjacent pseudogene with 97% homology to *SBDS* is also present on chromosome 7. Pseudogenes are copies of genes, created in ancestral duplication events, with mutations that render them nonfunctional. The *SBDS* pseudogene is fully transcribed into mRNA, but the deviations from the true *SBDS* sequence prevent the proper translation of pseudogene mRNA. Shwachman-Diamond syndrome typically arises through a process of "gene conversion," whereby a recombination event replaces portions of the normal *SBDS* gene with the homologous, defective pseudogene sequences, leading to a marked reduction in protein expression [Nakashima 2004]. Essentially, then, Shwachman-Diamond syndrome arises due to the reactivation of sequences that have been duplicated and corrupted on an evolutionary time scale.

SBDS codes for a protein that localizes to the nucleolus and binds ribosomal RNA [Austin 2005, Ganapathi 2007]. Based on these findings and comparative studies involving yeast and other organisms, the *SBDS* gene product appears to function in the maturation of the 60s ribosomal subunit and mitotic spindle stabilization [Austin 2008, Menne 2007]. The protein also associates with nucleophosmin, mutations of which characterize a subset of acute myeloid leukemias [Ganapathi 2007]. *SBDS* mutations may render the cell susceptible to Fas-mediated apoptosis through an unclear mechanism, perhaps accounting for the development of bone marrow failure [Watanabe 2008].

Chromosomal abnormalities often arise in Shwachman-Diamond syndrome, most commonly i(7q), monosomy 7, 7q translocations, and del(20q). The significance of these specific abnormalities is surprisingly divergent. Shwachman-Diamond patients may harbor i(7q) or del(20q) mutations for long periods with few hematologic consequences [Dror 2002], and in some cases these clones may become undetectable over time [Smith 2002]. In contrast, patients with chromosome 7 abnormalities *other* than i(7q) may present with or progress to an overt myeloid malignancy [Dror 2005]. The basis for these apparently distinct clinical courses remains unclear, as does the connection, if any, between pseudogene conversion of *SBDS* on chromosome 7 and the frequency of structural abnormalities of the same chromosome. However, it has been suggested that karyotypic instability, perhaps reflecting the role of normal SBDS in the mitotic spindle, is part of the natural history of Shwachman-Diamond syndrome [Austin 2009, Maserati 2009].

The diagnosis of Shwachman-Diamond syndrome has traditionally relied upon the coexistence of exocrine pancreatic insufficiency and bone marrow failure. However, pancreatic function tends to improve over time, and the bone marrow manifestations may be mild or intermittent, significantly complicating the diagnosis, especially in patients lacking additional physical abnormalities. The prominence of the pancreatic symptomatology dictates that Pearson syndrome and cystic fibrosis enter the differential diagnosis. Genetic testing via sequencing of the most frequently affected *SBDS* exons is available **sidebar 11.1**.

[11.3.2] **Severe Congenital Neutropenia and Cyclic Neutropenia**

Severe congenital neutropenia is an umbrella term that encompasses several clinically and pathophysiologically distinct entities. The severe congenital neutropenia syndromes typically present in infancy with profound neutropenia or agranulocytosis, which renders the patient susceptible to life-threatening infection.

Kostmann provided the first description of severe congenital neutropenia in 1956. These original cases showed an autosomal recessive pattern of inheritance. Subsequently it was realized that

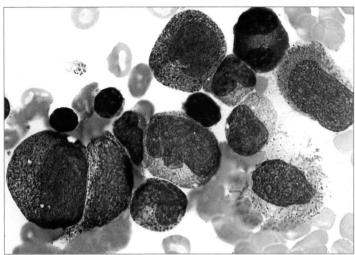

i11.4 *Bone marrow aspirate smear from a patient with severe congenital neutropenia showing marked reduction of granulocytic lineage including only rare myeloblasts and promyelocytes. (Wright) (courtesy P Izadi)*

most cases of severe congenital neutropenia in fact represent autosomal dominant mutations of genes that were not affected in the patients originally identified by Kostmann. Thus, most would restrict the eponym *Kostmann syndrome* specifically to autosomal recessive cases of severe congenital neutropenia. Mutations of *HAX1*, which encodes an anti-apoptotic mitochondrial protein, cause the Kostmann form of severe congenital neutropenia [Dale 2009].

Cyclic neutropenia is also a constitutional neutropenia syndrome, distinguished clinically by the approximately 21-day periodicity of the decline in ANC. Cyclic neutropenia is due to mutations in the *ELANE* (also known as *ELA2*) gene, the same gene affected in most cases of non-cyclic autosomal dominant severe congenital neutropenia; thus, we describe these related entities together. The genetic basis for the phenotypic heterogeneity of these syndromes is addressed in more detail in **sidebar 11.2**.

Affected infants usually come to attention with severe infections in the setting of ANC in the range of $0\text{-}0.2 \times 10^3/\mu L$ $(0\text{-}0.2 \times 10^9/L)$. During an acute infection, however, there may be a slight reactive elevation in the ANC, potentially complicating recognition of constitutional neutropenia. The variability in ANC characteristic of cyclic neutropenia may also present a challenge to clinical diagnosis, but serial complete blood count (CBC) monitoring over a period of weeks to months provides strong evidence for or against cyclic neutropenia. There is often concomitant monocytosis and eosinophilia, thought to represent a compensatory response to neutropenia.

The bone marrow findings in cases of severe congenital neutropenia are striking, but nonspecific. The peripheral neutropenia is paralleled by a granulocytic hypoplasia or even aplasia [Foucar 2008]; of those myeloid cells present, few represent stages of maturation later than the promyelocyte or myelocyte **i11.4**. Unfortunately, an identical left-shifted granulocytic hypoplasia may also be seen in neutropenia of

[sidebar 11.2] **Severe Congenital Neutropenia and the Unfolded Protein Response**

In cases of severe congenital neutropenia, the morphologic impression of a deficiency in neutrophilic maturation reflects the underlying genetic lesions. Some 70% to 90% of cases of severe congenital neutropenia are caused by mutations in one allele of the neutrophil elastase gene, *ELANE* (*ELA2*), which codes for a component of the primary granules [Alter 2007, Bohn 2007]. The same gene is affected in cyclic neutropenia. The subsets of mutations giving rise to severe congenital neutropenia and cyclic neutropenia are largely distinct, implying a genotype-phenotype correlation that remains, at present, obscure in mechanism [Horwitz 2007].

The connection between *ELANE* mutations and disease is complicated by the finding that mice completely lacking in *ELANE* showed no abnormalities in granulopoiesis [Belaaouaj 1998]. It now appears that *ELANE* mutations may induce apoptosis though the so-called "unfolded protein response," in which the detection of significant protein misfolding in the endoplasmic reticulum triggers cell death in a manner analogous to apoptosis following irreparable genetic damage [Grenda 2007, Xia 2008]. Thus, it is the specific properties of the mutated protein, rather than a simple loss of function, or haploinsufficiency, that appears to be responsible for the disease. Some have suggested that the degree of activation of the unfolded protein response in the setting of different *ELANE* mutations may account for the distinct cyclic and non-cyclic phenotypes [Berliner 2008].

Mutations of other genes have also been implicated in constitutional neutropenia, including *HAX1*, encoding an antiapoptotic mitochondrial protein, in autosomal recessive Kostmann syndrome; rarely, *GFI1*, a zinc finger transcription factor that regulates *ELANE* expression; and *WAS*, the gene encoding the Wiskott-Aldrich syndrome protein; and *G6PC3*, which codes for glucose-6-phophatase catalytic subunit 3 [Dale 2009, Germeshausen 2008, Kazanjian 2006].

Very rare cases due to a mutation in *CSF3R*, the gene coding for the G-CSF receptor, have also been described; these G-CSF mutated cases, unsurprisingly, do not show a clinical response to the standard G-CSF therapy. These uncommon constitutional *CSF3R* mutations must be distinguished from the acquired *CSF3R* mutations that may arise during G-CSF treatment in cases of severe congenital neutropenia due to other mutations [Berliner 2004].

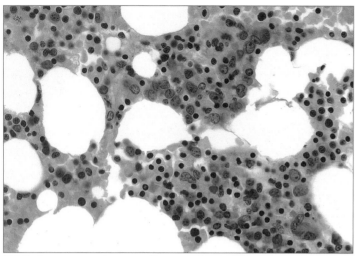

i11.5 *Bone marrow clot section illustrates a loss in cellularity secondary to a profound drug-induced agranulocytosis. Note absence of maturing granulocytic cells. (H&E)*

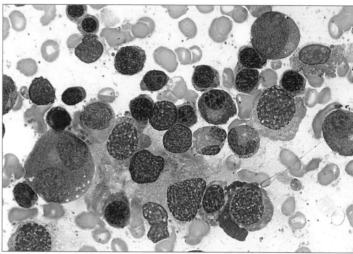

i11.6 *This bone marrow aspirate smear is from a child with severe congenital neutropenia, which is characterized by a "maturation arrest" picture with strikingly enlarged and frequently multinucleated promyelocytes. (Wright)*

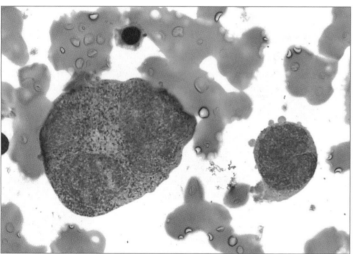

i11.7 *This bone marrow aspirate smear illustrates the pronounced enlargement and multinucleation of promyelocytes that characterize severe congenital neutropenia. (Wright)*

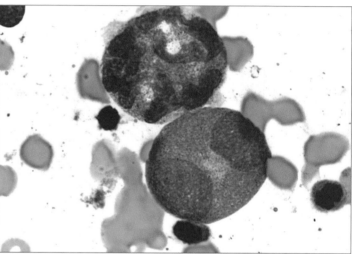

i11.8 *This bone marrow aspirate smear illustrates multinucleation of mature and immature granulocytic cells in a patient with severe congenital neutropenia (see i11.7). (Wright)*

extrinsic etiology i11.5. Indeed, such a picture is often seen in primary autoimmune neutropenia, an important differential diagnostic consideration in neutropenic children. Some cases of Kostmann syndrome show characteristic binucleated or multinucleated promyelocytes, a finding that helps to narrow the differential diagnosis when present i11.6, i11.7, i11.8. Of note, these constitutional neutropenia syndromes show changes only in the granulocytic lineage. If multilineage hypoplasia is present, then other etiologies, particularly Shwachman-Diamond syndrome and Fanconi anemia, become more likely. Finally, cyclic neutropenia is unique among the constitutional neutropenias in that the granulocytic aplasia/neutropenia is followed by a predictable hematopoietic rebound characterized by myeloid hyperplasia and full maturation. In the blood a wave of monocytosis often precedes neutrophil recovery i11.9. Thus, bone marrow

evaluation in these cases must be performed in the context of the long-term trends in peripheral neutrophil count i11.10, i11.11, i11.12.

Treatment with granulocyte colony-stimulating factor (G-CSF) produces a dramatic recovery of the ANC, and has transformed severe congenital neutropenia from a disease fatal in early childhood to a more chronic disease i11.13, i11.14. However, the risk of progression to myelodysplastic syndrome (MDS) and acute myeloid leukemia (AML) in severe congenital neutropenia is substantial, with an incidence of 21% at only 10 years of follow-up [Rosenberg 2006]. The development of leukemia is associated with acquired mutations in the gene encoding the G-CSF receptor (*CSF3R*) and the duration and intensity of G-CSF therapy [Ancliff 2003, Donadieu 2005]. Some have speculated that long-term G-CSF treatment in this setting may confer a proliferative

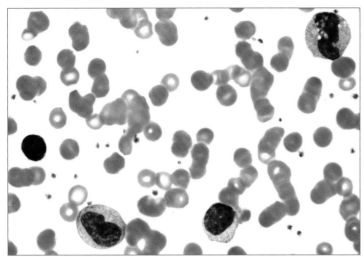

i11.9 *Peripheral blood smear showing increased circulating monocytes preceding neutrophil recovery in patient with cyclic neutropenia at nadir. (Wright)*

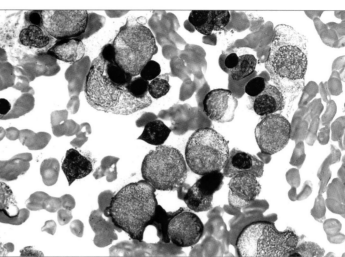

i11.10 *Bone marrow aspirate smear with markedly reduced and left-shifted granulocytic lineage in a patient with cyclic neutropenia at nadir. (Wright)*

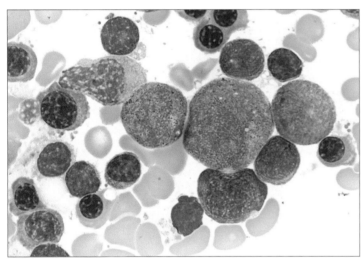

i11.11 *This bone marrow aspirate smear from a patient with cyclic neutropenia illustrates myeloid "maturation arrest" in that only isolated myeloblasts and promyelocytes are evident. (Wright)*

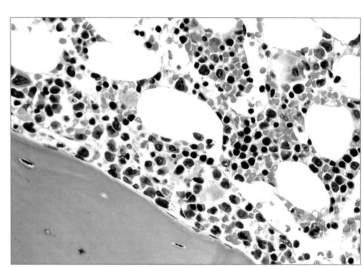

i11.12 *Bone marrow core biopsy specimen showing reduced and left-shifted granulocytic cells with a paratrabecular localization. (H&E)*

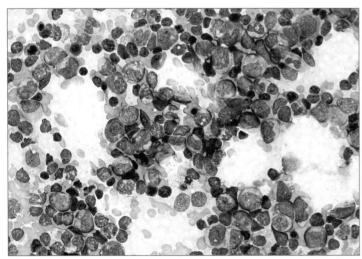

i11.13 *Bone marrow aspirate smear showing marked hypercellularity with intact neutrophilic maturation in a patient with severe congenital neutropenia receiving granulocyte colony-stimulating factor treatment. (Wright) (courtesy J Choi, MD)*

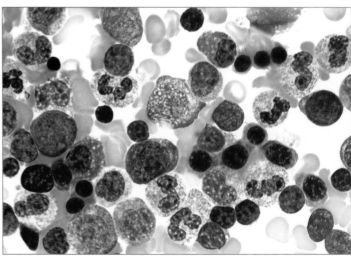

i11.14 *Bone marrow aspirate smear from a patient with cyclic neutropenia receiving granulocyte colony-stimulating factor treatment that shows abundance of mature neutrophils. (Wright)*

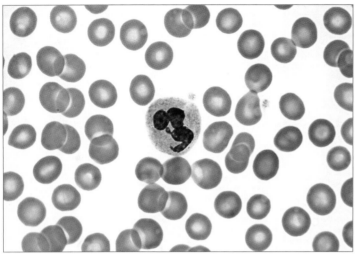

i11.15 *Peripheral blood smear showing neutrophil with thin internuclear strands in a patient with myelokathexis. (Wright) (courtesy S Kroft, MD)*

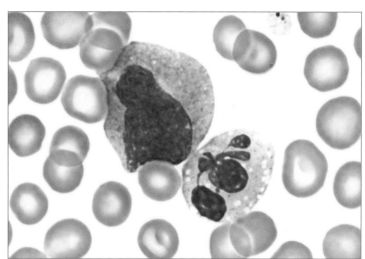

i11.16 *Peripheral blood smear with myelokathexis showing elongated and markedly thin internuclear strands. (Wright) (courtesy S Kroft, MD)*

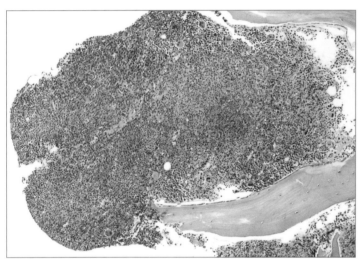

i11.17 *Bone marrow core biopsy specimen showing marked hypercellularity in a 23-year-old woman with myelokathexis. (H&E) (courtesy S Kroft, MD)*

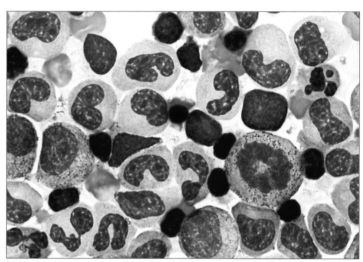

i11.18 *Bone marrow aspirate smear showing marked hypercellularity and right-shifted granulopoiesis in a patient with myelokathexis. (Wright) (courtesy S Kroft, MD)*

advantage upon those cells acquiring leukemogenic genetic or cytogenetic abnormalities [Welte 2009]. In contrast, cyclic neutropenia does not appear to share this significant risk of progression to MDS or AML [Dale 2003, Xia 2008]. Interestingly, even after achieving an adequate complement of neutrophils, patients are susceptible to infection and sepsis, suggesting that a subtle deficiency of neutrophilic function persists despite treatment-induced cellular maturation [Donini 2007].

[11.3.3]   **Myelokathexis and WHIM Syndrome**

In contrast to Shwachman-Diamond syndrome and the constitutional neutropenias, in which neutrophilic production is compromised, myelokathexis causes an inherited neutropenia in which granulocytic production and maturation remain intact. However, mature neutrophils are not released from the bone marrow (*kathexis* = retention).

Neutrophils are thus hypermature, with overly condensed nuclei and prominent nuclear irregularities, including degenerative changes such as nuclear fragmentation and "string" formation (ie, long thin strands of chromatin connecting nuclear lobes) **i11.15**, **i11.16**. Degenerative cytoplasmic vacuoles are also present. Those granulocytes that do not escape the bone marrow undergo intramedullary apoptosis. The bone marrow is hypercellular, with an accumulation of "right-shifted" mature granulocytes (again, in sharp contrast to the pattern seen in other constitutional neutropenias) **i11.17**, **i11.18**, **i11.19**, **i11.20**. Myelokathexis characteristically occurs as a component of WHIM syndrome (warts, hypogammaglobulinemia, infections, myelokathexis), which is caused by mutations in the gene encoding chemokine receptor *CXCR4* (an important regulator of neutrophil release

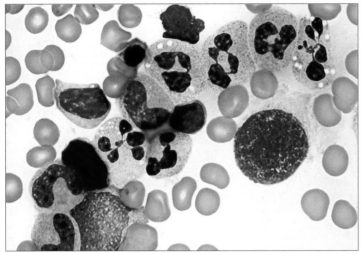

i11.19 *Bone marrow aspirate smear showing numerous neutrophils with thin internuclear filamentous strands in a patient with myelokathexis. (Wright) (courtesy S Kroft, MD)*

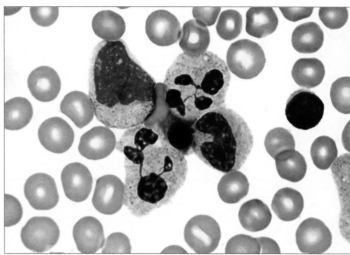

i11.20 *Thin filamentous internuclear strands within neutrophils in bone marrow aspirate smear from a patient with myelokathexis. (Wright) (courtesy S Kroft, MD)*

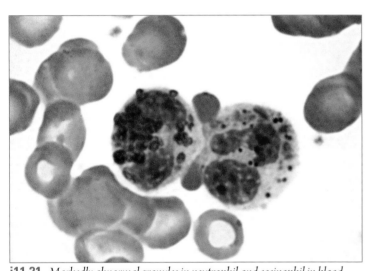

i11.21 *Markedly abnormal granules in neutrophil and eosinophil in blood smear from a patient with Chédiak-Higashi syndrome. (Wright) (courtesy P Izadi)*

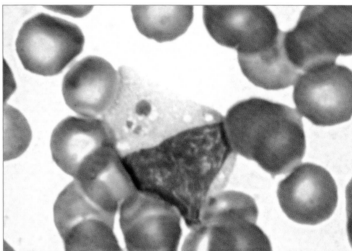

i11.22 *Enlarged granule in large granular lymphocyte in blood smear from a patient with Chédiak-Higashi syndrome. (Wright) (courtesy R Brynes, MD)*

from the bone marrow) or by dysfunction of its regulatory protein GRK3 [Balabanian 2008, Eash 2009].

[11.3.4] **Constitutional Neutropenia due to Intracellular Trafficking Abnormalities**

Constitutional neutropenia may also arise as part of a larger constellation of symptoms in the setting of abnormal intracellular trafficking. Some subtypes of Griscelli syndrome and Hermansky-Pudlak syndrome produce neutropenia in addition to T/NK-cell and platelet dysfunction, respectively. Chédiak-Higashi syndrome causes neutropenia via a similar trafficking defect, secondary to mutations in the *LYST* gene [Kaplan 2008]. Key features on examination of the peripheral smear, including abnormal inclusions in lymphocytes and neutrophils, aid in diagnosing the cause of neutropenia in this setting

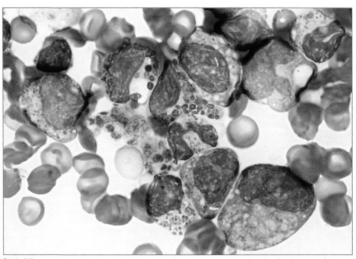

i11.23 *Bone marrow aspirate smear from a patient with Chédiak-Higashi syndrome showing abnormal granules in mature and immature myeloid cells. (Wright) (courtesy R Brynes, MD)*

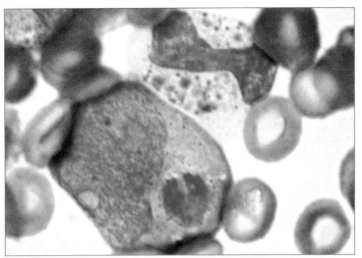

i11.24 *Immature myeloid cell with markedly enlarged abnormal granule in bone marrow aspirate smear from a patient with Chédiak-Higashi syndrome. (Wright) (courtesy R Brynes, MD)*

i11.21, i11.22. The bone marrow is typically hypercellular with strikingly abnormal granulation, even in nongranulocytic cells such as large granular lymphocytes i11.23, i11.24. In addition, the presence of systemic signs and symptoms, such as partial albinism, neurologic deficits, or abnormalities in other hematopoietic lineages, allow these syndromes to be distinguished from isolated constitutional neutropenia.

[11.3.5] **Constitutional Neutropenia Due to Miscellaneous Syndromes**

Inherited immunodeficiency syndromes such as hyper immunoglobulin (Ig) M syndrome and common variable immunodeficiency may also cause neutropenia, presumably through immune dysregulation and antibody-mediated destruction [Cham 2002]. Immunoglobulin subset analysis is often indicated in the workup of pediatric chronic neutropenia [James 2006]. Inherited neutropenia is also seen in Barth syndrome (an X-linked disorder of lipid metabolism) and glycogen storage disease type Ib [Dale 2009].

[11.4] **Neutropenia of Extrinsic Etiology**

In cases of neutropenia of extrinsic etiology, we must consider both initiating causes and proximate mechanisms. Drug-induced agranulocytosis, for example, is an initiating event that may occur via several subsequent mechanisms, including direct toxic insult from drug metabolites and immune-mediated processes. A complete description of a given case of neutropenia, then, would detail both the initiating causative event and the direct means by which the cytopenia is produced. As we will see, however, in many cases of neutropenia even extensive clinicopathologic correlation will fail to identify one or both of these elements. The relationship between direct mechanisms and ultimate causes of neutropenia is illustrated in t11.6, which can also serve as a quick reference for directed reading within this section.

[11.4.1] **General Morphologic Considerations in Neutropenia of Extrinsic Etiology**

Bone marrow morphologic findings are quite variable in cases of neutropenia and agranulocytosis, depending on the etiology and clinical setting t11.7. First, before one jumps to a consideration of the myeloid lineage, it is important to assess the specimen for the presence of dysplasia in all lineages and for increased numbers of lymphocytes i11.25. These findings would tend to implicate MDS and T-cell large granular lymphocytic (T-LGL) leukemia, respectively, in the etiology of the neutropenia. Cytogenetic analysis and

t11.6 Interplay between Initiating Causes (Left) and Direct Mechanisms (Top) of Neutropenia and Agranulocytosis of Secondary Etiology

	Toxic	Immune	Direct Infection of Progenitor	Increased Utilization	Passive Sequestration	Increased Margination	Cytokine Modulation	Direct Neutrophilic Activation	Inhibitor of Unclear Nature
Drug-induced	X	X							
Auto-immune		X			X		X	X	
Allo-immune		X							
Infection		X	X	X	X	X	X	X	
T-cell large granular lymphocytic leukemia		X				X	X	X	
Artificial membrane-induced (eg, dialysis)						X		X	
Neonates of hypertensive mother									X
Chronic idiopathic							X		

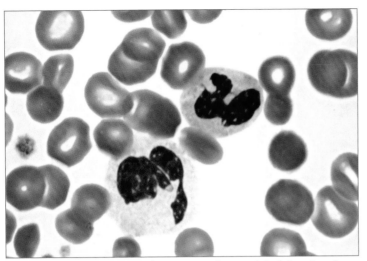

i11.25 *Peripheral blood smear showing normal neutrophil side by side with a hypogranular neutrophil in a patient with myelodysplasia. (Wright)*

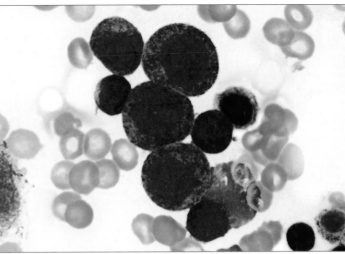

i11.26 *Bone marrow aspirate smear showing so-called maturation arrest at the myelocyte stage of maturation in the bone marrow aspirate smear from a patient with possible autoimmune neutropenia of infancy. (Wright)*

immunohistochemistry for CD34 and CD3 provide key support in the consideration of these processes.

In general, changes to the myeloid series in cases of neutropenia or agranulocytosis are quantitative rather than qualitative and depend on the mechanism of the insult to myelopoiesis. If there is a peripheral cause of neutropenia, including increased utilization, sequestration, or selective antibody-mediated destruction of mature granulocytes, then central myelopoiesis will remain intact and a compensatory myeloid hyperplasia will result. In contrast, if myelopoiesis itself is impaired, for example via

direct toxic effect, direct infection, or autoimmune attack on progenitor cells, then myeloid hypoplasia may be seen. In this situation, those precursors present may be limited to early stages of maturation, so that no maturation is detected past the promyelocyte or early myelocyte stage i11.26. This phenomenon has been labeled *maturation arrest*, but this term is to be discouraged because it may wrongly imply an intrinsic deficit in the ability of the cell to differentiate, as is seen in an acute leukemia. In fact, this appearance of arrested maturation indicates that the extrinsic pathologic mechanism at work

t11.7 Morphologic Approach to Isolated Neutropenia in Adults

Bone Marrow Morphology	Consider	Next Step
Increased lymphocytes/LGLs	T-LGL leukemia	Immunophenotyping for CD3, CD57, TIA-1
		Molecular clonality studies
Myeloid hypoplasia or aplasia	Drug toxicity / toxic insult	Correlate with drugs commonly implicated in neutropenia and agranulocytosis t11.9, p 222
	Autoimmune processes	Clinical correlation for symptoms
		Serology for rheumatoid factor, ANA
	Infection (with direct suppression of myeloid progenitors)	Clinical correlation
		Evaluate for toxic changes on peripheral smear
	Late onset of constitutional neutropenia	See t11.4 and t11.5
Myeloid hyperplasia	Infection (with peripheral destruction/ consumption of neutrophils)	Clinical correlation
		Evaluate for toxic changes on peripheral smear
	Altered distribution (especially splenomegaly)	Clinical correlation
	Autoimmune processes	Clinical correlation for symptoms
		Serology for rheumatoid factor, ANA
	Myelokathexis	Evaluate for cellular degenerative changes
		Assess for presence of warts and hypogammaglobulinemia (WHIM syndrome)

ANA = antinuclear antibodies; LGL = large granular lymphocytes; WHIM = warts, hypogammaglobulinemia, infections, myelokathexis

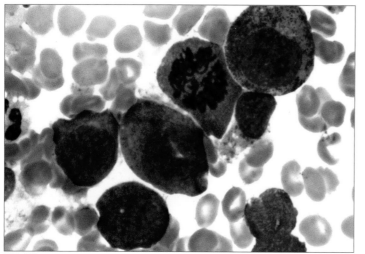

i11.27 *Prominent granulocyte colony-stimulating factor effect in bone marrow aspirate smear showing left shift, prominent Golgi, and prominent granulation. (Wright)*

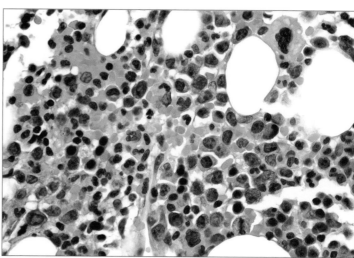

i11.28 *Bone marrow core biopsy section from a patient receiving granulocyte colony-stimulating factor treatment showing left shift of granulocytic lineage. (H&E)*

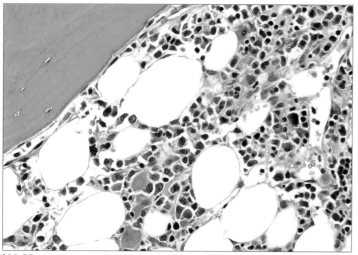

i11.29 *Bone marrow core biopsy specimen from a patient with diabetes mellitus (taking numerous medications) and agranulocytosis shows only paratrabecular immature granulocytic cells. (H&E)*

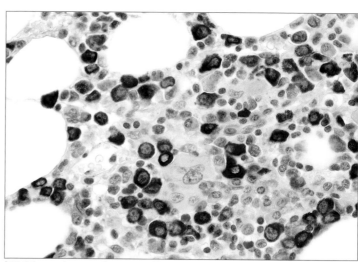

i11.30 *Myeloperoxidase stain of bone marrow core biopsy specimen showing immature granulocytic cells in a patient with diabetes mellitus with medication-induced agranulocytosis. (myeloperoxidase)*

is applicable to the more mature cells, which are either selectively destroyed or rapidly released into the blood.

The quantity of myeloid precursors can provide an important clue as to the mechanism (although not the ultimate cause) of the neutropenia. However, some caution should be used, because neutropenia and agranulocytosis are "moving targets" in terms of temporal evolution. For example, if there is an insult to myelopoiesis that decreases the number of granulocytic precursors, bone marrow examination at that moment would produce a hypoplastic picture. If, however, the causative agent is removed—for example, the discontinuation of the responsible drug—then a regenerative wave of myeloid maturation will occur, resulting in myeloid hyperplasia or a "pseudo-maturation arrest" picture.

G-CSF is often administered to patients with neutropenia, and it is critical to determine whether cytokine therapy has been initiated; this situation can cause significant diagnostic challenges because G-CSF treatment can create a wave of granulocytic production that might closely mimic a neoplastic process. Myeloid precursors under the influence of endogenous or exogenous G-CSF adopt a strikingly hypergranular appearance i11.27. This feature, combined with the absence of maturing granulocytes, may lead to a mistaken impression of involvement by acute promyelocytic leukemia i11.28. Morphologic distinction between these processes hinges on the realization that the hypergranular promyelocytes seen in severe neutropenia are normal in every respect other than granularity. In contrast, acute promyelocytic leukemia usually involves prominent nuclear abnormalities and cellular irregularities, including the presence of Auer rods.

Major Mechanisms of Extrinsic Neutropenia

Keeping in mind the difference between proximate mechanisms and initiating causes of secondary neutropenia, we will briefly consider the direct mechanisms by which extrinsic neutropenia and agranulocytosis may arise.

[sidebar 11.3] Neutrophilic Susceptibility to Drug Toxicity

Myeloperoxidase is a potent source of oxidative capacity in the neutrophil, and many drugs, in particular the primary arylamines, may be oxidized by MPO to form reactive metabolites and free radicals [Mason 1995, Uetrecht 1995a]. Many agranulocytosis-associated drugs have been shown to be metabolized in this manner, forming free radical metabolites that are either trapped by glutathione or form protein adducts with cellular constituents [Lai 1999, 2000, Liu 2000, Mason 1995, Parrish 1997, Uetrecht 1994, 1995b]. The connection between agranulocytosis and neutrophil-dependent drug metabolism has been most fully explored in the case of clozapine, the atypical antipsychotic drug associated with a significant incidence of agranulocytosis. Mass spectrometry shows that clozapine is metabolized by and covalently bound to neutrophils, a process that is abolished with increasing concentrations of glutathione [Frimat 1997, Liu 1995]. Neutrophils and granulocytic precursors incubated with clozapine show increased expression of apoptosis-associated proteins [Husain 2006, Loeffler 2003]. Intriguingly, neutrophils from subjects with a history of clozapine-induced agranulocytosis are more susceptible to toxicity than are neutrophils from normal controls and patients who have tolerated clozapine therapy [Tschen 1999].

This attractive hypothesis (ie, metabolism of certain drugs by MPO leads to free radical damage and apoptosis) likely explains only a portion of the drug toxicity that may lead to agranulocytosis. Indeed, the covalent modification of cellular components seems to alter the proteins sufficiently that they may, in some cases, become the target of immune attack. Some studies also implicate toxic damage to the bone marrow stromal environment as a potential mechanism of drug-induced agranulocytosis [Aizawa 1997, Guest 1999, Nabeshima 1997, Pereira 2006]. Rapidly proliferating granulocytes may also be especially susceptible to drugs that alter cellular metabolic and synthetic pathways. Thus, it would appear that different mechanisms of neutropenia may be at work in different patients, underscoring that the toxic effects of these drugs are diverse and complex in origin.

Unfortunately, these mechanisms of granulocytic toxicity do not explain the idiosyncratic nature of the phenomenon. In other words, why doesn't everyone who receives these drugs develop agranulocytosis in a predictable manner? Some evidence suggests that genetic polymorphisms may constrain the degree of neutropenia that an individual experiences in response to a common drug-related challenge. First, certain polymorphisms may influence baseline myelopoietic capacity. A multiethnic study recently found that a single nucleotide polymorphism (SNP) in the *ELANE* gene is associated with a significantly lower average ANC [Grann 2008a]. Second, the possession of specific HLA alleles may render some patients susceptible to drug-induced neutropenia via increased binding of drug-modified peptide fragments, as has been suggested in the cases of levamisole- and methimazole-induced agranulocytosis [Mosyagin 2004, Ostrousky 2003]. Third, SNPs in genes related to drug metabolism may either decrease the efficiency of drug clearance, thus augmenting the concentration of drug, or increase the efficiency of chemical modifications that produce metabolites associated with toxic damage [Mosyagin 2004, Ostrousky 2003]. Drug-induced agranulocytosis may therefore occur in a "multihit" process, requiring both a causative drug *and* a susceptible individual [Tesfa 2009].

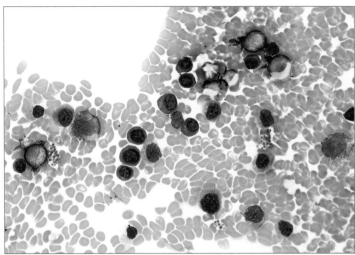

i11.31 *Bone marrow aspirate smear showing marked reduction in granulocytic cells and marked increase in plasma cells and immunoblasts in a patient developing agranulocytosis after illicit use of levamisole-tainted cocaine. (Wright)*

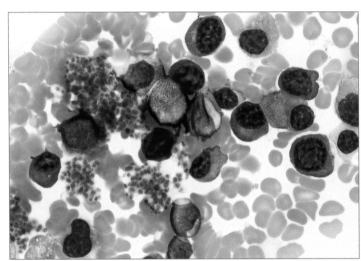

i11.32 *Bone marrow aspirate smear showing only rare granulocytic precursor and abundant plasma cells in a patient developing agranulocytosis after illicit use of levamisole-tainted cocaine. (Wright)*

Direct Granulocytic Toxicity

Certain drugs, especially those used for chemotherapeutic purposes, are reliably associated with secondary neutropenia and pancytopenia. These drugs act by suppressing global cellular functions, and therefore the effects are not specific to hematopoietic cells; however, the high rate of proliferation of bone marrow precursors renders these cells relatively susceptible **i11.29, i11.30**. These effects are, in most cases, logical and predictable and unlikely to generate clinical concern as to the origin of the neutropenia. More likely to cause concern is the idiosyncratic granulocytic toxicity that can develop unexpectedly during the course of therapy with certain drugs. In some cases, this granulocytic toxicity is secondary to myeloperoxidase-dependent metabolism of the drug to reactive intermediates **sidebar 11.3**.

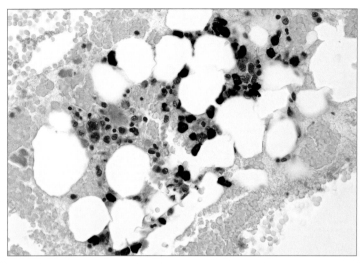

i11.33 *Myeloperoxidase stain of bone marrow clot section from a patient developing agranulocytosis secondary to illicit use of levamisole-tainted cocaine showing only isolated immature granulocytic cells. (myeloperoxidase)*

t11.8 Human Neutrophil Antigens (HNA), with Standardized Nomenclature

Antigen Group	CD Name	Antigen	Glycoprotein
HNA-1*	CD16b	HNA-1a	Fcγ receptor IIIb
		HNA-1b	
		HNA-1c	
HNA-2	CD177	HNA-2	NB1
HNA-3	–	HNA-3a	GP 70-95
HNA-4	CD11b	HNA-4a	MAC-1
HNA-5	CD11a	HNA-5a	LFA-1

*HNA-1 antibodies are the most frequently detected in neonatal alloimmune neutropenia, primary autoimmune neutropenia, and secondary autoimmune neutropenia; patients with primary autoimmune neutropenia often develop HNA-1a or 1b specificity, while secondary autoantibodies are more likely to be pan-HNA-1 reactive

References: [Berliner 2008, Bruin 1999, 2005, Bux 2008]

Antibody-Mediated Damage

Antineutrophil antibodies arise through processes broadly similar to those responsible for the generation of pathologic antibody responses in general [Capsoni 2005]. Alloimmune reactivity may develop after a transfusion or in the perinatal setting. Molecular mimicry subsequent to exposure to microbial antigens has been postulated. Antineutrophil antibodies are associated with systemic autoimmune syndromes, especially rheumatoid arthritis and systemic lupus erythematosus, and may also be seen in large granular lymphocytic leukemia.

Drug-initiated antibody responses occur via at least 3 mechanisms i11.31, i11.32, i11.33. First, the drug itself may act as a hapten, in which case antibodies bind to neutrophils only in the presence of the drug. This phenomenon has been described for aminopyrine, penicillin, and several antithyroid drugs [Watts 2009]. Second, circulating immune complexes, as seen in quinidine therapy, may be deposited on the neutrophil [Stroncek 1995]. Third, modification of self-antigens by drug exposure is thought to be a mechanism of drug-induced neutropenia [Siraki 2007, 2008].

Regardless of ultimate cause, these antineutrophil antibodies produce neutropenia by fixing complement and/or opsonizing the target cells for reticuloendothelial phagocytosis. It is noteworthy that some of the common antigen targets listed in t11.8 are also expressed on bone marrow granulocytic progenitors, thus rendering the central pool of maturing granulocytes susceptible to similar immune-mediated destruction [Harmon 1984]. Clinical testing for specific antineutrophil antibodies is discussed in sidebar 11.4.

Excessive Complement Activation

While most cases of immune-mediated neutropenia are antibody-dependent, excessive complement activity can

[sidebar 11.4] Antineutrophil Antibody Testing

While red blood cell antibodies are routinely identified in clinical practice, testing for antineutrophil antibodies is performed less frequently. Nevertheless, an understanding of the nature and the limitations of this esoteric assay becomes important when working up a case of neutropenia of unknown etiology, especially when primary autoimmune neutropenia is a diagnostic consideration. The granulocyte agglutination test (GAT) is analogous to the agglutination reactions universally used in red blood cell typing and blood banking, in which agglutination of the cells indicates the presence of antibody. The direct or indirect granulocyte immunofluorescence test (GIFT) uses fluorescently labeled antihuman IgG to detect the presence of antibodies bound to neutrophils; using serum samples of known specificity, neutrophils may also be "typed" by this method t11.8. In the monoclonal antibody-specific immobilization of granulocyte antigens test (MAIGA), monoclonal antibody to neutrophil-specific antigens allows purification on an affinity column or solid phase, after which the presence or absence of human antibody is determined [Berliner 2004]. In addition, direct immunofluorescence and flow cytometric techniques have been described [Lane 2008, Yamada 2002]. It should be noted that "antineutrophil antibodies" may sometimes be abbreviated as "ANA," a usage that can cause unfortunate confusion with "antinuclear antibodies," a separate and distinct entity.

While these tests are useful, there are several barriers to interpretation. In patients with very severe neutropenia or agranulocytosis, there may be too few circulating neutrophils on which to perform these tests, limiting their sensitivity. Neutrophils are notoriously fragile, and often aggregate spontaneously in vivo, again hindering the process. Perhaps most importantly, neutrophils may naturally bind antibody nonspecifically through their abundant Fc receptors, thus decreasing the specificity of the test. Similarly, the presence of immune complexes deposited on the surface of the neutrophil may cause a false-positive result. An understanding of these limitations is essential in the proper interpretation of these assays. In particular, repeat testing may be necessary to establish a definitive diagnosis [Capsoni 2005].

In contrast to testing for the antibodies in t11.8, investigation of antibodies directed at cytoplasmic neutrophilic antigens, such as c-ANCA and p-ANCA, is generally less useful, as the pathologic antibody recognition is occurring on the cell surface. Antinuclear antibodies and rheumatoid factor assays, however, can be extremely helpful. These tests will *not* detect potential surface neutrophil-specific antibodies, but they may aid in establishing a diagnosis of rheumatoid arthritis or systemic lupus erythematosus, 2 entities that are associated with secondary neutropenia.

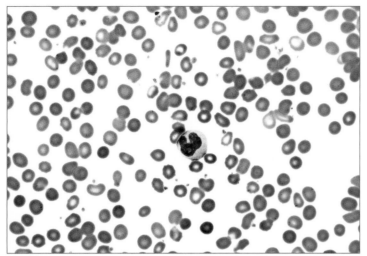

i11.34 *Peripheral blood smear in a patient with advanced AIDS showing severe neutropenia; the patient is receiving granulocyte colony-stimulating factor therapy. (Wright)*

i11.35 *Bone marrow core biopsy specimen showing abnormal megakaryocytes and reduced granulocytic lineage in a patient with advanced AIDS is receiving granulocyte colony-stimulating factor therapy. (H&E)*

itself cause neutropenia, largely via neutrophil aggregation and adherence to the endothelial surfaces, often in the pulmonary vasculature [Watts 2009]. This phenomenon is the central mechanism of neutropenia following exposure of blood to artificial membranes (eg, apheresis or hemodialysis) and may also contribute to neutropenia during anaphylaxis and septicemia [Bergh 1991, Watts 2009]. Streptokinase administration produces abrupt complement activation that may cause transient neutropenia [Frangi 1994].

Direct Infection of Progenitor Cells

Just as infection by parvovirus is an important cause of erythroblastopenia, direct infection of immature granulocytes can, in some cases, lead to impaired granulopoiesis. This is best described in the setting of cytomegalovirus (CMV) infection. CMV may directly infect and remain latent in progenitor cells, leading to suppression of myelopoiesis [Li 2007, Sindre 1996, Sing 1990]. Indeed, the myeloid-associated antigen CD13 appears to facilitate CMV binding and entry into the cell [Soderberg 1993]. Certain CMV genotypes are associated with increased severity of myelosuppression [Randolph-Habecker 2002]. Similarly, CMV may depress hematopoiesis by direct infection of stromal cells and alteration of the bone marrow microenvironment [Randolph-Habecker 2002, Simmons 1990].

The human immunodeficiency virus (HIV) often causes neutropenia via a multifactorial process that is thought to include direct progenitor cell infection i11.34, i11.35, i11.36. However, while CD34+ cells possess the necessary viral receptors and are indeed capable of viral infection [Sloand 2004], some evidence suggests that direct infection may not be the only mechanism of proliferative impairment and neutropenia [Molina 1990]. One study reports abnormal progenitor cell function in HIV– infants of HIV+ mothers,

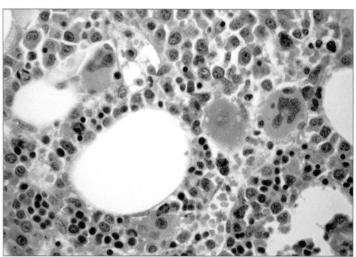

i11.36 *Bone marrow core biopsy specimen from a patient with advanced AIDS who is receiving granulocyte colony-stimulating factor therapy. The specimen shows increased CD34+ immature granulocytic cells. (immunoperoxidase for CD34)*

implying that direct infection is not necessary to adversely impact granulopoiesis [Nielsen 2001].

Epstein-Barr virus (EBV), hepatitis, and parvovirus can also produce direct progenitor cell infection and bone marrow suppression [Watts 2009]. While the effects are not typically limited to the granulocytic series, cases of isolated neutropenia or agranulocytosis have been described in association with these viruses [Barlow 2000, Brkic 1998, Honda 2000, Istomin 2004, Savard 2006, Sing 1993, Sumimoto 1990]. Other in vitro data suggest that the measles virus can directly infect early myelomonocytic progenitors [Helin 1999], but the clinical relevance of this finding is unclear.

Inflammatory Cytokines

Hematopoiesis is exquisitely sensitive to cytokine signaling, as detailed in Chapter 1, p 7. One mechanism of neutropenia, then, appears to be the production of particular cytokines in amounts sufficient to alter the kinetics of hematopoiesis. Altered production of cytokines (especially IFN-γ and TNF-α) may play a role in neutropenia due to infections, as well as in the nebulous entity of chronic idiopathic neutropenia discussed later. Conceptually, it seems counterintuitive that cytokines produced during inflammation would suppress hematopoiesis and therefore produce, by virtue of decreased granulocyte production, an immuno-compromised state. However, the effects of cytokines are pleiotropic by tissue type, and, in the context of the bone marrow microenvironment, these molecules are likely to be important inhibitors of proliferation that ensure orderly and regular maturation of progenitors [Selleri 1995, 1996]. It is only in pathologic states, for example, the presence of activated T-cells in the marrow or the development of significant distant inflammation, that these regulatory networks may become disturbed.

Increased Peripheral Demand or Altered Distribution

In contrast to the pathophysiologically complex mechanisms outlined previously, neutropenia may arise from a simple imbalance of supply and demand. Neutrophils may be physically consumed in the course of fighting infection, and may also adhere to endothelial surfaces that have been altered or damaged in the course of viral infection [Dale 2006]. The pulmonary microvasculature is an important site for normal neutrophilic margination [Doerschuk 1987], but systemic neutrophilic activation produces a dramatic increase in the number of neutrophils accumulating in this location (ie, the "marginating pool"), likely as a result of cytoskeletal alterations and decreased deformability of the activated neutrophils [Inano 1992, Yoshida 2006]. Thus, neutrophilic depletion from the circulation may be either a direct or indirect consequence of significant systemic inflammation.

Conditions that produce splenomegaly may result in splenic sequestration of neutrophils. Neutropenia in this setting is typically accompanied by thrombocytopenia and/or anemia.

[11.4.3] Major Initiating Causes of Extrinsic Neutropenia

Having considered the major mechanisms of secondary neutropenia, we may now turn to the initiating clinical causes, each of which may involve more than one mechanism. This concept is illustrated in t11.6, which also serves as a summary of this section.

Drug-Induced Neutropenia and Agranulocytosis

Beginning in 1931 with aminopyrine, an analgesic that was then contained in a number of patent medications, the roster of drugs associated with significant neutropenia and/

t11.9 Selected Drugs Frequently Implicated in Agranulocytosis (Excluding Chemotherapeutic Agents)*

Drug Class	Prominent Drugs Associated with Agranulocytosis
Analgesics	Dipyrone, ibuprofen
Antiarrythmics	Procainamide, quinidine
Antibiotics	Ampicillin, cefotaxime, oxacillin, penicillin G, quinine
Anticonvulsants	Phenytoin
Antirheumatics	Levamisole
Antithyroid drugs	Propylthiouracil
Gastrointestinal drugs	Cimetidine
Psychotropic drugs	Clozapine, chlorpromazine

*This is a selected list; well over 100 drugs have been linked to the development of neutropenia and/or agranulocytosis
For a complete list, the reader is referred to the comprehensive meta-analysis from which this table is adapted

Reference: [Andersohn 2007]

or agranulocytosis has steadily expanded. Well over 100 drugs currently in clinical use have been associated with neutropenia. However, drug-induced agranulocytosis is a rare and idiosyncratic event, making it challenging to document both its overall incidence and the drugs most commonly implicated. Population-based studies estimate the incidence of drug-induced agranulocytosis at roughly 3.5 cases per million, with a fatality rate of 7% [Ibanez 2005]. Males and females are equally affected, with a wide range of affected ages. The mean duration of neutropenia is 8 days, during which 68% of patients experience a localized or systemic infectious complication, followed by complete recovery in 86% of cases [Andersohn 2007]. There has been a significant decrease in the case fatality rate over the past 40 years in patients treated both with and without G-CSF, perhaps because of improved antibiotic coverage and intensive care support [Andersohn 2007]. The most frequently implicated drugs are listed in t11.9.

It is important to bear in mind that prescribed medications are not the only sources of drug exposure in patients. Unregulated alternative or herbal remedies may contain unadvertised compounds, and even illicit drugs may be contaminated with foreign substances [Behrman 2008]. Cocaine cut or contaminated with levamisole, for example, represents an underappreciated etiology of otherwise unexplained agranulocytosis i11.31, i11.32, i11.33 [Zhu 2009, Czuchlewski 2010].

Clinically, the level of myelosuppression induced by the drug may be quite variable. Certain drugs, such as clozapine, are so strongly associated with neutropenia that proactive monitoring of the ANC is standard of care during therapy. In these cases, the neutropenia may be moderate, but true

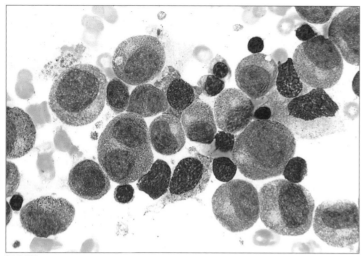

i11.37 *Bone marrow aspirate smear shows a prominent wave of promyelocytic regeneration during early recovery in a patient with drug-induced agranulocytosis. (Wright)*

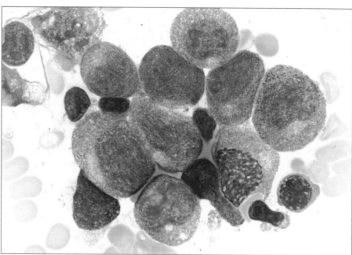

i11.38 *A pale paranuclear Golgi zone characterizes regenerating promyelocytes on this bone marrow aspirate smear (see **i11.37**). (Wright)*

agranulocytosis may also develop during therapy with these agents. Idiosyncratic reactions, on the other hand, tend to be associated with abrupt and dramatic clinical presentations of true agranulocytosis. It is tempting to speculate that these clinical differences might be manifestations of the different underlying mechanisms discussed earlier.

As a practical matter, it may be difficult to produce iron-clad proof that a given drug is responsible for a given case of neutropenia or agranulocytosis. There is often a significant time lag between initial administration of the drug and the decline in ANC, ranging from 19-60 days in most cases [Andersohn 2007]. The time lag upon reintroduction of the drug may be on the order of 6-12 weeks [Safferman 1992]. Curiously, the ANC occasionally shows a transient increase in the period immediately preceding agranulocytosis [Alvir 1995]. Thus, the temporal connection between drug administration and neutropenia may be obscure. Widespread polypharmacy, especially in older patients, can also complicate the investigation for the responsible agent. If a given drug is strongly suspected of causing a patient's neutropenia, then prudence dictates that the drug be discontinued or substituted, as clinically permissible. Even recovery of the ANC after such an action would provide only circumstantial evidence of causation **i11.37, i11.38, i11.39**. The presence of specific drug-dependent antibodies may definitively implicate a drug [Stroncek 1993], but these assays are not routinely performed.

Neutropenia and Autoimmune Disease

While immune-mediated destruction of granulocytes may play a role in neutropenia of many, if not most, clinical etiologies, it is most central to the pathogenesis of neutropenia in the setting of autoimmune disease.

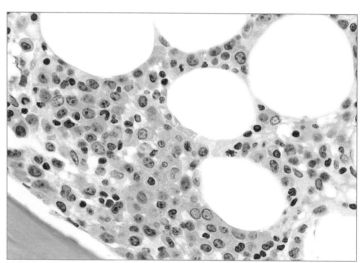

i11.39 *Bone marrow biopsy section from the same patient depicted in **i11.38** illustrates a broad paratrabecular cuff of immature granulocytic cells, which characterizes the early regeneration process; only sparse mature neutrophils are evident. (H&E)*

Primary autoimmune neutropenia. Primary autoimmune neutropenia (ie, neutropenia as the sole manifestation of autoimmunity) typically affects children and for this reason is also known as *autoimmune neutropenia of childhood, autoimmune neutropenia of infancy*, and, in light of its clinical course, *benign neutropenia of childhood*. In contrast, autoimmune neutropenia in adults arises almost exclusively in the setting of broad autoimmune syndromes such as systemic lupus erythematosus (SLE).

In primary autoimmune neutropenia, isolated moderate to severe neutropenia develops, typically between the ages of 5 and 15 months, and usually due to the presence of anti-HNA-1 antibodies **t11.8**, p 220 [Bruin 2005, Bux 1998]. The bone marrow in children with primary autoimmune neutropenia often shows granulocytic hyperplasia with intact maturation.

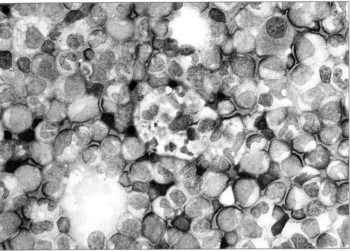

i11.40 *Bone marrow imprint smear shows striking granulocytic hyperplasia with intact maturation in a 7-month-old infant with autoimmune neutropenia of infancy. Although subtle, an increase in macrophages is also evident admixed with these granulocytic cells (see* i11.41*). (Wright)*

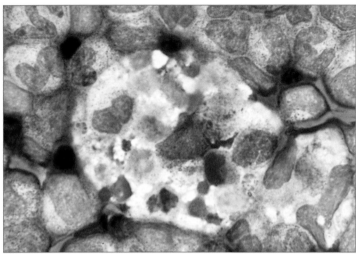

i11.41 *Pronounced phagocytosis of neutrophils by macrophages is evident on this imprint smear. The variable nuclear appearance of these ingested cells suggests that longstanding and ongoing neutrophil phagocytosis is a contributing cause of neutropenia in this infant (see* i11.40*). (Wright)*

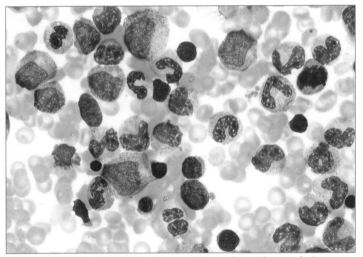

i11.42 *This aspirate smear illustrates granulocytic hyperplasia in the bone marrow of a neutropenic patient with Felty syndrome. Note intact maturation with mild left shift. (Wright)*

Ingestion of neutrophils by macrophages may be prominent i11.40, 11.41. The neutropenia undergoes spontaneous remission in almost all cases after 7-24 months, but the duration of neutropenia depends on the initial strength of the antibody response [Bux 1998, Kobayashi 2002]. Titers of antineutrophil antibodies often decrease in the period preceding recovery of the ANC [Lyall 1992]. Although infectious complications occur, these are usually less severe than might be expected for a given degree of neutropenia. Serious infections such as sepsis or meningitis occur in 12% of patients, and prophylactic antibiotics may be administered to further limit morbidity [Bruin 2005, Capsoni 2005]. Given that syndromes of inherited neutropenia are an important element of the differential diagnosis in these cases, confirmatory testing for antineutrophil antibodies should be strongly considered (see **sidebar 11.4**, p 220).

Secondary autoimmune neutropenia. In contrast to the unique clinical features of primary autoimmune neutropenia, neutropenia in the setting of other autoimmune disorders (ie, secondary autoimmune neutropenia) is nonspecific and likely multifactorial in etiology.

Neutropenia may develop during the course of rheumatoid arthritis, often due to Felty syndrome and/or LGL leukemia ("T-LGL Leukemia–Associated Neutropenia," p 226, and Volume 2, Chapters 21 and 33) i11.42. While antineutrophil antibodies may be present, passive immune complex deposition, splenomegaly, and the production of inflammatory cytokines that inhibit granulopoiesis are also thought to contribute to rheumatoid arthritis-associated neutropenia [Berliner 2004]. Given the strong association of rheumatoid arthritis, neutropenia, and T-LGL leukemia, careful assessment of LGL numbers and clonality should always be considered in the neutropenic patient with rheumatoid arthritis.

Neutropenia is seen in up to half of all patients with SLE and antineutrophil antibodies play an important role, likely affecting both peripheral neutrophils and maturing granulocytic precursors [Berliner 2004]. SLE-associated antineutrophil antibodies are heterogeneous in specificity [Chen 2004].

Alloimmune Neutropenia

Neonatal alloimmune neutropenia is analogous in mechanism to hemolytic disease of the newborn and neonatal alloimmune thrombocytopenia. Fetal neutrophils cross the placenta, eliciting production of maternal antibodies to unfamiliar paternally-derived neutrophil antigens. These antibodies then cross the placenta and effect neutropenia

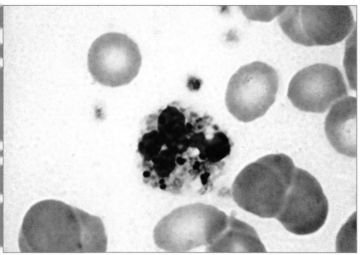

i11.43 *Peripheral blood smear showing rare neutrophil with ingested bacteria in septic, neutropenic patient. (Wright)*

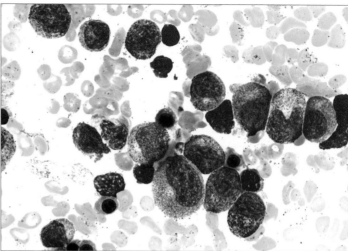

i11.44 *Bone marrow aspirate smear showing left-shifted granulopoiesis in patient with T-cell large granular lymphocytic leukemia and associated neutropenia. (Wright)*

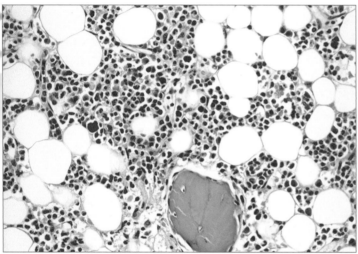

i11.45 *Bone marrow core biopsy section from a patient with left-shifted granulopoiesis and T-cell large granular lymphocytic leukemia–associated neutropenia. (H&E)*

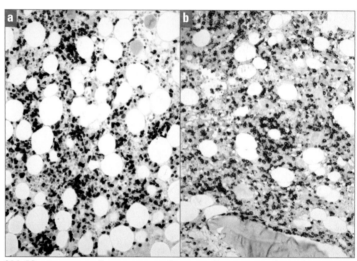

i11.46 *Composite of immunoperoxidase stains for CD3 **a** and CD8 **b** in a patient with T-cell large granular lymphocytic leukemia with associated left-shifted granulopoiesis and neutropenia. (immunoperoxidase for CD3 and CD8)*

during fetal development and early infancy. Neonatal alloimmune neutropenia may occur during a first pregnancy [Fung 2003]. The degree of neutropenia varies, and G-CSF administration may be necessary in severe cases [Gilmore 1994]. Neutrophil counts normalize by 11 weeks on average, as fetal levels of maternal IgG wane [Berliner 2004].

Infection-Associated Neutropenia

While drug-induced neutropenia dominates the differential diagnosis in adults with isolated neutropenia, infection is a more frequent cause of neutropenia in children. However, infection may produce neutropenia at any age. The mechanisms by which this occurs include direct viral infection of progenitor cells, increased utilization of neutrophils at the site of infection, sequestration due to splenomegaly or generalized neutrophilic activation,

increased binding of neutrophils to infected or altered endothelial cells, immune attack via molecular mimicry of foreign antigens, the production of bone marrow suppressive inflammatory cytokines, and even hemophagocytosis due to systemic macrophage activation (see **t11.6**, p 216). Infection by virtually any organism can produce neutropenia by some combination of these mechanisms. However, transient neutropenia in children is consistently produced by viral infections, including nonspecific viral gastroenteritis and respiratory tract infections [Phillips 1992].

Neutropenia in this setting is mild and usually clinically inconsequential. In contrast, more severe and prolonged neutropenia is typically seen in the uncommon instances in which progenitor cell capacity is directly affected, by either direct infection or the production of cross-reactive antibodies.

If a bacterial infection develops in a patient subsequently diagnosed with severe neutropenia or agranulocytosis, consideration should be given to the possibility that the infection is not the primary cause of the neutropenia, but rather the consequence of neutropenia due to other etiologies. This relationship may be difficult to sort out, but as a general rule, bacterial infections *may* cause neutropenia, but severe neutropenia *often* causes severe bacterial infections (especially involving skin, oropharynx, or the perirectal soft tissue) i11.43.

T-LGL Leukemia–Associated Neutropenia

Although often implicated in rheumatoid arthritis–associated neutropenia, T-LGL leukemia may also develop independent of any rheumatologic condition i11.44, i11.45, i11.46. T-LGL leukemia and its related entity, Felty syndrome, are described in detail in Chapters 21 and 33. At least 3 main mechanisms of neutropenia have been postulated or demonstrated in T-LGL leukemia. First, antineutrophil antibodies may be produced, in particular against the eukaryotic elongation factor-1A-1 (eEF1A-1) [Ditzel 2000]. Second, immune complexes are consistently present in Felty syndrome, and when deposited on neutrophils, the cells may undergo apoptosis or become activated, which increases their tendency to marginate [Berliner 2004]. Finally, clonal T-LGLs constitutively express Fas ligand, an apoptosis-inducing molecule that is normally expressed by T-LGLs only upon activation. Neutrophils express substantial amounts of Fas (CD95), the receptor for Fas that triggers apoptosis upon binding of Fas ligand [Liles 1996]. Thus, increased availability of Fas ligand, whether directly on the surface of the T-LGLs or cleaved into the circulation from the surface of these cells, appears to be a major factor in T-LGL leukemia-associated neutropenia [Liu 2000].

Nonimmune Chronic Idiopathic Neutropenia

In some cases of chronic neutropenia in adults, no initiating cause can be identified. Nonimmune chronic idiopathic neutropenia is a diagnosis of exclusion and is rendered only in the absence of therapy with suspect drugs, antineutrophil antibodies, systemic autoimmune phenomena, infection, nutritional deficiency, myelodysplasia, and T-LGL leukemia. The pathogenesis of neutropenia in these cases is unclear. Significant alterations in cytokine levels at the level of the bone marrow microenvironment may lead to increased apoptosis of granulocytic precursors, but the ultimate cause of these changes remains unexplained [Palmblad 2008, Pyrovolaki 2007].

Miscellaneous Causes of Neutropenia

The categories listed herein encompass the vast majority of cases of neutropenia. Rare miscellaneous etiologies have also been described, but these are less likely to be encountered in practice. Newborns of hypertensive (and/or preeclamptic) mothers show prolonged neutropenia of unknown etiology that places them at increased risk for infection [Gray 1999]. Neutropenia in this setting appears to arise due to a placentally derived inhibitor of G-CSF that is present in cord blood, but the exact identity or nature of this substance is unknown [Guner 2007, Koenig 1991, Zuppa 2002]. Exposure of blood to artificial membranes, as occurs in apheresis, heart-lung bypass and dialysis, may activate complement and lead to increased margination in the pulmonary vasculature [Watts 2009], as described earlier.

[11.5] Clues and Caveats

1. Neutropenia may be intrinsic or extrinsic in etiology.
2. Extrinsic neutropenia is substantially more common than intrinsic neutropenia in all age groups.
3. Most cases of intrinsic neutropenia arise from heritable constitutional neutropenia syndromes.
4. Shwachman-Diamond syndrome (*SBDS* mutation) and severe constitutional neutropenia/cyclic neutropenia (usually *ELANE* mutation) are classic causes of intrinsic neutropenia.
5. Primary autoimmune neutropenia and neonatal alloimmune neutropenia are unique extrinsic neutropenias of childhood.
6. Secondary neutropenia and agranulocytosis may arise through multiple direct mechanisms, singly or in combination.
7. Mechanisms may be shared by dissimilar initiating causes of neutropenia.
8. T-LGL leukemia and MDS should be ruled out in every case of unexplained neutropenia.
9. Neutropenia in children is often secondary to infection, while in adults it is often drug induced.
10. Many drugs have been associated with the development of neutropenia and/or agranulocytosis. If a neutropenic patient is taking such a drug, it should be stopped or substituted, if clinically feasible.
11. While investigation of systemic infection is best carried out by the clinician, the pathologist may consider immunohistochemical and in situ hybridization techniques to evaluate for viral infection in the marrow.
12. Physical examination and laboratory investigation should be undertaken to investigate possible systemic autoimmune syndromes.
13. Specialized testing for the presence of specific antineutrophil antibodies is available and can be used to investigate possible primary or secondary autoimmune etiologies of neutropenia.

14. If a reactive neutropenia resolves, then it is almost certainly due to a transient insult to myelopoiesis such as drug toxicity or infection. If it lingers or recurs, then immune-mediated mechanisms become more likely.

15. In general, myeloid hyperplasia in the setting of neutropenia indicates a peripheral survival or distribution defect, while myeloid hypoplasia implicates impaired production.

16. Supportive care of the severely neutropenic patient, including prophylactic broad-spectrum antibiotics, is essential in reducing morbidity and mortality.

17. G-CSF therapy often successfully increases the ANC, regardless of the etiology of neutropenia.

[11.6] References

Aizawa S, Nakano M, Yaguchi M, et al [1997] Possible involvement of bone marrow stromal cells in agranulocytosis caused by vesnarinone treatment. *Acta Haematol* 98:140-146.

Alter BP [2007] Diagnosis, genetics, and management of inherited bone marrow failure syndromes. *Hematology (Am Soc Hematol Educ Program)* 2007:29-39.

Alvir JM, Lieberman JA, Safferman AZ [1995] Do white-cell count spikes predict agranulocytosis in clozapine recipients? *Psychopharmacol Bull* 31:311-314.

Ancliff PJ, Gale RE, Liesner R, et al [2003] Long-term follow-up of granulocyte colony-stimulating factor receptor mutations in patients with severe constitutional neutropenia:implications for leukaemogenesis and therapy. *Br J Haematol* 120:685-690.

Andersohn F, Konzen C, Garbe E [2007] Systematic review: Agranulocytosis induced by nonchemotherapy drugs. *Ann Intern Med* 146:657-665.

Austin KM, Leary RJ, Shimamura A [2005] The Shwachman-Diamond SBDS protein localizes to the nucleolus. *Blood* 106:1253-1258.

Austin KM, Gupta ML, Coats SA, et al [2008] Mitotic spindle destabilization and genomic instability in Shwachman-Diamond syndrome. *J Clin Invest* 118:1511-1518.

Balabanian K, Lagane B, Pablos JL, et al [2005] WHIM syndromes with different genetic anomalies are accounted for by impaired CXCR4 desensitization to CXCL12. *Blood* 105:2449-2457.

Balabanian K, Levoye A, Klemm L, et al [2008] Leukocyte analysis from WHIM syndrome patients reveals a pivotal role for GRK3 in CXCR4 signaling. *J Clin Invest* 118:1074-1084.

Barlow GD, McKendrick MW [2000] Parvovirus B19 causing leucopenia and neutropenia in a healthy adult. *J Infect* 40:192-195.

Behrman AD [2008] Luck of the draw: common adulterants found in illicit drugs. *J Emerg Nurs* 34:80-82.

Belaaouaj A, McCarthy R, Baumann M, et al [1998] Mice lacking neutrophil elastase reveal impaired host defense against gram-negative bacterial sepsis. *Nat Med* 4:615-618.

Bellanne-Chantelot C, Clauin S, Leblanc T, et al [2004] Mutations in the *ELA2* gene correlate with more severe expression of neutropenia: a study of 81 patients from the French Neutropenia Register. *Blood* 103:4119-4125.

Bergh K, Olsen PO, Halgunset J, Iversen OJ [1991] Complement activation and pulmonary dysfunction in experimental *Escherichia coli* septicaemia. *Acta Anaesthesiol Scand* 35:267-274.

Berliner N [2008] Lessons from constitutional neutropenia: 50 years of progress in understanding myelopoiesis. *Blood* 111:5427-5432.

Berliner N, Horwitz M, Loughran TP, Jr [2004] Constitutional and acquired neutropenia. *Hematology (Am Soc Hematol Educ Program)* 2004:63-79.

Bohn G, Welte K, Klein C [2007] Severe constitutional neutropenia: new genes explain an old disease. *Curr Opin Rheumatol* 19:644-650.

Boocock GR, Morrison JA, Popovic M, et al [2003] Mutations in SBDS are associated with Shwachman-Diamond syndrome. *Nat Genet* 33:97-101.

Brkic S, Aleksic-Dordevic M, Belic A, et al [1998] Agranulocytosis as a complication of acute infectious mononucleosis. *Med Pregl* 51:355-358.

Bruin M, Dassen A, Pajkrt D, et al [2005] Primary autoimmune neutropenia in children: a study of neutrophil antibodies and clinical course. *Vox Sang* 88:52-59.

Bruin MC, von dem Borne AE, Tamminga RY, et al [1999] Neutrophil antibody specificity in different types of childhood autoimmune neutropenia. *Blood* 94:1797-1802.

Burroughs L, Woolfrey A, Shimamura A [2009] Shwachman-Diamond syndrome: a review of the clinical presentation, molecular pathogenesis, diagnosis, and treatment. *Hematol Oncol Clin North Am* 23:233-248.

Bux J [2008] Human neutrophil alloantigens. *Vox Sang* 94:277-285.

Bux J, Behrens G, Jaeger G, Welte K [1998] Diagnosis and clinical course of autoimmune neutropenia in infancy: analysis of 240 cases. *Blood* 91:181-186.

Capsoni F, Sarzi-Puttini P, Zanella A [2005] Primary and secondary autoimmune neutropenia. *Arthritis Res Ther* 7:208-214.

Cham B, Bonilla MA, Winkelstein J [2002] Neutropenia associated with primary immunodeficiency syndromes. *Semin Hematol* 39:107-112.

Chen M, Zhao MH, Zhang Y, Wang H [2004] Antineutrophil autoantibodies and their target antigens in systemic lupus erythematosus. *Lupus* 13:584-589.

Czuchlewski DR, Brackney M, Ewers C, et al [2010] Clinicopathologic features of agranulocytosis in the setting of levamisole-tainted cocaine. *Am J Clin Pathol* 133:466-472.

Dale D [2006] Neutropenia and neutrophilia. In: Lictman M, Beutler E, Kipps T, et al, eds. *Williams Hematology.* 7th ed. New York: McGraw; 823-834.

Dale DC, Cottle TE, Fier CJ, et al [2003] Severe chronic neutropenia: Treatment and follow-up of patients in the Severe Chronic Neutropenia International Registry. *Am J Hematol* 72:82-93.

Dale DC, Link DC [2009] The many causes of severe constitutional neutropenia. *N Engl J Med* 360:3-5.

Ditzel HJ, Masaki Y, Nielsen H, et al [2000] Cloning and expression of a novel human antibody-antigen pair associated with Felty's syndrome. *Proc Natl Acad Sci USA* 97:9234-9239.

Doerschuk CM, Allard MF, Martin BA, et al [1987] Marginated pool of neutrophils in rabbit lungs. *J Appl Physiol* 63:1806-1815.

Dokal I, Vulliamy T [2008] Inherited aplastic anaemias/bone marrow failure syndromes. *Blood Rev* 22:141-153.

Donadieu J, Leblanc T, Bader Meunier B, et al [2005] Analysis of risk factors for myelodysplasias, leukemias, and death from infection among patients with constitutional neutropenia. Experience of the French Severe Chronic Neutropenia Study Group. *Haematologica* 90:45-53.

Donini M, Fontana S, Savoldi G, et al [2007] G-CSF treatment of severe constitutional neutropenia reverses neutropenia but does not correct the underlying functional deficiency of the neutrophil in defending against microorganisms. *Blood* 109:4716-4723.

Dror Y [2005] Shwachman-Diamond syndrome. *Pediatr Blood Cancer* 45:892-901.

Dror Y, Durie P, Ginzberg H, et al [2002] Clonal evolution in marrows of patients with Shwachman-Diamond syndrome: a prospective 5-year follow-up study. *Exp Hematol* 30:659-669.

Eash KJ, Means JM, White DW, Link DC [2009] CXCR4 is a key regulator of neutrophil release from the bone marrow under basal and stress granulopoiesis conditions. *Blood* 113:4711-4719.

Foucar K, Viswanatha D, Wilson C [2008] Bone marrow failure disorders. In: King D, Gardner W, Sobin L, et al, eds. *Non-Neoplastic Disorders of Bone Marrow (AFIP fascicle).* Washington, DC: American Registry of Pathology; 221-248.

Frangi D, Gardinali M, Conciato L, et al [1994] Abrupt complement activation and transient neutropenia in patients with acute myocardial infarction treated with streptokinase. *Circulation* 89:76-80.

Frimat B, Gressier B, Odou P, et al [1997] Metabolism of clozapine by human neutrophils: evidence for a specific oxidation of clozapine by the myeloperoxidase system with inhibition of enzymatic chlorination cycle. *Fundam Clin Pharmacol* 11:267-274.

Fung YL, Pitcher LA, Willett JE, et al [2003] Alloimmune neonatal neutropenia linked to anti-HNA-4a. *Transfus Med* 13:49-52.

Ganapathi KA, Austin KM, Lee CS, et al [2007] The human Shwachman-Diamond syndrome protein, SBDS, associates with ribosomal RNA. *Blood* 110:1458-1465.

Geaghan S [2008] Normal blood values: Selected health-associated values for neonatal, pediatric, and adult populations. In: Greer JP, Foerster J, Rodgers G, et al, eds. *Wintrobe's Clinical Hematology*. 12th ed. Philadelphia: Lippincott Williams & Wilkins; 2584-2594.

Germeshausen M, Grudzien M, Zeidler C, et al [2008] Novel HAX1 mutations in patients with severe constitutional neutropenia reveal isoform-dependent genotype-phenotype associations. *Blood* 111:4954-4957.

Gilmore MM, Stroncek DF, Korones DN [1994] Treatment of alloimmune neonatal neutropenia with granulocyte colony-stimulating factor. *J Pediatr* 125:948-951.

Grann VR, Bowman N, Joseph C, et al [2008a] Neutropenia in 6 ethnic groups from the Caribbean and the U.S. *Cancer* 113:854-860.

Grann VR, Ziv E, Joseph CK, et al [2008b] Duffy (Fy), DARC, and neutropenia among women from the United States, Europe and the Caribbean. *Br J Haematol* 143:288-293.

Gray PH, Rodwell RL [1999] Neonatal neutropenia associated with maternal hypertension poses a risk for nosocomial infection. *Eur J Pediatr* 158:71-73.

Grenda DS, Murakami M, Ghatak J, et al [2007] Mutations of the ELA2 gene found in patients with severe constitutional neutropenia induce the unfolded protein response and cellular apoptosis. *Blood* 110:4179-4187.

Guest I, Uetrecht J [1999] Drugs that induce neutropenia/agranulocytosis may target specific components of the stromal cell extracellular matrix. *Med Hypotheses* 53:145-151.

Guner S, Yigit S, Cetin M, et al [2007] Evaluation of serum granulocyte colony-stimulating factor levels in infants of preeclamptic mothers. *Turk J Pediatr* 49:55-60.

Harmon DC, Weitzman SA, Stossel TP [1984] The severity of immune neutropenia correlates with the maturational specificity of antineutrophil antibodies. *Br J Haematol* 58:209-215.

Helin E, Salmi AA, Vanharanta R, Vainionpaa [1999] Measles virus replication in cells of myelomonocytic lineage is dependent on cellular differentiation stage. *Virology* 253:35-42.

Hershman D, Weinberg M, Rosner Z, et al [2003] Ethnic neutropenia and treatment delay in African American women undergoing chemotherapy for early-stage breast cancer. *J Natl Cancer Inst* 95:1545-1548.

Honda K, Ishiko O, Tsujimura A, et al [2000] Neutropenia accompanying parvovirus B19 infection after gynecologic surgery. *Acta Haematol* 103:186-190.

Horwitz MS, Duan Z, Korkmaz B, et al [2007] Neutrophil elastase in cyclic and severe constitutional neutropenia. *Blood* 109:1817-1824.

Hsieh MM, Everhart JE, Byrd-Holt DD, et al [2007] Prevalence of neutropenia in the U.S. population: age, sex, smoking status, and ethnic differences. *Ann Intern Med* 146:486-492.

Husain Z, Almeciga I, Delgado JC, et al [2006] Increased FasL expression correlates with apoptotic changes in granulocytes cultured with oxidized clozapine. *Toxicol Appl Pharmacol* 214:326-334.

Ibanez L, Vidal X, Ballarin E, Laporte JR [2005] Population-based drug-induced agranulocytosis. *Arch Intern Med* 165:869-874.

Inano H, English D, Doerschuk CM [1992] Effect of zymosan-activated plasma on the deformability of rabbit polymorphonuclear leukocytes. *J Appl Physiol* 73:1370-1376.

Istomin V, Sade E, Grossman Z, et al [2004] Agranulocytosis associated with parvovirus B19 infection in otherwise healthy patients. *Eur J Intern Med* 15:531-533.

James RM, Kinsey SE [2006] The investigation and management of chronic neutropenia in children. *Arch Dis Child* 91:852-858.

Kaplan J, De Domenico I, Ward DM [2008] Chédiak-Higashi syndrome. *Curr Opin Hematol* 15:22-29.

Kazanjian A, Gross EA, Grimes HL [2006] The growth factor independence-1 transcription factor: new functions and new insights. *Crit Rev Oncol Hematol* 59:85-97.

Kelly DL, Kreyenbuhl J, Dixon L, et al [2007] Clozapine underutilization and discontinuation in African Americans due to leucopenia. *Schizophr Bull* 33:1221-1224.

Kobayashi M, Nakamura K, Kawaguchi H, et al [2002] Significance of the detection of antineutrophil antibodies in children with chronic neutropenia. *Blood* 99:3468-3471.

Koenig JM, Christensen RD [1991] The mechanism responsible for diminished neutrophil production in neonates delivered of women with pregnancy-induced hypertension. *Am J Obstet Gynecol* 165:467-473.

Lai WG, Gardner I, Zahid N, Uetrecht JP [2000] Bioactivation and covalent binding of hydroxyfluperlapine in human neutrophils: implications for fluperlapine-induced agranulocytosis. *Drug Metab Dispos* 28:255-263.

Lai WG, Zahid N, Uetrecht JP [1999] Metabolism of trimethoprim to a reactive iminoquinone methide by activated human neutrophils and hepatic microsomes. *J Pharmacol Exp Ther* 291:292-299.

Lane SW, Hassell P, Kennedy GA, et al [2008] Characterization of the bone marrow immunofluorescence test in childhood autoimmune neutropenia. *Int J Lab Hematol* 31:567-571.

Lehmann H, Henry J [2007] SI units. In: McPherson R, Pincus M, eds. *Henry's Clinical Diagnosis and Management by Laboratory Methods*. 21st ed. Philadelphia: Saunders Elsvier; 1404-1418.

Li XF, Wang QW, He ZX, et al [2007] Human cytomegalovirus induces apoptosis of human promyelocytic leukemic cells via direct infection in vitro. *Zhongguo Shi Yan Xue Ye Xue Za Zhi* 15:63-66.

Liles WC, Kiener PA, Ledbetter JA, et al [1996] Differential expression of Fas (CD95) and Fas ligand on normal human phagocytes: implications for the regulation of apoptosis in neutrophils. *J Exp Med* 184:429-440.

Liu ZC, Uetrecht JP [1995] Clozapine is oxidized by activated human neutrophils to a reactive nitrenium ion that irreversibly binds to the cells. *J Pharmacol Exp Ther* 275:1476-1483.

Liu ZC, Uetrecht JP [2000] Metabolism of ticlopidine by activated neutrophils: implications for ticlopidine-induced agranulocytosis. *Drug Metab Dispos* 28:726-730.

Loeffler S, Fehsel K, Henning U, et al [2003] Increased apoptosis of neutrophils in a case of clozapine-induced agranulocytosis: a case report. *Pharmacopsychiatry* 36:37-41.

Lyall EG, Lucas GF, Eden OB [1992] Autoimmune neutropenia of infancy. *J Clin Pathol* 45:431-434.

Mason DY, Cordell JL, Brown MH, et al [1995] CD79a: a novel marker for B-cell neoplasms in routinely processed tissue samples. *Blood* 86:1453-1459.

Maserati E, Pressato B, Valli R, et al [2009] The route to development of myelodysplastic syndrome/acute myeloid leukaemia in Shwachman-Diamond syndrome: the role of ageing, karyotype instability, and acquired chromosome anomalies. *Br J Haematol* 145:190-197.

Mayr FB, Spiel AO, Leitner JM, et al [2007] Ethnic differences in plasma levels of interleukin-8 (IL-8) and granulocyte colony-stimulating factor (G-CSF). *Transl Res* 149:10-14.

Menne TF, Goyenechea B, Sanchez-Puig N, et al [2007] The Shwachman-Bodian-Diamond syndrome protein mediates translational activation of ribosomes in yeast. *Nat Genet* 39:486-495.

Molina JM, Scadden DT, Sakaguchi M, et al [1990] Lack of evidence for infection of or effect on growth of hematopoietic progenitor cells after in vivo or in vitro exposure to human immunodeficiency virus. *Blood* 76:2476-2482.

Mosyagin I, Dettling M, Roots I, et al [2004] Impact of myeloperoxidase and NADPH-oxidase polymorphisms in drug-induced agranulocytosis. *J Clin Psychopharmacol* 24:613-617.

Nabeshima R, Aizawa S, Nakano M, et al [1997] Effects of vesnarinone on the bone marrow stromal cell-dependent proliferation and differentiation of HL60 cells in vitro. *Exp Hematol* 25:509-515.

Nakashima E, Mabuchi A, Makita Y, et al [2004] Novel SBDS mutations caused by gene conversion in Japanese patients with Shwachman-Diamond syndrome. *Hum Genet* 114:345-348.

Nielsen SD, Jeppesen DL, Kolte L, et al [2001] Impaired progenitor cell function in HIV-negative infants of HIV-positive mothers results in decreased thymic output and low CD4 counts. *Blood* 98:398-404.

Ostrousky O, Meged S, Loewenthal R, et al [2003] NQO2 gene is associated with clozapine-induced agranulocytosis. *Tissue Antigens* 62:483-491.

Palmblad J, Papadaki HA [2008] Chronic idiopathic neutropenias and severe constitutional neutropenia. *Curr Opin Hematol* 15:8-14.

Parrish DD, Schlosser MJ, Kapeghian JC, Traina VM [1997] Activation of CGS 12094 (prinomide metabolite) to 1,4-benzoquinone by myeloperoxidase: implications for human idiosyncratic agranulocytosis. *Fundam Appl Toxicol* 35:197-204.

Pereira A, Dean B [2006] Clozapine bioactivation induces dose-dependent, drug-specific toxicity of human bone marrow stromal cells: a potential in vitro system for the study of agranulocytosis. *Biochem Pharmacol* 72:783-793.

Phillips AD, Shah AR, Walker-Smith JA [1992] Neutrophil response to mucosal infection. *J Med Microbiol* 36:318-320.

Pyrovolaki K, Mavroudi I, Papadantonakis N, et al [2007] Transforming growth factor-beta1 affects interleukin-10 production in the bone marrow of patients with chronic idiopathic neutropenia. *Eur J Haematol* 79:531-538.

Randolph-Habecker J, Iwata M, Torok-Storb B [2002] Cytomegalovirus mediated myelosuppression. *J Clin Virol* 25 Suppl 2:S51-56.

Rezvani K, Flanagan AM, Sarma U, et al [2001] Investigation of ethnic neutropenia by assessment of bone marrow colony-forming cells. *Acta Haematol* 105:32-37.

Rosenberg PS, Alter BP, Bolyard AA, et al [2006] The incidence of leukemia and mortality from sepsis in patients with severe constitutional neutropenia receiving long-term G-CSF therapy. *Blood* 107:4628-4635.

Ruggiero C, Metter EJ, Cherubini A, et al [2007] White blood cell count and mortality in the Baltimore Longitudinal Study of Aging. *J Am Coll Cardiol* 49:1841-1850.

Safferman AZ, Lieberman JA, Alvir JM, Howard A [1992] Rechallenge in clozapine-induced agranulocytosis. *Lancet* 339:1296-1297.

Savard M, Gosselin J [2006] Epstein-Barr virus immunossuppression of innate immunity mediated by phagocytes. *Virus Res* 119:134-145.

Selleri C, Maciejewski JP, Sato T, Young NS [1996] Interferon-gamma constitutively expressed in the stromal microenvironment of human marrow cultures mediates potent hematopoietic inhibition. *Blood* 87:4149-4157.

Selleri C, Sato T, Anderson S, et al [1995] Interferon-gamma and tumor necrosis factor-alpha suppress both early and late stages of hematopoiesis and induce programmed cell death. *J Cell Physiol* 165:538-546.

Shimamura A [2006] Shwachman-Diamond syndrome. *Semin Hematol* 43:178-188.

Simmons P, Kaushansky K, Torok-Storb B [1990] Mechanisms of cytomegalovirus-mediated myelosuppression: Perturbation of stromal cell function vs direct infection of myeloid cells. *Proc Natl Acad Sci USA* 87:1386-1390.

Sindre H, Tjoonnfjord GE, Rollag H, et al [1996] Human cytomegalovirus suppression of and latency in early hematopoietic progenitor cells. *Blood* 88:4526-4533.

Sing GK, Prior S, Fernan A, Cooksley G [1993] Hepatitis B virus differentially suppresses myelopoiesis and displays tropism for immature hematopoietic cells. *J Virol* 67:3454-3460.

Sing GK, Ruscetti FW [1990] Preferential suppression of myelopoiesis in normal human bone marrow cells after in vitro challenge with human cytomegalovirus. *Blood* 75:1965-1973.

Siraki AG, Bonini MG, Jiang J, et al [2007] Aminoglutethimide-induced protein free radical formation on myeloperoxidase: a potential mechanism of agranulocytosis. *Chem Res Toxicol* 20:1038-1045.

Siraki AG, Deterding LJ, Bonini MG, et al [2008] Procainamide, but not N-acetylprocainamide, induces protein free radical formation on myeloperoxidase: a potential mechanism of agranulocytosis. *Chem Res Toxicol* 21:1143-1153.

Sloand E, Groopman J [2004] Acquired immunodeficiency syndrome. In: Greer J, Rodgers G, Foerster J, et al, eds. *Wintrobe's Clinical Hematology.* 11th ed. Philadelphia: Lippincott Williams & Wilkins; 1875-1892.

Smith A, Shaw PJ, Webster B, et al [2002] Intermittent 20q- and consistent i(7q) in a patient with Shwachman-Diamond syndrome. *Pediatr Hematol Oncol* 19:525-528.

Soderberg C, Giugni TD, Zaia JA, et al [1993] CD13 (human aminopeptidase N) mediates human cytomegalovirus infection. *J Virol* 67:6576-6585.

Stroncek DF [1993] Drug-induced immune neutropenia. *Transfus Med Rev* 7:268-274.

Stroncek DF, Herr GP [1995] The chemical and immunoglobulin structural features necessary for reactions of quinine-dependent antibodies to neutrophils. *Transfusion* 35:247-253.

Sumimoto S, Kasajima Y, Hamamoto T, et al [1990] Agranulocytosis following infectious mononucleosis. *Eur J Pediatr* 149:691-694.

Tesfa D, Keisu M, Palmblad J [2009] Idiosyncratic drug-induced agranulocytosis: possible mechanisms and management. *Am J Hematol* 84:428-434.

Tschen AC, Rieder MJ, Oyewumi LK, Freeman DJ [1999] The cytotoxicity of clozapine metabolites: implications for predicting clozapine-induced agranulocytosis. *Clin Pharmacol Ther* 65:526-532.

Uetrecht JP [1995a] Myeloperoxidase as a generator of drug-free radicals. *Biochem Soc Symp* 61:163-170.

Uetrecht JP, Ma HM, MacKnight E, McClelland R [1995b] Oxidation of aminopyrine by hypochlorite to a reactive dication: possible implications for aminopyrine-induced agranulocytosis. *Chem Res Toxicol* 8:226-233.

Uetrecht JP, Zahid N, Whitfield D [1994] Metabolism of vesnarinone by activated neutrophils: implications for vesnarinone-induced agranulocytosis. *J Pharmacol Exp Ther* 270:865-872.

Watanabe KI, Ambekar C, Wang H, et al [2008] SBDS-deficiency results in specific hypersensitivity to Fas stimulation and accumulation of Fas at the plasma membrane. *Apoptosis* 1:77-89.

Watts R [2009] Neutropenia. In: Greer J, Foerster J, Rodgers G, et al, eds. *Wintrobe's Clinical Hematology.* 12th ed. Philadelphia: Lippincott Williams & Wilkins; 1527-1547.

Welte K, Zeidler C [2009] Severe congenital neutropenia. *Hematol Oncol Clin North Am* 23:307-320.

Xia J, Link DC [2008] Severe constitutional neutropenia and the unfolded protein response. *Curr Opin Hematol* 15:1-7.

Yamada S, Yasui K, Shinozaki K, et al [2002] Detection of neutrophil-associated immunoglobulin using flow cytometry in autoimmune neutropenia of infancy. *Pediatr Int* 44:269-272.

Yoshida K, Kondo R, Wang Q, Doerschuk CM [2006] Neutrophil cytoskeletal rearrangements during capillary sequestration in bacterial pneumonia in rats. *Am J Respir Crit Care Med* 174:689-698.

Zhu NY, Legatt DF, Turner AR [2009] Agranulocytosis after consumption of cocaine adulterated with levamisole. *Ann Intern Med* (e-pub ahead of print).

Zuppa AA, Girlando P, Florio MG, et al [2002] Influence of maternal preeclampsia on recombinant human granulocyte colony-stimulating factor effect in neutropenic neonates with suspected sepsis. *Eur J Obstet Gynecol Reprod Biol* 102:131-136.

Megakaryocytic/Platelet Disorders

Kaaren Reichard, MD

This chapter focuses on the morphologic features of hereditary and reactive qualitative and quantitative disorders of megakaryocytes and platelets and associated comparison with neoplastic disorders. A succinct presentation of the differential diagnostic possibilities and key tips for diagnosis are emphasized. Bone marrow morphologic findings are our focus; however, peripheral blood features are also addressed because many of these disorders often present with an abnormality of platelet size and/or number.

This chapter first presents normal megakaryopoiesis, platelet/megakaryocytic morphology, and megakaryocytic topography in the bone marrow. This is followed by the workup of megakaryocytic/platelet abnormalities in the peripheral blood and classification of megakaryocytic/platelet disorders.

Most cases of thrombocytopenia and thrombocytosis are reactive in nature. However, rare constitutional disorders and relatively infrequent myeloid neoplasms should always be considered. Integration of the clinical data with the hematologic, laboratory, morphologic, and genetic findings is critical for complete interpretation of qualitative and quantitative megakaryocytic/platelet disorders. See Chapters 13, 14, 16, 17, and 18 for comprehensive discussions of myeloid neoplasms, myeloproliferative neoplasms, myelodysplastic syndromes, myelodysplastic/myeloproliferative neoplasms, and acute myeloid leukemias.

[12.1] Brief Overview of Megakaryopoiesis and Thrombopoiesis

Megakaryocytes originate from pluripotent hematopoietic stem cells, which ultimately commit to the megakaryocytic lineage via a committed progenitor cell (see Chapter 1). Thrombopoietin, the ligand for the *MPL* receptor, plays a key role in megakaryocyte development from progenitor cells and appears to be the key regulator [Kaushansky 1994, 2008, 2009, Kuter 1994, Solar 1998].

Hematopoietic stem cells and progenitor cells are not readily identifiable morphologically in bone marrow; however, their immunophenotypic features provide for routine identification by flow cytometry (Lin–/c-Kit+/Sca-1+/CD34– and Lin–/c-Kit+/Sca-1+/CD34+, respectively) [Weissman 2008]. Megakaryocytic precursors become evident at the megakaryocyte/erythroid progenitor stage (Lin–/c-Kit+/Sca-1–/CD34–/FcγR–) with subsequent definitive identification by acquisition of megakaryocytic associated antigens (CD41, CD42b, CD31, von Willebrand factor, Mpl 1) i12.1.

In normal bone marrow, megakaryoblasts are inconspicuous and difficult to identify with certainty, though blasts with cytoplasmic blebbing and shedding are likely candidates i12.2. Megakaryocytes mature via a unique process termed *endomitosis,* which involves repeated DNA replication without cell division, resulting in a multilobulated cell [Nagata 1997, Papadantonakis 2008, Ravid 2002, Vitrat 1998, Zimmet 2000]. With maturation, normal megakaryocytes become readily identifiable in the bone marrow due to their multilobulation and resultant giant size compared with other marrow hematopoietic cells i12.3, i12.4. As a result of the repeated DNA duplication, megakaryocytes are polyploid and, on average, show 16N ploidy.

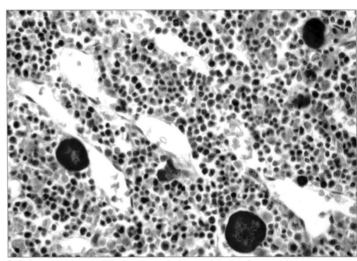

i12.1 *Immunoperoxidase staining for CD42b highlights megakaryocytes in this bone marrow core biopsy. Note the perisinusoidal localization. (immunoperoxidase for CD42b)*

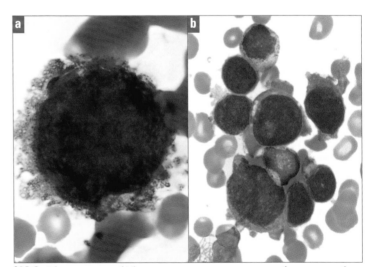

i12.2 *This composite of 2 bone marrow aspirate smears, one from a normal patient* a *and one from a patient with acute megakaryoblastic leukemia* b *highlights normal immature megakaryocytes with prominent cytoplasmic shedding and nearby platelets* a *in comparison to leukemic megakaryoblasts, which also exhibit cytoplasmic blebs. (Wright)*

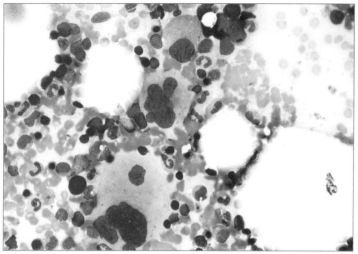

i12.3 *This bone marrow aspirate smear from a normal bone marrow shows a spectrum of megakaryocytic maturation. Note that the top megakaryocyte is the smallest and most immature and shows no nuclear lobation, while the middle and bottom megakaryocytes show progressive increase in nuclear lobation and overall size. (Wright)*

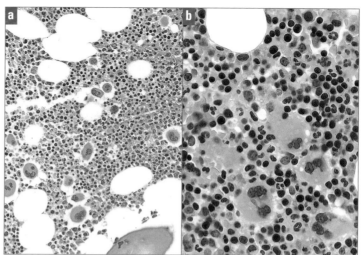

i12.4 *A spectrum of megakaryocytic size is evident on these bone marrow biopsy sections from a patient with chronic immune thrombocytopenia (ITP). (H&E)*

However, megakaryocytes with 32N or 64N can be induced in cases of increased thrombopoietin (THPO) stimulation as a result of thrombocytopenia [Raslova 2007, Zimmet 2000].

Megakaryocytes show characteristic voluminous, finely granular cytoplasm reflecting the presence of numerous organelles, cytoskeletal components, other molecules, and granules i12.5 [Kaushansky 2008]. Platelets form from proplatelets, which are pseudopodial projections of megakaryocytic cytoplasm [Balduini 2008, Italiano 1999, Li 2001, Patel 2005]. Adults produce 10^{11} platelets per day, which can increase 20-fold in times of need [Kaushansky 2008].

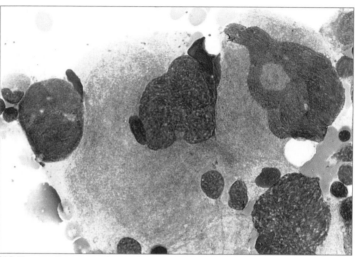

i12.5 *Megakaryocytic hyperplasia with an occasional megakaryoblast (left) is evident on this bone marrow aspirate smear from a patient with immune thrombocytopenia. (Wright)*

[12.2] Overview of Megakaryocytic Number, Topography, and Morphology in Bone Marrow

Megakaryocytes are readily identified in bone marrow aspirate smears and in clot and core biopsy sections. They number on average one to 4 per 40× magnification in an adult bone marrow tissue section and are predominantly individually distributed i12.6. Even in situations in which megakaryocytes are increased (eg, immune thrombocytopenia) or in the normally generously cellular bone marrows from children, megakaryocytes remain largely individually dispersed i12.7, i12.8.

Megakaryocytic location in the bone marrow is unique, as they typically reside adjacent to the bone marrow sinuses to enable direct shedding of platelets into the peripheral circulation i12.1 [Foucar 2008, Tavassoli 1989]. From this strategic perisinusoidal site, megakaryocytes extend organelle-rich segments of cytoplasm to produce proplatelets/platelets and allow transmigration of other hematopoietic elements

through the cytoplasm (emperipolesis) directly into the circulation i12.9, i12.10 [Hartwig 2003, Tavassoli 1989]. This abluminal location by megakaryocytes may be difficult to appreciate in most hematoxylin and eosin–stained bone marrow biopsy sections but is highlighted by immunostains for endothelium (CD31/CD34) or in cases with megakaryocytes in the sinus itself i12.11. Each megakaryocyte may extend from 6-20 proplatelets and ultimately give rise to 1,000-3,000 platelets [Hartwig 2003, Stenberg 1989, Tavassoli 1989].

Megakaryocyte cytomorphology is best assessed using the bone marrow aspirate smears and paraffin-embedded clot and core biopsy sections in combination. One caveat in assessing megakaryocytic morphology on tissue sections is that the lobation of a megakaryocyte may be underestimated, raising concern for myelodysplasia due to sectioning through these large cells. Either a significant number of

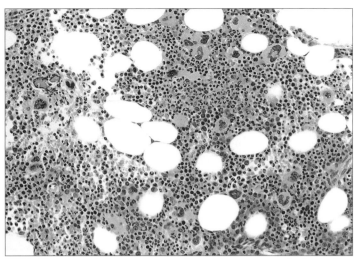

i12.6 *This image of a bone marrow core biopsy shows occasional individually dispersed mature-appearing megakaryocytes. (H&E) (courtesy P Armell, MD)*

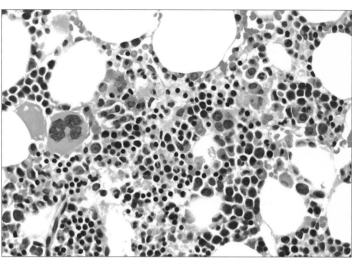

i12.7 *Bone marrow biopsy section from a patient with primary immune thrombocytopenia; note increased megakaryocytes. (H&E)*

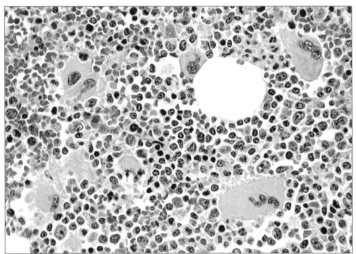

i12.8 *This bone marrow clot section is from a neonate with thrombocytopenia. Note overall cellularity of approximately 90% and abundant megakaryocytes, which are primarily individually dispersed. (H&E)*

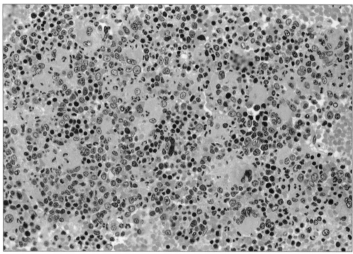

i12.9 *Markedly increased megakaryocytes are evident on this bone marrow clot section from a 10-month-old infant with chronic immune thrombocytopenia since 3 months of age. Note the tremendous increase in megakaryocytes. Also note that many of these megakaryocytes contain neutrophils within their cytoplasm, so-called emperipolesis. (H&E)*

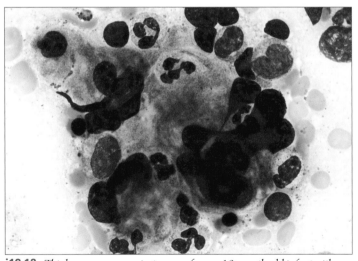

i12.10 *This bone marrow aspirate smear from a 10-month-old infant with chronic immune thrombocytopenia shows not only significantly increased megakaryocytes, but numerous neutrophils within the cytoplasm within these megakaryocytes, so-called emperipolesis. (Wright)*

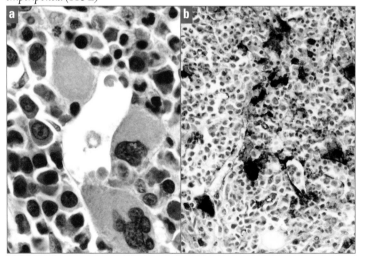

i12.11 *The perisinusoidal (abluminal) localization of megakaryocytes is readily apparent on both H&E and immunoperoxidase staining for CD31 in this composite of bone marrow core biopsy sections. (H&E and immunoperoxidase for CD31)*

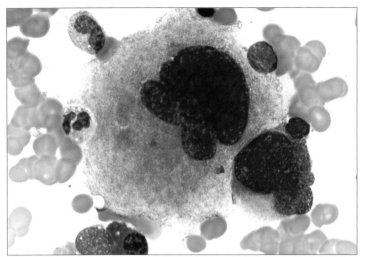

i12.12 *An immature megakaryocyte (right) is immediately adjacent to a fully mature megakaryocyte on this bone marrow aspirate smear. Note basophilic cytoplasm of immature megakaryocyte. (Wright)*

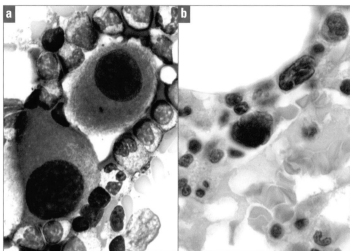

i12.13 *This composite highlights megakaryocytes with reduced nuclear lobation, a feature that can be seen in myelodysplasia **a** as well as in chronic human immunodeficiency virus (HIV-1) infection **b**. Note the deeply pyknotic nucleus with denuded cytoplasm associated with chronic HIV-1 infection **b**. (Wright and H&E)*

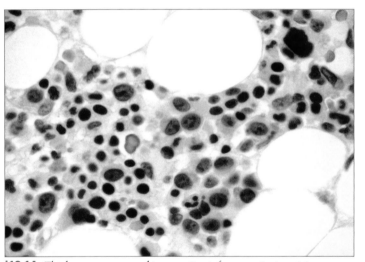

i12.14 *This bone marrow core biopsy section is from a patient receiving valproic acid therapy and shows megakaryocyte dysplasia in which megakaryocytes exhibit reduced lobulation and pyknotic nuclei. (H&E) (courtesy T Elghetany, MD)*

the megakaryocytes should show a similar appearance, or monolobated and small megakaryocytes should be seen on the concurrent bone marrow aspirate smears or touch preparations. Distinguishing immature (young) megakaryocytes from small, monolobated forms is critical, since the youngest megakaryocytes are normally monolobated.

Maturing megakaryocytes are normally pleomorphic and show a spectrum of morphologic appearances (see **i12.3**, **i12.4**). Some megakaryocytes are of larger size with numerous nuclear lobulations, while others are smaller with fewer lobulations. Of note are relatively small megakaryocytes (30-50 μm in diameter), which have a deeper basophilic cytoplasm and monolobated nucleus occupying >80% of the cytoplasm **i12.12**; see also **i12.5**. These immature (young) megakaryocytes should not be confused with the

monolobated megakaryocytes seen in myelodysplastic syndromes (MDS) or the pyknotic megakaryocytes seen in patients with human immunodeficiency virus (HIV-1), other viral infections, or immune thrombocytopenia (ITP) **i12.13**.

The atypical megakaryocytic morphologic features seen in myeloid malignancies are shown in **t12.1**. When >10% of bone marrow megakaryocytes exhibit any of these features, one should consider a primary myeloid neoplasm. Individual variation in megakaryocytic morphology is neither sensitive nor specific for myeloid neoplasia in and of itself. Therefore, integration of the concurrent clinical findings, hematologic parameters, and other marrow features is key to establishing a diagnosis of a myeloid neoplasm. For example, megakaryocyte "dysplasia" may be associated with valproic acid use **i12.14** (for a complete discussion of MDS see Chapter 16; for a discussion of MPN see Chapter 14).

Although megakaryocytic clustering is predominantly a feature of a primary myeloid neoplasm, it is often transiently seen in regenerative bone marrow sections **i12.15**, **i12.16**. Loose clusters of 3-4 megakaryocytes may sometimes be seen after recombinant colony-stimulating factor therapy. Thus, while clustering of megakaryocytes is generally seen in a myeloid malignancy, evaluation for and consideration of a non-neoplastic process is necessary.

Circulating megakaryocytic nuclei (devoid of cytoplasm) and circulating intact megakaryocytes may be seen in physiologically normal pediatric and adult individuals and are not necessarily indicative of a myeloid neoplasm **i12.17** [Hansen 1978, Wilde 1997, Woods 1992]. They are best appreciated at the feathered edge of the slide and may be more noticeable in acutely ill individuals with systemic stress reactions (eg, myocardial

t12.1 Atypical Megakaryocytic Morphology in Myeloid Malignancies

Megakaryocytic Feature/Illustrative Disease (*listed by size of megakaryocytes [smallest to largest]*)		Comments
Monolobation/CML	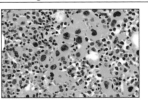	Smallest mean megakaryocyte size May mimic MDS megakaryocytes Perform *BCR-ABL1* testing Regenerating megakaryocytes may show a predominance of monolobated forms
Monolobation/MDS	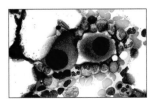	Non-lobated megakaryocyte nuclei common Overall megakaryocyte size characteristically low Perform cytogenetics to evaluate for del(5q)
Separate nuclei/MDS	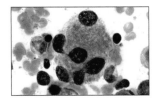	Lack of connection between nuclear lobes; a feature of neoplastic megakaryocytes Failure of normal endomitosis
Enlarged and hyperchromatic nucleus/PMF	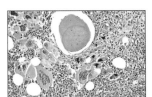	Pleomorphic megakaryocytes with heterogeneous range in cell size from small to large, but overall increased Marked clustering of megakaryocytes May see intrasinusoidal distribution in PMF
Enlarged and hyperlobulated/ET	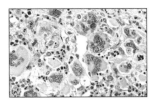	Largest mean megakaryocyte size May see prominent emperipolesis Striking hyperlobation of most megakaryocytes typical of ET Megakaryocytes uniformly markedly enlarged Clustering prominent
Clustering of >3 megakaryocytes without intervening hematopoietic cells	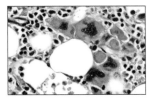	Megakaryocyte clustering typical in MDS and MPN Clustering may also be seen in early regeneration after therapy/toxic insult
Intrasinusoidal megakaryocytes with/without other hematopoietic cells	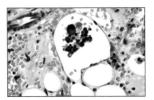	Intrasinusoidal megakaryocytes indicative of extramedullary hematopoiesis Common feature of MPN Often seen in dilated sinuses
Circulating megakaryocyte nuclei or micromegakaryocytes	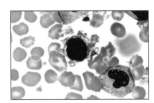	Not definitive for a myeloid disorder May see in non-neoplastic situations, but more prominent in MPN Micromegakaryocytes in blood in CML May show nuclear atypia reflecting underlying neoplasm

CML = chronic myelogenous leukemia; ET = essential thrombocythemia; MDS = myelodysplastic syndrome; MPN = myeloproliferative neoplasm; PMF = primary myelofibrosis

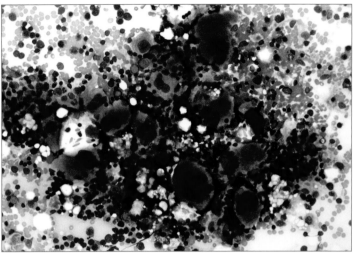

i12.15 *This bone marrow aspirate smear from a patient with acute lymphoblastic leukemia on day 2 of induction therapy shows a striking increase in megakaryocytes, which virtually fill the bone marrow particle. (Wright)*

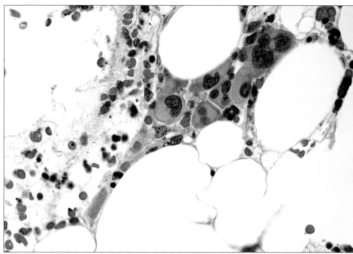

i12.16 *This bone marrow core biopsy shows damaged stroma and prominently clustered megakaryocytes as evidence of early regeneration after induction chemotherapy for acute leukemia. (H&E)*

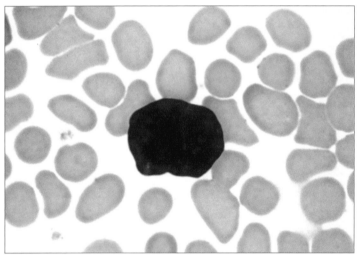

i12.17 *This peripheral blood smear from a normal newborn shows a circulating megakaryocyte nucleus. Megakaryocyte nuclei are generally more apparent at the feathered edge. (Wright)*

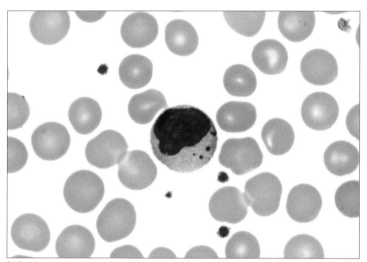

i12.18 *Morphologically normal platelets are evident on this peripheral blood smear. Note the relative uniform size of these platelets as well as the abundant cytoplasmic granules. (Wright)*

infarction, infection, etc). In neoplastic myeloid diseases (particularly myeloproliferative neoplasms), integration of clinical history, hematologic indices, and morphology of other cell lineages is necessary to exclude a reactive condition.

[12.3] **Overview of Platelet Morphology, Platelet Number, and Approach to Platelet Abnormalities on the Peripheral Blood Smear**

Platelets form from proplatelets, which are cytoplasmic projections of mature megakaryocytes. They number, on average, $150\text{-}400 \times 10^3/\mu L$ ($150\text{-}400 \times 10^9/L$) in the peripheral blood and have a mean platelet volume of 6.8-12.4 (varies depending on gender, ethnicity, and automated hematology analyzer). Their major function is

promoting hemostasis by leading to the formation of blood clots. They are anucleate, similar to normal terminally differentiated red blood cells. Their life span ranges from 7-12 days.

On a well-stained peripheral blood smear, platelets are variably sized, ranging from 2-4 μm in diameter, with numerous purple granules i12.18. One may reasonably estimate the platelet count by enumerating the number of platelets in a 100× oil objective field and multiplying by 2.

Abnormal size and/or granulation of platelets often provide the initial clue to an underlying platelet abnormality. Qualitative platelet disorders are generally recognized by abnormal platelet aggregation studies, von Willebrand testing, and/or bleeding times. Assessment of quantitative platelet abnormalities often begins with complete blood count, review of the blood smear, and correlation with clinical information.

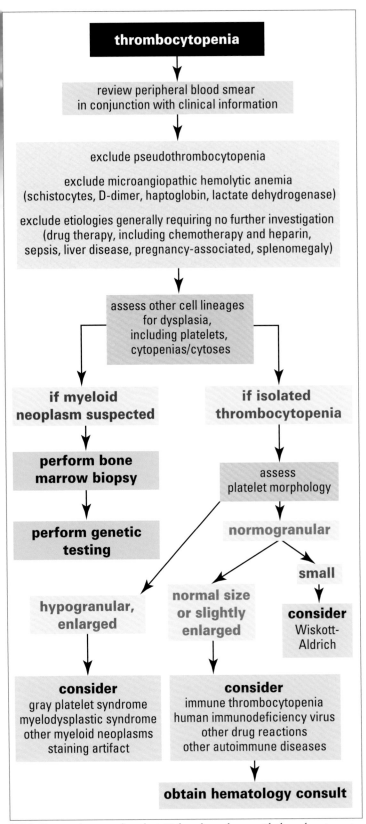

f12.1 *Practical approach to the initial workup of cases with thrombocytopenia.*

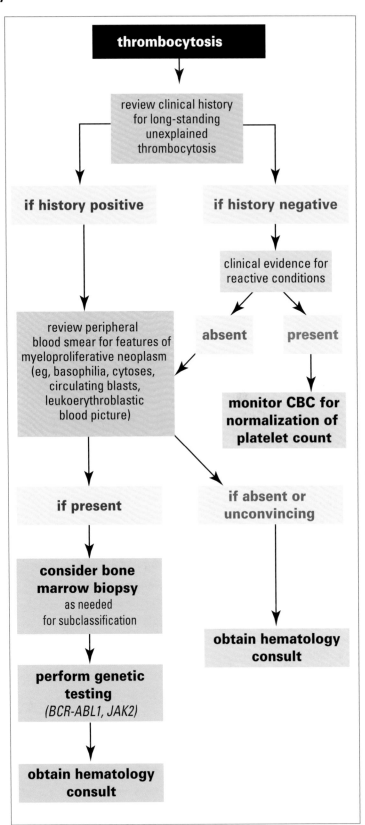

f12.2 *Practical approach to the initial workup of cases with thrombocytosis.*

One of the main objectives in cases with quantitative platelet abnormalities is to determine when further testing is needed (eg, bone marrow examination). The most common causes of thrombocytopenia are non-neoplastic and acquired, and can generally be diagnosed without performing a bone marrow

biopsy. The same is true for thrombocytosis. A practical approach to the workup of cases with thrombocytopenia and thrombocytosis is shown in **f12.1** and **f12.2**. These figures also incorporate abnormal platelet size and granulation where appropriate (see also **t12.2**).

t12.2 Approach to Blood Smears with Abnormal Platelet Morphology and/or Size

Parameter	Comments
Hypogranular	Exclude staining artifact
	Evaluate other lineages for possible primary myeloid neoplasm
	Gray platelet syndrome (thrombocytopenia and large size)
Normal granulation	
If large	*Common:*
	Platelet consumption (eg, ITP) either central or peripheral
	Rare:
	MHY9 disorders (May-Hegglin anomaly, Fechtner, Epstein and Sebastian syndromes)
	Paris-Trousseau/Jacobsen syndromes
	Mediterranean macrothrombocytopenia
	Bernard-Soulier
	Platelet-type VWD
	GATA1-related thrombocytopenia with dyserythropoiesis
If small	*Rare:*
	Wiskott-Aldrich syndrome
	X-linked thrombocytopenia

ITP = immune thrombocytopenia; VWD = von Willebrand disease

The first step in the evaluation of thrombocytopenia is to exclude spurious thrombocytopenia. Pregnancy-associated, drug-associated, and liver disease-associated thrombocytopenia are also common and generally require no further investigation in the proper clinical context. One must always consider the possibility of a microangiopathic hemolytic process (eg, thrombotic thrombocytopenic purpura, hemolytic uremic syndrome), which would require emergent treatment. Review of the blood smear for schistocytes is crucial, in addition to assessing coagulation studies, D-dimer, fibrinogen, and serum levels of hemoglobin and lactate dehydrogenase (LDH). The second step is to assess the other cell lineages for clues to a possible myeloid neoplasm (eg, dysplasia, other cytopenias/cytoses, unexplained circulating blasts). If isolated thrombocytopenia, assess platelet morphology with subsequent workup as needed f12.1.

Thrombocytosis may be the result of a primary myeloid neoplasm or a reactive condition. Although reactive conditions are much more common, distinction from a neoplastic condition is critical, as the patient with a myeloid neoplasm is at risk for thrombotic/hemorrhagic sequelae. The clinical history (no recent surgery, trauma, infection, etc) and physical findings (eg, presence or absence of splenomegaly)

are useful in making this distinction in collaboration with the other complete blood count findings (other cytoses, unexplained circulating blasts, dysplasia, and basophilia favor a primary myeloid neoplasm) f12.2. Genetic studies (eg, JAK2 mutation, chromosome analysis) may be needed in challenging cases. In general, the degree of thrombocytosis is a poor discriminator between neoplasia and reactive states as both may show platelet counts above/below $1,000 \times 10^3/\mu L$ ($1,000 \times 10^9/L$).

If there is clinical evidence for non-neoplastic thrombocytosis, no further workup is generally necessary aside from the monitoring/treatment of the underlying condition. If it is unclear whether the thrombocytosis is reactive, a review of the peripheral blood smear for other features of a primary myeloproliferative neoplasm and a hematology consult may be obtained for further guidance and workup.

[12.4] Classification of Non-Neoplastic Platelet/Megakaryocytic Disorders

There are several approaches to the classification of megakaryocytic/platelet disorders. These include categorization based on constitutional vs acquired conditions, quantitative abnormalities and abnormal morphology. Our approach to classification is based on alterations in the platelet count and concomitant presence of normal, increased, or decreased megakaryocytes in the bone marrow. Such a classification is then further divided based on a constitutional vs an acquired etiology. t12.3 and t12.4 summarize our approach for thrombocytopenic patients, while t12.5 and t12.6 summarize thrombocytosis.

[12.5] Acquired Thrombocytopenic Disorders

Thrombocytopenia is most commonly the result of an acquired, nonclonal condition in both children and adults and is generally defined as a platelet count $<150 \times 10^3/\mu L$ ($<150 \times 10^9/L$) [Rivers 2009]. A decreased platelet count may be the consequence of pseudothrombocytopenia (spurious thrombocytopenia), inadequate production by megakaryocytes (generally due to diminished/absent megakaryocytes in the marrow), intramedullary loss of platelets (as in myelodysplasia), or platelet consumptive processes t12.3 and t12.4. Most non-neoplastic etiologies are associated with normal or increased bone marrow megakaryocytes. In these disorders, the primary mechanism is overwhelmingly a platelet survival defect; however, a notable exception is intramedullary cell death seen in megaloblastic anemia.

Pseudothrombocytopenia, also known as spurious thrombocytopenia, must be excluded as a cause of a decreased platelet count. It can be caused by various phenomena, several

t12.3 Congenital Megakaryocytic Disorders with Thrombocytopenia

Disorder	Comments
Normal/Increased Megakaryocytes in Bone Marrow	
Bernard-Soulier	Defect in platelet adhesion
	Giant platelets
	Autosomal recessive
	Mutations in *GPIBA, GP1BB, GP9*
MYH9 related diseases (May-Hegglin anomaly, Fechtner, Epstein, and Sebastian)	Large platelets
	Autosomal dominant
	22q12–13 (*MYH9* gene)
Gray platelet syndrome	Mostly recessive
	Enlarged platelets lacking α-granules
	Myelofibrosis
	Molecular abnormality undefined
X-linked *GATA1* macrothrombocytopenia with dyserythropoiesis	Nonlobulated or hypolobulated megakaryocytes
	Large platelets
	GATA1 (Xp11.23) mutation
Mediterranean macrothrombocytopenia	Large platelets
	Autosomal dominant
	GP1BA mutation [Savoia 2001]
Wiskott-Aldrich syndrome	Microthrombocytopenia
	Hypolobulated megakaryocytes
	WAS gene mutation
Paris-Trousseau syndrome (related variant Jacobsen syndrome)	Nonlobulated or hypolobulated megakaryocytes
	Giant α granules
	FLI1 (Paris-Trousseau)
	11q23.3 deletion
Autosomal dominant thrombocytopenia with incomplete megakaryocytic differentiation	Nonlobulated or hypolobulated megakaryocytes
Familial platelet disorder with predisposition to AML with *RUNX1* mutations	
Decreased/Absent Megakaryocytes in Bone Marrow	
Fanconi anemia	Usually autosomal recessive
	Dysmorphic features (see Chapter 7 for more details)
Thrombocytopenia with absent radii (TAR)	Autosomal recessive
	Large deletion 1q21
Congenital amegakaryocytic thrombocytopenia	Progresses to trilineage bone marrow failure
	Autosomal-recessive form now known to be due to mutations in the thrombopoietin receptor gene, *MPL*
	Cases with radio-ulnar synostosis associated with specific mutations of *HOXA11* (7p15-14)
X-linked amegakaryocytic thrombocytopenia	Small platelets
	WAS gene
Dyskeratosis congenita	Multiple defective genes involved in telomere maintenance
Shwachman-Diamond syndrome	Often progresses to trilineage bone marrow failure
	SBDS gene
Cyclic thrombocytopenia	Rare
	Intermittent amegakaryocytosis parallels thrombocytopenia

AML = acute myeloid leukemia

References: [Althaus 2009, Ballmaier 2009, Bosticardo 2009, Breton-Gorius 1995, Clauser 2009, Drachman 2000, Fox 2009, Geddis 2009, Hadjkacem 2009, Kirito 2008, Klopocki 2007, Michaud 2002, Nurden 2007, 2008, Ochs 2008, Redman 2008, Rivers 2009, Tubman 2007, White 2007a, 2007b]

t12.4 Acquired Megakaryocytic Disorders with Thrombocytopenia

Non-Neoplastic Disorders

Normal/Increased Megakaryocytes

ITP
SLE, collagen vascular disease
Drug-induced (heparin, quinine, other)
HIV-1
Other infections
Neonatal alloimmune thrombocytopenia
Post-transfusion purpura
Microangiopathic hemolytic anemia (HUS, TTP, DIC, pregnancy associated)
Hypersplenism (including liver disease)
Liver disease
Megaloblastic anemia
Turbulent blood flow (hemangiomas, cardiac valve abnormalities)
Regeneration after therapy/toxic insult

Decreased/Absent Megakaryocytes

Aplastic anemia
Potent chemotherapy
Toxic injury
Radiation
Infection, mainly viral
Drug suppression (chloramphenicol [trilineage aplasia], chlorothiazide, estrogen, prednisone, and alcohol can selectively suppress megakaryocyte lineage)

Neoplastic Disorders

Normal/Increased Megakaryocytes

Primary myeloid neoplasm (MDS, MPN, MDS/MPN, acute megakaryoblastic leukemia) (see Chapters 14, 16, 17, 18)

Decreased Megakaryocytes

Paroxsymal nocturnal hemoglobinuria (some cases)
Bone marrow involvement by infiltrative lesion: metastatic tumor, leukemia, lymphoma

ITP = immune thrombocytopenia; SLE = systemic lupus erythematosus; HIV = human immunodeficiency virus; HUS = hemolytic uremic syndrome; TTP = thrombotic thrombocytopenic purpura; DIC = disseminated intravascular coagulation; MDS = myelodysplastic syndrome; MPN = myeloproliferative neoplasm

References: [Cines 2009a, 2009b, George 2009, Rodeghiero 2009, Witters 2008]

t12.5 Constitutional Megakaryocytic Disorders with Thrombocytosis

Disorder	Comments
Familial thrombocytosis*	Mutations in either the thrombopoietin gene (THPO) on chromosome 3 or, more rarely, the thrombopoietin receptor gene (MPL) on chromosome 1
Transient abnormal myelopoiesis, Down syndrome associated	Mutations in GATA1 gene

*Also known as hereditary thrombocytosis

References: [Brink 2006, Dame 2005, Kaushansky 1994, Liu 2008, Moliterno 2004, Percy 2009, Schafer 2004, Tecuceanu 2006, Webb 2007, Wiestner 1998, Wiestner 2000]

t12.6 Acquired Megakaryocytic Disorders with Thrombocytosis

Non-Neoplastic Disorders

Normal/Increased Megakaryocytes

Reactive conditions due to stress, trauma, infection, inflammatory condition, surgery, physical injury, burn, autoimmune disorders

Iron deficiency anemia

Postsplenectomy

Chronic hemolysis, blood loss

Occult malignancy

Neoplastic Disorders

Normal/Increased Megakaryocytes

Primary myeloid neoplasms (MPN, MDS/MPN, MDS with isolated del(5q), acute megakaryoblastic leukemia)*

*Less commonly megakaryocytes are decreased; several of these disorders, particularly MPN/MDS and acute megakaryoblastic leukemia may also show thrombocytopenia (see t12.4)
MPN= myeloproliferative neoplasm; MDS = myelodysplastic syndrome

of which are readily identifiable in a well-stained peripheral blood smear [Er 2009, Zandecki 2007]. Platelet satellitism i12.19 and platelet clumping i12.20 are well-known causes of pseudo-thrombocytopenia. The former is recognized by platelets forming a circumferential ring around circulating neutrophils; both processes may be in vitro phenomena resulting from antiplatelet antibodies reacting with platelets in blood drawn into ethylenediaminetetraacetic acid (EDTA) [Bartels 1997, Bizzaro 1995, Morselli 1999, Pegels 1982, Peters 1998]. As a result of platelet agglutination, an automated hematology analyzer does not recognize the platelet clumps and thus yields an abnormally low platelet count.

[12.5.1] **Increased/Normal Bone Marrow Megakaryocytes**
Idiopathic/immune thrombocytopenia is a classic example of a platelet survival disorder with a compensatory increase in megakaryocytes in the bone marrow [Cines 2009a, Cines 2002, Cooper 2006, Nugent 2009, Palaniappan 2009, Provan 2010, Psaila 2008, Schech 2006]. ITP has recently been proposed to stand for **I**mmune **T**hrombocyto**P**enia to reflect its immune-mediated mechanism of action, discounting purpura, which is unusual in the typical case [Rodeghiero 2009]. ITP is an acquired disorder in which platelet surface antigens become targets of autoantibodies, resulting in excessive platelet clearance as well as some degree of impairment of megakaryocytic production [Bromberg 2006, McMillan 2007]. Individuals of all ages are affected, including newborns. In children the disorder tends to be self-limited and may follow immunizations or viral infections.

The hallmark peripheral blood features include marked isolated thrombocytopenia—assuming no blood loss—(platelet count $<20 \times 10^3/\mu L$ [$<20 \times 10^9/L$] if untreated)

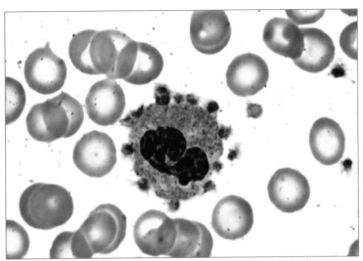

i12.19 *Striking platelet satellitism is evident in this peripheral blood smear, likely the consequence of the anticoagulant ethylenediamine tetraacetic acid. (Wright)*

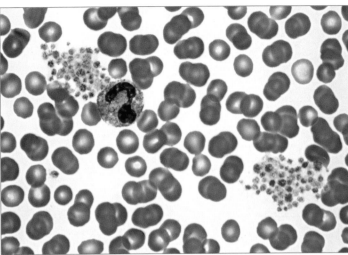

i12.20 *Prominent platelet clumping is evident on this peripheral blood smear. Platelet clumping is a major cause of spurious thrombocytopenia. (Wright)*

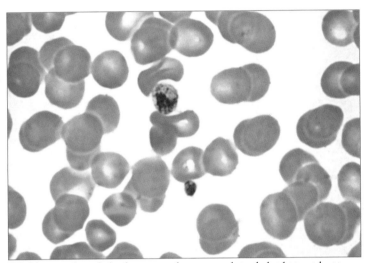

i12.21 *An enlarged platelet proximal to a normal-sized platelet is evident in this peripheral blood smear from a 51-year-old female with immune thrombocytopenia. (Wright)*

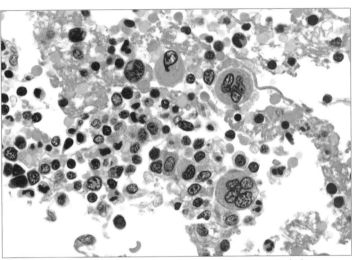

i12.22 *Increased megakaryocytes showing a spectrum in size, including more immature, non-lobated forms, are evident on this bone marrow clot section from a patient with immune thrombocytopenia. (H&E)*

with increased large/giant platelets **i12.21**. The bone marrow displays megakaryocytic hyperplasia with increased immature megakaryocytes admixed with more mature forms **i12.22**, **i12.23** [Bromberg 2006, Dameshek 1946, McMillan 2007, Pisciotta 1953, Thiele 1991]. The megakaryocytes are evenly distributed throughout the marrow without cluster formation. Scattered, small, pyknotic-appearing megakaryocytes may be noted similar to those seen in bone marrow sections from HIV-1+ patients **i12.23a**. In most cases of otherwise straightforward ITP, antiplatelet antibodies are revealed, and a bone marrow examination is not typically indicated. In cases of refractory ITP (eg, lack of appropriate treatment response or persistent thrombocytopenia after a procedure such as splenectomy), a bone marrow examination may be considered in children before initiating corticosteroid therapy and in adults [Psaila 2008]. Gene expression profiling studies have revealed an ITP-specific

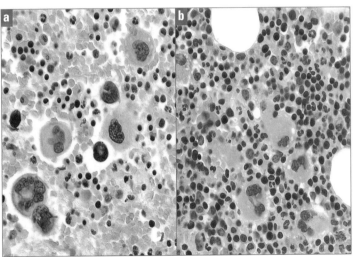

i12.23 *A spectrum of megakaryocytic size, including pyknotic forms, is evident on these bone marrow biopsy sections from patients with immune thrombocytopenia. The erythroid hyperplasia **b** is secondary to iron deficiency. (H&E)*

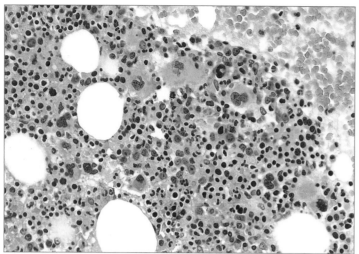

i12.24 *The spectrum of megakaryocytic hyperplasia and dysplasia common to patients with acquired immunodeficiency syndrome is illustrated on this bone marrow clot section. (H&E)*

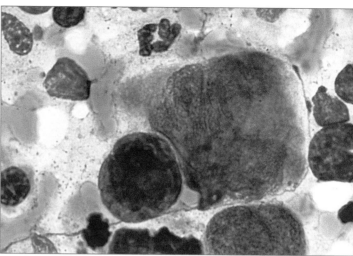

i12.25 *Denuded megakaryocytes are encountered on this bone marrow aspirate smear from a patient with acquired immunodeficiency syndrome. (Wright) (courtesy R Brynes, MD)*

profile with many genes overlapping with other autoimmune disorders such as systemic lupus erythematosus (SLE) [Sood 2008]. Recently it was proposed that an activating *FCGR2C* genotype may predispose to ITP, arguing that genetic differences likely contribute to disease predisposition [Breunis 2008].

In secondary immune-mediated thrombocytopenia, particularly those associated with autoimmune/collagen vascular disease, other bone marrow morphologic findings may be seen in addition to megakaryocytic hyperplasia. These include polyclonal plasmacytosis, interstitial lymphoid aggregates, and lipogranulomas (see Chapter 34) [Hunt 2009, Vlasoff 2006]. In drug-induced immune thrombocytopenia, platelet destruction is most often due to drug-induced antibodies [Aster 1999, George 2009]. Heparin-induced thrombocytopenia (HIT) is caused by heparin-dependent antibodies. Interestingly, despite the thrombocytopenia, HIT is a strong risk factor for both arterial and venous thromboses [Hassell 2008, Warkentin 2007].

Human immunodeficiency virus 1 infection warrants special commentary given its quite distinctive bone marrow features in florid infection. For a complete discussion of the marrow findings see Chapter 33. Chronic thrombocytopenia is relatively common in individuals with HIV-1 (~10% of cases), and the degree of platelet reduction generally parallels the severity of the infection [Scaradavou 2002]. The mechanisms contributing to low platelets are twofold [Cines 2009b, Li 2005, Nardi 2001, Zucker-Franklin 1989]

1. immune-mediated peripheral destruction
2. impaired production of platelets due to HIV-1 specific infection of megakaryocytes

The megakaryocytic morphology is unique in HIV-1, characterized by pyknotic and often dysplastic megakaryocytes i12.24, i12.25. Pyknotic megakaryocytes are distinctive with minimal cytoplasm and a dark, smudged nucleus. Such

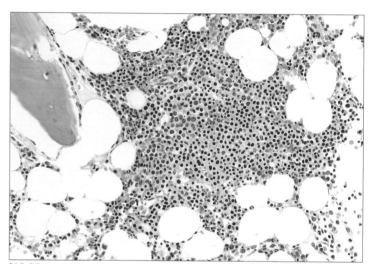

i12.26 *Low magnification of a bone marrow biopsy section from a child with acquired amegakaryocytosis is shown. (H&E)*

megakaryocytes have also been referred to as naked megakaryocytes and most likely reflect virus-induced apoptosis. In HIV-1, the megakaryocytes may occasionally form loose clusters. If significant clustering or frankly dysplastic forms are noted, strong consideration must be given to a primary myeloid neoplasm. In HIV-1, the megakaryocytes are generally normal or slightly increased in number, the latter particularly if there is an associated ITP-like picture [Scaradavou 2002].

[12.5.2] **Decreased Bone Marrow Megakaryocytes**

Acquired pure amegakaryocytic/thrombocytopenic disorders are rare with only a limited number of reports in the literature to date [Hoffman 1991]. They occur generally as the result of viral infections, drug/toxin exposure, immune-mediated phenomena, underlying tumor such as T-cell large granular lymphocytic leukemia, or as a presenting component of aplastic anemia or, less likely, MDS i12.26, i12.27, 12.28

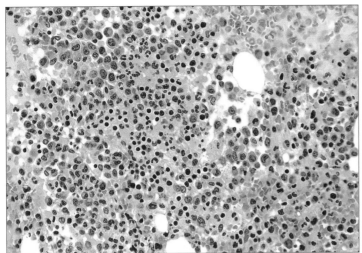

i12.27 *This bone marrow clot section depicts erythroid and granulocytic clustering, which suggests recovery from a bone marrow insult in a patient with acquired amegakaryocytosis. (H&E)*

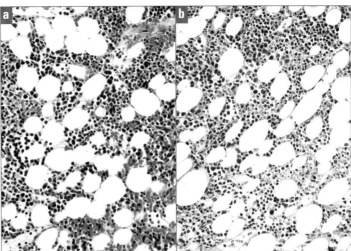

i12.28 *This composite of bone marrow clot and bone marrow core biopsy sections is from a patient with an acquired amegakaryocytic process associated with abnormal cytogenetics likely representing myelodysplasia. The absence of megakaryocytes is confirmed with immunohistochemical staining for CD42b* **b**. *(H&E and immunoperoxidase for CD42b)*

[Agarwal 2006, Benedetti 1994, Felderbauer 2004, Hoffman 1991, Lai 2008, Niparuck 2008, Stoll 1981].

Autoantibodies to c-mpl have also been implicated in rare patients with autoimmune disease and acquired amegakaryocytosis [Katsumata 2003]. While the majority of drugs including chemotherapeutic agents generally induce a panmyelosuppression, a few offending drugs may selectively target the megakaryocytic lineage in some cases (mycophenolate, valproate, chlorothiazide, estrogen, prednisone, and alcohol) [Bartakke 2008, Bulchandani 2007, Hoffman 1991].

Amegakaryocytosis may be seen in association with infections such as parvovirus B19, Epstein-Barr virus (EBV), cytomegalovirus (CMV), HIV-1, and hepatitis C [Bhattacharyya 2005, Liebman 2008, Xiao 2006]. In general, both HIV-1 and parvovirus tend to exhibit preserved megakaryopoiesis, but in some cases all hematopoietic lineages may be affected [Bhattacharyya 2005]. Given the marked improvement in some cases of acquired amegakaryocytosis with immunosuppressive agents, an immune-mediated, cytotoxic etiology has been implicated [Niparuck 2008].

[12.6] Constitutional Thrombocytopenic Disorders

[12.6.1] Amegakaryocytic/Decreased Bone Marrow Megakaryocytes

Constitutional thrombocytopenic disorders with amegakaryocytosis/decreased megakaryocytes are listed in **t12.3** [Geddis 2006, Geddis 2009]. For disorders associated with multilineage bone marrow failure, a complete discussion is provided in Chapter 7. In amegakaryocytic disorders, platelet counts are usually $<20 \times 10^3/\mu L$ ($<20 \times 10^9/L$), and platelet size is typically normal or slightly small. The different inherited entities may be categorized based on whether the

amegakaryocytosis is an isolated finding (thrombocytopenia with absent radii [TAR], congenital amegakaryocytic thrombocytopenia [CAMT], X-linked amegakaryocytic thrombocytopenia, and some cases of cyclic thrombocytopenia), or part of a multilineage bone marrow failure syndrome (eg, Fanconi anemia, dyskeratosis congenita, and Shwachman-Diamond syndrome). Although TAR and CAMT share similar features, including isolated thrombocytopenia, reduced or absent marrow megakaryocytes, impaired responsiveness to THPO, and high plasma THPO levels, they can be distinguished based on absent radii in TAR and *MPL* mutations in CAMT **i12.29, i12.30** [Fox 2009, Geddis 2009]. Rare reports describe either constitutional or acquired cyclic thrombocytopenia with intermittent amegakaryocytosis [Apostu 2008, Fogarty 2005, Go 2005, Zent 1999]. A recent assessment of cyclic thrombocytopenia using a mathematical model suggests that a slower relative growth rate of megakaryocytes, in conjunction with an increased random destruction of platelets, are the significant contributing factors to the platelet fluctuations [Apostu 2008]. The genetic basis of many of these disorders is becoming increasingly elucidated **t12.3** (see Chapter 7).

[12.6.2] Preserved/Increased Bone Marrow Megakaryocytes

Congenital thrombocytopenic disorders characterized by preserved megakaryopoiesis are listed in **t12.3**. These entities, in large part, are characterized by unusually large platelets (so-called giant platelet syndromes) and include Bernard-Soulier, May-Hegglin, gray platelet syndrome (GPS), and others [Althaus 2009, Nurden 2007, Nurden 2009b]. The platelets in these

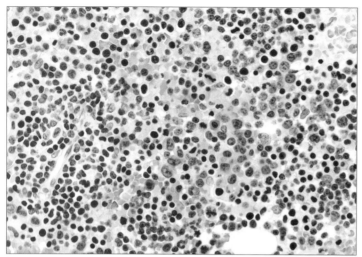

i12.29 *This bone marrow clot section shows a virtual absence of megakaryocytes in a patient with likely familial amegakaryocytosis. (H&E)*

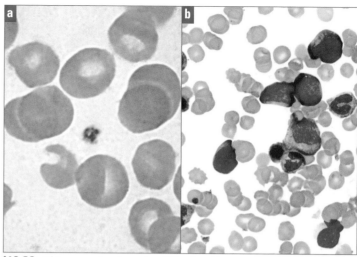

i12.30 *This composite of peripheral blood and bone marrow aspirate smear from a patient with thrombocytopenia with absent radii shows reduced numbers but morphologically normal platelets within the peripheral blood **a** and a virtual absence of megakaryocytes from the bone marrow **b**. (Wright) (courtesy P Izadi)*

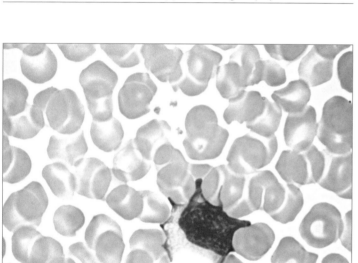

i12.31 *This blood smear from a patient with Wiskott-Aldrich syndrome shows microthrombocytes. (Wright)*

disorders show various qualitative abnormalities, including poor platelet function and adhesion abnormalities. Wiskott-Aldrich syndrome is distinguished by microthrombocytopenia and poorly lobulated megakaryocytes **i12.31**, **i12.32**, in addition to eczema and immunodeficiency. GPS is a unique disorder with overall normal platelets (with some enlarged forms) but with a characteristic lack of granulation due to absence of α granules **i12.33** [Nurden 2007]. A *GATA1* gene mutation has been linked to a family with GPS, suggesting a subset of GPS disorders that are X-linked [Tubman 2007]. GPS megakaryocytes are for the most part unremarkable in morphology, but occasional hypolobulated and hyperlobulated forms may be seen; bone marrow fibrosis is common **i12.34**.

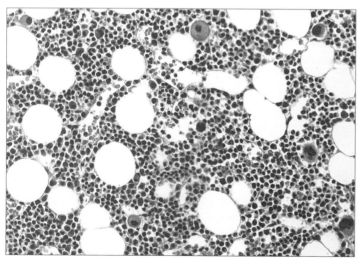

i12.32 *This bone marrow core biopsy section from a patient with Wiskott-Aldrich syndrome shows normal numbers of megakaryocytes, which are morphologically abnormal. Note characteristic small megakaryocyte size and reduced nuclear lobation. (H&E)*

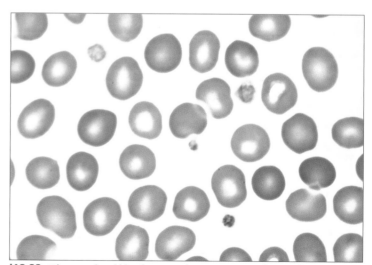

i12.33 *This peripheral blood smear is from a patient with gray platelet syndrome. Note absence of granules within certain platelets, which are somewhat enlarged. (Wright) (courtesy C Sever, MD)*

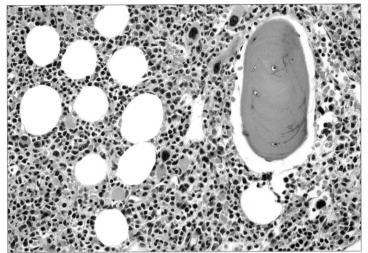

i12.34 *This bone marrow core biopsy section from a patient with gray platelet syndrome shows abundant, individually dispersed megakaryocytes, a fair proportion of which show nuclear hypolobation. Moderate fibrosis was also documented by reticulin stain in this case of gray platelet syndrome. (H&E) (courtesy C Sever, MD)*

[12.7] Special Considerations

[12.7.1] Neonatal Thrombocytopenia and Gestational Thrombocytopenia

About 5% of healthy babies have thrombocytopenia, so-called benign neonatal thrombocytopenia. These infants are not at risk for hemorrhage and recover spontaneously. Cases of benign neonatal thrombocytopenia are excluded from further discussion in this section. Thrombocytopenia in the neonatal (perinatal) period is relatively common, contributing to approximately 25%-35% of admissions to intensive care units in one study [Murray 2002b, Roberts 2008b, Sola-Visner 2009]. Although the list of potential etiologies is long, the biggest contributors are infection, immune-mediated destruction, and impaired megakaryopoiesis **t12.7** [Roberts 2003a, Roberts 2008a]. In addition, the time to onset of thrombocytopenia may play a key role in the underlying etiology **t12.7**. The impaired megakaryocytic production may be in part due to the fact that neonatal megakaryocytes tend to be smaller, although mature, and produce fewer overall platelets [Levine 1996, Mattia 2002, Olson 1992]. Findings from a recent study suggest that thrombocytopenic neonates can increase the number, but not the size, of their megakaryocytes in the bone marrow [Sola-Visner 2007]. Chronic intrauterine hypoxia is the most common cause of thrombocytopenia in preterm neonates and is generally associated with maternal placental insufficiency due to hypertension or diabetes [Murray 2002a, Roberts 2003b]. Gestational thrombocytopenia is discussed in Chapter 31.

t12.7 Causes of Neonatal Thrombocytopenia*

Fetal	Immune-mediated (including rare severe HDN, NAIT, maternal SLE, maternal ITP)
	Congenital infection (eg, CMV, enterovirus, toxoplasma, rubella, HIV-1)
	Aneuploidy (eg, trisomies 13, 18, 21)
	Maternal medication, other maternal factors
	Constitutional disorder
Early onset neonatal (<72 hours)	Gestational thrombocytopenia
	Placental insufficiency/chronic hypoxia (eg, pregnancy-induced hypertension, diabetes)
	Bacterial infection
	Disseminated intravascular coagulation
	Immune-mediated
	Rare: congenital infection, bone marrow replacement (eg, congenital leukemia), Kasabach-Merritt syndrome, metabolic disease, constitutional disorder (either restricted to megakaryocytic lineage or multilineage)
Late onset neonatal (>72 hours)	Sepsis developing at a later time
	Necrotizing enterocolitis
	Rare: all others

*Gestational thrombocytopenia is also commonly encountered and often a management challenge
CMV = cytomegalovirus; HIV = human immunodeficiency virus; HDN = hemolytic disease of the newborn due to maternal anti-Rh antibodies; ITP = immune thrombocytopenia; NAIT = neonatal alloimmune thrombocytopenia; SLE = systemic lupus erythematosus

References: [Gerth 2009, Kato 2009, Roberts 2003a]

[12.8] Constitutional and Acquired Thrombocytotic Disorders

Thrombocytosis, like thrombocytopenia, is most commonly the result of an acquired, nonclonal condition in both children and adults [Mantadakis 2008, Schafer 2001, Skoda 2009]. Top etiologies include a secondary phenomenon due to serious trauma, injury, burn, postsplenectomy status, and iron deficiency anemia (albeit the thrombocytosis in iron deficiency is less pronounced than in the other conditions listed).

Constitutional thrombocytotic disorders are exceedingly rare **t12.5**. There are 2 main causes of hereditary thrombocytosis involving mutations in either the *THPO* gene on chromosome 3 or, more rarely, the THPO receptor gene (*MPL*) on chromosome 1 [Dame 2005, Kaushansky 1994, Liu 2008, Moliterno 2004, Percy 2009, Schafer 2004, Tecuceanu 2006, Wiestner 1998, 2000]. THPO normally binds to its receptor on circulating platelets. Any unbound THPO promotes megakaryocytic proliferation and production of platelets. Thus, as a consequence of thrombocytosis, less THPO is available for megakaryopoiesis [Schafer 2004]. In the setting of familial mutations, constitutive activation occurs, contributing to sustained thrombocytosis. Another cause of constitutional

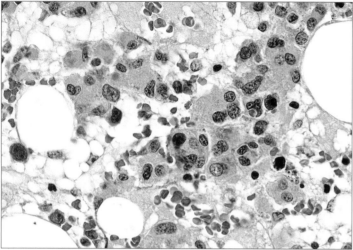

i12.35 *This bone marrow clot section from a patient with acute myeloid leukemia (AML) undergoing induction chemotherapy shows a striking megakaryocytic hyperplasia with clustering. The original AML did not have a megakaryocytic component, and these megakaryocytes were presumed to be regenerative. (H&E)*

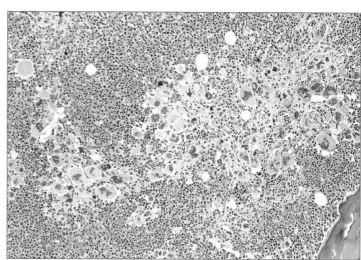

i12.36 *Striking megakaryocyte clustering is evident at low magnification on a bone marrow biopsy section from a patient with essential thrombocythemia. (H&E)*

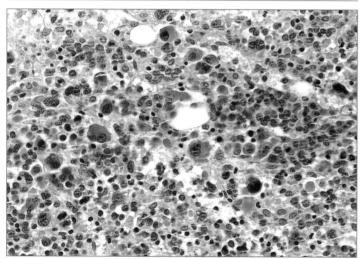

i12.37 *Bone marrow biopsy section illustrates that megakaryocytes are a component of acute leukemia demonstrating multilineage differentiation. Note increase in blast forms in addition to morphologically obvious dysplastic megakaryocytes. (H&E)*

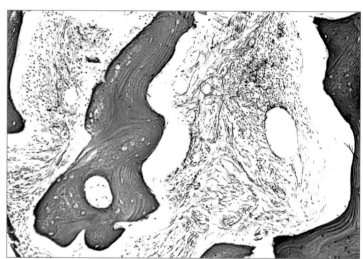

i12.38 *Marked reticulin fibrosis is evident on a bone marrow biopsy section from a patient with primary myelofibrosis. (reticulin) (courtesy C Leith, MD)*

thrombocytosis is transient abnormal myelopoiesis, which is seen in the early weeks of life of patients with Down syndrome [Brink 2006, Webb 2007]. For further discussion of this disorder see Chapters 18 and 30.

Acquired causes of thrombocytosis are much more common than those of congenital origin and include etiologies such as secondary reactions to trauma, stress, and infections t12.6 [Schafer 2004]. In children, infections are the most common cause of thrombocytosis, followed by trauma, hypoxemia, and autoimmune disorders [Dame 2005, Sutor 1995]. Reactive thrombocytosis in the setting of infection is likely driven in part to multiple cytokines and factors including elevated IL-6 and thrombopoietin [Hollen 1991, Ishiguro 2002, Kaushansky 1995].

In most instances of thrombocytosis, obtaining a good clinical history will reveal the etiology, and bone marrow examination is not necessary. In reactive cases in which a bone marrow biopsy is performed, cellularity is normal and megakaryocytes are normal to slightly increased in number without abnormal clustering or morphology. This is in contrast to acquired clonal disorders in which atypical megakaryocyte morphology and clustering is routinely observed. Occasionally, megakaryocytic clustering is seen in non-neoplastic bone marrow scenarios (eg, after recovery after injury/insult or chemotherapy). Rarely, striking megakaryocytic hyperplasia with clustering may be identified early in the treatment of acute myeloid leukemia i12.35 [Rosenthal 1991].

Overall, when comparing neoplastic vs non-neoplastic bone marrow sections from thrombocytotic individuals, the former conditions generally show increased cellularity, increased reticulin/collagen fibrosis, and overt clustering of

t12.8 Comparison of Blood and Bone Marrow Findings in Reactive and Neoplastic Thrombocytotic Disorders

Reactive Thrombocytosis	Thrombocytotic Myeloproliferative Neoplasms
Causes include inflammatory conditions, rebound after bone marrow suppression, postsplenectomy, posttrauma, and iron deficiency	Causes include chronic myelogenous leukemia, BCR-ABL1+, polycythemia vera, essential thrombocythemia and primary myelofibrosis
Variably sized platelets with some enlarged forms	Blood picture variable; some cases with extreme platelet pleomorphism and others exhibit predominance of uniformly enlarged forms; circulating megakaryocytes common
Bone marrow cellularity usually normal or slightly increased	Bone marrow typically, often markedly, hypercellular
Storage iron generally normal, except in iron deficiency	Storage iron may be absent, especially in polycythemia vera
No increase in reticulin fibers	Reticulin fibers often increased; most dramatic reticulin fibrosis in primary myelofibrosis
Megakaryocytes normal or mildly to moderately increased	Megakaryocytes often markedly increased
Megakaryocyte size normal to slightly increased	Megakaryocytes variably pleomorphic with many large forms, except in chronic myelogenous leukemia
Clustering of megakaryocytes in minority of cases; no diffuse sheets of megakaryocytes	Prominent megakaryocyte clustering; diffuse sheets of megakaryocytes in some cases
Other lineages usually normal	Multilineage abnormalities in blood and bone marrow
Low risk of thrombosis or hemorrhage	Thrombosis/hemorrhage risk substantial
Normal spleen size	Splenomegaly
Increased acute phase reactants/cytokines	No increase in acute phase reactants or cytokines
Normal karyotype	Clonal cytogenetic abnormalities common

References: [Tefferi 2007, Tefferi 2008, Thiele 2005]

megakaryocytes, or the presence of many megakaryocytes with clearly abnormal morphology i12.36, i12.37, 12.38. Sclerotic bone, intrasinusoidal hematopoiesis, and dilated sinuses may also be seen. Acquired clonal disorders with thrombocytosis mainly include the myeloproliferative neoplasms but also some MDSs and refractory anemia with ring sideroblasts and thrombocytosis. A comparison of blood and bone marrow findings in reactive and neoplastic thrombocytotic disorders is presented in t12.8.

[12.9] Potential Morphologic Mimics of Megakaryocytes in Bone Marrow and Differential Diagnosis

Those familiar with bone marrow examination are keenly aware of potential morphologic mimics of megakaryocytes. Most commonly, the presence of any type of multinucleated cell prompts consideration of several diagnostic possibilities t12.9. In particular, with clustered or atypical megakaryocytes or in the presence of significant fibrosis, it may be morphologically difficult to distinguish amongst these various entities; ancillary studies such as immunohistochemistry are hugely helpful i12.39, i12.40, i12.41, i12.42, i12.43, i12.44, 12.45.

t12.9 Differential Diagnosis of Multinucleated and/or Giant Cells in Bone Marrow

Cell Type	Strategies to Distinguish
Megakaryocyte	In abnormal conditions (regenerative or neoplastic), may be clustered and associated with varying degrees of fibrosis
	IHC positivity for CD41, CD42b, and CD61 helpful
Non-hematopoietic large cell neoplasm	Clinical history of malignancy
	IHC markers confirm epithelial, mesenchymal, melanocytic, etc. origin
Reed-Sternberg cell	CD30, CD15, PAX-5 weak+ in association with characteristic lymphohistiocytic fibrotic lesion
Histiocytes	May form collections (granulomas) or be singly distributed as in hemophagocytosis
	May contain polarizable material
	Positive for CD68 and CD163
Multilobulated lymphoma cells	May form discrete lesions or be singly distributed
	Generous use of immunohistochemistry will reveal cell lineage

IHC = immunohistochemistry

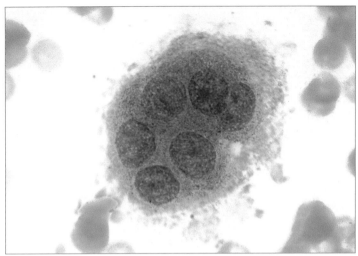

i12.39 *A typical osteoclast with multiple discrete nuclei and granular cytoplasm on a bone marrow aspirate smear. (Wright)*

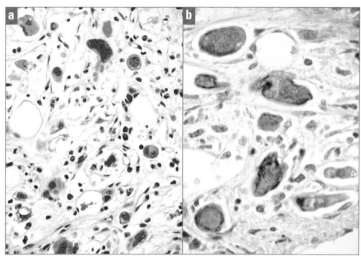

i12.40 *This composite of H&E **a** and immunoperoxidase for keratin 7 **b** is from a bone marrow core biopsy section from a patient with metastatic carcinoma with numerous individual multinucleated carcinoma cells mimicking megakaryocytes. The patient had a history of breast carcinoma. (H&E and immunoperoxidase for keratin 7)*

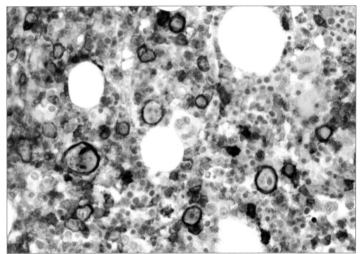

i12.41 *Immunohistochemical staining for CD3 on this bone marrow core biopsy section shows large positive anaplastic large cell lymphoma cells adjacent to negative megakaryocytes of similar overall size. Anaplastic large cell lymphoma in bone marrow can mimic megakaryocytes, especially since these tumor cells are typically individually dispersed. (immunoperoxidase for CD3) (courtesy R Macaulay, MD)*

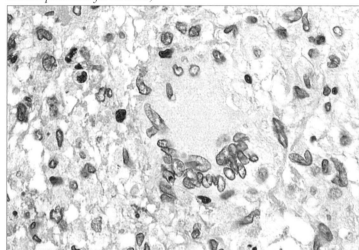

i12.42 *A Touton-type giant cell is apparent within this massive granuloma on a bone marrow biopsy section from a patient with acquired immunodeficiency syndrome. Note the striking multinucleation forming a ring at the periphery of the cytoplasm. (H&E)*

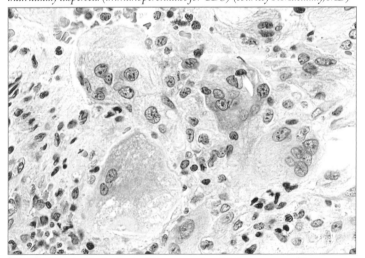

i12.43 *A foreign-body giant cell is apparent on this bone marrow biopsy section. (H&E)*

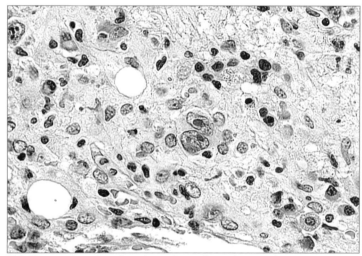

i12.44 *A multinucleated Reed-Sternberg cell is evident on a bone marrow biopsy section from an HIV-1+ patient with extensive bone marrow replacement by Hodgkin lymphoma. (H&E)*

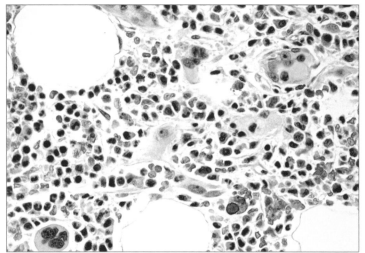

i12.45 *This bone marrow core biopsy section shows sinusoidal infiltration by metastatic neuroblastoma. These defined nests of tumor cells can mimic megakaryocytes (upper right). (H&E)*

[12.10] Clues and Caveats

1. Knowledge of normal platelet and megakaryocytic number and morphology is critical to diagnose abnormalities.

2. Congenital causes of thrombocytopenia are rare compared with their acquired counterparts, and can be further subdivided based on normal/increased or decreased megakaryocytes. When increased, the megakaryocytes are not overtly clustered and do not exhibit dysplastic features.

3. Prominent clustering of megakaryocytes with small or large forms with bizarre nuclei should prompt consideration for a primary myeloid neoplasm.

4. Congenital thrombocytopenias tend to manifest with amegakaryocytosis and may be isolated to the megakaryocytic lineage (eg, TAR) or be part of a multilineage disorder (eg, Fanconi anemia).

5. Thrombocytosis is by far most commonly seen as a reactive phenomenon secondary to stress, trauma, infection.

6. Congenital thrombocytosis is exceedingly rare with most reports focusing on familial cohorts.

7. In ITP, megakaryocytes are increased and are predominated by smaller, more immature forms.

8. HIV-1 characteristically exhibits small, "naked" megakaryocytes, but these are not specific and may be seen in other reactive conditions (viral infection, ITP) or myelodysplasia.

9. Perinatal thrombocytopenia is common and usually due to infection, immune-mediated destruction, or impaired megakaryopoiesis.

10. Circulating megakaryocytes and megakaryocytic nuclei may be seen in both children and adults and do not equate with a myeloid disorder.

11. Acquired amegakaryocytosis is rare; it is most often seen in viral infections, drug/toxin exposure, or an immune-mediated process.

12. Morphologic destruction of megakaryocytes from other "giant cells" in the bone marrow may require immunohistochemical studies.

[12.11] Acknowledgments

The author acknowledges the photographic contributions of P Izadi, P Armell, MD, T Elghetany, MD, R Macaulay, MD, and C Sever, MD.

[12.12] References

Agarwal N, Spahr JE, Werner TL, et al [2006] Acquired amegakaryocytic thrombocytopenic purpura. *Am J Hematol* 81:132-135.

Althaus K, Greinacher A [2009] MYH9-related platelet disorders. *Semin Thromb Hemost* 35:189-203.

Apostu R, Mackey MC [2008] Understanding cyclical thrombocytopenia: a mathematical modeling approach. *J Theor Biol* 251:297-316.

Aster RH [1999] Drug-induced immune thrombocytopenia: an overview of pathogenesis. *Semin Hematol* 36:2-6.

Balduini A, Pallotta I, Malara A, et al [2008] Adhesive receptors, extracellular proteins and myosin IIA orchestrate proplatelet formation by human megakaryocytes. *J Thromb Haemost* 6:1900-1907.

Ballmaier M, Germeshausen M [2009] Advances in the understanding of congenital amegakaryocytic thrombocytopenia. *Br J Haematol* 146:3-16.

Ballmaier M, Germeshausen M, Schulze H, et al [2001] c-mpl mutations are the cause of congenital amegakaryocytic thrombocytopenia. *Blood* 97:139-146.

Bartakke S, Abdelhaleem M, Carcao M [2008] Valproate-induced pure red cell aplasia and megakaryocyte dysplasia. *Br J Haematol* 141:133.

Bartels PC, Schoorl M, Lombarts AJ [1997] Screening for EDTA-dependent deviations in platelet counts and abnormalities in platelet distribution histograms in pseudothrombocytopenia. *Scand J Clin Lab Invest* 57:629-636.

Benedetti F, de Sabata D, Perona G [1994] T suppressor activated lymphocytes (CD8+/DR+) inhibit megakaryocyte progenitor cell differentiation in a case of acquired amegakaryocytic thrombocytopenic purpura. *Stem Cells* 12:205-213.

Bhattacharyya J, Kumar R, Tyagi S, et al [2005] Human parvovirus B19-induced acquired pure amegakaryocytic thrombocytopenia. *Br J Haematol* 128:128-129.

Bizzaro N, Brandalise M [1995] EDTA-dependent pseudothrombocytopenia. Association with antiplatelet and antiphospholipid antibodies. *Am J Clin Pathol* 103:103-107.

Bosticardo M, Marangoni F, Aiuti A, et al [2009] Recent advances in understanding the pathophysiology of Wiskott-Aldrich syndrome. *Blood* 113:6288-6295.

Breton-Gorius J, Favier R, Guichard J, et al [1995] A new congenital dysmegakaryopoietic thrombocytopenia (Paris-Trousseau) associated with giant platelet α-granules and chromosome 11 deletion at 11q23. *Blood* 85:1805-1814.

Breunis WB, van Mirre E, Bruin M, et al [2008] Copy number variation of the activating FCGR2C gene predisposes to idiopathic thrombocytopenic purpura. *Blood* 111:1029-1038.

Brink DS [2006] Transient leukemia (transient myeloproliferative disorder, transient abnormal myelopoiesis) of Down syndrome. *Adv Anat Pathol* 13:256-262.

Bromberg ME [2006] Immune thrombocytopenic purpura—the changing therapeutic landscape. *N Engl J Med* 355:1643-1645.

Bulchandani D, Nachnani J, Belt R, Hinton S [2007] Acquired pure megakaryocytic aplasia: report of a single case treated with mycophenolate mofetil. *Am J Hematol* 82:650-651.

Cines DB, Blanchette VS [2002] Immune thrombocytopenic purpura. *N Engl J Med* 346:995-1008.

Cines DB, Bussel JB, Liebman HA, Luning Prak ET [2009a] The ITP syndrome: pathogenic and clinical diversity. *Blood* 113:6511-6521.

Cines DB, Liebman H, Stasi R [2009b] Pathobiology of secondary immune thrombocytopenia. *Semin Hematol* 46:S2-14.

Clauser S, Cramer-Borde E [2009] Role of platelet electron microscopy in the diagnosis of platelet disorders. *Semin Thromb Hemost* 35:213-223.

Cooper N, Bussel J [2006] The pathogenesis of immune thrombocytopaenic purpura. *Br J Haematol* 133:364-374.

Dame C, Sutor AH [2005] Primary and secondary thrombocytosis in childhood. *Br J Haematol* 129:165-177.

Dameshek W, Miller E [1946] The megakaryocytes in idiopathic thrombocytopenic purpura, a form of hypersplenism. *Blood* 1:27-52.

Drachman JG, Jarvik GP, Mehaffey MG [2000] Autosomal dominant thrombo-cytopenia: incomplete megakaryocyte differentiation and linkage to human chromosome 10. *Blood* 96:118-125.

Er TK, Ruiz Gines MA [2009] Interpretation of the flag of platelet clumping from the Coulter LH 750. *Platelets* 20:68-69.

Felderbauer P, Ritter PR, Mattern D, et al [2004] Acquired pure megakaryocytic aplasia: a separate haematological disease entity or a syndrome with multiple causes? *Eur J Haematol* 72:451-454.

Fogarty PF, Stetler-Stevenson M, Pereira A, Dunbar CE [2005] Large granular lymphocytic proliferation-associated cyclic thrombocytopenia. *Am J Hematol* 79:334-336.

Foucar K [2008] Non-neoplastic megakaryocytic lineage disorders. In: King D, Gardner W, Sobin L, et al, eds. *Non-Neoplastic Disorders of Bone Marrow (AFIP fascicle)*. Washington, DC: American Registry of Pathology; 177-220.

Fox NE, Chen R, Hitchcock I, et al [2009] Compound heterozygous c-Mpl mutations in a child with congenital amegakaryocytic thrombocytopenia: functional characterization and a review of the literature. *Exp Hematol* 37:495-503.

Geddis AE [2006] Inherited thrombocytopenia: congenital amegakaryocytic thrombocytopenia and thrombocytopenia with absent radii. *Semin Hematol* 43:196-203.

Geddis AE [2009] Congenital amegakaryocytic thrombocytopenia and thrombocy-topenia with absent radii. *Hematol Oncol Clin North Am* 23:321-331.

George JN, Aster RH [2009] Drug-induced thrombocytopenia: pathogenesis, evaluation, and management. *Hematology Am Soc Hematol Edu Program* 2009:153-158.

Gerth J, Schleussner E, Kentouche K, et al [2009] Pregnancy-associated thrombotic thrombocytopenic purpura. *Thromb Haemost* 101:248-251.

Go RS [2005] Idiopathic cyclic thrombocytopenia. *Blood Rev* 19:53-59.

Hadjkacem B, Elleuch H, Gargouri J, Gargouri A [2009] Bernard-Soulier syndrome: novel nonsense mutation in *GPIbeta* gene affecting GPIb-IX complex expression. *Ann Hematol* 88:465-472.

Hansen M, Pedersen NT [1978] Circulating megakaryocytes in blood from the antecubital vein in healthy, adult humans. *Scand J Haematol* 20:371-376.

Hartwig J, Italiano J, Jr [2003] The birth of the platelet. *J Thromb Haemost* 1:1580-1586.

Hassell K [2008] Heparin-induced thrombocytopenia: diagnosis and management. *Thromb Res* 123Suppl1:S16-21.

Hoffman R [1991] Acquired pure amegakaryocytic thrombocytopenic purpura. *Semin Hematol* 28:303-312.

Hollen CW, Henthorn J, Koziol JA, Burstein SA [1991] Elevated serum interleukin-6 levels in patients with reactive thrombocytosis. *Br J Haematol* 79:286-290.

Hunt K, Salama M, Sever C, Foucar K [2009] Characterization of collagen vascular disease-associated bone marrow changes by morphologic and immunohisto-chemical assessment. *Mod Pathol* 22Suppl1:268A Abstract [1218].

Ishiguro A, Suzuki Y, Mito M, et al [2002] Elevation of serum thrombopoietin precedes thrombocytosis in acute infections. *Br J Haematol* 116:612-618.

Italiano JE Jr, Lecine P, Shivdasani RA, Hartwig JH [1999] Blood platelets are assembled principally at the ends of proplatelet processes produced by differen-tiated megakaryocytes. *J Cell Biol* 147:1299-1312.

Kato R, Shinohara A, Sato J [2009] ADAMTS13 deficiency, an important cause of thrombocytopenia during pregnancy. *Int J Obstet Anesth* 18:73-77.

Katsumata Y, Suzuki T, Kuwana M, et al [2003] Anti-c-Mpl (thrombopoietin receptor) autoantibody-induced amegakaryocytic thrombocytopenia in a patient with systemic sclerosis. *Arthritis Rheum* 48:1647-1651.

Kaushansky K [1995] Thrombopoietin: the primary regulator of platelet production. *Blood* 86:419-431.

Kaushansky K [2008] Historical review: megakaryopoiesis and thrombopoiesis. *Blood* 111:981-986.

Kaushansky K [2009] Determinants of platelet number and regulation of thrombo-poiesis. *Hematology Am Soc Hematol Edu Program* 2009:147-152.

Kaushansky K, Lok S, Holly RD, et al [1994] Promotion of megakaryocyte progenitor expansion and differentiation by the c-Mpl ligand thrombopoietin. *Nature* 369:568-571.

Kirito K, Sakoe K, Shinoda D, et al [2008] A novel RUNX1 mutation in familial platelet disorder with propensity to develop myeloid malignancies. *Haematologica* 93:155-156.

Klopocki E, Schulze H, Strauss G, et al [2007] Complex inheritance pattern resembling autosomal recessive inheritance involving a microdeletion in thrombocytopenia-absent radius syndrome. *Am J Hum Genet* 80:232-240.

Kuter DJ, Beeler DL, Rosenberg RD [1994] The purification of megapoietin: a physiological regulator of megakaryocyte growth and platelet production. *Proc Natl Acad Sci USA* 91:11104-11108.

Lai DW, Loughran TP, Jr [2008] Maciejewski JP, et al. Acquired amegakaryocytic thrombocytopenia and pure red cell aplasia associated with an occult large granular lymphocyte leukemia. *Leuk Res* 32:823-827.

Levine RF, Olson TA, Shoff PK, et al [1996] Mature micromegakaryocytes: an unusual developmental pattern in term infants. *Br J Haematol* 94:391-399.

Li J, Kuter DJ [2001] The end is just the beginning: megakaryocyte apoptosis and platelet release. *Int J Hematol* 74:365-374.

Li Z, Nardi MA, Karpatkin S [2005] Role of molecular mimicry to HIV-1 peptides in HIV-1-related immunologic thrombocytopenia. *Blood* 106:572-576.

Liebman HA [2008] Viral-associated immune thrombocytopenic purpura. *Hematology Am Soc Hematol Educ Program* 2008:212-218.

Liu K, Kralovics R, Rudzki Z, et al [2008] A de novo splice donor mutation in the thrombopoietin gene causes hereditary thrombocythemia in a Polish family. *Haematologica* 93:706-714.

Mantadakis E, Tsalkidis A, Chatzimichael A [2008] Thrombocytosis in childhood. *Indian Pediatr* 45:669-677.

Mattia G, Vulcano F, Milazzo L, et al [2002] Different ploidy levels of megakaryocytes generated from peripheral or cord blood CD34+ cells are correlated with different levels of platelet release. *Blood* 99:888-897.

McMillan R [2007] The pathogenesis of chronic immune thrombocytopenic purpura. *Semin Hematol* 44:S3-S11.

Michaud J, Wu F, Osato M, et al [2002] In vitro analyses of known and novel *RUNX1/AML1* mutations in dominant familial platelet disorder with predisposition to acute myelogenous leukemia: implications for mechanisms of pathogenesis. *Blood* 99:1364-1372.

Moliterno AR, Williams DM, Gutierrez-Alamillo LI, et al [2004] Mpl Baltimore: a thrombopoietin receptor polymorphism associated with thrombocytosis. *Proc Natl Acad Sci USA* 101:11444-11447.

Morselli M, Longo G, Bonacorsi G, et al [1999] Anticoagulant pseudothrombocy-topenia with platelet satellitism. *Haematologica* 84:655.

Murray NA [2002a] Evaluation and treatment of thrombocytopenia in the neonatal intensive care unit. *Acta Paediatr Suppl* 91:74-81.

Murray NA, Howarth LJ, McCloy MP, et al [2002b] Platelet transfusion in the management of severe thrombocytopenia in neonatal intensive care unit patients. *Transfus Med* 12:35-41.

Nagata Y, Muro Y, Todokoro K [1997] Thrombopoietin-induced polyploidization of bone marrow megakaryocytes is due to a unique regulatory mechanism in late mitosis. *J Cell Biol* 139:449-457.

Nardi M, Tomlinson S, Greco MA, Karpatkin S [2001] Complement-independent, peroxide-induced antibody lysis of platelets in HIV-1-related immune thrombo-cytopenia. *Cell* 106:551-561.

Niparuck P, Atichartakarn V, Chuncharunee S [2008] Successful treatment of acquired amegakaryocytic thrombocytopenic purpura refractory to corticosteroids and intravenous immunoglobulin with antithymocyte globulin and cyclosporin. *Int J Hematol* 88:223-226.

Nugent D, McMillan R, Nichol JL, Slichter SJ [2009] Pathogenesis of chronic immune thrombocytopenia: increased platelet destruction and/or decreased platelet production. *Br J Haematol* 146:585-596.

Nurden AT, Fiore M, Pillois X, Nurden P [2009a] Genetic testing in the diagnostic evaluation of inherited platelet disorders. *Semin Thromb Hemost* 35:204-212.

Nurden AT, Nurden P [2007] The gray platelet syndrome: clinical spectrum of the disease. *Blood Rev* 21:21-36.

Nurden P, Nurden AT [2008] Congenital disorders associated with platelet dysfunctions. *Thromb Haemost* 99:253-263.

Nurden AT, Viallard JF, Nurden P [2009b] New-generation drugs that stimulate platelet production in chronic immune thrombocytopenic purpura. *Lancet* 373:1562-1569.

Ochs HD, Filipovich AH, Veys P, et al [2008] Wiskott-Aldrich syndrome: diagnosis, clinical and laboratory manifestations, and treatment. *Biol Blood Marrow Transplant* 15:84-90.

Olson TA, Levine RF, Mazur EM, et al [1992] Megakaryocytes and megakaryocyte progenitors in human cord blood. *Am J Pediatr Hematol Oncol* 14:241-247.

Palaniappan G, Jennings W [2009] Idiopathic thrombocytopenic purpura. *Mod Med* 106:69-73.

Papadantonakis N, Makitalo M, McCrann DJ, et al [2008] Direct visualization of the endomitotic cell cycle in living megakaryocytes: differential patterns in low and high ploidy cells. *Cell Cycle* 7:2352-2356.

Patel SR, Hartwig JH, Italiano JE, Jr [2005] The biogenesis of platelets from megakaryocyte proplatelets. *J Clin Invest* 115:3348-3354.

Pegels JG, Bruynes EC, Engelfriet CP, von dem Borne AE [1982] Pseudothrombocytopenia: an immunologic study on platelet antibodies dependent on ethylene diamine tetra-acetate. *Blood* 59:157-161.

Percy MJ, Rumi E [2009] Genetic origins and clinical phenotype of familial and acquired erythrocytosis and thrombocytosis. *Am J Hematol* 84:46-54.

Peters M, Heyderman RS, Klein NJ [1998] Platelet satellitism. *N Engl J Med* 339:131-132.

Pisciotta AV, Stefanini M, Dameshek W [1953] Studies on platelets. X. Morphologic characteristics of megakaryocytes by phase contrast microscopy in normals and in patients with idiopathic thrombocytopenic purpura. *Blood* 8:703-723.

Provan D, Stasi R, Newland AC, et al [2010] International consensus report on the investigation and management of primary immune thrombocytopenia. *Blood* 115:168-186.

Psaila B, Bussel JB [2008] Refractory immune thrombocytopenic purpura: current strategies for investigation and management. *Br J Haematol* 143:16-26.

Raslova H, Kauffmann A, Sekkai D, et al [2007] Interrelation between polyploidization and megakaryocyte differentiation: a gene profiling approach. *Blood* 109:3225-3234.

Ravid K, Lu J, Zimmet JM, Jones MR [2002] Roads to polyploidy: the megakaryocyte example. *J Cell Physiol* 190:7-20.

Redman R, Shunkwiler SM, Harris NS, et al [2008] Sebastian syndrome with abnormal platelet response to ristocetin. *Lab Hematol* 14:19-23.

Rivers A, Slayton WB [2009] Congenital cytopenias and bone marrow failure syndromes. *Semin Perinatol* 33:20-28.

Roberts IA, Murray NA [2003a] Neonatal thrombocytopenia: causes and management. *Arch Dis Child Fetal Neonatal Ed* 88:F359-364.

Roberts IA, Murray NA [2003b] Thrombocytopenia in the newborn. *Curr Opin Pediatr* 15:17-23.

Roberts IA, Murray NA [2008a] Neonatal thrombocytopenia. *Semin Fetal Neonatal Med* 13:256-264.

Roberts IA, Stanworth S, Murray NA [2008b] Thrombocytopenia in the neonate. *Blood Rev* 22:173-186.

Rodeghiero F, Stasi R, Gernsheimer T, et al [2009] Standardization of terminology, definitions and outcome criteria in immune thrombocytopenic purpura of adults and children: report from an international working group. *Blood* 113:2386-2393.

Rosenthal NS, Farhi DC [1991] Dysmegakaryopoiesis resembling acute megakaryoblastic leukemia in treated acute myeloid leukemia. *Am J Clin Pathol* 95:556-560.

Savoia A, Balduini CL, Savino M, et al [2001] Autosomal dominant macrothrombocytopenia in Italy is most frequently a type of heterozygous Bernard-Soulier syndrome. *Blood* 97:1330-1335.

Scaradavou A [2002] HIV-related thrombocytopenia. *Blood Rev* 16:73-76.

Schafer AI [2001] Thrombocytosis and thrombocythemia. *Blood Rev* 15:159-166.

Schafer AI [2004] Thrombocytosis. *N Engl J Med* 350:1211-1219.

Schech SD, Brinker A, Shatin D, Burgess M [2006] New-onset and idiopathic thrombotic thrombocytopenic purpura: incidence, diagnostic validity, and potential risk factors. *Am J Hematol* 81:657-663.

Skoda RC [2009] Thrombocytosis. *Hematology Am Soc Hematol Edu Program* 2009:159-167.

Sola-Visner MC, Christensen RD, Hutson AD, Rimsza LM [2007] Megakaryocyte size and concentration in the bone marrow of thrombocytopenic and nonthrombocytopenic neonates. *Pediatr Res* 61:479-484.

Sola-Visner M, Sallmon H, Brown R [2009] New insights into the mechanisms of nonimmune thrombocytopenia in neonates. *Semin Perinatol* 33:43-51.

Solar GP, Kerr WG, Zeigler FC, et al [1998] Role of c-mpl in early hematopoiesis. *Blood* 92:4-10.

Sood R, Wong W, Gotlib J, et al [2008] Gene expression and pathway analysis of immune thrombocytopenic purpura. *Br J Haematol* 140:99-103.

Stenberg PE, Levin J [1989] Mechanisms of platelet production. *Blood Cells* 15:23-47.

Stoll DB, Blum S, Pasquale D, Murphy S [1981] Thrombocytopenia with decreased megakaryocytes. Evaluation and prognosis. *Ann Intern Med* 94:170-175.

Sutor AH [1995] Thrombocytosis in childhood. *Semin Thromb Hemost* 21:330-339.

Tavassoli M, Aoki M [1989] Localization of megakaryocytes in the bone marrow. *Blood Cells* 15:3-14.

Tecuceanu N, Dardik R, Rabizadeh E, et al [2006] A family with hereditary thrombocythaemia and normal genes for thrombopoietin and c-Mpl. *Br J Haematol* 135:348-351.

Tefferi A, Vardiman JW [2007] The diagnostic interface between histology and molecular tests in myeloproliferative disorders. *Curr Opin Hematol* 14:115-122.

Tefferi A, Vardiman JW [2008] Classification and diagnosis of myeloproliferative neoplasms: the 2008 World Health Organization criteria and point-of-care diagnostic algorithms. *Leukemia* 22:14-22.

Thiele J, Kvasnicka HM, Orazi A [2005] Bone marrow histopathology in myeloproliferative disorders—current diagnostic approach. *Semin Hematol* 42:184-195.

Thiele J, von Ammers E, Wagner S, et al [1991] Megakaryocytopoiesis in idiopathic thrombocytopenic purpura: a morphometric and immunohistochemical study on bone marrow biopsies with special emphasis on precursor cells. *Hematol Pathol* 5:75-82.

Tubman VN, Levine JE, Campagna DR, et al [2007] X-linked gray platelet syndrome due to a GATA1 Arg216Gln mutation. *Blood* 109:3297-3299.

Vitrat N, Cohen-Solal K, Pique C, et al [1998] Endomitosis of human megakaryocytes are due to abortive mitosis. *Blood* 91:3711-3723.

Vlasoff D, Morice W [2006] Non-neoplastic bone marrow pathology associated with autoimmune disorders. *Mod Pathol* 19Suppl1:250A Abstract [1162].

Warkentin TE [2007] Heparin-induced thrombocytopenia. *Hematol Oncol Clin North Am* 21:589-607, v.

Webb D, Roberts I, Vyas P [2007] Haematology of Down syndrome. *Arch Dis Child Fetal Neonatal* Ed 92:F503-507.

Weissman IL, Shizuru JA [2008] The origins of the identification and isolation of hematopoietic stem cells, and their capability to induce donor-specific transplantation tolerance and treat autoimmune diseases. *Blood* 112:3543-3553.

White JG [2007a] Platelet pathology in carriers of the X-linked *GATA1* macrothrombocytopenia. *Platelets* 18:620-627.

White JG [2007b] Platelet storage pool deficiency in Jacobsen syndrome. *Platelets* 18:522-527.

Wiestner A, Padosch SA, Ghilardi N, et al [2000] Hereditary thrombocythaemia is a genetically heterogeneous disorder: exclusion of TPO and MPL in 2 families with hereditary thrombocythaemia. *Br J Haematol* 110:104-109.

Wiestner A, Schlemper RJ, van der Maas AP, Skoda RC [1998] An activating splice donor mutation in the thrombopoietin gene causes hereditary thrombocythaemia. *Nat Genet* 18:49-52.

Wilde NT, Burgess R, Keenan DJ, Lucas GS [1997] The effect of cardiopulmonary bypass on circulating megakaryocytes. *Br J Haematol* 98:322-327.

Witters P, Freson K, Verslype C, et al [2008] Review article: blood platelet number and function in chronic liver disease and cirrhosis. *Aliment Pharmacol Ther* 27:1017-1029.

Woods MJ, Landon CR, Wagner BE, et al [1992] Isolation of circulating megakaryocytes in man. *Med Lab Sci* 49:252-258.

Xiao Y, Lin W, Liu Q, et al [2006] Direct infection of colony forming unit-megakaryocyte by human cytomegalovirus contributes the pathogenesis of idiopathic thrombocytopenic purpura. *J Huazhong Univ Sci Technolog Med Sci* 26:555-557.

Zandecki M, Genevieve F, Gerard J, Godon A [2007] Spurious counts and spurious results on haematology analysers: a review. Part I: platelets. *Int J Lab Hematol* 29:4-20.

Zent CS, Ratajczak J, Ratajczak MZ, et al [1999] Relationship between megakaryocyte mass and serum thrombopoietin levels as revealed by a case of cyclic amegakaryocytic thrombocytopenic purpura. *Br J Haematol* 105:452-458.

Zimmet J, Ravid K [2000] Polyploidy: occurrence in nature, mechanisms, and significance for the megakaryocyte-platelet system. *Exp Hematol* 28:3-16.

Zucker-Franklin D, Cao YZ [1989] Megakaryocytes of human immunodeficiency virus-infected individuals express viral RNA. *Proc Natl Acad Sci USA* 86:5595-5599.

Conceptual Overview of Myeloid Neoplasms

Kathryn Foucar, MD

The successful diagnosis of a myeloid neoplasm requires an integrated multidisciplinary approach spanning basic frontline clinical evaluation to complex esoteric molecular genetic testing **t13.1, t13.2**. Consternation may arise from both the sheer number of specific myeloid neoplasms in the 2008 World Health Organization (WHO) classification (>50) and the complexity of molecular genetic testing required to establish many of these diagnoses [Vardiman 2008, 2009]. Consequently a systematic approach is essential, acknowledging that esoteric testing, although important, complements rather than replaces more routine diagnostic and prognostic information **t13.2**. The 2008 WHO classification of myeloid neoplasms highlights the expanding role of pathologists in clinical practice. No longer is a final diagnostic "label" sufficient. Instead, the pathologist must expand this diagnostic workup to include prognostic information as well as molecular/genetic information that may justify targeted therapy [Baldus 2007, Mrozek 2004].

[13.1]   Pathologic Objectives

Goals for the practicing pathologist now include successfully identifying and communicating to clinicians and patients a distinct biologic entity within the broad categories of myeloid neoplasms, in conjunction with information relevant to targeted therapy, possible treatment resistance, disease monitoring, and outcome prediction. Further testing could even include predictions of susceptibility to subsequent therapy-related neoplasms [Ellis 2008, Ng 2005, Rund 2005, Seedhouse 2007]. If a definitive diagnosis cannot be made, the pathologist should recommend additional tests that could potentially resolve diagnostic uncertainty.

t13.1   Key Clinical Data Relevant to Myeloid Neoplasms

Family history of hematologic disorders

Constitutional hematopoietic disorder——Down syndrome, Fanconi anemia, etc

Underlying disorder that could mimic myeloid neoplasm (collagen vascular disease, infection—notably HIV-1)

Medication, homeopathic remedies, or toxic exposures that could impact hematopoiesis (zinc-induced copper deficiency)

Careful assessment for possible cytokine (growth factor) therapy

Exposure to chemotherapy and/or radiation therapy

Duration and pattern of hematologic abnormality: stable vs progressive; single vs multilineage

Physical findings: splenomegaly, hepatomegaly, lymphadenopathy, skin lesions, petechiae, gum infiltrates, other pathologic sites

Laboratory evaluation for nutritional deficiency, LDH, other testing as appropriate

HIV-1 = human immunodeficiency virus; LDH = lactate dehydrogenase

t13.2   Integrative Diagnostic Approach to Myeloid Neoplasms

Clinical information (see **t13.1**)	History
	Physical examination
	Laboratory assessment
	Radiologic assessment
Hematologic assessment	CBC and differential
	Intact vs failed hematopoiesis
	Morphologic assessment of all lineages
	Reticulocyte count
	Iron, folate, cobalamin assessment as appropriate
	Other tests as needed, eg, PNH screening, cerruloplasmin
Bone marrow evaluation	Correlate with blood findings (smears)
	Quantitate blasts and determine blast lineage (smears)
	Apply cytochemical stains as needed for blast lineage determination (smears)
	Evaluate all hematolymphoid lineages for qualitative and quantitative abnormalities (smears, biopsy for megakaryocytes)
	Use specific criteria to assess dysplasia in all hematopoietic lineages (smears, biopsy)
	Evaluate cellularity, bone, stroma, sinuses, megakaryocytes, other hematopoietic lineage architecture (biopsy)
	Estimate blasts on core biopsy for concordance/discordance with smears
	Immunohistochemical staining as needed (biopsy, clot sections)
Flow cytometric immunophenotyping	Assess for proportion and lineage of immature cells
	Assess patterns of antigen coexpression
	Use sufficiently broad panel to detect aberrant antigen expression
Genetic assessment	Conventional cytogenetics to detect chromosomal translocations, deletions, duplications
	FISH for cryptic translocations and deletions
	Targeted FISH for rapid detection of genetic abnormality in advance of conventional karyotype
	Polymerase chain reaction for myeloid neoplasm-related gene mutations
Final integrated report	Synthesize and integrate all parameters
	Provide evidence supporting specific WHO entity
	Recommendations for additional evaluations to resolve diagnostic uncertainty

CBC = complete blood count; FISH = fluorescence in situ hybridization; PNH = paroxysmal nocturnal hemoglobinuria; WHO = World Health Organization

t13.3 Hemogram Data in Myeloid Neoplasms*

Finding	Comments
Pancytopenia (anemia, absolute neutropenia, and thrombocytopenia)	Supports hematopoietic failure (ineffective hematopoiesis)
	Prototypic of MDS and many AMLs
	Cytopenias generally more pronounced in AML
Isolated cytopenia (other counts normal)	Prototypic of low-grade MDS
Cytosis(es) (erythrocytosis, neutrophilia, thrombocytosis)	Elevations in single or multiple hematopoietic lineages characteristic of MPN (effective hematopoiesis)
Hybrid cytosis/cytopenias	Prototypic of MDS/MPN and some AMLs
Absolute neutrophilia	Prototypic of MPN, especially pronounced in CML and CNL
Absolute basophilia	Prototypic of MPN, notably CML, especially if pronounced (>2.0 × 10⁹/L)
	May be seen in other myeloid neoplasms
Absolute eosinophilia	Prototypic of myeloid neoplasms with *PDGFRA*, *PDGFRB*, and *FGFR1* mutations and systemic mastocytosis
	Also seen in other myeloid neoplasms, but less pronounced
Absolute monocytosis	Prototypic of MDS/MPN and some types of AML
Low WBC count	Prototypic of MDS and selected AMLs
Marked leukocytosis	>300 × 10³/µL (>300 × 10⁹/L) prototypic of CML; may occur in occasional AML
	>100 × 10³/µL (>100 × 10⁹/L) in CML, MPN, CNL, CEL, MDS/MPN, AML

*Reflects only myeloid neoplasms; there are many other possible causes of these complete blood count aberrations
AML = acute myeloid leukemia; CEL = chronic eosinophilic leukemia; CML = chronic myelogeneous leukemia; CNL = chronic neutrophilic leukemia; MDS = myelodysplastic syndrome; MPN = myeloproliferative neoplasm; WBC = white blood cell count

t13.4 Blood Smear Features of Myeloid Neoplasms*

Finding	Comments
Anisopoikilocytosis	Nonspecific, but may be pronounced in some MDS and AML cases
Polychromasia	Elevated in MPN, especially polycythemia vera
	Reduced in MDS, AML, and most MDS/MPN
Macrocytosis (not related to polychromasia)	Common in MDS
Hypogranular and/or hyposegmented neutrophils	Common in MDS, some types of MDS/MPN and AML
Atypical monocytic cells	Must distinguish monoblasts and promonocytes from more mature forms
	Prototypic of several MDS/MPN and some AMLs
Dysplastic eosinophils (hypogranular, nuclear segmentation abnormalities)	Not a reliable feature of a myeloid neoplasm
	May be seen in myeloid neoplasms with *PDGFRA/B* and *FGFR1* mutations
	Occasional feature in other myeloid neoplasms (eg, mastocytosis)
Blast/blast equivalents	Categorize by type, percentage
	Often low percentage in MPN, many MDS subtypes, many MDS/MPN subtypes
	Highest proportion in AML
	Blast count may be higher in bone marrow than in blood

*Reflects only myeloid neoplasms; there are many other possible causes of these blood smear abnormalities
AML = acute myeloid leukemia; MDS = myelodysplastic syndrome; MPN = myeloproliferative neoplasm

[13.2] Classification

Myeloid neoplasms are subcategorized into 5 broad groups [Vardiman 2008]:

1. Myeloproliferative neoplasms (MPN)
2. Myeloid (and lymphoid) neoplasms associated with eosinophilia and abnormalities of *PDGFRA*, *PDGFRB*, and *FGFR1*
3. Myelodysplastic/myeloproliferative neoplasms (MDS/MPN)
4. Myelodysplastic syndromes (MDS)
5. Acute myeloid leukemias and related neoplasms

In addition, acute leukemias of ambiguous lineage include some myeloid-related neoplasms. All of these diagnostic groups are based on de novo disease presentations, though chronic myeloid neoplasms may transform over time into more aggressive disorders.

[13.3] Diagnostic Considerations

Subsequent chapters in this book will provide specific diagnostic strategies for individual myeloid neoplasms, while the current chapter provides a "broad strokes" approach, helping the diagnostician determine if a myeloid neoplasm is likely, and, if so, what general type. The complete blood count (CBC) data and blood smear review can go a long way toward answering both of these questions t13.3, t13.4, i13.1.

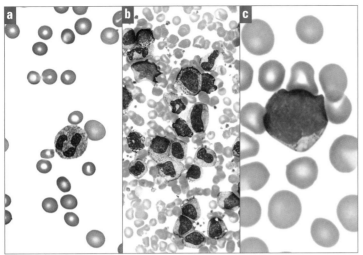

i13.1 *This composite illustrates the typical blood features of myelodysplasia* **a**, *a myeloproliferative neoplasm* **b**, *and acute myeloid leukemia* **c**. *Note that pancytopenia is present in the patient with myelodysplasia (ineffective hemato-poiesis). Myeloproliferative neoplasms are characterized by high cell counts (effective hematopoiesis). Acute myeloid leukemias have a highly variable white blood cell count (8.6 × 10³/μL [8.6 × 10⁹/L] in this case), while anemia and thrombocytopenia are typical. (Wright)*

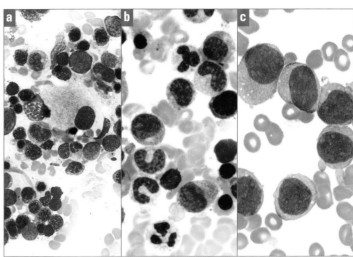

i13.2 *This composite of bone marrow aspirate smears shows a comparison of myelodysplasia* **a**, *a myeloproliferative neoplasm* **b**, *and acute myeloid leukemia* **c**. *Note that maturation is intact in myelodysplasia and especially in myeloproliferative neoplasms, where mature cells predominate. Blasts predominate in the case of acute myeloid leukemia illustrated. (Wright)*

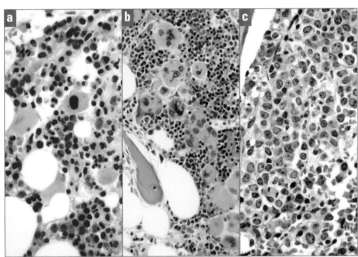

i13.3 *This comparison composite of bone marrow core biopsy sections from patients with myelodysplasia* **a**, *a myeloproliferative neoplasm* **b**, *and acute myeloid leukemia* **c**. *Note that maturation is intact in myelodysplasia and myeloproliferative neoplasms, while the bone marrow is effaced by blasts in the case of acute myeloid leukemia. (H&E)*

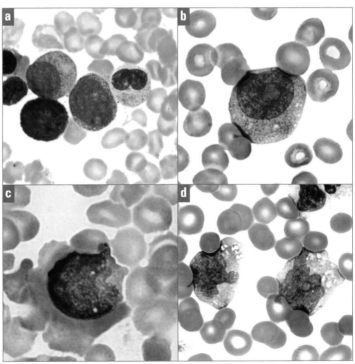

i13.4 *This composite shows morphologic features of a myeloblast* **a**, *a monoblast* **b**, *a megakaryoblast* **c**, *and a promonocyte* **d**. *The promonocyte differs from the monoblast in that there is some nuclear folding, but the nucleus retains features of immaturity, including nucleoli. The megakaryoblast illustrated is nondescript and could not be identified based on morphologic features alone. (Wright)*

In general, a bone marrow examination and specialized testing are pursued when clinical, CBC, and morphologic features of the blood smear suggest that a myeloid neoplasm is a strong diagnostic consideration. In some cases the blood alone is diagnostic; specialized flow cytometric, cytogenetic, and molecular tests can all be performed on blood if the abnormal cell population is sufficiently represented. Nonetheless, bone marrow examination is frequently performed to assess myeloid neoplasms and confirm blood

findings; **t13.5** and **t13.6** list key features to assess on aspirate smears and core biopsies **i13.2**, **i13.3**.

t13.7 denotes the types of blasts and blast equivalents **i13.4** [Mufti 2008]. Accurate quantification of these cells by morphology

t13.5 Bone Marrow Aspirate Features in Myeloid Neoplasms

Finding	Comments
Hypercellularity	Common in all categories of myeloid neoplasms
Increased megakaryocytes	Common in MPN, MDS, some MDS/MPN
	Dysplasia best assessed on core biopsy
Reduced megakaryocytes	Seen in many types of AML
Intact hematopoietic lineage maturation	Prototypic of MPN, but also generally present in MDS and MDS/MPN
Left-shifted myeloid maturation	Common in AML
	May be seen in high-grade MDS, MDS/MPN
Blasts/blast equivalents (see t13.7)	Must determine lineage and percentage
	Note any distinctive features of blasts (may be clue to genotype)
	≥20% in AML (note some exceptions)
	<20% in MDS, MDS/MPN, and MPN
Erythroid lineage	Erythroblasts not included in blast percentage (exception: acute erythroid leukemia)
	If erythroid cells exceed 50% of all HP cells, proportion of myeloid blasts ≥20% based on percentage of non-erythroid cells in several AML subtypes
	Many types of erythroid dysplasia may be useful in diagnosis and subclassification
Assess all HP lineages for dysplasia, degree of maturation, and proportion among HP cells	Useful in MDS and AML in particular
	Note distinctive features (may be clue to genotype)
Assess mast cells, lymphocytes, and plasma cells	Mast cells may be component of myeloid neoplasm

AML = acute myeloid leukemia; MDS = myelodysplastic syndrome; MPN = myeloproliferative neoplasm; HP = hematopoietic

t13.6 Bone Marrow Core Biopsy Findings in Myeloid Neoplasms

Finding	Comments
Hypercellularity	Typical in all myeloid neoplasms
Hypocellularity	Rare cases of hypocellular MDS and AML
	In advanced PMF, the hematopoietic cavity is effaced by fibrosis with marked hypocellularity
Prominent bony abnormalities	Characteristic of MPN, especially PMF and systemic mastocytosis
Dilated sinuses containing myeloid cells	Characteristic of MPN, especially PMF
Increased megakaryocytes	Characteristic of MPN and MDS
	Also present in some MDS/MPN and rare AMLs
Hyperlobated megakaryocytes (often in clusters)	Characteristic of MPN, especially ET and PMF
	Also present in some MDS/MPN
Pleomorphic megakaryocytes (often in clusters)	Characteristic of MPN, especially PMF
Hypolobated megakaryocytes	Typical in CML and many MDS
	Hallmark of MDS with isolated del(5q)
	Also present in some AMLs
Prominent fibrosis	Often present in MPN, especially PMF and systemic mastocytosis
	Occasionally seen in all other types of myeloid neoplasms
ALIP	Often seen in MDS
	MPO+ with variable CD34+
	May see collections of blasts in MPN or MDS/MPN, especially if transforming
Large sheets of blasts	AML or transformation of other myeloid neoplasm to AML

ALIP = abnormal localization of immature precursors; AML = acute myeloid leukemia; ET = essential thrombocytopenia; MDS = myelodysplastic syndrome; MPN = myeloproliferative neoplasm; MPO = myeloperoxidase; PMF = primary myelofibrosis

with or without cytochemical staining is essential in the diagnosis of myeloid neoplasms. Lineage and stage of maturation can also be validated by flow cytometric immunophenotyping, a valuable adjunct to morphologic assessment. All of the blast/blast equivalents listed in t13.7 have distinctive immunophenotypic profiles. Markers of immaturity include weak CD45 expression often in conjunction with

CD34, CD117, or possibly TdT expression. Although blast percentage is readily available by flow cytometric immunophenotyping, this is not a substitute for morphologic blast delineation. In fact, the blast percentage can readily be either overestimated (due to standard lysis of erythroid cells) or underestimated (in hemodilute second aspirate) by flow cytometric immunophenotyping. Even more importantly, reliance on CD34 expression for blast quantification will fail to detect monoblasts, promonocytes, promyelocytes, erythroblasts, and megakaryoblasts, which are typically CD34–. Some myeloblasts may even be CD34–.

t13.7 Blasts and Blast Equivalents in Myeloid Neoplasms

Morphologic Type	Cytochemistry	Comments
Myeloblast	MPO	Both agranular and granular types
		Included in all blast percentages
Promyelocytes	MPO	Blast equivalent in APL only
Monoblasts	NSE	Voluminous cytoplasm
		Included in all blast percentages
Promonocytes	NSE	Blastic nuclear features, but some folding, nucleoli
		Included in all blast percentages
Megakaryoblasts	None commonly used	Included in all blast percentages
		Must be distinguished from differentiating megakaryocytes, which are *not* included in blast count, even if monolobate
Erythroblasts	PAS (not commonly used)	Only included in blast percentage in acute erythroid leukemia; erythroblasts must predominate
Other blastic cells	Variable	Metastatic neoplasms, notably neuroblastoma, retinoblastoma, and rhabdomyosarcoma—can mimic acute leukemia, especially on smears

APL = acute promyelocytic leukemia; MPO = myeloperoxidase;
NSE = non-specific esterase cytochemical stain; PAS = periodic acid Schiff

t13.8 Myeloid Neoplasms Defined by Cytogenetic Molecular Features*

Disorder	Defining Genetic Feature
MDS (one type)	Isolated del(5q)
CML	*BCR-ABL1*
Myeloid neoplasms with eosinophilia (3 types)	Mutations/rearrangements of *PDGFRA*, *PDGFRB*, *FGFR1*
AML with specific recurring abnormality (9 types)	*RUNX1-RUNX1T1*
	CBFB-MYH11
	PML-RARA
	MLLT3-MLL
	DEK-NUP214
	RPN1-EVI1
	RBM15-MKL1
	Mutated *NPM1* (provisional)
	Mutated *CEBPA* (provisional)

*Many other genetic abnormalities identified in myeloid neoplasms, but these do not define specific entities
AML = acute myeloid leukemia; CML = chronic myelogenous leukemia; MDS = myelodysplastic syndrome

References: [Vardiman 2008, Vardiman 2009]

Flow cytometric immunophenotyping is an excellent modality for lineage delineation. Myeloid lineage antigens include CD33, CD13, CD15, and myeloperoxidase. Glycophorin highlights erythroid cells. CD36 and CD64 are useful in monocytic lineage delineation, while CD41, CD42b, and CD61 highlight megakaryocytic cells [Vardiman 2008, Vardiman 2009]. A sufficiently broad immunophenotypic panel must be used to detect aberrant patterns of antigen expression, which is particularly useful in MDS, MDS/MPN, and AML. Flow cytometric immunophenotyping can also be used for monitoring for both response to therapy and minimal residual disease (see Chapter 36).

Generally morphologic, cytochemical, immunohisto-chemical, and flow cytometric immunophenotyping data are available shortly after bone marrow examination, facilitating integration of this information into the initial diagnosis. The genetic information is often delayed, although fluorescence in situ hybridization (FISH) testing requires only an overnight incubation and is generally available sooner than either conventional cytogenetics or polymerase chain reaction (PCR). Because genetic testing provides definitive diagnostic "proof" of many myeloid neoplasms, critical prognostic information for many neoplasms, and may even identify patients for targeted therapy, molecular/genetic testing is essential in virtually all myeloid neoplasms. In fact, these genetic data often provide the basis for the subclassification of myeloid neoplasms **t13.8**. For example, constitutive activation of protein tyrosine kinases is a genetic hallmark of MPN and myeloid neoplasms with eosinophilia and abnormalities of *PDGFRA/B* and *FGFR1*, while mutations in the *RAS/MAPK* pathway are notable in many MDS/MPN cases [Bain 2007, Orazi 2008, Quintas-Cardama 2009, Reilly 2008]. In AML, cooperating class I and class II mutations are often detected. Class I mutations, including *FLT3* and *c-KIT* mutations, result in constitutive tyrosine kinase activation, and promote proliferation and cell survival. Class II mutations involve transcription factors (*RUNX1, RARA, NPM1,* etc) that impair maturation programs [Falini 2007, Renneville 2008, Schlenk 2008]. Gene deletions, common in MDS and some AMLs, result in haploinsufficiency and other genetic

t13.9 Testing Recommendations for Myeloid Disorders

Diagnosis under Consideration	CBC and Differential	Morphology Review*	Flow Cytometry	Targeted FISH	Full Karyotyping	Other Molecular (Specify)
MDS MDS/MPN	Y	Y	S Utility in detecting aberrant antigen profiles Blast quantification may not be accurate May be useful in monocytic lineage assessment	S If suboptimal cytogenetics† BCR-ABL1 if cytogenetically normal	Y	S JAK2 may be helpful in some MDS/MPN and can confirm clonality
MPN, non-CML	Y	Y	S Limited utility unless blasts substantially increased	S BCR-ABL1 if cytogenetically normal PDGFRA (eos)	S Exclude t(9;22) (q34;q11), 5q33 (PDGFRB), or 8p11(FGFR1) rearrangements	S JAK2, BCR-ABL1; must exclude CML
CML	Y	Y	X in chronic phase Y if blasts increased (acute leukemia panel)	S BCR-ABL1 if cytogenetically normal or failed	Y	Y JAK2 in selected circumstances Q; BCR-ABL1 for monitoring treatment response
Myeloid disease with PDGFRA/B and FGFR1	Y (eos)	Y	Not generally needed unless blasts increased	PDGFRA; BCR-ABL1 if cytogenetically normal or failed	Y	S For detection of occult fusion genes
AML	Y	Y	Y (comprehensive acute leukemia panel)	S PML-RARA for STAT result CBFB rearrangement if questionable inv(16)	Y Alert lab to possible inv(16) if morphology suggestive	S FLT3, NPM1 if karyotypically normal, other circumstances Q; PML-RARA, etc in selected circumstances Other as needed

*Morphologic, hematologic review should guide all specialized testing

†Suboptimal = <20 metaphases, poor quality staining, banding, or spreading

AML = acute myeloid leukemia; CML = chronic myelogenous leukemia; MDS = myeloproliferative disorders; MPN = myeloproliferative neoplasms

S = Sometimes recommended in specific circumstances; factor in clinical issues such as patient age, comorbidities, likelihood of therapy

Q = Quantitative reverse transcriptase polymerase chain reaction

X = No, not recommended; not necessary for diagnosis, but may be needed in selected cases to exclude other differential diagnostic considerations

Y = Yes, necessary in all or almost all circumstances

aberrations [Bernasconi 2007, Haase 2007]. Therefore, a "positive" genetic result not only secures the diagnosis of a clonal myeloid neoplasm, but also provides essential prognostic and potential therapeutic information.

A wealth of specialized tests could be used potentially in the assessment of a hematologic specimen. However, in addition to being costly, each of these specialized tests has some limitation(s). Before a "one size fits all" type of testing strategy is adopted, careful consideration should be given to unique patient circumstances as well as the likelihood that a given esoteric test will be "value added." The results of specialized tests can even be misleading. For example, conventional cytogenetics will be normal in a bone marrow specimen in which the target neoplastic cell is absent or present in very low numbers. Thus the normal karyotype does *not* reflect the genotype of the neoplasm. Similarly, many genetic abnormalities are karyotypically cryptic and are detectable only with either FISH or molecular testing. Thus, even specimens with sufficient neoplastic cells may yield a normal conventional karyotype, despite possessing a significant genetic aberration. Suggested testing recommendations and considerations for the assessment of myeloid disorders are presented in **t13.9** and **t13.10**.

t13.10 Additional Suggestions/Considerations for Specialized Testing Strategies

Consider limiting specialized testing workup if patient is very elderly, debilitated, or *not* a candidate for therapy (discuss with clinician)

If CBC *morphology* is prototypic/clear cut, much more targeted workup for the likely disorder is warranted

Protocol requirements may result in additional mandatory specialized testing at diagnosis and for subsequent MRD monitoring

If morphology and IHC/flow cytometric immunophenotyping are *negative* for a given cell population, further FISH and karyotyping is *not* cost effective; molecular studies may still be warranted *if* assessing for possible MRD

Recommendations apply to the most common scenarios; exceptions are appropriate for more unique clinical circumstances

CBC = complete blood count; FISH = fluorescence in situ hybridization; IHC = immunohistochemistry; MRD = minimal residual disease

[13.4] References

Bain BJ, Fletcher SH [2007] Chronic eosinophilic leukemias and the myeloproliferative variant of the hypereosinophilic syndrome. *Immunol Allergy Clin North Am* 27:377-388.

Baldus CD, Mrozek K, Marcucci G, Bloomfield CD [2007] Clinical outcome of de novo acute myeloid leukaemia patients with normal cytogenetics is affected by molecular genetic alterations: a concise review. *Br J Haematol* 137:387-400.

Bernasconi P, Klersy C, Boni M, et al [2007] World Health Organization classification in combination with cytogenetic markers improves the prognostic stratification of patients with de novo primary myelodysplastic syndromes. *Br J Haematol* 137:193-205.

Ellis NA, Huo D, Yildiz O, et al [2008] MDM2 SNP309 and TP53 Arg72Pro interact to alter therapy-related acute myeloid leukemia susceptibility. *Blood* 112:741-749.

Falini B, Nicoletti I, Martelli MF, Mecucci C [2007] Acute myeloid leukemia carrying cytoplasmic/mutated nucleophosmin (NPMc+ AML): biologic and clinical features. *Blood* 109:874-885.

Haase D, Germing U, Schanz J, et al [2007] New insights into the prognostic impact of the karyotype in MDS and correlation with subtypes: evidence from a core dataset of 2,124 patients. *Blood* 110:4385-4395.

Mrozek K, Heerema NA, Bloomfield CD [2004] Cytogenetics in acute leukemia. *Blood Rev* 18:115-136.

Mufti GJ, Bennett JM, Goasguen J, et al [2008] Diagnosis and classification of Myelodysplastic Syndrome: International Working Group on Morphology of myelodysplastic syndrome (IWGM-MDS) consensus proposals for the definition and enumeration of myeloblasts and ring sideroblasts. *Haematologica* 93:1712-1717.

Ng A, Taylor GM, Wynn RF, Eden OB [2005] Effects of topoisomerase 2 inhibitors on the MLL gene in children receiving chemotherapy: a prospective study. *Leukemia* 19:253-259.

Orazi A, Germing U [2008] The myelodysplastic/myeloproliferative neoplasms: myeloproliferative diseases with dysplastic features. *Leukemia* 22:1308-1319.

Quintas-Cardama A, Cortes J [2009] Molecular biology of *bcr-abl1*-positive chronic myeloid leukemia. *Blood* 113:1619-1630.

Reilly JT [2008] Pathogenetic insight and prognostic information from standard and molecular cytogenetic studies in the *BCR-ABL*-negative myeloproliferative neoplasms (MPNs). *Leukemia* 22:1818-1827.

Renneville A, Roumier C, Biggio V, et al [2008] Cooperating gene mutations in acute myeloid leukemia: a review of the literature. *Leukemia* 22:915-931.

Rund D, Krichevsy S, Bar-Cohen S, et al [2005] Therapy-related leukemia: clinical characteristics and analysis of new molecular risk factors in 96 adult patients. *Leukemia* 19:1919-1928.

Schlenk RF, Dohner K, Krauter J, et al [2008] Mutations and treatment outcome in cytogenetically normal acute myeloid leukemia. *N Engl J Med* 358:1909-1918.

Seedhouse C, Russell N [2007] Advances in the understanding of susceptibility to treatment-related acute myeloid leukaemia. *Br J Haematol* 137:513-529.

Vardiman J, Brunning R, Arber D, et al [2008] Introduction and overview of the classification of the myeloid neoplasms. In: Swerdlow S, Campo E, Harris N, et al, eds. *WHO Classification of Tumours: Pathology & Genetics: Tumours of Haematopoietic and Lymphoid Tissues.* Lyon, France: IARC Press; 18-30.

Vardiman JW, Thiele J, Arber DA, et al [2009] The 2008 revision of the WHO classification of myeloid neoplasms and acute leukemia: rationale and important changes. *Blood* 114:937-951.

Myeloproliferative Neoplasms

Kaaren Reichard, MD

Since the second edition of this book in 2001, several significant genetic discoveries and changes to the classification of myeloproliferative neoplasms (MPNs) have been made **t14.1**. Arguably, the discovery of *JAK2*-activating mutations in 2005 has had the greatest impact to date on MPN classification and diagnosis [Baxter 2005, James 2005, Kralovics 2005, Levine 2005]. MPNs comprise a broad spectrum of neoplastic disorders that are characterized by abnormal, clonal excess proliferation with complete maturation of one or more of the myeloid cell lineages (erythroid, megakaryocytic, granulocytic, neutrophilic eosinophilic, and mast cells) (eg, "effective hematopoiesis").

This chapter focuses on providing the necessary diagnostic morphologic clues in the diagnosis of MPN. The use of specialized testing techniques is also important in the work-up of these neoplasms but is applied differentially depending on the case type. The successful diagnosis of MPNs requires a systemic approach with the integration of clinical, hematologic, laboratory, morphologic and genetic parameters **t14.2**. The reader is referred to Chapter 13 for comparisons of the prototypic hematologic, morphologic and bone marrow features among all myeloid neoplasms. As delineated in Chapter 13, each category of myeloid neoplasm exhibits prototypic hemogram, blood and bone marrow morphology and core biopsy features.

[14.1] Incidence and Pathogenesis of MPNs

MPNs are rare, with an aggregate incidence of approximately 6.0-10.0 cases per 100,000 people [Johansson 2006, Rollison 2008]. Variations in the reported incidence rates are likely due to geographic and/or ethnic differences [Rohrbacher 2009]. While MPNs occur predominantly in older adults, they also occur rarely in young children and adolescents. Chronic

t14.1 Recent Significant Advances in the Classification of MPNs

Incorporation of *JAK2* mutation testing into the MPN diagnostic algorithms

Mast cell disease included as a subcategory of MPN

Cases of chronic eosinophilic leukemia with genetic aberrations involving *FGFR1*, *PDGFRA* and *PDGFRB* placed into a separate category (see Chapter 15)

Chronic idiopathic myelofibrosis now termed *primary myelofibrosis*

The term *myeloproliferative neoplasm* replaces *myeloproliferative disorder*

MPN = myeloproliferative neoplasm

t14.2 Approach to the Diagnosis of an MPN

Clinical and hematologic features	Comprehensive clinical evaluation and history (including family history/pedigree)
	Document persistent cytosis(es)
	Exclude non-MPN causes for cytosis(es)
Blood and bone marrow features	Morphologic assessment of hyperplastic lineages; no or minimal granulocytic/erythroid dysplasia (in good-quality specimens)
	Assessment of bone marrow architecture for dilated sinuses, intrasinusoidal hematopoiesis, megakaryocytic clustering, and atypia
	Blast enumeration
	Assessment for reticulin/collagen fibrosis
	Assessment of bone for osteosclerosis/osteopenia
Conventional cytogenetics	Should be performed to identify recurring genetic abnormalities indicative of a particular disorder and/or for appropriate classification [eg, t(9;22) (for CML), abnormalities of 5q31-q33 (*PDGFRB*), 8p11 (*FGFR1*), or 4q12 (*PDGFRA*)]
FISH	Perform *BCR-ABL1* to assess for CML if cytogenetics is normal or suboptimal
	Perform *FIP1L1-PDGFRA* in eosinophilia cases
Flow cytometry	Role is not well defined; largely unnecessary; may be useful to determine blast lineage in leukemic transformation
	Not required for blast enumeration (problematic)
Genetics	Perform *JAK2* V617F, *JAK2* exon 12, *MPL*, and *KIT* D816V mutation analyses on a case-by-case basis
Diagnostic interpretation	Requires integration of clinical, hematologic, morphologic, and genetic findings
	Provide WHO 2008 subtype:
	chronic myelogenous leukemia, *BCR-ABL1*+
	polycythemia vera
	primary myelofibrosis (aka chronic idiopathic myelofibrosis, myeloid metaplasia with myelofibrosis)
	essential thrombocythemia
	chronic neutrophilic leukemia
	chronic eosinophilic leukemia, not otherwise specified
	systemic mastocytosis and mast cell leukemia
	myeloproliferative neoplasm, unclassifiable

MPN = myeloproliferative neoplasm; CML = chronic myelogenous leukemia; FISH = fluorescence in situ hybridization

myelogenous leukemia (CML) is the most common MPN diagnosed in children (2.5% of all childhood leukemias) [Kurosawa 2009, Nakatani 2008, Teofili 2009]. Familial clustering of MPNs has been observed, and distinction from sporadic MPN in childhood may be challenging (see **[14.6]** "Familial MPNs," p 310) [Landgren 2008, Rumi 2008].

The pathophysiology of MPNs is quite complex and varies significantly depending on the disease subtype. However, MPNs all share a common stem cell-derived clonal myeloproliferation, which is in many cases attributable to activation of intracellular signaling pathways by mutated protein tyrosine kinases; sidebar 14.1 discusses the pathogenesis of several tyrosine kinases known to be abnormal in MPN, including the *JAK2* mutation and *BCR-ABL1* fusion. The stem cell origin of the classic MPNs has been established by demonstrating clonal involvement of B-, T-, and natural killer cells in addition to the myeloid cells [Bellanne-Chantelot 2006, Buschle 1988, Delhommeau 2007, Larsen 2007, Reeder 2003, Tefferi 1995a]. Scientific evidence indicates that the acquisition of known genetic changes (eg, *JAK2* and *BCR-ABL1*) is secondary and occurs in the setting of an already-existing predisposing state. Endothelial cells in MPN patients lack clonality [Piaggio 2009].

[14.2] Prognostic Factors in MPNs

The prognostic features in MPNs vary depending on the disease subtype. As a consequence, these are discussed primarily within each individual disease section. In general, transformation to acute leukemia and/or myelofibrosis is associated with an adverse or inferior outcome in essential thrombocythemia (ET), polycythemia vera (PV), and primary myelofibrosis (PMF). Vascular events such as thrombosis and hemorrhage are also adverse prognostic features in ET and PV [Cervantes 2008, Passamonti 2008a]. Both higher leukocyte counts and *JAK2* allele burden may be linked to thrombotic events in ET and PV [Marchetti 2008]. In PMF, several predictive models of prognosis and survival exist [Cervantes 2009]. In systemic mastocytosis, outcome is predicated on the degree of bone marrow failure and type of associated clonal hematological non-mast cell lineage disease if present [Pardanani 2009]. In chronic eosinophilic leukemia, not otherwise specified (CEL, NOS), prognosis is often linked to the extent of organ/tissue damage from the intravascular/intracardiac release of eosinophilic cationic, fibrinolytic proteins.

[14.3] Hematologic Features and Minimal Diagnostic Criteria

The constellation of unexplained single or multilineage "cytosis," hypercellular bone marrow with panmyelosis, intact maturation, abnormal (often clustered) megakaryocytes,

dilated sinuses with intrasinusoidal hematopoiesis, usually normal blast count, and varying degrees of fibrosis and osteosclerosis typifies an MPN at presentation. The prototypic findings of an MPN in peripheral blood and bone marrow are listed in **t14.3**.

[14.3.1] Blast Enumeration

The percent blasts in blood and bone marrow includes myeloblasts, monoblasts, promonocytes, and megakaryoblasts, although myeloblasts are by far the most frequent blast type in MPN. Lymphoblasts may occur in blast phase of CML (~20% of cases) but are otherwise very rare in MPNs. Blasts are counted as a percent of total nucleated cells, although lymphocytes, plasma cells, and mast cells should be excluded in patients with underlying lymphoid/plasma cell/mast cell neoplasms [Vardiman 2008a].

[14.3.2] Hematopoietic Lineage and Architecture Assessment

One of the main challenges in the diagnosis of MPN is to determine that the single or multilineage "cytosis" is not the result of a confounding non-neoplastic process (see **[14.8]** "Differential Diagnosis," p 311). This may be particularly vexing for the diagnostician lacking salient clinical, laboratory or genetic data. Most often, careful examination of an adequate and technically satisfactory blood smear, bone marrow aspirate, and bone marrow core biopsy will allow for the correct diagnosis to be established. Brief tips helpful in assigning lineage involvement are shown in **t14.4**. In addition to various cytoses (granulocytosis, thrombocytosis, or erythrocytosis), the peripheral blood may reveal basophilia, circulating megakaryocytes, and rare blasts **i14.1, i14.2, i14.3, i14.4, i14.5, i14.6, i14.7**. In longstanding MPN with fibrosis, teardrop erythrocytes and leukoerythroblastosis are typical with large, highly atypical megakaryocytic fragments **i14.2, i14.3, i14.7**. On bone marrow aspirate smears, MPNs are characterized by hypercellularity, intact maturation with normal myeloblast percentages, absent dysplasia in erythroid and granulocytic lineages, and increased megakaryocytes **i14.8, i14.9**. For inaspirable specimens, touch preparations may be helpful.

A variety of features on bone marrow biopsy sections are used to categorize MPN, especially megakaryocyte morphology, histotopography, type of hematopoietic lineage involvement, bony changes, and fibrosis **t14.3, i14.10, i14.11**. Of particular importance in reaching "definitive" criteria for MPN is the megakaryocytic morphology and architectural clustering. Megakaryocytes range from small to giant, with varying degrees of nuclear lobulation, maturation, and hyperchromasia among the different MPNs **i14.12, i14.13, i14.14, i14.15, i14.16, i14.17**. Particularly for CML, ET, and

Myeloproliferative Neoplasms from a Molecular Perspective

In 1951, William Dameshek, the preeminent hematologist of his time and a founding editor of *Blood*, published "Some speculations on the myeloproliferative syndromes," in which he suggested that myeloproliferative neoplasms (MPNs) "are all somewhat variable manifestations of proliferative activity of the bone marrow cells, perhaps due to a hitherto undiscovered stimulus" [Dameshek 1951, Tefferi 2008a]. Almost 60 years later, his speculation has proven prescient. The "hitherto undiscovered stimuli" in many (though not all) cases of MPN have been indentified and harnessed for diagnostic molecular assays. In this section we very briefly consider the molecular topography, the pathophysiologic consequences, and the diagnostic utility of these changes, all of which bear upon tyrosine kinase-signaling pathways.

Perhaps the most celebrated of these tyrosine kinases is the *BCR-ABL1* translocation observed in all cases of CML. The *ABL1* breakpoint consistently falls adjacent to exon 2 (often called a2). The *BCR* breakpoint is more variable. In the vast majority of cases of CML, the breakpoints fall within the major breakpoint region, M-BCR, juxtaposing either exon 13 or 14 of *BCR* to exon 2 of *ABL1* (e13a2 or e14a2) in the spliced chimeric mRNA. (These fusions are also referred to, using an alternative system for identifying the exons, as b2a2 or b3a2.) This arrangement leads to the production of a protein with a molecular weight of 210 kilodaltons, termed the p210. Rare cases of CML use the minor breakpoint (m-BCR, which is often seen in childhood Ph+ B-ALL), generating the e1a2 fusion and the p190 protein; these cases of CML tend to show a predominantly monocytic proliferation. Finally, some CML cases with predominance of mature neutrophils or marked thrombocytosis are characterized by usage of the μ-BCR, resulting in e19a2 (or c3a2) fusion and a p230 protein. From this, the diagnostician should draw 3 important conclusions:

1. The detection of the *BCR-ABL1* translocation is not pathognomonic for CML, as it also occurs in poor risk ALL and some cases of de novo AML.
2. The detection of *BCR-ABL1* is an absolute requirement for the diagnosis of CML. Though the fusion usually gives rise to the traditional Philadelphia chromosome, rarely, it may involve variant translocations or be detectable only by FISH or molecular analysis. Regardless, it must be present for a diagnosis of CML.
3. All 3 forms of the *BCR-ABL1* fusion can occur in CML. The M-BCR break is expected, though rare cases use the m-BCR (more monocytic phenotype) or the μ-BCR (more neutrophilic/thrombocythemic phenotype). Despite some historical confusion, all of these are now considered to be bona fide CML.

In the early 1990s, Brian Druker began screening signal transduction inhibitors for in vitro activity against CML. One compound, which had been rationally designed to occupy the ATP binding site of the *ABL1* tyrosine kinase, had the remarkable property of inhibiting growth of CML cells, but not normal cells [Druker 1996]. In 1998, Druker administered the first dose of the compound, imatinib mesylate, in a phase I trial, to "Bud," a patient with CML. Bud's wife "Yvonne" later described the effect:

"He started taking this STI-571, which is Gleevec, and [in] about 17 days, he was back down in his normal range on his white blood count, and he's been normal ever since. And this is just an important thing—what a breakthrough, I don't know what else to call it."

On imatinib, CML patients persist for long periods of time without hematologic, cytogenetic, or (in some cases) molecular evidence of disease, though crucially, the drug only abrogates the growth advantage provided by the BCR-ABL1 chimeric protein and does not actually eliminate the clone. A 3 $\log_{10}$ reduction in transcript levels is the goal of therapy, and after prolonged treatment, complete disappearance of detectable transcripts is not unexpected [Branford 2007, Hochhaus 2009]. Long-term monitoring of CML patients by quantitative molecular techniques is necessary to guard against rising levels of transcripts (generally a 0.5-1 $\log_{10}$ increase over at least 2 consecutive analyses) that may signal the development of imatinib resistance. Since resistance often arises upon the acquisition of mutations to *ABL1* that render the tyrosine kinase insensitive to the drug, sequencing of the *ABL1* kinase domain is indicated to detect such mutations. In some cases, altering the dose or switching to an alternative tyrosine kinase inhibitor can re-establish effective therapy. In other cases, most importantly the T315I mutation, the mutated protein is rendered resistant to all currently known agents [Quintas-Cardama 2008].

The centrality of altered tyrosine kinase activity in MPNs was further established in 2005 when several research teams turned their attention to the *BCR-ABL1*– MPNs. Drawing on the example of *BCR-ABL1* in CML and working under the hypothesis that aberrant tyrosine kinase activity could also be at work in PV, 4 teams independently and almost simultaneously discovered the *JAK2* V617F mutation [Baxter 2005, James 2005, Kralovics 2005, Levine 2005, Tefferi 2008a]. JAK proteins are intracellular tyrosine kinases that associate with cell surface receptors, which themselves lack tyrosine kinase activity. The V617F mutation prevents an autoinhibitory domain of JAK2 from performing its normal negative regulatory function, leading to constitutive activation of the protein. JAK2 normally associates with the receptor for erythropoietin, thus neatly explaining the connection between the mutation and the polycythemic phenotype. Soon thereafter, it was recognized that approximately 50% of ET and PMF cases also carry the *JAK2* V617F. (The exact detection rate varies somewhat by study, with some groups finding the mutation in up to 72% of ET and 57% of PMF [Levine 2007].) Analysis for this mutation is now among the most frequently requested molecular diagnostic assays. We would emphasize a few points regarding this test. *JAK2* V617F is not specific for a *BCR-ABL1*– MPN, as it is present in some cases of MDS, MDS/MPN, and AML. Conversely, *JAK2* V617F is not sensitive for a *BCR-ABL1*– MPN, as relatively rare cases of PV and substantial numbers of ET and PMF will be negative. Nevertheless, in a patient with the clinical and morphologic stigmata of an MPN, the presence of the mutation assists in clinching the diagnosis and ruling out reactive cytoses. The "allele burden" (the ratio of mutated to wild-type *JAK2*) is higher in PV and some cases of PMF, though this parameter alone is not diagnostic of the specific subtype of MPN [Hussein 2009a]. It has recently been recognized that most cases of PV lacking the V617F mutation (which falls in exon 14) instead carry mutations scattered across a range of possible sites in exon 12. Thus, a JAK2 mutation in either the V617F or a variant is present in virtually all cases of PV. Many laboratories now offer reflex analysis for exon 12 mutations on samples found to be negative for the more common V617F. Similarly, a small number (<10%) of cases of JAK2– PMF and ET instead harbor activating mutations at codon 515 of *MPL*, which encodes the thrombopoietin receptor [Abdel-Wahab 2009]. *MPL* mutation analysis is also a useful adjunct to *JAK2* testing in selected cases.

Mastocytosis is yet another major category of MPN tied etiologically to an altered tyrosine kinase. *KIT*, which encodes the cell surface receptor for stem cell factor, is mutated in many cases of mastocytosis. The detection rate depends on the clinical characteristics of the disease (ie, cutaneous vs systemic) and the methodology employed. With highly sensitive techniques, approximately 95% of cases of systemic mastocytosis can be shown to carry the most common *KIT* D816V mutation [Akin 2006]. The detection rate with techniques of moderate sensitivity is lower, and mutations elsewhere in the gene are not infrequently observed. *KIT* mutations are also present in other disease processes, including a large subset of core binding factor AML. Thus, as with the tests described above, *KIT* mutation analysis is neither completely sensitive nor totally specific for a diagnosis of mastocytosis, but in the correct clinical setting serves as a valuable aid to diagnosis—fulfilling, in this case, one of the "minor" diagnostic criteria. Detection of the D816V mutation is also clinically important, since such cases respond poorly to imatinib therapy.

The remarkable progress in understanding the molecular underpinnings of the MPNs, and particularly the success of imatinib, may lend itself to premature triumphalism. Much remains to be understood, especially in the realm of the *BCR-ABL1*– MPNs. How, for example, can we account for the presence of one common mutation in 3 quite distinct phenotypic diseases? What changes are at work in those cases found to be negative for both *JAK2* and *MPL* mutations? Though it would appear that Dameshek's "undiscovered stimulus" is largely related to aberrant tyrosine kinase signaling, recent research has in fact documented a surprising degree of underlying molecular heterogeneity in these neoplasms [Kralovics 2008]. In the coming years, molecular testing for MPNs will increasingly reflect this evolving complexity.

t14.3 Prototypic Blood and Bone Marrow Features of MPNs

Blood	Comments
Unexplained erythrocytosis	Typical of PV
Unexplained non-toxic neutrophilic leukocytosis with left shift	Most pronounced in CML
	Insignificant granulocytic dysplasia in early disease
Unexplained thrombocytosis	Typical of ET, but may be seen in CML, early PMF and PV
	May see circulating bare megakaryocyte nuclei, micromegakaryocytes, huge megakaryocyte cytoplasmic fragments
Unexplained leukoerythroblastosis	Typical of PMF; may be present in PV and CML
Basophilia	Most pronounced in CML; mild or absent in other MPNs
Eosinophilia	May be seen in a variety of MPNs: CML, mastocytosis, CEL
Circulating blasts	Usually <2% unless disease in evolution
Circulating mast cells	Exceedingly rare except in mast cell leukemia

Bone Marrow	Comments
Cellularity	Typically hypercellular with intact HP lineage maturation
	Some disorders with multilineage hyperplasia (panmyelosis)
Blasts	<20%
Dysplasia	Minimal/absent in the granulocyte and erythroid lineages
	Abnormal (often increased) megakaryocytes with spectrum of appearances: small, mononuclear ("dwarf") forms, enlarged hyperlobated forms, large forms with dark/bizarre nuclei, maturation defects
Architecture	Abnormal localization of megakaryocytes common
	Increased, often clustered megakaryocytes with atypical features (see "dysplasia" above) (see t14.4)
	Benign lymphoid nodules, notably in PMF
	Dilated sinuses with intrasinusoidal hematopoiesis, notably in PMF
Bone marrow stroma and bone	Varying degrees of reticulin and/or collagen fibrosis
	Osteosclerosis most evident in PMF and SM
	Neoangiogenesis in all MPN
Mast cells	Assess for atypical morphology (spindled or immature) and formation of compact aggregates in core biopsy; aberrant immunophenotype
	May be underrepresented on differential cell counts because of concentration within dense particles
	May be inaspirable in fibrotic lesions

CEL = chronic eosinophilic leukemia; CML = chronic myelogenous leukemia; ET = essential thrombocythemia; HP = hematopoietic; MPN = myeloproliferative neoplasm; PMF = primary myelofibrosis; PV = polycythemia vera; SM = systemic mastocytosis

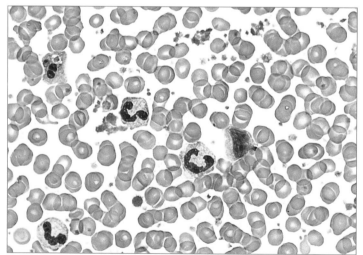

i14.1 *This peripheral blood smear shows a myeloproliferative neoplasm with neutrophilia, basophilia, and thrombocytosis. Elevated cell counts are characteristic of myeloproliferative neoplasms. (Wright)*

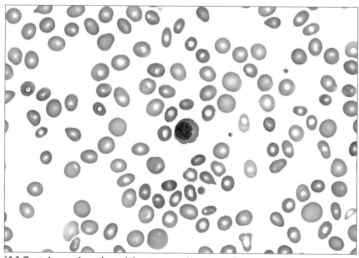

i14.2 *Advanced myeloproliferative neoplasms are characterized by anemia with teardrop erythrocytes as seen in this case of post-polycythemic myelofibrosis. Note nucleated red blood cell. (Wright)*

t14.4 Lineage Assessment in MPNs

Lineage	Clinical/Lab	Blood	Bone Marrow
Erythroid	Serum EPO level reduced	Erythrocytosis	Erythroid hyperplasia/ predominance
		RBCs usually normochromic/normocytic; may be microcytic hypochromic if concurrent iron deficiency anemia	Intact maturation but often left shift
		Circulating nucleated RBCs in leukoerythroblastic reaction	
Neutrophilic	G-CSF level reduced	Leukocytosis with left shift/myelocyte bulge in CML	Granulocytic hyperplasia
			Intact maturation
		Absence of dysplasia and toxic change (except in some cases of CNL)	
Megakaryocytic	Thrombopoietin level reduced	Thrombocytosis	Megakaryocyte hyperplasia
		Marked platelet anisocytosis	Striking clustering, atypia
		Hypogranularity of platelets	CML: small hypolobated
		Circulating megakaryocytic nuclei and cytoplasmic fragments	ET: large/giant, hyperlobulated, intact maturation
			PMF: pleomorphic, hyperchromatic, abnormal maturation, pyknotic
			PV: usually enlarged and somewhat hyperlobated
Eosinophil	Serum tryptase may be modestly elevated	Eosinophilia	Hypereosinophilia
		Eosinophil dysplastic features common; not specific for neoplasia	Variety of bone marrow appearances due to large number of MPN and non-MPN disease entities that may exhibit eosinophilia (see t14.25 and Chapter 15)
Basophil		Basophilia most prominent in CML; mild in other MPNs	Basophils and precursors may be increased in CML
Mast cell	Serum tryptase typically substantially increased	Rarely circulate except in MCL	Mast cell aggregates; target lesions
		Features of associated clonal hematologic non-mast cell lineage disease may predominate	Focal or diffuse infiltrate (often associated with osteosclerosis)
			Highly variable if associated clonal hematologic non-mast cell lineage disease present (ranges from acute leukemia, other myeloid neoplasms to lymphoid/plasma cell neoplasms)

CML = chronic myelogenous leukemia; CNL = chronic neutrophilic leukemia; EPO = erythropoietin; G-CSF = granulocyte colony-stimulating factor; ET = essential thrombocythemia; MCL = mast cell leukemia; MPN = myeloproliferative neoplasm; PMF = primary myelofibrosis; PV = polycythemia vera

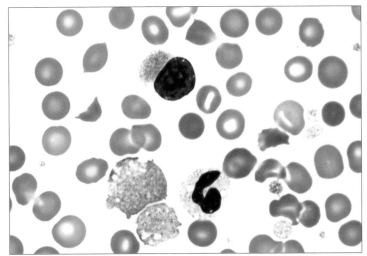

i14.3 *Circulating megakaryocytes are common in patients with myeloproliferative neoplasms. In addition, giant platelets and fragments of megakaryocyte cytoplasm are also common findings in myeloproliferative neoplasms. (Wright)*

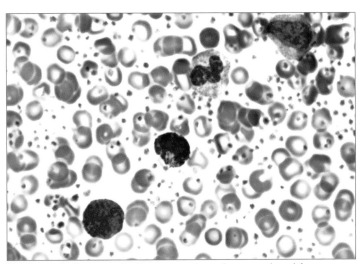

i14.4 *Markedly increased cell counts may be evident in myeloproliferative neoplasms such as this case of chronic myelogenous leukemia in which the platelet count exceeded 5 million. (Wright)*

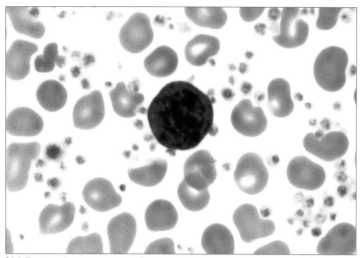

i14.5 *Circulating micromegakaryocytes are common in chronic myelogenous leukemia. (Wright)*

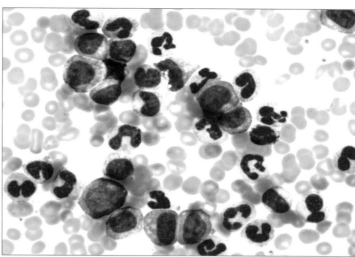

i14.6 *Leukocytosis is a common finding in myeloproliferative neoplasms and is most dramatic in chronic myelogenous leukemia. Note striking leukocytosis with predominance of mature neutrophils although a left shift to blasts is evident. (Wright)*

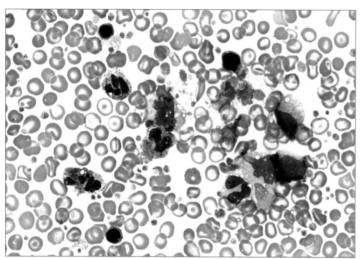

i14.7 *In longstanding myeloproliferative neoplasms, the peripheral blood picture can become markedly pathologic. Note the leukoerythroblastic blood picture, huge megakaryocyte cytoplasmic fragments, thrombocytosis, and red blood cell changes associated with both iron deficiency and splenectomy in iron-deficient polycythemia vera. (Wright)*

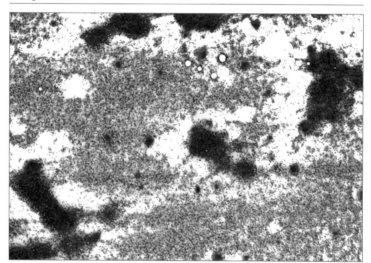

i14.8 *This low magnification of a bone marrow aspirate smear shows the characteristic hypercellularity with increased megakaryocytes that typifies a myeloproliferative neoplasm. (Wright)*

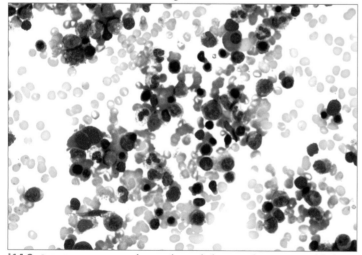

i14.9 *Intact maturation and normal morphology are characteristic of the bone marrow aspirate smears in myeloproliferative neoplasms. (Wright)*

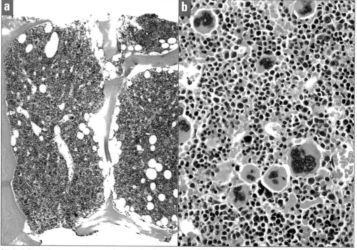

i14.10 *This composite shows the low- **a** and high-magnification **b** appearance of a bone marrow core biopsy in a myeloproliferative neoplasm. Note hypercellularity, dilated sinuses, and increased and clustered megakaryocytes. Some megakaryocytes have hyperlobated nuclei. (H&E)*

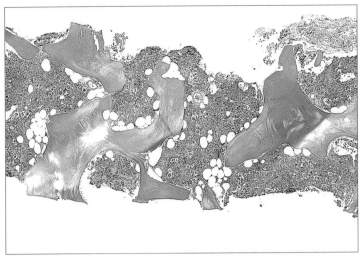

i14.11 *This bone marrow core biopsy section shows primary myelofibrosis. Note striking osteosclerosis. Bony trabeculae should always be evaluated to assess for features of a possible myeloproliferative neoplasm. (H&E)*

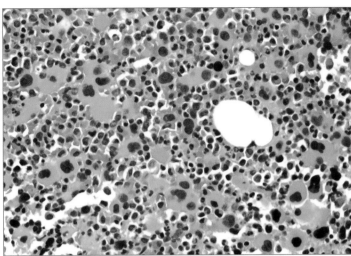

i14.12 *A striking increase in small monolobated megakaryocytes is evident on this bone marrow core biopsy section in chronic myelogenous leukemia. It is essential to evaluate megakaryocyte features in myeloproliferative neoplasms. (H&E)*

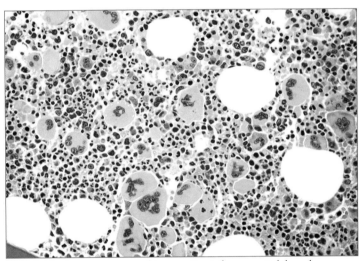

i14.13 *This bone marrow core biopsy section is from essential thrombocythemia. Note markedly increased and clustered giant megakaryocytes, many of which show nuclear hyperlobation. (H&E)*

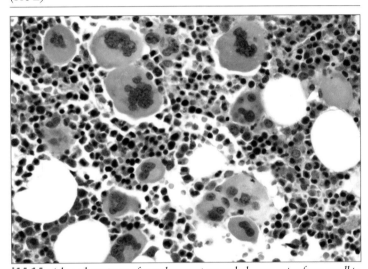

i14.14 *A broad spectrum of megakaryocyte morphology ranging from small to markedly enlarged and hyperlobulated megakaryocytes is evident on this bone marrow core biopsy section of primary myelofibrosis. (H&E)*

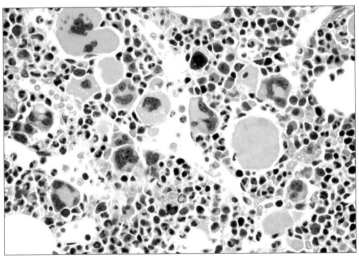

i14.15 *A strikingly dramatic range in megakaryocyte size is evident in this bone marrow core biopsy in primary myelofibrosis. Note dilated sinuses. (H&E)*

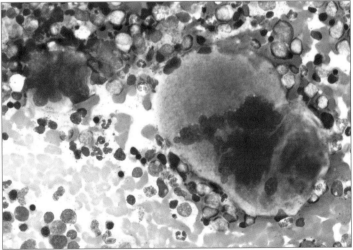

i14.16 *A markedly hyperlobated megakaryocyte is evident on this bone marrow aspirate smear in essential thrombocythemia. (Wright)*

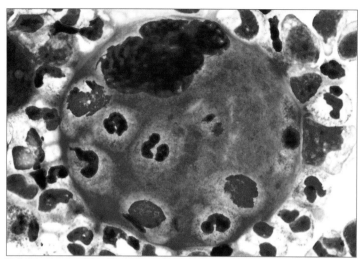

i14.17 *Neutrophils often migrate through the cytoplasm of markedly enlarged megakaryocytes in patients with myeloproliferative neoplasms as seen on this bone marrow aspirate smear. (Wright)*

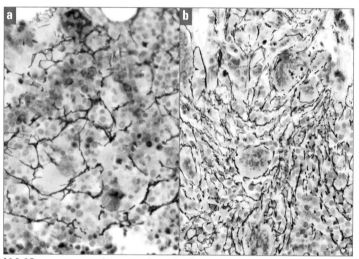

i14.18 *A spectrum of severity of reticulin fibrosis is highlighted in this composite from 2 myeloproliferative neoplasms. Mild reticulin fibrosis a is compared to moderate reticulin fibrosis b. Reticulin fibers tend to surround megakaryocytes. (reticulin)*

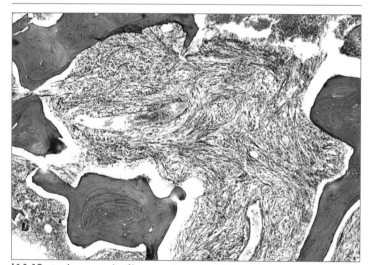

i14.19 *Striking reticulin fibrosis with associated osteosclerosis is evident in this bone marrow core biopsy section in advanced primary myelofibrosis. (reticulin)*

PMF, the megakaryocyte morphology is quite distinctive in well-established cases. In early phases of ET and prefibrotic PMF, megakaryocyte morphology may overlap, although typical hyperlobulated and staghorn-like nuclei in ET and pleomorphic megakaryocytes in PMF have been reported as discriminating features [Thiele 1999, 2006b]. Moderate to marked degrees of reticulin fibrosis are useful to support PMF or advanced PV vs ET i14.18, i14.19. Immunohistochemistry can be used to assess the hematopoietic architecture, which is frequently abnormal in well-established MPN, and to document normal blast percentages and neoangiogenesis (see [14.4] "Specialized Studies in MPNs").

[14.3.3] **Minimal Diagnostic Criteria**

Based on an integrative approach, a definitive diagnosis of MPN is possible in many cases t14.5. This is most readily facilitated in the well-established cases by integrating the hematologic findings with the bone marrow appearance. However, in earlier stages of disease, a diagnostic "gray zone" may occur between MPN and reactive states [Kvasnicka 2009, Tefferi 2008b]. In such scenarios, the typical clinical and hematologic findings of MPN may be absent or minimal. However, the detection of a *JAK2, MPL,* or similar mutation may be sufficient to exclude a reactive process. While *JAK2* mutations cannot discriminate PV from ET and PMF, it must also be remembered that a small proportion of other myeloid disorders and myelodysplastic syndrome (MDS) may show a similar mutation. Therefore, while one may be capable of identifying MPNs at an earlier or prodromal stage, review of the peripheral blood and bone marrow morphologic features is still required to definitively place it in the MPN category. In rare cases that exhibit persistent/unexplained borderline or high blood cell count(s), lack a genetic abnormality, and show an overall unremarkable bone marrow, the term "idiopathic cytosis of uncertain significance" (ICSUS) may be useful. Close clinical follow-up is required, and repeat bone marrow biopsy is reasonable if clinical symptoms or hematologic parameters worsen.

[14.4] **Specialized Studies in MPNs**

[14.4.1] **Conventional Cytogenetics**

In MPNs, there is to date only one disease-defining genetic mutation evident at the conventional cytogenetic (CC) level: t(9;22)(q34;q11.2) (the Philadelphia chromosome) in CML. CC should be performed in every case of possible CML to confirm the presence of the Philadelphia chromosome or variant and to reveal any additional cytogenetic abnormalities that could indicate disease progression (clonal evolution).

t14.5 Minimal Diagnostic Criteria in the Classic MPNs (CML, PV, ET, PMF)

Definitive Diagnosis of MPN

Sustained cytosis(es)

Reactive causes of cytosis(es) excluded

Hypercellular bone marrow with single or multilineage hyperplasia with intact maturation

Abnormal megakaryocyte morphology and histotopography

<20% blasts

With/without a clonal cytogenetic or molecular abnormality*

Presumptive Diagnosis of PV

JAK2 V617F mutation positive[†] and

Low/normal serum erythropoietin level

OR

JAK2 V617F mutation negative

Unexplained low serum erythropoietin level

JAK2 exon 12 mutation positive and/or sufficient bone marrow features

Presumptive Diagnosis of MPN[‡]

Normal/borderline high cell count(s)

Reactive causes of cytosis(es) excluded

Hypercellular bone marrow with single or multilineage hyperplasia with intact maturation; abnormal megakaryocyte morphology and histotopography

Cytogenetic and molecular genetic studies normal

OR

Normal, borderline or elevated cell count(s)

Bone marrow morphology not definitive

Presence of clonal cytogenetic abnormality or molecular mutation compatible with MPN (eg, *BCR-ABL1*, *JAK2*)

in all instances

Reactive causes of cytosis(es) excluded

No monocytosis

Blasts <20%

Idiopathic CytoSis of Uncertain Significance (ICSUS)

Unexplained, persistent cytosis(es)

Other causes of cytosis(es) excluded

Normal blast percentage

Cytogenetic and molecular genetic studies normal

Nondiagnostic bone marrow features

*BCR-ABL1 fusion or Philadelphia chromosome required for diagnosis of CML
[†]JAK2 V617F mutation is not specific for MPN; rare in other myeloid disorders
[‡]Excludes PMF, which does not require an elevated cell count for diagnosis
CML = chronic myelogenous leukemia; ET = essential thrombocythemia; MPN = myeloproliferative neoplasm; PMF = primary myelofibrosis; PV = polycythemia vera

References: [Ganly 2007, Kvasnicka 2010, Michiels 2004, Steensma 2005, Szpurka 2006, Tefferi 2008b, Thiele 2008a, 2008b, 2008c, Vardiman 2008b]

t14.6 Genetic Findings in MPNs

Finding	Comment	Frequency
t(9;22)(q34;q11.2)	*BCR-ABL1* molecular fusion Diagnostic of CML in context of MPN	100% of CML
del(20q)	Not specific for MPN	<10%
del(13q)	Not specific for MPN	<5%
del(5q)	Not specific for MPN	<5%
+8, +9	Not specific for MPN	<10%
Abnormalities of chromosome 1	Not specific for MPN	<30%
JAK2 V617F mutation	Not specific for MPN	>95% PV ~50% ET/PV
JAK2 exon 12	PV	~2%
MPL mutation	Not specific for MPN subtype	≤10% of ET, PMF
KIT mutation	Systemic mastocytosis D816V mutation most common	>90% of SM cases
TET2 mutation	Not specific for MPN May be late event linked to progression	17% of PMF 16% of PV 5% of ET

CML = chronic myelogenous leukemia; ET = essential thrombocythemia; MPN = myeloproliferative neoplasm; PMF = primary myelofibrosis; PV = polycythemia vera; SM = systemic mastocytosis

References: [Caramazza 2010, Cross 2008, Hussein 2009a, Pardanani 2006, Saint-Martin 2009, Schaub 2010; Tefferi 2009a, 2009b, 2009c, Vardiman 2009b]

In the classic *BCR-ABL1*– MPNs (eg, ET, PV and PMF), either CC or FISH should be performed to exclude CML in all cases. Rare cases of CML with the p230 fusion product will be missed in molecular laboratories that do not utilize a long-template primer set. Subsequent additional fluorescence in situ hybridization (FISH) or molecular studies for suspected cryptic or submicroscopic aberrations (eg, *JAK2* mutation, *FIP1L1-PDGFRA* fusion) may be performed on an individual case basis. While all 8 World Health Organization (WHO) MPN subtypes derive from a sustained clonal myeloproliferation, their phenotypic variability is likely the result of different genotype profiles. The more common cytogenetic and/or molecular abnormalities are detailed in **t14.6**.

[14.4.2] **Fluorescence In Situ Hybridization (FISH)**

FISH plays a limited role in the work-up of MPNs in the setting of an otherwise optimal cytogenetic study. The exceptions to this rule include the occasional cryptic *BCR-ABL1* in CML (~5% of cases) and the need to exclude a submicroscopic *PDGFRA* abnormality in cases of neoplastic eosinophilia.

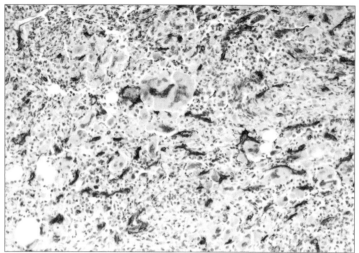

i14.20 *Striking neoangiogenesis is highlighted by CD34 immunoperoxidase staining in this bone marrow core biopsy section in a myeloproliferative neoplasm. (immunoperoxidase for CD34)*

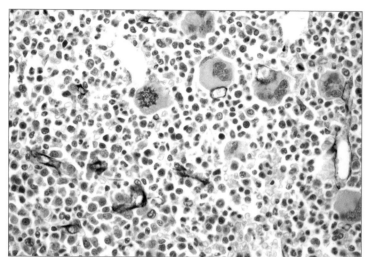

i14.21 *High magnification of an immunoperoxidase stain for CD34 in a myeloproliferative neoplasm shows increased small blood vessels but no significant increase in blasts. (immunoperoxidase for CD34)*

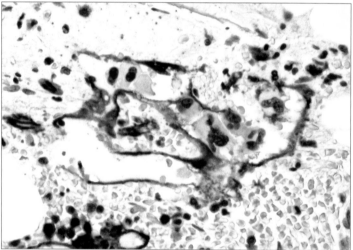

i14.22 *Markedly dilated sinuses with intrasinusoidal hematopoietic cells are highlighted by immunoperoxidase staining for CD34 in this bone marrow core biopsy section in an advanced myeloproliferative neoplasm. (immunoperoxidase for CD34)*

[14.4.3] Molecular Genetic Tests in MPN

Molecular testing for submicroscopic mutations in *JAK2, MPL, KIT,* and *TET2* plays a significant role in the work-up of MPNs, especially *JAK2* mutation assessment. The frequency of these mutations is listed in **t14.6**. The *JAK2* mutation has transformed the diagnosis of MPNs, but is not specific by itself for a particular subtype of MPN and is also seen in non-MPN myeloid neoplasms. While none of the listed genetic abnormalities are specific for a disease entity, the *KIT* mutation is quite characteristic of systemic mastocytosis.

[14.4.4] Special Stains in MPN

Stains for reticulin and collagen should be considered, especially in cases in which bone marrow aspiration is compromised, since the degree of fibrosis may correlate with a more aggressive disease course (see **appendix** for protocols and Chapter 4 for grading scales).

[14.4.5] Immunophenotyping in MPN

Immunohistochemistry for CD34, myeloperoxidase, and various megakaryocyte antigens plays a valuable role in the evaluation of MPNs, particularly in the setting of a fibrotic bone marrow with suboptimal, hemodilute, or inadequate aspirate smears. In such cases, although CD34 and/or CD117 are not a perfect substitute for the morphologic blast count, they may provide the best assessment in a bone marrow core biopsy for degree of immaturity. CD34 highlights blasts as well as neoangiogenesis and dilated sinuses **i14.20, i14.21, i14.22** [Boveri 2008, Gianelli 2007]. CD42b and CD31 reveal the often increased, atypical, and clustered megakaryocytes **i14.23, i14.24**. Hemoglobin A and myeloperoxidase show mostly intact erythroid colonies and granulocytic maturation, although a spectrum of changes may be seen, particularly in advanced stages of disease **i14.25, i14.26, i14.27**. Other immunohistochemical markers of reported diagnostic significance include pSTAT-3, pSTAT-5, and MPL [Aboudola 2007, Gibson 2008, Grimwade 2009, Mesa 2002, Teofili 2007c, Yoon 2000]. Often, reduced expression of pSTAT-3 and pSTAT-5 is seen in PMF, whereas increased expression is seen in PV. Increased MPL expression is seen in megakaryocytes and total bone marrow cells in MPN [Bock 2004]. These changes are typically most marked in megakaryocytes but are also seen variably in the other hematopoietic lineages. Newer markers to highlight basophils include BB1 (basogranulin) [Agis 2006]. Tryptase readily identifies mast cells.

The role of flow cytometric immunophenotyping (FCI) in stable MPN is not well-defined, and in most cases flow cytometry is not necessary. However, aberrant antigen

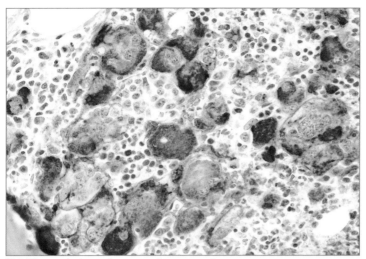

i14.23 *Marked megakaryocyte clustering and a prominent range in megakaryocyte size are both highlighted by immunoperoxidase staining for CD42b in this bone marrow core biopsy section in a myeloproliferative neoplasm. (immunoperoxidase for CD42b)*

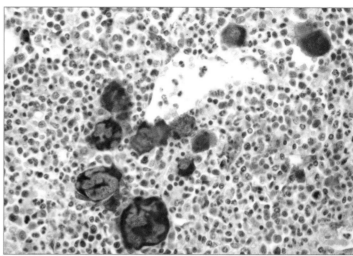

i14.24 *Megakaryocyte clustering adjacent to a dilated sinus is evident in this bone marrow core biopsy in a myeloproliferative neoplasm. Note broad range in megakaryocyte size and nuclear lobation. (immunoperoxidase for CD42b)*

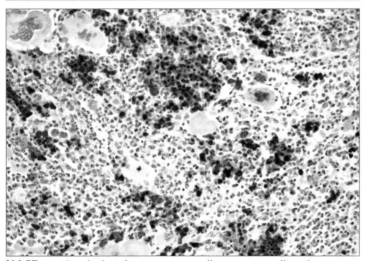

i14.25 *Erythroid colony formation is generally intact, especially early in myeloproliferative neoplasms as highlighted in this bone marrow core biopsy section. (immunoperoxidase for hemoglobin A)*

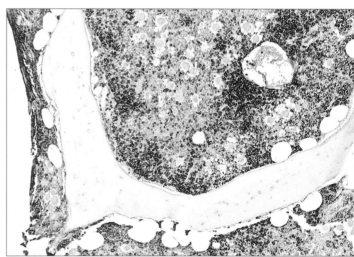

i14.26 *At low magnification of this bone marrow core biopsy section, normal localization of granulocytic precursors is evidenced by the myeloperoxidase positivity adjacent to bony trabeculae. (immunoperoxidase for myeloperoxidase)*

expression patterns may be detected on the blasts and myeloid lineage cells, which could potentially be supportive of a myeloid neoplasm in borderline diagnostic/presumptive MPN cases [Feng 2010]. The utility of FCI is most evident in cases of transformation in which determination of the lineage of the blasts (myeloid vs lymphoid) is of diagnostic and potentially therapeutic importance.

[14.4.6] **Paroxysmal Nocturnal Hemoglobinuria Studies**

Paroxysmal nocturnal hemoglobinuria (PNH) studies do not play a significant role in MPN. In a recent study looking at only 5 cases of myelofibrosis, no PNH clones were identified [Wang 2009].

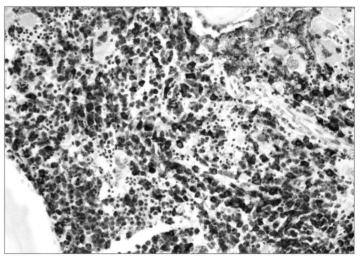

i14.27 *Abnormal localization of immature granulocytic cells, which are strikingly increased and confluent, away from bony trabeculae is evident in this bone marrow core biopsy section in primary myelofibrosis. (immunoperoxidase for myeloperoxidase)*

t14.7 Comparative Blood/Bone Marrow Morphologic and Genetic Features of Selected Myeloproliferative Neoplasms*

Feature	CML	ET	PV	PMF
Peripheral blood cytosis	**Prominent, increased granulocytic and basophilic lineage**	**Mild to marked thrombocytosis (platelets ≥450 to >1×10⁹/L)** **Cytosis generally restricted to megakaryocytic lineage**	**May see trilineage cytoses, but erythroid lineage most distinctive**	Thrombocytosis common; leukocytosis in early phase
LE reaction with teardrop red cells	Infrequent	Infrequent	Infrequent, unless spent phase	**Prominent in fibrotic PMF**
Blasts	<5% at diagnosis Blast phase ≥20% Accelerated phase 5%-19% Any lineage including lymphoblasts	<5% at diagnosis Blastic transformation rare[†]	<5% at diagnosis Blastic transformation rare[†]	<5% at diagnosis Blastic transformation rare[†]
Predominant lineage of myeloproliferation	**Granulocytic**	**Megakaryocytic**	**Erythroid**	All myeloid
Mast cells	Usually decreased	Rarely increased or clustered or spindled	Rarely increased or clustered or spindled	Rarely increased or clustered or spindled
Megakaryocyte morphology	**Small, hypolobated, monolobated**	**Increased, markedly enlarged, hyperlobulated** **Often see emperipolesis**	Loose collections of somewhat hyperlobated megakaryocytes	**Increased, pleomorphic megakaryocytes; often clustered**
Bone morphology	Often normal	Often normal	**Osteosclerosis in fibrotic phase**	**Osteosclerosis in advanced disease**
Bone marrow sinuses	Normal to slightly dilated	Normal to slightly dilated	Normal to moderately dilated	**Usually moderately to markedly dilated with intrasinusoidal HP**
Fibrosis	None to mild at diagnosis May indicate accelerated phase	None to minimal	Minimal at presentation; marked in spent phase	**Prominent in fibrotic phase**
Genetics/other	**BCR-ABL1+** Disease evolution: additional Ph+ chromosome, +8, iso17q, +19	*JAK2* V617F activating mutation, ~50%	*JAK2* V617F activating mutation, ~95%	*JAK2* V617F activating mutation, ~50%

*Key differentiating features are highlighted in bold
[†]Except in setting of prior cytotoxic therapy and/or radiation
abnl = abnormality; BM = bone marrow; CEL = chronic eosinophilic leukemia; CML = chronic myelogenous leukemia; CNL = chronic neutrophilic leukemia; ET = essential thrombocythemia; HP = hematopoiesis; PB = peripheral blood; PMF = primary myelofibrosis; PV = polycythemia vera; WBC = white blood cell

References: [Bain 2008a, 2008b, Horny 2008, Kvasnicka 2008, Thiele 2008a, 2008b, 2008c, Vardiman 2008b]

[14.5] Classification

The purpose of any classification system is to segregate diseases into distinct clinicopathologic entities that have well-defined natural histories, disease courses and/or possible therapeutic targets. In the realm of the MPNs, this is particularly relevant given the wide range in outcome, median survival rates, risk of disease evolution, and susceptibility to particular drug therapies. While the diagnosis of ET, PV, PMF, CML, and systemic mastocytosis (SM) can generally be comfortably made by integrating clinical, morphologic and genetic features, chronic eosinophilic leukemia and chronic neutrophilic leukemia can be more challenging [Tefferi 2006a]. In

t14.7 Comparative Blood/Bone Marrow Morphologic and Genetic Features of Selected Myeloproliferative Neoplasms* (Continued)

Feature	Mastocytosis	CNL	CEL
Peripheral blood cytosis	Rare to see circulating mast cells except in mast cell leukemia	Neutrophilic leukocytosis **Neutrophils ≥25 × 10⁹/L** May have toxic appearance Immature neutrophilic precursors <10% of WBCs No dysplasia	Eosinophilia ≥1.5 × 10⁹/L Variable dysplasia
LE reaction with teardrop red cells	Infrequent	Rare	Rare
Blasts	<5%; if an associated clonal non-mast cell lineage disorder present, then blasts may be increased	Rare in blood Not increased in BM	Blasts >2% in PB or >5% in BM if no clonal genetic abnormality, but <20% overall
Predominant lineage of myeloproliferation	**Mast cells**	Neutrophils	Eosinophils
Mast cells	**Focal, compact dense aggregates Spindled, atypical morphology**	Not increased or clustered or atypical	Not increased or clustered or atypical
Megakaryocyte morphology	Usually normal unless associated myeloid neoplasm	Normal; may be hyperlobated and clustered	Usually normal; may be hyperlobated and clustered
Bone morphology	Osteosclerosis common	Normal	Usually normal
Bone marrow sinuses	Usually normal	Normal	Normal
Fibrosis	**Prominent, particularly in association w/mast cell aggregates and osteosclerosis**	Uncommon	Occasionally seen; generally mild
Genetics/other	*KIT* D816V mutation (or variant)	Normal genetics in 90% of cases Must exclude non-neoplastic disorders Must exclude neutrophilic variant of CML	Diagnosis of exclusion; must exclude another MPN with eosinophilia **Must exclude abnormalities of *PDGFRA, PDGFRB, FGFR1, BCR-ABL1*, inv16**

*Key differentiating features are highlighted in bold
†Except in setting of prior cytotoxic therapy and/or radiation
abnl = abnormality; BM = bone marrow; CEL = chronic eosinophilic leukemia; CML = chronic myelogenous leukemia; CNL = chronic neutrophilic leukemia; ET = essential thrombocythemia; HP = hematopoiesis; PB = peripheral blood; PMF = primary myelofibrosis; PV = polycythemia vera; WBC = white blood cell

References: [Bain 2008a, 2008b, Horny 2008, Kvasnicka 2008, Thiele 2008a, 2008b, 2008c, Vardiman 2008b]

some cases, the complete criteria for a distinct MPN cannot be established, and a diagnosis of MPN, unclassifiable, is utilized.

Useful peripheral blood and bone marrow morphology and genetic features for differentiating the various classic myeloproliferative neoplasms are listed in t14.7. Given the unique genetic features of CML and potential for tyrosine kinase inhibitor (TKI)-targeted therapy, assessment for the Philadelphia chromosome or *BCR-ABL1* fusion should be performed in all suspected myeloid neoplasms. The WHO 2008 diagnostic criteria for the classic *BCR-ABL1–* MPNs have been updated to include the significant discovery of *JAK2* mutations in a substantial fraction of these disorders t14.8.

t14.8 WHO 2008 Diagnostic Criteria for Polycythemia Vera, Essential Thrombocythemia, and Primary Myelofibrosis

Criteria	Polycythemia Vera	Essential Thrombocythemia	Primary Myelofibrosis
Major criteria	Hgb >18.5 g/dL (men); Hgb >16.5 g/dL (women) *or** Presence of *JAK2* V617F or similar mutation	Platelets ≥450 × 10⁹/L Bone marrow: megakaryocytic proliferation with enlarged forms, mature morphology; absent or minimal granulocytic or erythroid proliferation Not meeting WHO 2008 criteria for any other myeloid neoplasm Presence of *JAK2* V617F or other clonal abnormality or exclusion of reactive thrombocytosis	Megakaryocytic proliferation, clustering, and atypia, with associated reticulin or collagen fibrosis; in absence of fibrosis (pre-fibrotic), megakaryocyte abnormalities seen with BM hypercellularity (granulocytic proliferation and often erythroid hypoplasia) Not meeting WHO 2008 criteria for any other myeloid neoplasm Presence of *JAK2* V617F or other clonal abnormality or exclusion of other causes of BM fibrosis
Minor criteria	Trilineage BM proliferation; hypercellular, panmyelosis Low EPO level Endogenous erythroid colony growth		Leukoerythroblastosis Increased serum LDH Anemia Splenomegaly
Establishment of diagnosis	Both major and 1 minor criteria First major and 2 minor criteria	Need all 4 major criteria	Need all 3 major and 2 minor criteria

*Hgb >17 g/dL (men) or >15 g/dL (women) if documented sustained 2 g/dL increase above the patient's baseline Hgb and not due to correction of iron deficiency, or Hgb or Hct >99th percentile of established reference range for age, sex, altitude, or red cell mass >25% above the normal average
BM = bone marrow; EPO = erythropoietin; Hct = hematocrit; Hgb = hemoglobin; LDH = lactate dehydrogenase; WHO = World Health Organization

References: [Haferlach 2008, Tefferi 2008b, 2009c, Thiele 2008b]

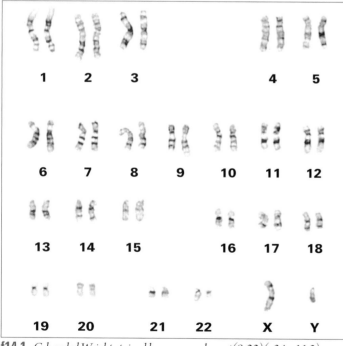

f14.1 *G-banded Wright-stained karyogram shows t(9;22)(q34;q11.2) in a case of chronic myelogenous leukemia in stable phase. The abnormal chromosomes 9 and 22 are on the right of the pairs.*

[14.5.1] **Chronic Myelogenous Leukemia, BCR-ABL1+**

CML is the prototypic MPN and is important to diagnosis, given the advances in patient overall survival due to targeted therapy **t14.9** [Druker 2006]. It is a clonal stem cell disorder that is always associated with the *BCR-ABL1* genetic fusion. The *BCR-ABL1* fusion is most often the result of reciprocal translocation between chromosomes 9 and 22, t(9;22)(q34;q11.2) **f14.1**. The resultant, small, derivative chromosome 22 harbors the native *BCR* juxtaposed to the *ABL1* oncogene. This genetic rearrangement underlies the pathogenesis of CML, which is due to constitutively activated tyrosine kinase activity **sidebar 14.1**.

The natural history of CML is classically triphasic (occasionally biphasic) with an initial chronic phase followed by accelerated phase and blast phase **t14.10**. Most patients are diagnosed in chronic phase with an insidious onset of disease **t14.9**. Approximately 1/3 of asymptomatic patients are diagnosed by detection of an elevated WBC count during a routine medical examination.

t14.9 Historical, Clinical, Epidemologic, and Prognostic Features in Chronic Myelogenous Leukemia, *BCR-ABL1*+

Historical features	First described by Bennett and Virchow in 1845
	Nowell and Hungerford identified the derivative (small) chromosome 22 in 1960
	In 1973 Rowley showed the derivative chromosome 22 was the result of a 9;22 reciprocal translocation [t(9;22)]
	In 1983 the genetic basis of t(9;22) involving *BCR* and *ABL1* was elucidated
	Targeted therapy (STI571) against *BCR-ABL1*
Clinical presentation	Most often chronic phase (see **t14.10**)
	~30% of patients are asymptomatic; detected on routine examination
	In symptomatic patients, splenomegaly and non-specific symptoms of fatigue, malaise, headache, and weight loss
Incidence/ epidemiology	1-2 cases per year per 100,000 population
	May occur at any age including childhood (median age: 53 years)
	Incidence in children in Western world: 1 per 1,000,000 children
	Clear association with prior radiation exposure
	No apparent inherited predisposition
Pathogenesis	*BCR-ABL1* genetic fusion (see **sidebar 14.1**)
Therapy	TKIs have revolutionized treatment by achieving durable clinical and cytogenetic remissions
	To date, only curative therapy is allogeneic stem cell transplantation
Prognosis	Moderate to marked fibrosis in accelerated phase (even in era of TKI therapy); reportedly associated with worse prognosis
	Clonal cytogenetic evolution associated with disease progression
	Blastic transformation associated with poor disease prognosis
	Detection of increasing *BCR-ABL1* molecular transcripts may indicate disease evolution, therapy resistance
	Historically (prior to TKIs), blast phase in virtually all patients (usually 3-7 years after diagnosis)
	With imatinib, current 5-year overall survival is 80%-95% with a marked decline in the incidence of blast phase

TKI = tyrosine kinase inhibitor

References: [Baccarani 2009, Bartram 1983, Bennett 1845, Bizzozero 1966, Buesche 2003, Corso 1995, Druker 2006, Irvine 2010; Millot 2005, Nowell 1960, Rowe 1984, Rowley 1973, Thiele 2000, Virchow 1845]

t14.10 Disease Phases of Chronic Myelogenous Leukemia, *BCR-ABL1*+

Stage	Features
Chronic phase	Myeloblasts <5%*† in blood and bone marrow
Accelerated phase‡	Persistent/increasing WBC and/or persistent/ progressive splenomegaly; not responsive to treatment
	Persistent thrombocytosis (plt >1000 × 10⁹/L) or thrombocytopenia (plt <100 × 10⁹/L); not responsive to therapy
	Clonal cytogenetic evolution
	≥20% basophils in the peripheral blood
	>10%-19% myeloblasts* in blood or bone marrow
	Progressive reticulin or collagen fibrosis commonly observed with large clusters of sheets of megakaryocytes
Blast phase‡ (acute leukemia transformation)	≥20% blasts (any lineage; see **t14.12**) in bone marrow or extramedullary site
	Focal significant clusters of blasts in bone marrow, which morphologically and immunophenotypically are "eye-catching" and expansile
	Dysplastic features predominantly in granulocytic series
	Clonal cytogenetic evolution

*Any percent lymphoblasts should raise concern for transformation
†In the era of tyrosine kinase inhibitor therapy and molecular monitoring, potential role of increasing transcript levels in predicting disease progression/impending evolution remains to be elucidated (see **sidebar 14.1**)
‡Clinical and morphologic parameters are often applied differently given the heterogeneity of disease features at these phases
WBC = white blood cell

Reference: [Vardiman 2008b]

Blood and Bone Marrow Findings

The hematologic and morphologic features in CML are highlighted in **t14.11**. Characteristic peripheral blood features that typify CML include a striking neutrophilic leukocytosis with left shift, <2% blasts, and invariable basophilia **i14.28, i14.29, i14.30, i14.31, i14.32**. The neutrophils and precursors do not typically show toxic changes or dysplasia; a "myelocyte bulge" is noted on differential count along with the predominance of neutrophils. Basophils are invariably increased and often degranulated. Eosinophils are frequently elevated but are not a dominant feature. Blasts typically have a myeloid appearance; however, if cells resembling

t14.11 Hematologic and Morphologic Features of Chronic Myelogenous Leukemia, *BCR-ABL1+*, in Chronic Phase*

Blood

Leukocytosis	WBC range (12-1,000 × 10⁹/L) (median 100)
	In children, median WBC count may be twice that of adults (250-750 × 10⁹/L)
	Marked increase in neutrophils and precursors; <2% blasts
	No dysplasia
Basophilia	Invariable finding
	Basophils often degranulated
Thrombocytosis	Present at diagnosis in most patients
	May be striking with platelet count >1000 × 10⁹/L
	Circulating micromegakaryocytes and bare nuclei seen
	Thrombocytopenia unusual
Monocytosis	May be present due to sheer numbers of WBCs, but account for <2%-3% of all WBCs
Eosinophilia	Not uncommon, but not a dominant feature
Erythrocytes	Essentially unremarkable
	Occasional normoblasts may be present

Bone Marrow

Cellularity	Markedly hypercellular, generally 100%
Hematopoiesis:	
Granulocytes	Striking granulocytic hyperplasia
	Progressive and complete maturation with predominance of neutrophils and myelocytes
	No significant dysplastic changes
	Blasts <5%
	Basophils inconspicuous in biopsy sections
	Precursor cells showing both eosinophil and basophil granules may be present
Megakaryocytes	Generally normal or increased in number
	Striking abnormal morphology; characteristic small, hypo-/monolobated forms (so-called dwarf or micromegakaryocytes)
	Occasionally form large clusters and sheets
Erythrocytes	Inconspicuous, but present with complete maturation
	Intact colonies, but inconspicuous secondary to striking granulocytic predominance
	No dysplasia
Histiocytes	Pseudo-Gaucher cells and sea-blue histiocytes frequent
	Derived from the leukemia clone
	Sea-blue histiocytes due to increased cell turnover
Fibrosis	Variable from minimal to marked
	Moderate to marked at diagnosis in ~25% of cases; may be linked to increased numbers of megakaryocytes and transformation
Bone	Generally unremarkable
	Rare lytic lesions

*For description of accelerated and blast phase see **t14.10**
WBC = white blood cell

References: [Anastasi 1998, Millot 2005, Vardiman 2008b, 2009a]

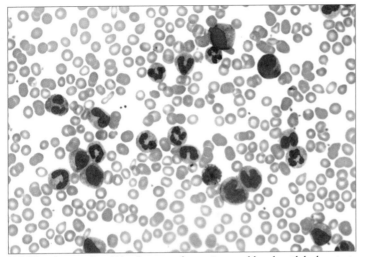

i14.28 *This peripheral blood smear is from a 2-year-old male with leukocytosis, basophilia and splenomegaly. Philadelphia chromosome positive chronic myelogenous leukemia was confirmed. Mature neutrophils predominate with 2% basophils and 1% myeloblasts. (Wright)*

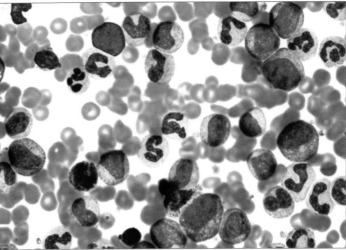

i14.29 *This proliferative blood smear is from a 55-year-old female with a WBC count of 349 × 10⁹/L. A diagnosis of chronic myelogenous leukemia was confirmed, and the proliferative blood features are characteristic of stable phase disease. (Wright)*

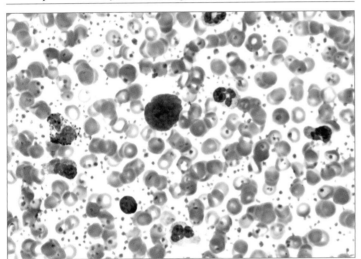

i14.30 *In this peripheral blood smear in chronic myelogenous leukemia, the platelet count exceeded 5 million. (Wright)*

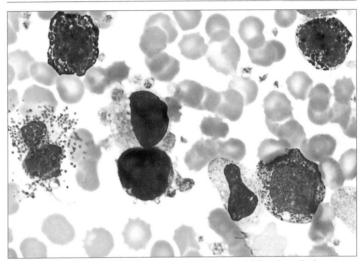

i14.31 *This peripheral blood smear from a 69-year-old female with chronic myelogenous leukemia shows numerous circulating micromegakaryocytes in conjunction with marked basophilia. (Wright)*

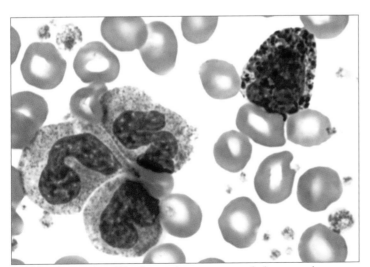

i14.32 *This peripheral blood smear from a patient with chronic myelogenous leukemia shows nontoxic neutrophils and basophilia. (Wright)*

lymphoblasts are seen, further assessment including immunophenotypic studies is necessary to exclude the possibility of disease evolution. The platelet count is generally elevated; atypical platelets, circulating megakaryocyte nuclei, and micromegakaryocytes are usual. Erythrocytes are essentially unremarkable.

Similar to the peripheral blood, CML displays characteristic bone marrow morphology. The bone marrow is markedly hypercellular (usually 100%) due to a granulocytic predominance with intact maturation. The granulocytes show minimal/absent toxic change and no dysplasia **i14.33** [Xu 2003]. Blasts are <5%. Pseudo-Gaucher cells and sea-blue histiocytes are readily identified in ~40% of cases **i14.33, i14.34**. The bone marrow core biopsy is hypercellular and demonstrates an expanded cuff of granulocyte precursors in their normal paratrabecular location. Increased interstitial neutrophils

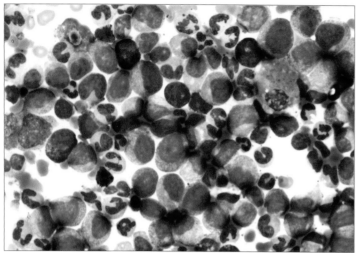

i14.33 *This bone marrow aspirate smear in chronic myelogenous leukemia shows a striking expansion of granulocytic lineage cells with intact maturation. Note sea-blue histiocyte (upper right). (Wright)*

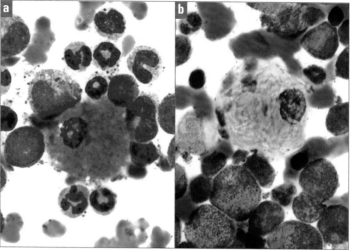

i14.34 *This bone marrow aspirate smear composite from 2 cases of chronic myelogenous leukemia shows the spectrum of histiocytes that can be seen in this disease. A sea-blue histiocyte is evident* **a**, *and a pseudo Gaucher histiocyte is present* **b**. *(Wright) (courtesy C Wilson, MD)*

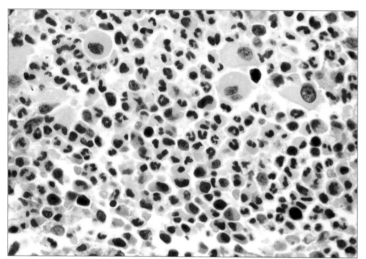

i14.35 *This bone marrow core biopsy in chronic phase chronic myelogenous leukemia highlights the marked hypercellularity with a predominance of mature granulocytic cells in conjunction with markedly increased and monolobated megakaryocytes. Blasts are not increased. (H&E)*

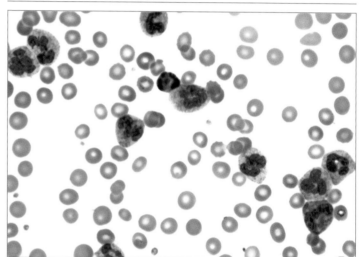

i14.36 *This peripheral blood smear in the neutrophilic variant of chronic myelogenous leukemia shows mature neutrophils with minimal left shift. (Wright)*

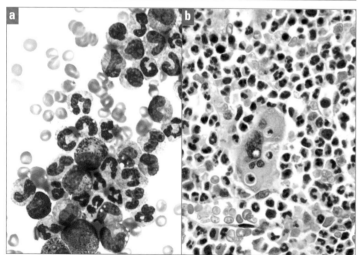

i14.37 *This bone marrow aspirate smear and bone marrow core biopsy composite in neutrophil-rich chronic myelogenous leukemia shows a striking granulocytic proliferation as well as an enlarged and somewhat hyperlobated megakaryocyte. (Wright and H&E)*

often predominate relative to the remaining erythroid islands **i14.35**. Megakaryocytes are normal to increased in number and are characteristically small and hypolobated **i14.35**. Occasionally, they may form variably sized clusters and exhibit more pleomorphism. Fibrosis is usually absent at diagnosis; cases exhibiting substantial fibrosis at presentation (up to 25% of cases) may indicate accelerated phase. In the neutrophilic variant of CML, which mimics chronic neutrophilic leukemia (CNL), some morphologic differences are noted, including toxic changes of neutrophils and large megakaryocytes **i14.36, i14.37**. This variant still displays the *BCR-ABL1* fusion, but involves an alternative breakpoint, resulting in a 230kD protein [Pane 1996].

In accelerated phase, which is inconsistently defined in the literature, a variety of morphological changes may be seen in peripheral blood and bone marrow **t14.10**. By definition,

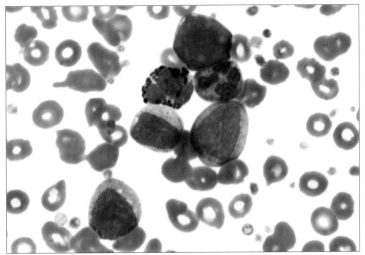

i14.38 *This peripheral blood smear is from a patient with chronic myelogenous leukemia in accelerated phase in which 10% myeloblasts and 20% basophils were noted. (Wright)*

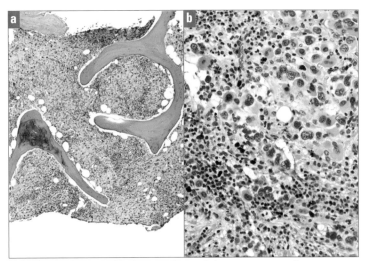

i14.39 *This low-* **a** *and high-magnification* **b** *bone marrow core biopsy composite shows chronic myelogenous leukemia in accelerated phase. Myeloblasts were increased and fibrosis was documented by reticulin stain. (H&E)*

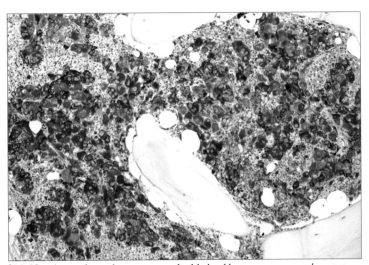

i14.40 *Sheets of megakaryocytes are highlighted by immunoperoxidase stain for CD42b in chronic myelogenous leukemia in accelerated phase. (immunoperoxidase for CD42b)*

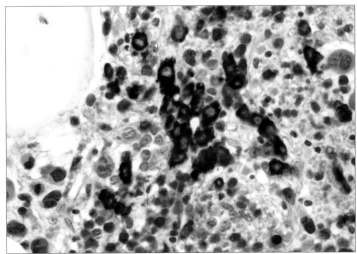

i14.41 *Abnormal localization of immature precursors is highlighted by myeloperoxidase staining in this bone marrow core biopsy section in chronic myelogenous leukemia in accelerated phase. (immunoperoxidase for myeloperoxidase)*

blasts account for <20%, and there are variable cytopenias, dysplastic changes, and increased basophils i14.38. The bone marrow core biopsy may show hypercellularity with sheets of megakaryocytes and prominent abnormal localization of immature granulocytic precursors (ALIP) i14.39, i14.40, i14.41. Progressive fibrosis may also characterize accelerated phase.

Overt blast phase generally means that ≥20% blasts are present in the peripheral blood and bone marrow, or discrete medullary and/or extramedullary foci of blasts are present i14.42, i14.43, i14.44, i14.45, i14.46, i14.47. A variety of phenotypes and genotypes may be evident in CML blast phase and are detailed in t14.12. Virtually any type of hematopoietic lineage may comprise blast phase, although myeloblasts are by far the most common. Lymphoid blast phase is usually of B-lineage i14.45. Megakaryoblastic blast

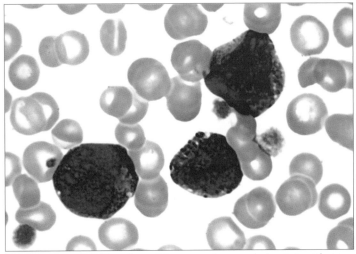

i14.42 *A basophilic blast phase of chronic myelogenous leukemia is evident in this peripheral blood smear. (Wright)*

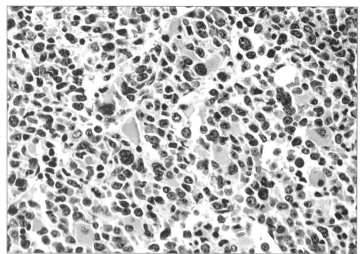

i14.43 *This bone marrow core biopsy in chronic myelogenous leukemia in blast phase shows marked predominance of immature cells in conjunction with markedly increased, hypolobated megakaryocytes. (H&E)*

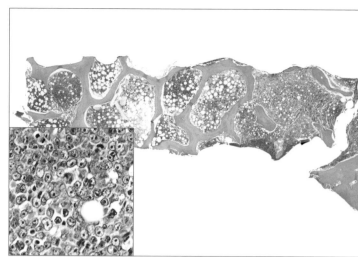

i14.44 *Low magnification of this bone marrow core biopsy in chronic myelogenous leukemia in blast phase shows focal patches of increased cellularity, which on high magnification (inset) are comprised of myeloblasts. (H&E) (courtesy J Said, MD)*

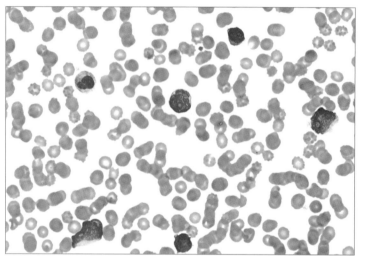

i14.45 *This peripheral blood smear shows chronic myelogenous leukemia in precursor B acute lymphoblastic phase. (Wright) (courtesy B Nelson, MD)*

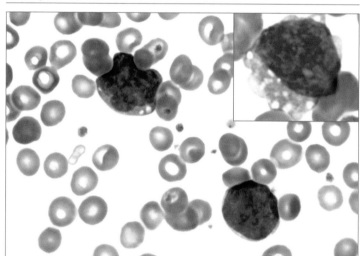

i14.46 *This peripheral blood smear composite shows chronic myelogenous leukemia in megakaryoblastic phase. (Wright) (courtesy M Irani, MD)*

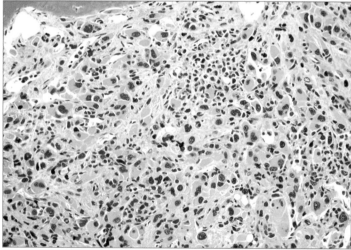

i14.47 *This bone marrow core biopsy in chronic myelogenous leukemia in megakaryoblastic phase shows virtually complete effacement of the bone marrow by abnormal megakaryocytes with a subtle infiltrate of blasts. (H&E) (courtesy M Irani, MD)*

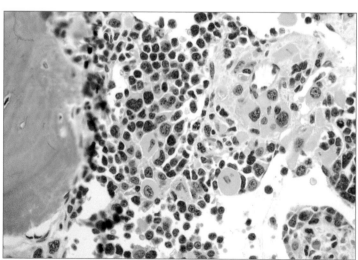

i14.48 *The combination of abnormal maturing megakaryocytes and sheets of blasts is evident at high magnification of this bone marrow core biopsy in chronic myelogenous leukemia in megakaryoblastic phase. (H&E) (courtesy M Irani, MD)*

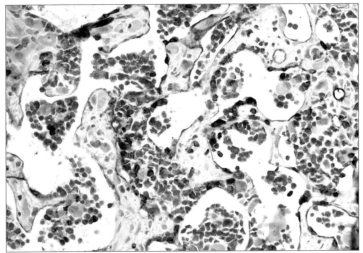

i14.49 *Immunoperoxidase staining for CD34 highlights markedly dilated sinuses as well as large collections of myeloblasts in this bone marrow core biopsy section in blast phase of chronic myelogenous leukemia. (immunoperoxidase for CD34) (courtesy M Irani, MD)*

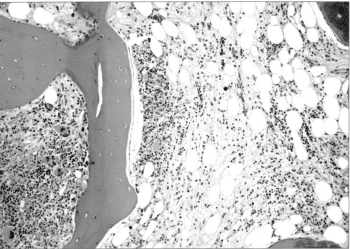

i14.50 *Foci of hypocellularity and fibrosis are evident on this bone marrow core biopsy section in a patient treated with imatinib for 5 years. Note areas of intact hematopoiesis in which megakaryocyte morphology is normal. (H&E) (courtesy C Sever, MD)*

t14.12 Chronic Myelogenous Leukemia, *BCR-ABL1+*, Blast Phase*

Lineage	Comments
Myeloid	~70%-80% of cases
	Additional Philadelphia chromosome, +8, +19, and iso(17q) seen most often
Lymphoid	~20%-30% of cases
	Mostly precursor B-cell type; rare precursor T-cell type
Megakaryoblastic	Associated with a translocation of the *EVI1* gene on chromosome 3q26
Erythroid	Rare, usually seen in conjunction with myeloid and megakaryoblastic phenotypes

Recurring Genetic Abnormalities (Other than *BCR-ABL1*)

inv(16)(p13q22)	Pathologic features resemble de novo disease (see Chapter 18)
t(8;21)(q22;q22)	
t(15;17)(q22;q21)	

*Most cases show cytogenetic of clonal evolution (see text); rare cases of concurrent myeloid and lymphoid lineage blasts, biphenotypic leukemia, and lineage switch

References: [Anand 2004, Chung 2006, 2008, Dorfman 1997, Khalidi 1998, Kim 2008a, Merzianu 2005, Oh 2009, Ohyashiki 1995, Oren 1999, Patel 2006, Reid 2009, Scolnik 1998, Wu 2006, Yin 2004, 2006]

phase of CML is well known and may rarely be the initial presentation i14.46, i14.47. The bone marrow biopsy shows numerous myeloblasts, which are highlighted by CD34, as well as numerous dysplastic megakaryocytes and megakaryoblasts i14.48, i14.49. Rarely, a *JAK2* positive non-CML MPN may develop after known CML [Mauro 2004].

In the era of TKI therapy, chronic phase CML bone marrow after therapy may exhibit some predictable features. These features include normalization of bone marrow cellularity and myeloid:erythroid (M:E) ratio [Frater 2003, Hasserjian 2002, McNamara 2003, Thiele 2005c]. Chapter 35 also discusses bone marrow morphology after imatinib therapy. Imatinib may cause a reversal of the initial reticulin fibrosis [Buesche 2007]. However, fibrosis may also be a consequence of long-term imatinib therapy i14.50. Stem cell transplantation (SCT) remains the only potential curative therapy for CML. Cases of CML that relapse post-SCT tend to behave more aggressively, harbor additional genetic abnormalities, and show resistance to therapy [Huang 2007].

Genetic Findings in CML

The cytogenetic and molecular genetic findings in CML are briefly summarized in **t14.13**. See **sidebar 14.1** for complete details on *BCR-ABL1* pathogenesis, molecular treatment, and monitoring. The genetic hallmark of CML is the Philadelphia chromosome, which is represented karyotypically by the derivative (small) chromosome 22 after a reciprocal translocation with chromosome 9 [t(9;22)(q34;q11.2)] **f14.1**. Rarely, a variant translocation or cryptic aberration is present. This genetic rearrangement results in the *BCR-ABL1* fusion gene. Depending on the available molecular testing, protocol requirement, or patient specifics, FISH and/or molecular (PCR-based) minimal residual disease monitoring may be

t14.13 Selected Key Tips Regarding Genetics in CML, BCR-ABL1+

The *BCR-ABL1* genetic fusion is the disease-defining abnormality

BCR-ABL1 is most often the result of the reciprocal translocation (9;22)(q34;q11.2) [aka Philadelphia chromosome (Ph)], although variant translocations can occur (with no effect on prognosis); a small fraction of cases may be cytogenetically cryptic

BCR is on chromosome 22; *ABL1* on chromosome 9

The finding of the Ph chromosome and/or *BCR-ABL1*+ fusion does not equate with CML; may be seen in rare cases of de novo AML and in B-ALL (25% of adults; 5% of children)

Conventional karyotyping should be performed in all cases to
1) document Ph chromosome,
2) identify any additional abnormalities at diagnosis that may herald impending disease transformation, or
3) establish a karyotypic fingerprint for future monitoring

FISH studies should be done to assess *BCR-ABL1* positivity in all suspected cases of CML in which conventional cytogenetics is negative

Molecular: 3 *BCR* breakpoints may occur, resulting in 3 fusion products of varying lengths: p210 (major), p190 (minor), and p230 (μ) (rare)

In the majority of cases of CML, the p210 is the fusion protein

Rarely, the p230 is seen and may show a predominance of neutrophils mimicking chronic neutrophilic leukemia

CML with the p190 is rare and associated with an inferior outcome

The p190 is most often associated with Ph+ ALL, but alternative splicing may show small amounts of this transcript in addition to p210 in CML

Clonal evolution in CML is a hallmark of disease progression; the most typical cytogenetic findings are an additional Ph chromosome, +8, +19, and iso(17q)

Genetic alterations identified in accelerated/blast phase of disease include *TP53, MYC, RAS, AML1*, and *EVI1* mutations

In rare follow-up cytogenetic studies of CML patients on TKI therapy, clonal abnormalities (in the absence of the Ph chromosome) may be identified and are of uncertain significance

Gene expression profiling may identify prognostic markers in CML

ALL = acute lymphocytic leukemia; AML = acute myeloid leukemia; CML = chronic myelogenous leukemia; TKI = tyrosine kinase inhibitor

References: [Kim 2008b, Melo 1996, Oehler 2009, van Rhee 1996, Verma 2009]

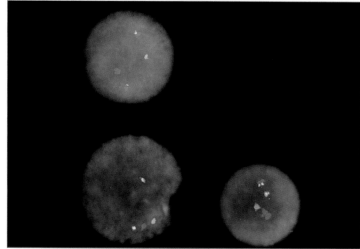

f14.2 *FISH for* BCR *and* ABL1 *(dual color, dual fusion probe set) shows the classic abnormal fusion pattern of 2 fused (yellow signals), 1 green signal, and 1 red signal indicating* BCR-ABL1 *fusion characteristic of chronic myelogenous leukemia.*

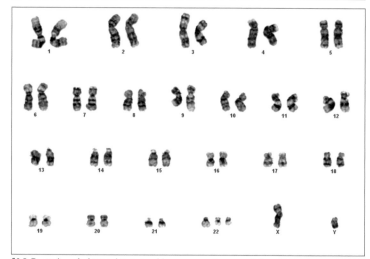

f14.3 *G-banded Wright-stained karyogram in case of chronic myelogenous leukemia in accelerated phase shows duplicate derivative 22 and translocation (9;22)(q34;q11.2).*

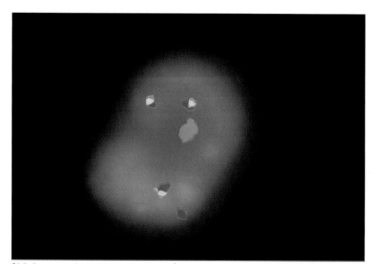

f14.4 *FISH for* BCR *and* ABL1 *(dual color, dual fusion probe set) shows 3* BCR-ABL1 *fusion signals (yellow) in this case of chronic myelogenous leukemia in blast phase.*

performed. In cases of suspected CML in which cytogenetics are normal, additional upfront FISH and/or molecular testing should be performed to assess for a cryptic *BCR-ABL1* **f14.2**. Disease evolution is often heralded by a combined progression of clinical, morphologic, and genetic features **t14.10**. The most common cytogenetic findings in myeloid blast transformation are acquisition of an additional Ph chromosome, +8, +19, or iso(17q) **f14.3, f14.4**. In lymphoid blast phase, these genetic features are often absent [Reid 2009]. Gene expression profiles may be used in the future to predict disease prognosis [Oehler 2009].

Unusual Disease Manifestations in CML

Unique presentations of CML are known and are important to recognize to minimize delay in diagnosis t14.14. These presentations may mimic both benign and malignant processes. CML presenting in blast phase should be a

t14.14 Unique Disease Manifestations of CML, BCR-ABL1+

Manifestation	Comments*
Normal or minimally elevated WBC count, but conspicuous, persistent basophilia	Exclude non-neoplastic basophilia
Leukocytosis dominated by mature neutrophils with little, if any, left shift	May mimic reactive condition (see Chapter 10)
	May mimic chronic neutrophilic leukemia (BCR-ABL1 p230 product)
Marked thrombocytosis with minimal/mild leukocytosis	May mimic secondary thrombocytosis (see Chapter 12) or essential thrombocythemia
	Evaluate closely for basophilia
	CML-type megakaryocytes in bone marrow
Leukocytosis with accompanying monocytosis	May mimic CMML, G-CSF, or reactive state (see Chapters 10 and 17)
	Evaluate for basophilia
	Dysplastic changes common in CMML
	CML-type megakaryocytes in bone marrow
Presentation in accelerated or blast phase without prior diagnosis of CML:	~5% of cases
	Megakaryoblastic leukemia well known
	Evaluate for underlying CML features: basophilia, dwarf megakaryocytes
	Distinction from de novo Ph+ AML may be difficult; less likely to have splenomegaly and basophilia
	Distinction from de novo Ph+ ALL may be difficult; lack of basophilia and presence of p190 may be helpful
morphologic features mimicking low blast count AML	Megakaryocytes may not be as prominent or atypical as in usual case of CML
	Basophilia may be inconspicuous
	Cytogenetics are critical
Extramedullary disease or lytic/other bony lesions	Rare, but clinically may mimic a variety of other disorders
	If neutrophilia is present in blood, do not assume it is due to underlying cytokine-mediated phenomena (eg, myeloma)

*In all cases, cytogenetic and BCR-ABL1 testing should be performed
AML = acute myeloid leukemia; CML = chronic myelogenous leukemia; CMML = chronic myelomonocytic leukemia; G-CSF = granulocyte colony-stimulating factor

References: [Campiotti 2007, Melo 1994, Pullarkat 2008, Soupir 2007]

consideration in patients with apparent de novo AML or ALL. Assessment for BCR-ABL1 is critical due to the potential for targeted therapy.

Differential Diagnosis of CML

Although the constellation of blood findings in CML is generally distinctive, the differential diagnosis includes reactive diseases (eg, leukemoid reaction) and other myeloid neoplasms. In general, reactive processes display toxic features and lack basophilia. Rarely, the WBC count may exceed $50 \times 10^9/L$ in a leukemoid reaction. In our opinion, if reasonable exclusion of underlying reactive disorders is performed or if the blood findings are persistent, then cytogenetic studies are clearly warranted. By definition, the detection of a Philadelphia chromosome or BCR-ABL1 fusion indicates CML in the appropriate morphologic setting (see t14.14 for discussion of Ph+ AML and Ph+ ALL).

[14.5.2]   **Polycythemia Vera (PV)**

PV is characterized by unregulated, autonomous, increased red blood cell production. The key clinical, epidemiologic, pathogenetic, and prognostic features are listed in t14.15. One of the major innovations in the diagnostic criteria for BCR-ABL1– MPNs is assessment for the JAK2 V617F mutation, which is present in a substantial number of cases of PV, ET, and PMF t14.6, t14.8, sidebar 14.1 [Baxter 2005, James 2005, Kralovics 2005, Levine 2005]. Important in PV pathogenesis is the fact that >95% of cases harbor the JAK2 V617F mutation, which is often homozygous. Some have argued that the presence of this JAK2 exon 14 mutation or the less common exon 12 mutation in conjunction with a low serum erythropoietin level may be all that is required for PV diagnosis.

Clinically and pathologically, PV may be categorized into 3 phases: early, polycythemic, and post-polycythemic (so-called spent phase). The early phase (aka "pre-polycythemic"/prodromal) may show a borderline or mild erythrocytosis. Occasionally, patients at this stage of disease may be identified at blood donation with an upper-limit hematocrit level; subsequent studies confirm JAK2 V617F mutation [Tagariello 2009]. Even though these pre-polycythemic patients do not exhibit the significant and diagnostic increase in red cell parameters required by the WHO 2008 criteria for PV, assessment of serum erythropoietin level and JAK2 V617F mutation status should be considered [Kvasnicka 2010]. The peripheral blood findings are largely within normal limits, although a mild increase in red blood cells may be seen. If thrombocytosis is present (~15% of cases), distinction from ET may be challenging [Thiele 2005b]. However, upon clinical follow-up, true polycythemia is manifest, confirming a diagnosis of PV [Thiele 2005b]. In such scenarios, bone marrow biopsy is most likely to be valuable, since the typical PV bone

t14.15 Key Features of PV

Clinical	Thrombosis; most events occur at diagnosis or in the 2 years prior; recurrence rate is ~5%-6% per patient/year
	Arterial thrombosis results in myocardial infarction, ischemic stroke, and peripheral arterial occlusion
	Venous thrombosis [eg, splanchnic vein thrombosis (SVT)]; 40% of patients with SVT not attributable to other causes harbor the *JAK2* V617F mutation
	Hemorrhage
	Splenomegaly 70%
	Hepatomegaly 40%
Incidence	Ranges from 0.1-2.6 per 100,000 persons/year
	Prevalence in the US is ~22/100,000 residents
Pathogenesis/genetics	Clonal stem cell disorder
	>95% of cases have *JAK2* V617F mutation; many of the remaining cases have a *JAK2* exon 12 mutation
Familial PV	Distinct from familial erythrocytosis, which is a single-lineage disorder (see Chapter 9)
	Demonstrates clonal hematopoiesis with clonality evident in all myeloid lineages; complex pattern of inheritance
	JAK2 V617F mutation seen in 55%-78% (lower than sporadic PV)
	May follow an autosomal dominant inheritance pattern
Prognosis/disease progression	2 basic types of disease progression:
	myelofibrotic phase (post-polycythemic myelofibrosis)
	development of acute leukemia
	Probability of postpolycythemic myelofibrosis evolution; 34% at 15 years
	Risk of leukemic transformation rare except in patients treated with cytotoxic regimens (~15%)
	Median life expectancy is 10 years
	Most mortality is associated with vascular events (nearly 50%); leukemic transformation (~15%)
	Leukocytosis may predict inferior survival and leukemia transformation
	Hemoglobin level, platelet, and leukocyte count may predict survival in post PV myelofibrosis

PV = polycythemia vera

References: [Alvarez-Larran 2009, Barbui 2009, Basquiera 2009, Cario 2009, De Stefano 2008, Gangat 2007a, 2008, Kralovics 2003, Ma 2008, Passamonti 2008b, Policitemia, Gls 1995]

t14.16 Blood and Bone Marrow Features in PV*

Peripheral Blood

Normochromic/normocytic red blood cells

Erythrocytosis with increased hemoglobin/hematocrit

Red blood cell morphology unremarkable except in cases with concomitant iron deficiency

Deeply basophilic reticulocytes and/or rare normoblasts may be present

Mild neutrophilic leukocytosis (WBC usually $<20 \times 10^9$/L) with rare left shift

Mild basophilia may be seen

Thrombocytosis; may be particularly prominent in prodromal phase or exaggerated by concurrent iron deficiency

Bone Marrow

Hypercellular

Panmyelosis with notable predominance of erythroid and megakaryocytic lineages

Complete and progressive maturation of all 3 hematopoietic lineages

Abnormal megakaryocyte morphology and architecture; variably hyperlobulated; not as pronounced hyperlobulation as in ET or as pleomorphic as in PMF

Reticulin fibrosis tends to be minimal or absent

Decreased, often absent iron stores

Post Polycythemic/Spent Phase

Leukoerythroblastosis

Overt bone marrow reticulin and collagen fibrosis

Osteosclerosis usually prominent

Blasts may increase, but <20%

Dilated sinuses with intrasinusoidal hematopoiesis

Decline in hematopoietic cells

Overall picture may be indistinguishable from advanced PMF; need prior documentation of PV diagnosis

*Prodromal (early) phase of PV shows similar bone marrow findings; peripheral blood may only demonstrate mild increase in red cell parameters
ET = essential thrombocythemia; PMF = primary myelofibrosis; PV = polycythemia vera; WBC = white blood cell

marrow features are generally sufficiently distinctive from those of ET **t14.16** [Kvasnicka 2010].

The peripheral blood and bone marrow findings in established PV are attributable to the bone marrow panmyelosis that occurs as a result of a clonal stem cell disorder, although excess erythrocyte production predominates **t14.16**. The peripheral blood exhibits increased red blood cells, which are most often normochromic/normocytic except in the setting of iron deficiency, in which hypochromic/microcytic red blood cells are seen **i14.51**, **i14.52**. Mild neutrophilia and/or basophilia are common

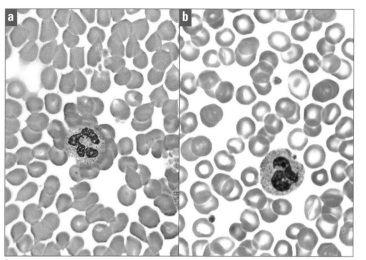

i14.51 *This peripheral blood smear composite is from 2 patients with polycythemia vera; iron stores are intact as reflected by normal red blood cell size and morphology in one case **a**, while iron deficient erythrocytes secondary to phlebotomy therapy are evident in another case **b**. (Wright)*

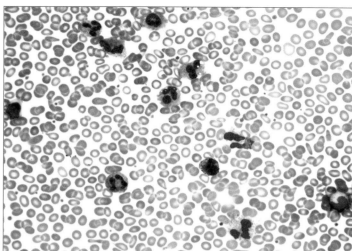

i14.52 *This peripheral blood smear shows iron deficient polycythemia vera. Note leukocytosis, neutrophilia, basophilia, and mild thrombocytosis in conjunction with hypochromic microcytic red blood cells. (Wright)*

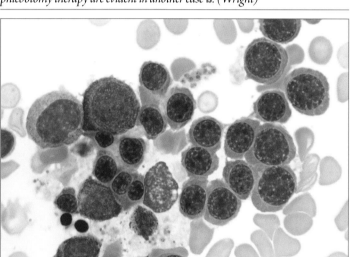

i14.53 *This bone marrow aspirate smear is from a patient with polycythemia vera. Note increased erythroid cells with little or no dysplasia. (Wright) (courtesy W Williams, MD)*

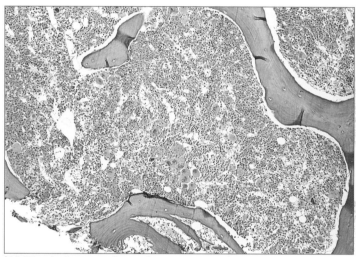

i14.54 *This low-magnification bone marrow core biopsy section in polycythemia vera shows normal bony trabeculae, dilated sinuses, hypercellularity, and increased megakaryocytes. (H&E)*

i14.52. Thrombocytosis may be present and, in early stages of PV, may require bone marrow examination or erythropoietin testing to discriminate from ET **t14.7, t14.8**.

The bone marrow findings in PV, polycythemic phase, are dominated by hypercellularity with a characteristic panmyelosis (expansion of all 3 bone marrow lineages) with a normal blast count (<5%). The erythroid and megakaryocytic proliferations tend to be most evident. In the bone marrow aspirate smear, the erythroid and granulocytic lineages show complete and progressive maturation without dysplasia **i14.53**. The bone marrow biopsy is typically hypercellular with dilated sinuses, increased megakaryocytes **i14.54**, and often erythroid hyperplasia **i14.55, i14.56**. Hemoglobin A immunohistochemistry highlights the erythroid predominance **i14.57**. Megakaryocyte pathology is the most striking finding. Megakaryocytes are increased, may be loosely clustered,

are often paratrabecular, and are typically enlarged and moderately hyperlobated, although there is a range in size **i14.55, i14.56**. Despite the substantial increase in megakaryocytes, reticulin fibrosis is absent or minimal. Iron stores may be absent in PV and are likely due to multiple factors, including sustained erythrocytosis and chronic blood loss if therapeutic phlebotomy has been initiated.

With progression to the fibrotic (spent) post-polycythemic phase of PV, the peripheral blood and bone marrow findings resemble remarkably those of advanced PMF **t14.16**. A leukoerythroblastic blood picture is common with moderate/marked reticulin/collagen fibrosis, dilated sinuses with intrasinusoidal hematopoiesis, and osteosclerosis **i14.58, i14.59, i14.60**. The diagnosis of spent phase PV requires a definitive prior diagnosis of PV, bone marrow fibrosis, and 2 or more of the following: anemia, leukoerythroblastic

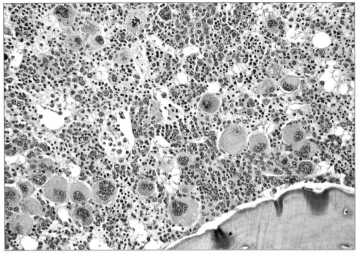

i14.55 *High magnification of this bone marrow core biopsy section in polycythemia vera shows increased and hyperlobated megakaryocytes. (H&E)*

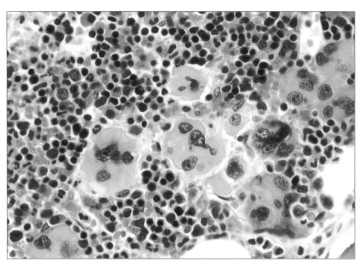

i14.56 *A cluster of hyperlobated megakaryocytes is evident in this bone marrow core biopsy section in polycythemia vera. Note increased erythroid cells. (H&E)*

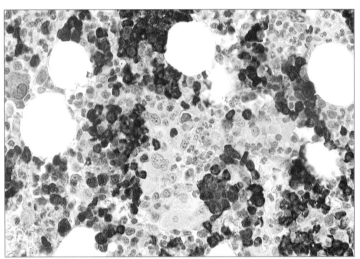

i14.57 *Increased erythroid colonies are evident on this bone marrow core biopsy section in polycythemia vera. (immunoperoxidase for hemoglobin A)*

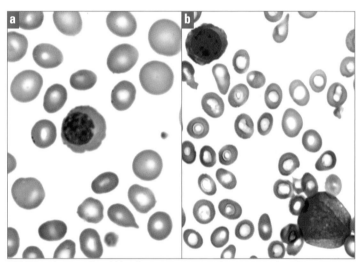

i14.58 *This peripheral blood smear composite shows post-polycythemic myelofibrosis. Note teardrop erythrocytes, nucleated red blood cells, and anemia. (Wright)*

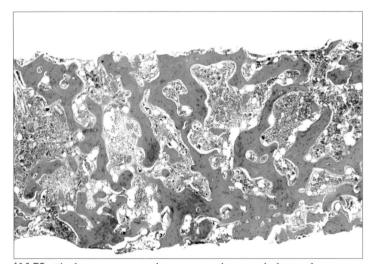

i14.59 *This bone marrow core biopsy section shows marked osteosclerosis, dilated sinuses, and fibrosis in post-polycythemic myelofibrosis. (H&E)*

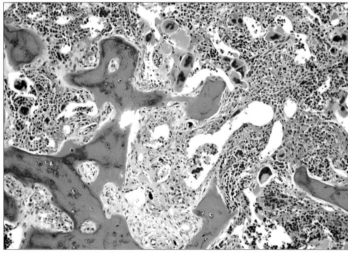

i14.60 *On high magnification, myelofibrosis, dilated sinuses containing megakaryocytes, and pleomorphic megakaryocytes are all evident in this bone marrow core biopsy section of post-polycythemic myelofibrosis. (H&E)*

blood picture; increasing splenomegaly and/or development of >10% weight loss in 6 months, night sweats, and fever (>37.5°C) [Thiele 2008a]. The percent blasts may increase from the polycythemic phase, but 20% or more is considered overt acute leukemic transformation.

Leukemic transformation in PV may arise as a natural sequela of the disease (rare, 2%-3% of cases) or as a consequence of prior cytotoxic therapy. The reported incidence of leukemic transformation varies depending on the study but is estimated to be up to 20% [Finazzi 2005, Marchioli 2005].

The median life expectancy of most patients with PV is 10 years and is mainly affected by disease-related complications such as vascular events and transformation to myelofibrosis or acute leukemia [Passamonti 2004].

No pathognomonic recurring genetic abnormality has been identified in PV. While a *JAK2* V617F mutation is by far the most frequent (>95%), it is not specific as it can be seen in the other MPNs **t14.6**. Cytogenetic abnormalities may be detected at diagnosis in up to 20% of patients, with +8, +9, del(20q), and trisomy (1q) being the most common, although, again, these are not disease specific [Reilly 2008]. With disease progression, 80% of cases show evidence of clonal evolution. Abnormalities of chromosome 7 and 13q have been linked to myelofibrotic disease evolution [Diez-Martin 1991, Swolin 1988]. In chemotherapy-related transformations, abnormalities of chromosomes 5 and 7 are common (see Chapter 18).

The differential diagnosis of PV includes congenital and reactive erythrocytotic disorders, including POEMS syndrome (polyneuropathy, organomegaly, endocrine abnormalities, monoclonal spike, and skin changes), familial erythrocytosis, and other myeloproliferative neoplasms **t14.7**. Secondary erythrocytosis results from appropriate or inappropriate excess erythropoietin production (see Chapter 9). These secondary erythrocytoses may be physiologic as a reaction to hypoxia or to the excess production of erythropoietin by a tumor. Causes of congenital erythrocytosis include high-oxygen-affinity hemoglobinopathies, methemoglobinemia, erythropoietin receptor mutations, as well as others [Patnaik 2009a]. Even though the hematologic abnormalities lie solely within the red cell lineage in reactive erythrocytoses, distinction from PV is not always straightforward, particularly in patients with other medical conditions, resulting in confounding factors such as peripheral basophilia (usually mild), circulating normoblasts, mild leukocytosis with left shift, or thrombocytosis. In such cases, direct communication with the clinician is indicated, and any further work-up (eg, *JAK2* mutation testing, erythropoietin level, bone marrow biopsy) should be based on the individual case.

[14.5.3] **Essential Thrombocythemia (ET)**

ET is a myeloproliferative neoplasm with morphologic and hematologic manifestations largely confined to the megakaryocytic lineage. The key clinical, epidemiologic, and pathogenetic features of ET are listed in **t14.17**. Although the WHO 2008 diagnostic criteria are relatively straightforward for ET, interobserver variability in assessing megakaryocyte

t14.17 Key Features of ET

Clinical	Most cases occur in the 5th and 6th decades with equal male to female ratio
	Microvascular disturbances occur in ~50% of patients at presentation (eg, thrombosis, hemorrhage), while the remainder are asymptomatic
	Presence of *JAK2* V617F mutation may be associated with increased risk of thrombotic events
	Increased risk of miscarriage (3-4 times the general population)
Incidence	Ranges from 0.6-2.5 per 100,000 persons/year; may be increasing with the use of WHO 2008 criteria
	Prevalence is ~24/100,000 residents in US
Pathogenesis/ genetics	50% of cases harbor the *JAK2* V617F mutation
	Mutations in *JAK2* exon 12 are not thought to occur
	Cytogenetic abnormalities uncommon at diagnosis (<10% of cases) and do not affect overall survival or risk of transformation
	~4% of cases harbor *MPL* mutation
	TET2 mutations are observed
	Leukemic progression very rare and involves the acquisition of additional genetic abnormalities
Childhood/ familial ET	Rare
	Incidence of *JAK2* V617F mutation and thrombosis lower than in adults
	Activating *MPL* mutation is most common cause
	Spontaneous megakaryocyte colony formation
	100% 10-year survival
Prognosis	Generally an indolent disorder
	Substantial increase in reticulin fibrosis over time places patients at increased risk of leukemic transformation
	Degree of anemia and level of thrombocytosis predict for increased risk of transformation
	Leukocytosis may be a risk factor for thrombosis

ET = essential thrombocythemia

References: [Barbui 2009, Beer 2009b, Campbell 2009, Carobbio 2007, Delhommeau 2009, Ding 2004, 2009a, Gangat 2007b, 2009, Girodon 2009, Higgs 2008, Larsen 2008, Ma 2008, Melillo 2009, Passamonti 2008a, Randi 2006, Rumi 2008, Sanchez 2006, Teofili 2007a, 2007b, 2009, Thiele 2008b]

morphology among expert hematopathologists is quite substantial t14.8 [Wilkins 2008]. This finding, although controversial, argues that distinguishing ET from prefibrotic myelofibrosis may be untenable in many circumstances [Thiele 2002, 2003a].

The characteristic peripheral blood and bone marrow findings in ET are detailed in t14.18. In classic ET, the peripheral blood findings are dominated by thrombocytosis, which ranges from modest to pronounced i14.61. The platelets exhibit anisocytosis, but marked agranularity/hypogranularity is uncommon i14.62. Circulating megakaryocytic nuclei and micromegakaryocytes may be seen. Concurrent iron deficiency may exist in young women or in patients with clinical or subclinical bleeding. In such cases, particularly with only mild thrombocytosis (platelet count 450-550 × 10^9/L), it is imperative to definitely exclude an uncomplicated iron deficiency. Although the WBC count may be moderately elevated, it rarely exceeds 30 × 10^9/L. Basophilia and eosinophilia are absent or minimal. Red blood cells are normal (unless concurrent iron deficiency), and a leukoerythroblastic blood picture is not seen.

Although bone marrow cellularity may be normal or only mildly increased, the platelet and megakaryocyte findings in ET are quite distinctive. In cases with marked thrombocytosis, numerous platelet clumps may mimic

particles in bone marrow aspirate smears at low magnification i14.63. Increased, markedly enlarged hyperlobulated megakaryocytes are prototypic of ET i14.64, i14.65. On the bone marrow core biopsy, if hypercellularity is seen, it is not as marked as in the other MPNs; cellularity is often normal in ET i14.66. Erythroid and granulocytic lineages are generally unremarkable but may be mildly increased. Megakaryocytes are frequently clustered, may be paratrabecular, and are occasionally present in large clusters i14.67. By comparison with the other myeloproliferative neoplasms, the megakaryocytes in ET are overall the largest in size, are markedly hyperlobulated, and show intact maturation. Intrasinusoidal and perisinusoidal hyperlobulated megakaryocytes are typical and often demonstrate emperipolesis of migrating neutrophils i14.68. Reticulin fibrosis is minimal to absent, which is a critical feature in the distinction from PMF.

t14.18 Blood and Bone Marrow Features in ET

Peripheral Blood

Platelets	Variable thrombocytosis (platelet count ≥450 to >1 × 10^{15}/L), striking anisocytosis including giant platelets, circulating megakaryocytic nuclei and micromegakaryocytes; significant platelet hypogranularity is not typical
Erythrocytes	Usually normal (except if concurrent iron deficiency); leukoerythroblastosis should not be observed
Granulocytes	Mild leukocytosis (rarely >30 × 10^9/L) may be seen, but is comprised mainly of neutrophilia without left shift; can see minimal basophilia and eosinophilia

Bone Marrow

Normal to mild hypercellularity

Erythroid and granulocytic lineages morphologically unremarkable; occasional mild granulocytic hyperplasia

Striking megakaryocytic hyperplasia and atypia; may see clustering and intrasinusoidal and perisinusoidal megakaryocytes with emperipolesis; megakaryocytes are large/giant, mature and uniform, markedly hyperlobulated

Absent/minimal reticulin fibrosis

Lymphoid nodules are rare to absent

Iron stores are normal (except in cases of iron deficiency)

Bone is within normal limits

ET = essential thrombocythemia

References: [Michiels 2002, Kvasnicka 2007, Thiele 2008b, Wilkins 2008]

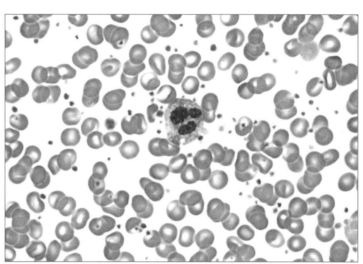

i14.61 *This peripheral blood smear shows essential thrombocythemia. Note striking increase in platelets with relatively unremarkable white blood cells and red blood cells. (Wright)*

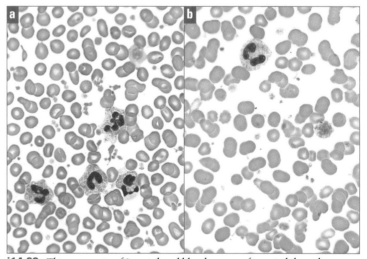

i14.62 *This composite of 2 peripheral blood smears of essential thrombocythemia shows a marked thrombocytosis in conjunction with neutrophilia. Note enlarged size of some platelets. (Wright)*

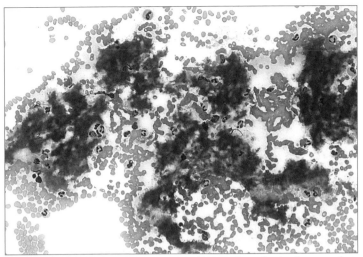

i14.63 *This bone marrow aspirate smear shows striking platelet clumping that mimics bone marrow particles in essential thrombocythemia. (Wright)*

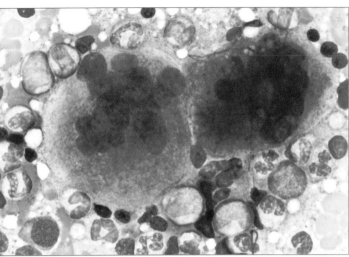

i14.64 *This bone marrow aspirate smear in essential thrombocythemia shows 2 markedly hyperlobated megakaryocytes. (Wright)*

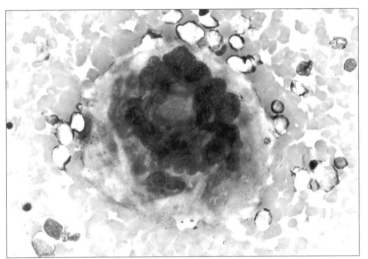

i14.65 *A markedly hyperlobated megakaryocyte is evident in this bone marrow aspirate smear of essential thrombocythemia. Note comparison to size of other hematopoietic cells. (Wright)*

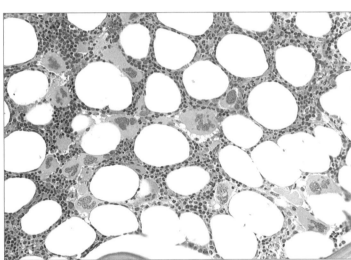

i14.66 *Cellularity is normal in this bone marrow core biopsy section in essential thrombocythemia. Note increased and hyperlobated megakaryocytes. (H&E)*

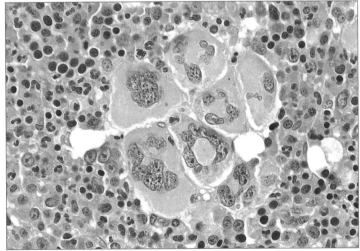

i14.67 *Markedly increased, clustered, and hyperlobated megakaryocytes are evident on this bone marrow core biopsy section in essential thrombocythemia. (H&E)*

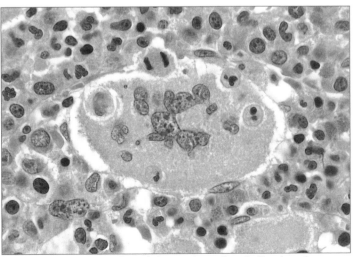

i14.68 *Neutrophils pass through the cytoplasm of markedly enlarged megakaryocytes on this bone marrow core biopsy section in essential thrombocythemia. (H&E)*

Blast phase (leukemic transformation) may occur as a late sequela of ET, but is uncommon (<5% of patients) and likely linked to prior chemotherapy [Passamonti 2009]. Most cases are acute myeloid leukemia.

Cytogenetic abnormalities at ET presentation are unusual, seen in <10% of cases **t14.17** [Gangat 2009]. There are no ET-specific recurring genetic abnormalities, but +8 and +9 most often are seen. The presence or absence of genetic abnormalities does not appear to correlate with an associated risk of disease progression or a worse survival. Cytogenetic evolution is seen in the rare cases of leukemic transformation.

The main differential diagnostic considerations for ET include reactive thrombocytosis, other myeloproliferative neoplasms, refractory anemia with ring sideroblasts and thrombocytosis (RARS-T), and rare myelodysplastic syndromes with thrombocytosis (eg, MDS with del5q). Causes of reactive thrombocytosis are diverse, usually readily clinically apparent, and are discussed in detail in Chapter 12. Exclusion of iron deficiency anemia is a must, since a mild thrombocytosis (usually not >550 × 10^9/L) is typical. Platelets in reactive disorders may show anisocytosis and even occasional circulating megakaryocytic nuclei (in the setting of severe trauma/surgery). However, the bone marrow is normocellular with normal to slightly increased numbers of morphologically normal megakaryocytes. Distinction of ET from the other MPNs can generally be accomplished by integrating clinical, hematologic, morphologic, and genetic findings **t14.7, t14.8**. Distinguishing ET from prefibrotic PMF may present a challenge in early disease; however, distinctive megakaryocytic morphologic differences in the bone marrow and assessment for osteosclerosis may be helpful **t14.19**. Distinction from MDS with thrombocytosis can generally be made by assessing for morphologic dysplasia (see Chapter 16), while RARS-T shows ring sideroblasts and anemia.

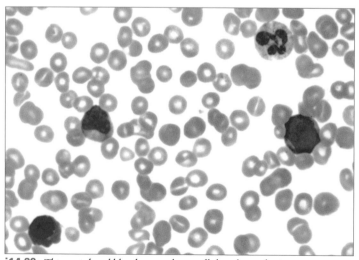

i14.69 *This peripheral blood smear shows cellular phase of primary myelofibrosis. Note leukoerythroblastic blood picture, but absence of teardrop erythrocytes. (Wright)*

t14.19 Clues to Aid in the Distinction of ET from Prefibrotic PMF and/or Early Phase PV*

Presence of *JAK2* V617F mutation accompanied by otherwise unexplained erythrocytosis and/or subnormal EPO level is good evidence in support of PV

Megakaryocytic morphology

ET	Uniform, giant, hyperlobulated megakaryocytes
PV	Loose collections of somewhat hyperlobated megakaryocytes
PMF	Small to giant pleomorphic megakaryocytes with cloud-like, bulbous and/or hyperchromatic nuclei

PMF megakaryocytes show hyperchromatic nuclei and a higher apoptotic fraction by immunohistochemistry assessment than ET

Granulocytic proliferation is considered a feature of early PMF, although may be seen in some cases of ET

*Significant interobserver variability among expert hematopathologists in reliably and consistently diagnosing ET has been observed
EPO = erythropoietin; ET = essential thrombocythemia; PMF = primary myelofibrosis; PV = polycythemia vera

References: [Florena 2009, Gianelli 2008, Kvasnicka 2007, Peterson 2008, Tefferi 2007a, 2007b, Thiele 2001, 2006a, 2006b, Wilkins 2008]

[14.5.4] **Primary Myelofibrosis (PMF)**

PMF is a clonal stem cell disorder characterized predominantly by megakaryocytic and granulocytic proliferation with intact maturation, progressive bone marrow fibrosis, splenomegaly, and extramedullary hematopoiesis. (Previous terminology includes chronic idiopathic myelofibrosis, myeloid metaplasia with myelofibrosis, and agnogenic myeloid metaplasia). Key clinical features are detailed in **t14.20**. Although rare, familial myelofibrosis exists and, in some cases, may have a rapidly progressive fatal disease course [Sheikha 2004].

The diagnostic criteria for PMF are detailed in **t14.8**. PMF is classically subcategorized into a cellular (pre-fibrotic) or fibrotic phase. The incidence of the pre-fibrotic phase of PMF is estimated at around 30% of PMF cases and is characterized by minimal to absent bone marrow fibrosis and intact hematologic indices, although the platelet count may be elevated (mimicking ET), and mild anemia may develop **i14.69**. With progression to the fibrotic phase, a leukoerythroblastic blood picture evolves with more atypical circulating platelets and megakaryocytes **t14.21**. Teardrop erythrocytes are also present **i14.70, i14.71, i14.72**.

The key bone marrow morphologic features in prefibrotic PMF include hypercellularity with increased,

t14.20 Key Clinical Features of PMF

Clinical	Up to 1/3 of patients may be asymptomatic at diagnosis
	Splenomegaly and often hepatomegaly
	Anemia, often requiring transfusion
	Predominantly a disease of older adults
	Hypermetabolic state leads to constitutional symptoms
	Gout due to hyperuricemia
Incidence	From 0.5-1.5 per 100,000 patients/year; M = F
Pathogenesis/genetics	*JAK2* V617F mutation seen in ~50% of cases; pathogenetic contribution not clear
	Karyotypic abnormalities identified in ~30% of patients at diagnosis
	Primary disease-causing mutation unknown
Childhood/familial PMF	Prevalence unknown
	Without extensive pedigree, may be difficult to distinguish childhood sporadic PMF vs familial
	It has been suggested that the natural history of childhood myelofibrosis differs from adults
	Clinical outcome varies from rapidly fatal to long-term survival >22 years
	JAK2 V617F mutation is up to 75% of patients and is acquired (similar to sporadic MPN)
Prognosis	Median survival 70-110 months
	Causes of death include infection and leukemic transformation
	IPSS based on 5 independent predictors of inferior survival: age >65 years, Hgb <10 g/dL, leukocyte count >25 × 10^9/L, circulating blasts ≥1%, and presence of constitutional symptoms
	New prognostic scoring system identifies 4 groups with clearly distinct differences with regard to survival
	Presence of 0, 1, 2, or ≥3 of above 5 parameters predicts median survival of 135, 95, 48, and 27 months
	Presence of normal karyotype, isolated del(13q) or del(20q) does not predict for worse outcome compared to any other abnormal karyotype
	Presence of *JAK2* V617F predicts for marked splenomegaly and leukemic transformation
	Low *JAK2* V617F allele burden may portend shortened survival
	Thrombotic events increased in patients with concomitant *JAK2* mutations and leukocytosis

IPSS = international prognostic scoring system; MPN = myeloproliferative neoplasm; PMF = primary myelofibrosis

References: [Altura 2000, Barbui 2010, Barosi 2007, Bellanne-Chantelot 2006, Cervantes 2009, Guglielmelli 2009, Hussein 2009b, 2009c, 2010, Morel 2010, Rumi 2007, Sheikha 2004, Vaidya 2009]

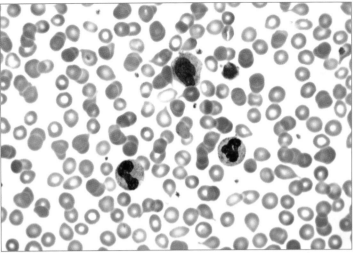

i14.70 *This peripheral blood smear shows primary myelofibrosis with a few teardrop erythrocytes in conjunction with a giant platelet, suggesting early reticulin fibrosis of the bone marrow. (Wright)*

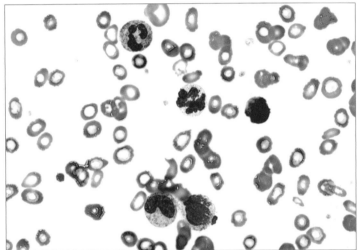

i14.71 *This peripheral blood smear shows end-stage primary myelofibrosis. Note marked anemia with teardrop erythrocytes and prominent left shift. (Wright)*

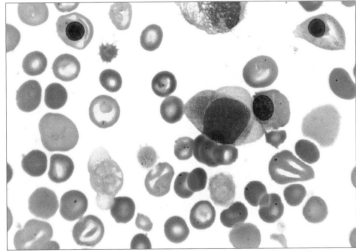

i14.72 *This peripheral blood smear shows end-stage primary myelofibrosis. Note nucleated red blood cells and circulating blasts, dysplastic platelets, and prominent erythrocyte anisopoikilocytosis. (Wright) (courtesy W Williams, MD)*

t14.21 Hematologic and Morphologic Features of PMF

Peripheral Blood

Component/Feature	Prefibrotic/Cellular Phase	Fibrotic PMF
Platelets	May see thrombocytosis (mimicking ET) Platelets abnormal, giant, hypogranular Circulating megakaryocytes	Thrombocytopenia with disease progression Circulating megakaryocytes typical
Red blood cells	Normal to mild anemia	Progressively more severe anemia with circulating normoblasts Leukoerythroblastic picture
White blood cells	Usually normal to mildly elevated May see subtle basophilia Blasts <2%	Variable count (15-30 × 10⁹/L) May see left shift in granulocytes Mild basophilia and/or eosinophilia in 10%-30% of cases Blasts variable (<5%)

Bone Marrow

Fibrosis	No significant increase in reticulin/collagen fibers	Clear-cut reticulin and/or collagen fibrosis ≥ grade 2 (scale 0-3)
Bone	Normal; minimal remodeling Early osteosclerosis	Progressive osteosclerosis Increased osteoclasts and osteoblastic activity
Cellularity/ hematopoiesis:	Usually hypercellular	Hypercellular early on; with progressive disease, fibrosis replaces hematopoiesis; foci of hypocellularity
Granulocytes	Granulocytic hyperplasia with intact maturation	Variable
Erythroids	Minimal dysplastic change Variable; may be decreased Intact maturation	Variable; progressive decrease with increasing fibrosis
Megakaryocytes	Increased, clustering and abnormal morphology Small to large, with cloud-like, bulbous and/or hyperchromatic nuclei	Strikingly abnormal; may form larger clusters and sheets
Blasts	<5%; no clusters	<10% generally; 10%-19% heralds disease progression
Sinuses	Variably dilated, abnormal megakaryocytes often perisinusoidal, paratrabecular	Dilated sinuses with prominent intrasinusoidal hematopoiesis (megakaryocytes predominate)
Stroma	Neoangiogenesis mild	Marked neoangiogenesis with progressive disease
Lymphoid nodules	May be seen in ~25% of cases	May be seen in ~25% of cases

ET = essential thrombocythemia; PMF= primary myelofibrosis

References: [Ahmed 2006, Bock 2005, Boruchov 2009, Kvasnicka 2010, Steurer 2007, Tefferi 2007b, 2009c, Thiele 2005a, 2006b, 2008c]

mildly left-shifted granulopoiesis, pleomorphic megakaryocytes, and variable osteosclerosis t14.21 i14.73. The megakaryocytes are both morphologically abnormal and show abnormal topography. Megakaryocytes are increased, clustered, and show striking pleomorphism ranging from small pyknotic forms to large forms with evidence of abnormal maturation i14.74. Blasts comprise <5% of cells and are not conspicuously clustered by morphology or CD34 immunohistochemistry. Neoangiogenesis is typical, as are lymphoid nodules (up to 1/3 of cases).

With progression to the fibrotic phase, clear-cut reticulin and/or collagen fibrosis, bony changes (osteosclerosis), and dilated sinuses with prominent intrasinusoidal hematopoiesis are evident i14.75, i14.76. The megakaryocytic atypia persists, and often large sheets of megakaryocytes develop i14.77. In advanced disease, bone marrow cellularity diminishes to small foci of residual cellularity; hematopoiesis may coexist with frank hypocellularity due to advanced fibrosis i14.77, i14.78, i14.79. Reticulin and collagen fibrosis is pronounced i14.80. Immunohistochemical stains for megakaryocyte-associated antigens highlight the marked atypia and pleomorphism i14.81. CD105 (or CD34) highlights the extent of microvascular density, which correlates with the degree of fibrosis and is an adverse prognosticator [Ponzoni 2004]. Bone marrow transplant offers the potential for cure by ablating the abnormal hematopoietic clone and restoring hematopoiesis. After cytoreductive therapy, varying degrees of gelatinous transformation, hypocellularity, and myelodysplastic features may be seen in PMF bone marrows [Thiele 2003b].

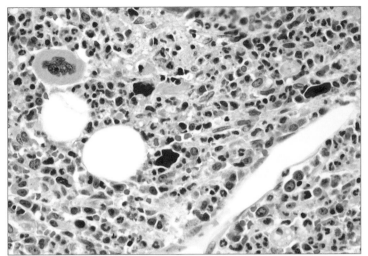

i14.73 *This bone marrow core biopsy section shows cellular phase of primary myelofibrosis. Note atypical megakaryocytes and dilated sinus. (H&E)*

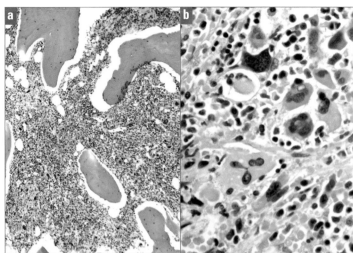

i14.74 *This composite shows the low- and high-magnification features of cellular phase primary myelofibrosis. Note osteosclerosis and increased, clustered, and atypical megakaryocytes. Some of the pleomorphic megakaryocytes have very dark nuclear chromatin. (H&E)*

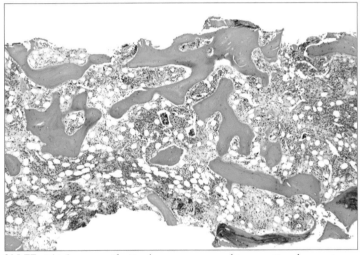

i14.75 *This low-magnification bone marrow core biopsy section shows primary myelofibrosis in early fibrotic phase with osteosclerosis, dilated sinuses, and intrasinusoidal hematopoietic cells. (H&E) (courtesy C Sever, MD)*

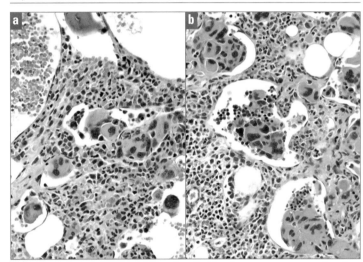

i14.76 *This composite highlights strikingly dilated sinuses containing abundant hematopoietic cells, notably megakaryocytes, in primary myelofibrosis. (H&E) (courtesy C Sever, MD)*

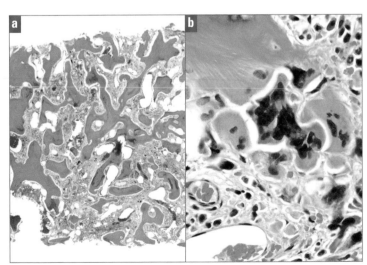

i14.77 *This low- **a** and high-magnification **b** view of a bone marrow core biopsy section shows advanced primary myelofibrosis exhibiting significant fibrosis, osteosclerosis, and markedly atypical and clustered megakaryocytes. (H&E)*

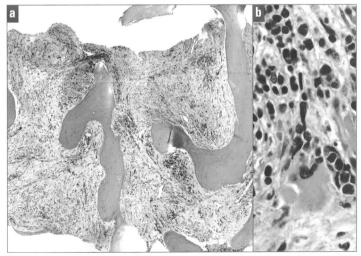

i14.78 *Only pockets of residual hematopoietic cells are evident at low **a** and high **b** magnification in this bone marrow core biopsy section in advanced primary myelofibrosis. (H&E)*

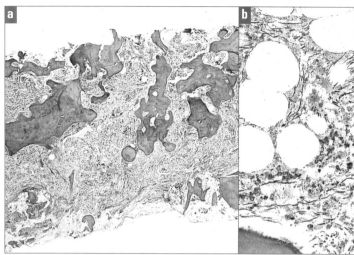

i14.79 *Hematopoiesis is essentially absent in this extensively fibrotic bone marrow core biopsy section in advanced primary myelofibrosis. Note striking osteosclerosis and prominent fibrosis. (H&E and reticulin) (courtesy W Williams, MD)*

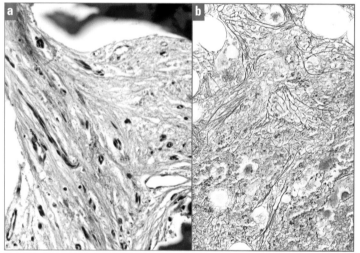

i14.80 *This composite shows advanced myelofibrosis consisting of both collagen fibrosis **a** and reticulin fibrosis **b**. (trichrome and reticulin)*

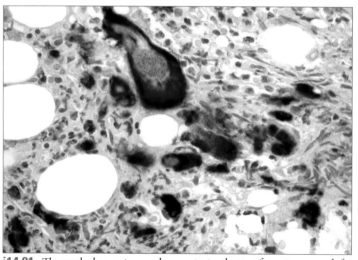

i14.81 *The marked range in megakaryocyte size that typifies primary myelofibrosis is highlighted in this bone marrow core biopsy section. (immunoperoxidase for CD42b)*

t14.22 Causes of Bone Marrow Osteosclerosis*

Mast cell disease

Metastatic tumor

Primary myelofibrosis

Paget disease

Osteosclerotic myeloma

Osteopetrosis

Previous fracture or biopsy site

Chronic renal failure-associated secondary hyperparathyroidism

Primary hyperparathyroidism

Hypervitaminosis A and D

Radiation

Fluorosis

Hepatitis C virus infection

Intravenous drug use

Storage disease

*For complete discussion of individual entities, see Chapters 14, 23, 27, 28, 29, 33, 34, and 35

References: [Barni 2006, Boruchov 2009, Diamond 1996, Hallanger Johnson 2007, Sanchez 2008, Schwartz 2008, Tefferi 2009c, Tolar 2004, Wenstrup 2002]

Differential Diagnosis of PMF

The differential diagnostic considerations for PMF are broad and include a variety of non-neoplastic and neoplastic diseases. It is optimal to consider differential diagnoses based on causes of myelofibrosis and/or osteosclerosis t14.22, t14.23.

Gray platelet syndrome can bear a striking resemblance to early fibrotic phase PMF, and although rare, it should be entertained as a diagnostic possibility when a diagnosis of MPN in a younger patient is being considered. Thrombocytopenia is the norm with abnormally large and hypogranular forms, which is not typical of MPN; however, the bone marrow can show MPN-like features, including mild reticulin fibrosis, dilated sinuses, and abnormal, mildly increased, loosely clustered megakaryocytes (see Chapter 12 for illustrations). Neither *JAK2* mutations nor significant splenomegaly are typical of gray platelet syndrome. Similarly, autoimmune disorders may also exhibit a leukoerythroblastic blood picture, bone marrow fibrosis, and increased megakaryocytes. However, peripheral cytopenias predominate rather than the elevated counts typical of MPN [Haas 2009, Pullarkat 2003, Rizzi 2004]. Furthermore, the clinical history of autoimmunity, positive laboratory tests for autoimmune disorders, and absence of genetic abnormalities allow distinction from PMF. Toxic injury to the bone marrow may demonstrate mild and rarely moderate reticulin fibrosis, with atypical megakaryocyte clusters during recovery. Hypercellularity would be unusual, although a granulocytic left shift could be seen early on. Colony-stimulating factor (eg, G-CSF)

t14.23 Causes of Bone Marrow Fibrosis

Etiology	Key Tip(s)
Neoplastic (see t28.3)	
Primary myelofibrosis	Osteosclerosis
	Dilated sinuses with intrasinusoidal hematopoiesis, leukoerythroblastosis
	Abnormal megakaryocytes with clustering and abnormal maturation
Mast cell disease	Osteosclerosis, diffuse lesions
	Target lesions
	Dense aggregates of tryptase positive mast cells
Other myeloid neoplasms with fibrosis	AML, MDS, MDS/MPN, acute megakaryoblastic leukemia (see t16.12)
Metastatic tumor	Non-hematopoietic tumor cell clusters
Hairy cell leukemia	Interstitial distribution
	"Fried-egg" morphology
Non-Hodgkin lymphoma (occasional)	Atypical single, large cells or sheets of any size cells
Hodgkin lymphoma	Usually see discrete lesions; may be diffuse
Myeloma (occasional)	Osteosclerosis; more common in POEMS syndrome (see Chapter 23)
	Clonal plasma cells
ALL (occasional)	Lymphoblasts by morphology and immunohistochemistry
T-LGL (occasional)	Large granular lymphocytes by morphology and immunophenotyping
Non-Neoplastic (see t28.3)	
Gray platelet syndrome	Thrombocytopenia, large pale platelets, reticulin fibrosis
	Younger age
Autoimmune myelofibrosis/ collagen vascular disease	Peripheral cytopenias, lymphocytic infiltration of marrow
	History of autoimmune disease
	Autoantibodies
	No splenomegaly
Osteopetrosis	Rare inherited disorder
	Detected at young age
	Key bony changes
Chronic renal failure	Osteitis fibrosis cystitica with advanced disease
	Variable bony remodeling progressive
Paget disease	Distinctive bone "mosaic" change
Fracture site/ previous biopsy site	Marked new bone formation
	History, rule out other causes of bony changes and fibrosis
Chronic infections	History, organisms possibly identified in bone marrow
Storage disease	Characteristic morphology of particular disease

ALL = acute lymphoblastic leukemia; AML = acute myeloid leukemia; MDS = myelodysplastic syndrome; MPN = myeloproliferative neoplasm; POEMS = polyneuropathy, organomegaly, endocrinopathy, M-protein, skin changes; T-LGL = T-cell large granular lymphocytic leukemia

References: [Abdel-Wahab 2009, Bass 2001, Bock 2008, Buesche 2007, Buhr 2003, Gruner 2003, Kuter 2007, Lim 2007, O'Malley 2005, Pullarkat 2003, Rameshwar 1998, Reilly 1997, Salgado 1992, Tefferi 1995b, Thiele 1997, Vega 2002]

can produce a transient hypercellular bone marrow, although clinical and medication history should allow for proper classification. Differential diagnostic considerations for osteosclerosis are listed in **t14.22**. Similarly, distinction of PMF from other fibrotic bone marrow neoplasms is delineated in **t14.23**.

[14.5.5] **Myeloproliferative Neoplasm, Unclassifiable**

Myeloproliferative neoplasm, unclassified (MPN-U), typifies a small group of MPN cases that otherwise defy subcategorization into CML, ET, PV, or PMF **t14.7**, **t14.8**, **i14.82**, **i14.83**, **i14.84**. In addition, a non-neoplastic disorder has

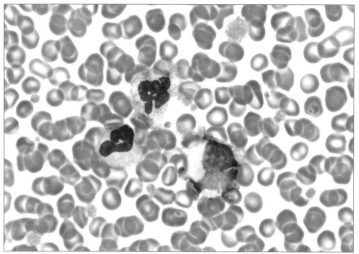

i14.82 *This peripheral blood smear shows leukocytosis, erythrocytosis, and moderate thrombocytosis. Note large platelets. Due to the hybrid features, a diagnosis of myeloproliferative neoplasm unclassifiable was made. (Wright) (courtesy C Sever, MD)*

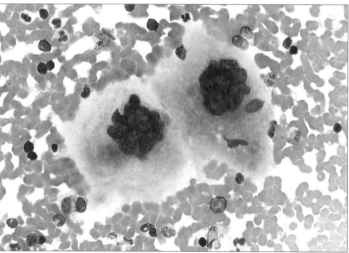

i14.83 *This bone marrow aspirate from a patient with a myeloproliferative neoplasm with hybrid features shows 2 hyperlobated megakaryocytes. (Wright) (courtesy C Sever, MD)*

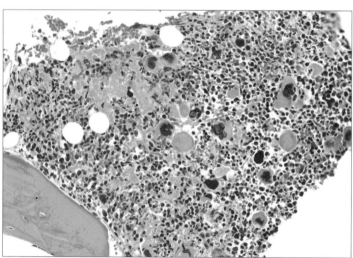

i14.84 *This bone marrow core biopsy section in a myeloproliferative neoplasm with hybrid features shows marked hypercellularity and increased variably hyperlobated megakaryocytes. The megakaryocytes are fairly uniform in size and are not strikingly hyperlobated. (H&E) (courtesy C Sever, MD)*

t14.24 Key Tips in the Bone Marrow Diagnosis of Myeloproliferative Neoplasms, Unclassifiable

Non-neoplastic disorders mimicking MPN should be completely excluded

Cytogenetic and molecular studies should be performed to identify:

a clonal abnormality, which would indicate a neoplasm (eg, *JAK2* V617F+ mutation)

recurrent abnormalities warranting alternative classification [eg, *BCR-ABL1*, abnormalities of *PDGFRA*, *PDGFRB*, *FGFR1*, inv16, t(8;21)]

Cases with suboptimal bone marrow biopsies, insufficient clinical, hematologic, or genetic data should *not* be arbitrarily placed in this category

Clear-cut dysplastic features of granulocytes or erythroid precursors and/or monocytosis should warrant consideration of a myelodysplastic syndrome or MPS/MPN

MPN = myeloproliferative neoplasm; MPS = myelodysplastic syndrome

been excluded. Cases often fall into this diagnostic category at 2 morphologic extremes:

1. early disease presentation (prepolycythemic PV, ET, and prefibrotic PMF)
2. end-stage disease with extensive fibrosis and osteosclerosis precluding recognition of the initial underlying MPN entity

Key diagnostic considerations in the potential diagnosis of MDS, unclassifiable, are listed in t14.24.

In early disease, the peripheral blood findings show variable peripheral thrombocytosis, leukocytosis with left shift, and basophilia, but specific criteria for the distinct MPN categories are not fulfilled i14.82. The bone marrow is often (but not always) hypercellular and aspirable i14.83. There is megakaryocytic proliferation and/or clustering, variable degrees of atypia, and no bony changes i14.84.

Cytogenetic and molecular studies are required to identify:

1. an abnormality that would indicate an alternative diagnosis (eg, *BCR-ABL1* positivity, abnormalities of *PDGFRA*, *PDGFRB*, and *FGFR1*)
2. the possible presence of a clonal abnormality, excluding a non-neoplastic disorder (eg, *JAK2* V617F mutation, +8)

If clear-cut dysplastic features or monocytosis are present, consideration of a hybrid myelodysplastic/myeloproliferative neoplasm is indicated (see Chapters 13 and 17).

t14.25 Key Diagnostic Features of CEL, NOS

Must Have

Sustained eosinophilia (eosinophils ≥1.5 × 10⁹/L)

Clonal genetic abnormality (excluding those below) **OR** blasts >2% in blood or >5% in bone marrow

Must Exclude

Recurring genetic abnormalities requiring alternate classification:

    BCR-ABL1 fusion/Philadelphia chromosome (CML)

    Rearrangement of *PDGFRA*, *PDGFRB*, or *FGFR1* (see Chapter 15 for complete details)

    inv(16)(p13.1;q22) (AML)

Another myeloproliferative neoplasm (eg, PV, ET, PMF, systemic mastocytosis)

An underlying cytokine-producing aberrant T-cell population

A reactive eosinophilia (eg, parasitic infection, hypersensitivity, allergy, Churg-Strauss syndrome, or similar disorder)

Other neoplastic disorders with accompanying eosinophilia: acute lymphoblastic leukemia with t(5;14), acute myeloid leukemia, MDS, MDS/MPN, lymphoma, carcinoma, melanoma

Terminology/Differential Diagnosis of CEL, NOS, after Exclusion of Above Entities

IHES: meets all criteria for CEL, NOS *except* no clonal abnormality detected, blasts <2% in blood and <5% in bone marrow, and there is evidence of eosinophil-mediated tissue/organ damage

Idiopathic hypereosinophilia: meets all criteria for IHES *except* no end organ/tissue damage

AML = acute myeloid leukemia; CEL, NOS = chronic eosinophilic syndrome, not otherwise specified; CML = chronic myelogenous leukemia; ET = essential thrombocythemia; IHES = idiopathic hypereosinophilic syndrome; MDS = myelodysplastic syndrome; MPN = myeloproliferative neoplasm; PMF = primary myelofibrosis; PV = polycythemia vera

References: [Bain 2008b, Helbig 2009, Lierman 2009, Tefferi 2009c, Valent 2009]

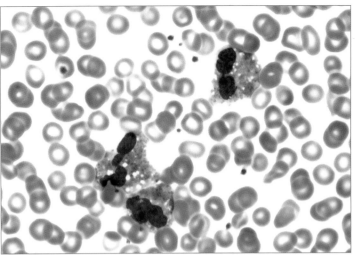

i14.85 *This peripheral blood smear shows chronic eosinophilic leukemia. Molecular genetic studies for various tyrosine kinase rearrangements and mutations were negative. (Wright) (courtesy C Sever, MD)*

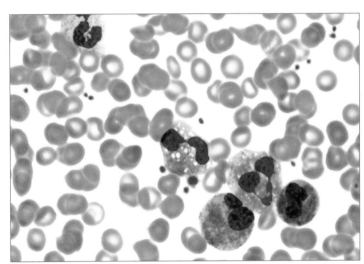

i14.86 *This peripheral blood smear shows marked eosinophilia ultimately diagnosed as chronic eosinophilic leukemia, not otherwise specified. No specific cytogenetic or molecular features were identified. (Wright) (courtesy C Sever, MD)*

[14.5.6] **Chronic Eosinophilic Leukemia, Not Otherwise Specified**

Chronic eosinophilic leukemia, not otherwise specified (CEL, NOS), is a type of myeloproliferative neoplasm characterized by sustained, clonal peripheral blood and bone marrow eosinophilia in which a reactive process or other well-defined recurrent genetic abnormality is excluded **t14.25** (see Chapter 15 for myeloid and lymphoid neoplasms with *PDGFRA*, *PDGFRB*, and *FGFR1* abnormalities) [Bain 2004, 2007, Martinelli 2007, Tefferi 2006b]. Chronic eosinophilias are uniquely challenging given the heterogeneous nature of disorders with eosinophilia and often confusing eosinophilia terminology **t14.25**. The key to diagnosing CEL, NOS is to exhaustively exclude all other diagnostic (reactive and neoplastic) possibilities [Gotlib 2010, Tefferi 2010]. This would include evaluation for particular genetic abnormalities that would otherwise

dictate an alternate classification [eg, abnormalities of *FGFR1* (5q33), *PDGFRA* (4q12), *PDGFRB* (8p11), inv(16), *BCR-ABL1* fusion].

Eosinophil morphology in eosinophilia is insufficient to reliably discriminate reactive from clonal disorders [Fletcher 2007]. The most remarkable peripheral blood feature is the eosinophilia with variable dysplastic features **i14.85, i14.86**. Neutrophilia without significant dysplasia may be evident, but blasts are <5%.

The bone marrow morphologic features in CEL, NOS necessarily *lack* features indicative of a distinct clinico-pathologic entity [eg, acute myeloid leukemia (AML), acute lymphoblastic leukemia (ALL), MPNs, systemic mastocytosis (SM)]. In CEL, NOS, the bone marrow aspirate smear is characteristically hypercellular with abundant eosinophils

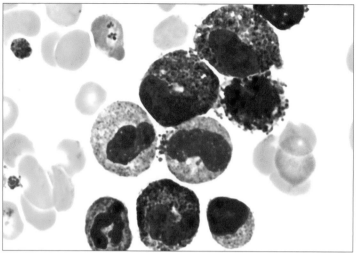

i14.87 *This bone marrow aspirate smear shows marked eosinophilia ultimately diagnosed as chronic eosinophilic leukemia, not otherwise specified, after all cytogenetic and molecular results were negative. The tryptase level was normal. (Wright) (courtesy C Sever, MD)*

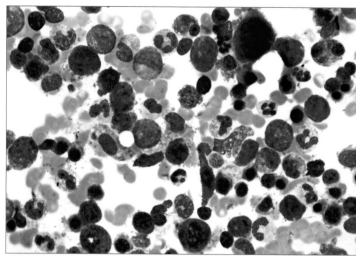

i14.88 *Low magnification of this bone marrow aspirate smear in chronic eosinophilic leukemia, not otherwise specified, shows increased granulocytic lineage cells, eosinophils, and abnormal megakaryocytes. (Wright) (courtesy C Sever, MD)*

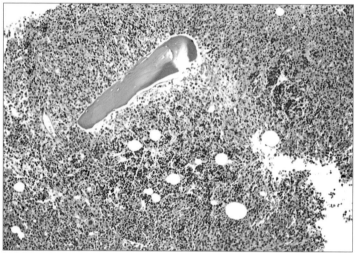

i14.89 *This bone marrow core biopsy section in chronic eosinophilic leukemia shows marked hypercellularity and normal bony trabeculae. (H&E) (courtesy C Sever, MD)*

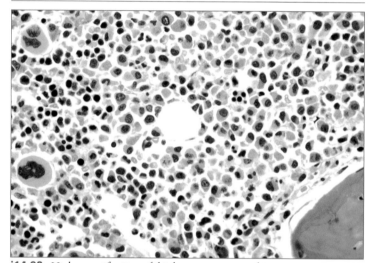

i14.90 *High magnification of this bone marrow core biopsy section in chronic eosinophilic leukemia, not otherwise specified, shows strikingly increased mature eosinophils in conjunction with abnormal megakaryocytes. (H&E) (courtesy C Sever, MD)*

and eosinophil precursors **i14.87, i14.88**. Occasional cases with abnormal megakaryocytes and increased myeloid precursors favor a primary hematopoietic neoplasm **i14.88**. The bone marrow core biopsy is hypercellular, with numerous eosinophils and often no significant bony changes **i14.89**. Abnormal megakaryocytes may be seen in conjunction with marked eosinophilia **i14.90**. A significant increase in blasts is not seen, although in a case lacking a genetic abnormality, either 2% peripheral blood or 5% bone marrow blasts are needed for the diagnosis. While dysplastic features in one or more of the marrow lineages have been reported, a myelodysplastic syndrome with prominent eosinophilia should be excluded. Marrow fibrosis is not surprising due to the reaction to released eosinophil granules, but is generally only mild. Tryptase immunohistochemistry is useful to confirm that mast cells are not increased or atypical **i14.91, i14.92**.

The differential diagnosis of CEL, NOS is huge and requires a methodical and exhaustive exclusion of numerous benign and neoplastic entities **t14.25**. In instances in which an underlying cause of eosinophilia is not readily evident, bone marrow morphologic studies, T-cell receptor gene rearrangement studies, flow cytometry (to detect increased blasts, clonal plasma cells, aberrant mast cells, abnormal T-cell clones, lymphoma), and genetics (cytogenetics and FISH/molecular for submicroscopic *FIP1L1-PDGFRA* fusion) may be needed. Rare cases of overt T-NHL in bone marrow can be masked by intense eosinophilia **i14.93**. The treatment of CEL, NOS has evolved in recent years and includes humanized anti-IL-5 antibodies and corticosteroids

[Gleich 2009, Lierman 2009, Rothenberg 2008].

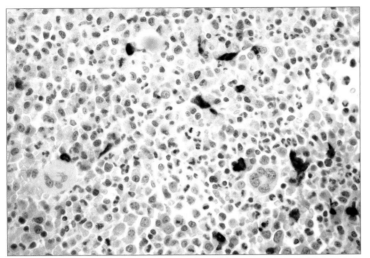

i14.91 *Mast cells are not increased as evidenced by immunoperoxidase staining for tryptase in this bone marrow core biopsy section in chronic eosinophilic leukemia. (immunoperoxidase for tryptase) (courtesy C Sever, MD)*

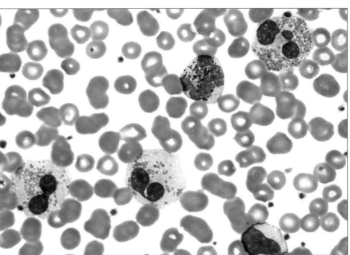

i14.92 *This peripheral blood smear is from a child with striking eosinophilia in conjunction with basophilia. Markedly increased mast cells were present in the bone marrow. (Wright) (courtesy J Mo, MD)*

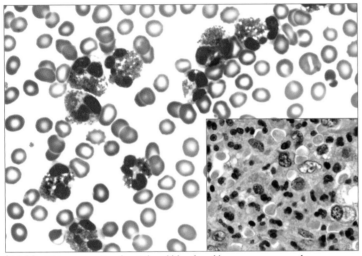

i14.93 *This composite of peripheral blood and bone marrow core biopsy section is from a patient with peripheral T-cell lymphoma who developed striking eosinophilia. The lymphoma cells in the bone marrow core biopsy section were morphologically occult, with individually dispersed large atypical cells (inset). (Wright and H&E)*

[14.5.7]   **Chronic Neutrophilic Leukemia (CNL)**

CNL is an exceedingly rare myeloproliferative neoplasm characterized by persistent peripheral blood neutrophilic and bone marrow granulocytic hyperplasia in conjunction with splenomegaly and less often hepatomegaly. CNL must be regarded as a diagnosis of exclusion. **t14.26** details the key clinical, morphologic, genetic and differential diagnostic features of CNL.

The peripheral blood shows a leukocytosis (WBC $\geq 25 \times 10^9/L$) consisting of an unexplained neutrophilia that lacks morphologic dysplasia, and with minimal left shift **i14.94**, **i14.95**. Toxic changes may be seen in some cases, and more common underlying etiologies, such as infection or colony-stimulating factor effect, must be excluded **i14.95**. Basophilia is usually absent, and red blood cells are typically unremarkable, although occasional normoblasts may be evident.

i14.94 *This peripheral blood smear shows chronic neutrophilic leukemia. Note marked predominance of mature neutrophils in conjunction with basophilia. Cytogenetic and FISH studies were negative. (Wright)*

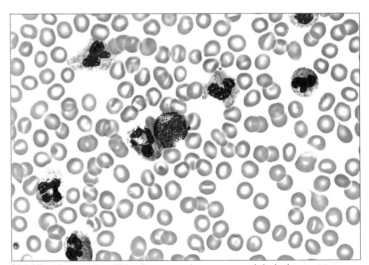

i14.95 *This peripheral blood smear in chronic neutrophilic leukemia. Note mild toxic changes of neutrophils, and minimal left shift. (Wright)*

t14.26 Key Features of CNL

Clinical	Generally seen in adults (average age 60 years, range from 20s to 80s) Splenomegaly Hepatomegaly Hyperuricemia with symptoms of gout Bleeding tendency
Morphology:	
Blood	Sustained WBC ≥25 × 10⁹/L; neutrophils and bands comprise >80% of the WBC; left-shifted granulocytes account for <10% of the WBC; blasts are <1% Toxic changes have been reported in some cases; must exclude reactive conditions Absence of dysplasia No significant basophilia or monocytosis Erythrocytes and platelets normal
Bone marrow	Hypercellular Granulocytic hyperplasia with neutrophilic predominance Complete and intact granulocytic maturation Blasts <5% of total nucleated cells Absence of granulocytic and erythroid dysplasia Megakaryocytes may be increased, atypical, and/or clustered May see neutrophilic phagocytosis by bone marrow histiocytes
Pathogenesis	Unknown CNL neutrophils may show insufficient response to typical external cytokine stimulation
Genetics	Conventional cytogenetics shows a normal karyotype in ~90% of cases; +8, +9, del20q reported Must exclude BCR-ABL1 fusion and abnormalities of PDGFRA, PDGFRB, FGFR1 JAK2 mutation reported; must exclude other MPN
Differential diagnosis:	CNL is a diagnosis of exclusion
Non-neoplastic considerations	Leukemoid reaction, underlying infection, inflammatory condition, autoimmune disorder, colony-stimulating factor effect, CNL-like blood and bone marrow picture due to underlying other hematopoietic malignancy (eg, myeloma, MGUS) or nonhematopoietic malignancy (eg, transitional cell carcinoma, hepatocellular carcinoma)
Neoplastic considerations	CML, particularly "neutrophilic variant"; p230 variant of BCR-ABL1 may be missed by molecular unless long-template PCR is performed BCR-ABL1– MPNs (see t14.7) CMML; monocytosis (monocytes > 1 × 10⁹/L) present; dysplastic changes of granulocytes usually present MDS: cytopenias and single or multilineage dysplasia are dominant features AML with maturation: blasts ≥20% unless t(8;21) or inv(16) present

AML = acute myeloid leukemia; CML = chronic myelogenous leukemia; CMML = chronic myelomonocytic leukemia; CNL = chronic neutrophilic leukemia; MDS = myelodysplastic syndrome; MGUS = monoclonal gammopathy of undetermined significance; MPN = myeloproliferative neoplasms

References: [Amato 2008, Bain 2008a, Bohm 2002, Dincol 2002, Elliott 2005, Haferlach 2008, Kako 2007, Mc Lornan 2005, Neureiter 2008, Noguchi 2001, Pane 1996, Patnaik 2009b, Reilly 2002, Shigekiyo 2008, Tilak 2007, Uemura 2009]

The bone marrow findings in CNL are non-specific and consist of hypercellularity due to granulocytic proliferation with intact and complete maturation. Blasts comprise <5% of total cells. Macrophage ingestion of neutrophils is often seen i14.96, i14.97. The core biopsy is hypercellular with dilated sinuses and increased granulocytes i14.98. Dysplastic changes of the granulocytic and erythroid lineages are absent, while megakaryocytes may be increased and show atypical morphology and/or clustering providing morphologic support for a myeloproliferative neoplasm i14.99. In some cases, core biopsy sections show abnormal localization of immature precursors. In addition, the ingested neutrophils within macrophages may closely mimic organisms on tissue sections i14.100.

Given that CNL is a rare entity with non-specific morphologic findings and normal cytogenetics in most cases, it is imperative that alternative diagnoses be considered and subsequently excluded t14.26. Reactive neutrophilias and leukemoid reactions with hypercellular bone marrow are commonly seen in reactive, infectious, or autoimmune (eg, rheumatoid) states, in G-CSF therapy or cytokine/chemokine-producing tumors, and in inflammatory conditions [Sakka 2006]. As an example, a paraneoplastic phenomenon producing a chronic neutrophilic leukemia-like blood and bone marrow picture may be seen in association with plasma cell dyscrasias (eg, myeloma) i14.101, i14.102. Rarely, CNL has been reported to coexist with myeloma [Dincol 2002]. The most important neoplastic disorder to exclude is CML, particularly

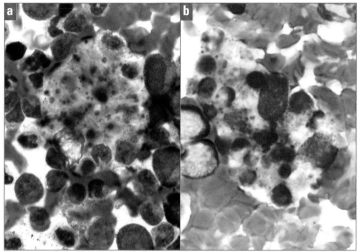

i14.96 *This composite of bone marrow aspirate smears shows chronic neutrophilic leukemia with striking ingestion of the neutrophils by macrophages. (Wright)*

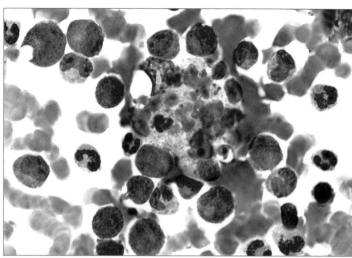

i14.97 *In addition to ingestion of neutrophils by macrophages, increased granulocytic lineage cells are also evident on this bone marrow aspirate smear in chronic neutrophilic leukemia. (Wright)*

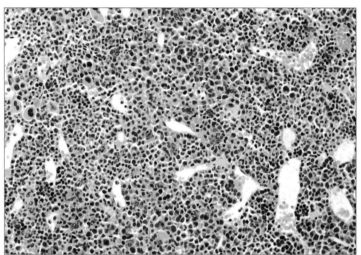

i14.98 *This bone marrow core biopsy section in chronic neutrophilic leukemia; note hypercellularity and dilated sinuses. (H&E)*

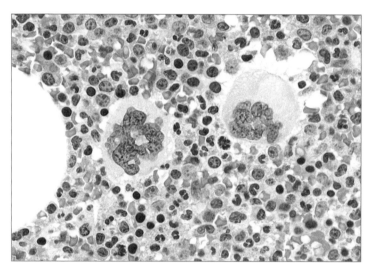

i14.99 *High magnification of a bone marrow core biopsy section in chronic neutrophilic leukemia shows markedly hyperlobated megakaryocytes. (H&E)*

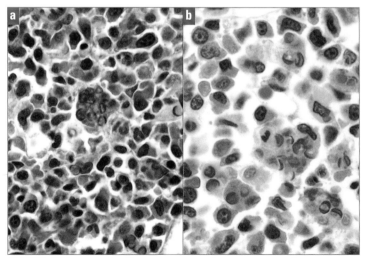

i14.100 *This composite of bone marrow core biopsy sections in chronic neutrophilic leukemia shows a striking predominance of neutrophilic lineage cells in conjunction with ingestion of neutrophils within macrophages, closely mimicking infectious organisms.*

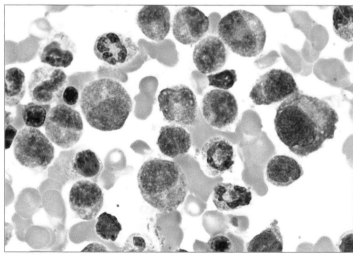

i14.101 *This bone marrow aspirate smear is from a patient with myeloma who developed a concurrent chronic neutrophilic leukemia-like process. Note abnormal plasma cell (right) admixed with tremendous numbers of toxic neutrophilic lineage cells. (Wright) (courtesy J Jones, MD)*

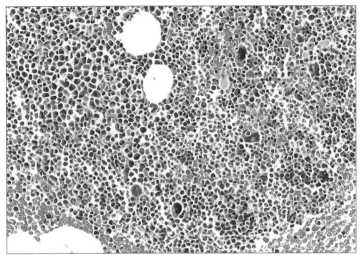

i14.102 *This bone marrow clot section is from a patient with myeloma who developed a chronic neutrophilic leukemia-like picture. Note hypercellularity, increased and hyperlobulated megakaryocytes, and subtle myelomatous infiltration. (H&E) (courtesy J Jones, MD)*

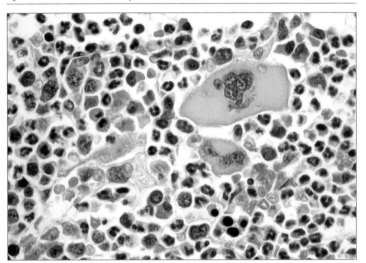

i14.103 *This bone marrow core biopsy section shows the neutrophilic variant of chronic myelogenous leukemia. Note markedly hyperlobulated megakaryocyte rather than the usual monolobate megakaryocytes that typify chronic myelogenous leukemia. Also note predominance of maturing granulocytic cells. (H&E)*

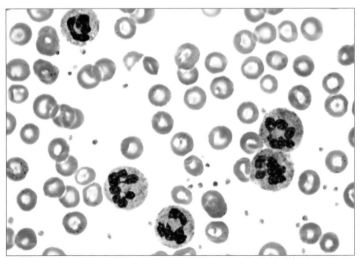

i14.104 *This peripheral blood smear is from a patient with bladder carcinoma who presented with a striking toxic neutrophilia likely secondary to chemokine production by the carcinoma. (Wright)*

the neutrophilic variant that shows a prominent mature neutrophilia **i14.103**. The Philadelphia chromosome/*BCR-ABL1* fusion is present, although it uses an alternative breakpoint (p230) [Pane 1996]. A CNL-like picture may be seen in the setting of nonhematopoietic tumors as well **i14.104**.

Demonstrating that CNL is, in fact, a clonal disorder of neutrophils is difficult but may be accomplished by X-inactivation pattern assays, progenitor cell assays, or by showing reduced apoptosis in the neoplastic neutrophils [Kobayashi 2002, Yanagisawa 1998]. The cytogenetic/FISH detection of +8, +9, and del(20q) confirms a neoplastic disorder but is not specific for any myeloid neoplasm. Therefore, definitive exclusion of more common entities such as myelodysplasia or other myeloproliferative neoplasms is warranted. Rare leukemic transformation of CNL has been reported [Amato 2008].

[14.5.8] **Systemic Mastocytosis (SM)**

Given the recent advances in the elucidation of abnormal tyrosine kinase activity in the pathogenesis of myeloproliferative neoplasms (eg, *JAK2, ABL1*) **sidebar 14.1**, SM, which is nearly always associated with the *KIT* gene D816V mutation, is now included under the umbrella of myeloproliferative neoplasms [Horny 2008]. In addition, the frequent association of SM with other clonal bone marrow disorders further supports this classification.

Mast cells are bone marrow-derived with broad functions, including immunologic and non-immunologic activities **t14.27** [Crivellato 2009, Galli 2005]. Mast cells proliferate and activate in response to a variety of factors, but most importantly in response to stimuli from the KIT receptor [Dobson 2008, Galli 2005]. Although bone marrow-derived, mast cell precursors home to their target tissues and mature at those specific tissue locations.

In normal bone marrow, mast cells comprise relatively few bone marrow nucleated cells but are readily identifiable, usually within particles, on aspirate smears, based on their striking, dark purple granules **i14.105**. Normal mast cells are round, have round to oblong nuclei, inconspicuous nucleoli, and numerous cytoplasmic granules that obscure the nucleus **i14.105, i14.106**. These granules are metachromatic by toluidine blue and Giemsa stains and, unlike basophils, exhibit cytoplasmic naphthol-ASD chloroacetate esterase positivity [Gotlib 2009, Parker 2000]. Because of the tissue-processing protocol, mast cell granules are often leached out and inconspicuous on tissue sections. Immunohistochemical studies for tryptase and CD117 can readily point out scattered mast cells in routine bone marrow biopsies **i14.106** [Agis 1996, van Daele 2009]. Although bone marrow-derived, mast cells are not seen normally in circulation but can be identified by sophisticated cell isolation techniques.

Mast cell proliferations can be generally categorized into non-specific reactive hyperplasia and clonal mast cell disease.

t14.27 Overview of Mast Cells

Origin	Bone-marrow derived cells
Homing	Mast cell precursors migrate to a variety of vascularized peripheral tissues; acquire mature phenotype in the target tissue
	Mainly located at the barrier to external environment (eg, skin, gut, lung)
	Mast cell specific phenotypes; granule contents based partly on target tissue
Production and maturation	Major cytokine is SCF, which acts via the KIT receptor
Function	Hypersensitivity reactions (immediate, delayed, cutaneous) (IgE-mediated)
	Inflammatory reactions
	Host defense against parasites, bacteria, viruses
	Component of autoimmune disease manifestation
	Angiogenesis
	Sustain B-cell expansion and promote IgA plasma cell production
Contents:	
preformed	Proteases: tryptases, chymases
	TNF
	Proteoglycans: histamine, chondroitin sulfate, heparin, serotonin
newly synthesized	Interleukins, prostaglandins, leukotrienes, cytokines (TNF, IFN), chemokines, growth factors (SCF, VEGF, GM-CSF)
Immunophenotype	Positive for tryptase, CD117, CD33, CD43, CD45
Morphology	Striking, dark purple cytoplasmic granules that obscure nucleus
Relationship to basophils	Recent proposal that both basophils and mast cells derive from a common bone marrow progenitor cell; however, each develops into its own distinct hematopoietic lineage
	Basophils and mast cells are both effectors of allergic reactions
	Both contain numerous granules and inflammatory mediators (eg, histamine)
	Both express IgE binding sites
	Basophils, unlike mast cells, express numerous interleukin binding sites

GM-GSF = granulocyte macrophage-colony-stimulating factor; IFN = interferon; SCF = stem cell factor; TNF = tumor necrosis factor; VEGF = vascular endothelial growth factor

References: [Agis 1996, Galli 2005, Kneilling 2009, Kovanen 2009, Merluzzi 2010, Metcalfe 2008, Valent 2009, van Daele 2009]

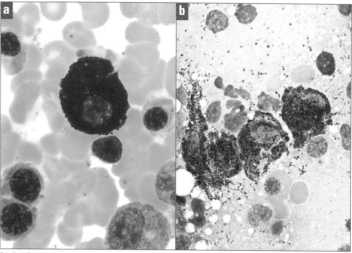

i14.105 *This composite shows a comparison of morphologic features of a normal mast cell **a** and mast cells in systemic mastocytosis **b**. Note spindled and somewhat degranulated appearance of neoplastic mast cells. (Wright)*

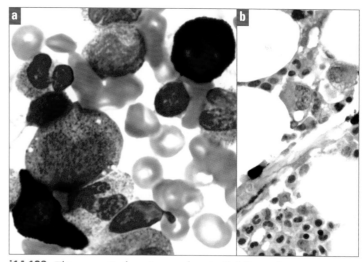

i14.106 *This composite shows increased mast cells following bone marrow injury. Note normal morphologic features on bone marrow aspirate smears **a** while tryptase staining of the bone marrow core biopsy **b** shows perivascular mast cells as well as individually dispersed mast cells. (Wright and immunoperoxidase for tryptase)*

Mast cell hyperplasia may be seen in the bone marrow after a variety of toxic or inflammatory exposures, such as chemotherapy **i14.106**. In such states, the mast cells exhibit normal morphology and immunophenotypic characteristics and do not form compact aggregates with fibrosis and/or osteosclerosis.

Mast cell disease is broadly subdivided into cases that mainly involve the skin (cutaneous mastocytosis) and cases that mainly involve the bone marrow (SM). The exact frequency of these disorders is difficult to determine with certainty. However, in adults, indolent SM is the most common bone marrow lesion [Horny 2009]. This is due to the fact that careful examination of the bone marrow in 80% of patients with cutaneous mastocytosis shows evidence of disease **t14.28**.

t14.28 Estimated Incidence of Mastocytosis in Adults*

Cutaneous mastocytosis

Indolent systemic mastocytosis[†]

Systemic mastocytosis with associated clonal hematological non-mast cell lineage disease (SM-AHNMD)[†]

Aggressive systemic mastocytosis[†]

Mast cell leukemia[†]

Mast cell sarcoma

Extracutaneous mastocytoma

*In descending order of frequency; excerpted from [Horny 2009]
[†]These diseases directly involve bone marrow

t14.29 Categorization of Bone Marrow Mastocytosis

Systemic mastocytosis (SM)

Variants:	Indolent SM
	SM-AHNMD
	Aggressive SM
	Mast cell leukemia

SM-AHNMD = systemic mastocytosis with associated clonal hematological non-mast cell lineage disease

Reference: [Horny 2008]

t14.30 Clinical, Physical, and Radiologic Features of Bone Marrow Mastocytosis*

Clinical:

Constitutional	Fatigue, weight loss, fever, GI disease
Cutaneous	Pruritus, dermatographia
Granule symptoms	Syncope, headache, tachycardia, respiratory distress, flushing
Physical	Splenomegaly[†], hepatomegaly[†], lymphadenopathy[†]
	SM may involve GI tract and other sites
Radiographic	Osteosclerosis, osteoporosis
	May be focal or diffuse
	Seen in almost 50% of symptomatic patients
Laboratory	Increased serum tryptase levels (usually ≥20 ng/mL)
Treatment	Imatinib resistant (KIT D816V mutation)
	Alternative TKIs [dasatinib and midostaurin (PKC412)] may be effective
	2-CDA and interferon alpha
Prognosis	Relates to the systemic mastocytosis variant (eg, indolent SM has near-normal life expectancy compared to mast cell leukemia, which is an aggressive disease)

*Variable depending on extent, activity, and subtypes of disease
[†]Organomegaly usually absent in indolent forms of disease
2-CDA = 2-chloroadenosine deaminase; GI = gastrointestinal; SM = systemic mastocytosis; TKI = tyrosine kinase inhibitor

References: [Cacace 2006, Gotlib 2009, Horny 2008, Ishii 2009, Kirsch 2008, Lee 2008, Lim 2009, Pettigrew 2009, Sperr 2009, Yoshida 2009]

t14.31 Hematologic and Morphologic Findings in Systemic Mastocytosis and Variants*

Hematology	Anemia (common), leukocytosis, eosinophilia (common), neutropenia, thrombocytopenia, basophilia (rare)
Morphology:	
Blood	Circulating mast cells exceedingly rare except in mast cell leukemia and cases of end-stage systemic mastocytosis
	Eosinophils show variable atypia
Bone marrow biopsy	Normocellular to hypercellular
	Focal, occasionally diffuse, compact/dense aggregates of mast cells

Four types of lesions:

1. paratrabecular: mast cells concentrated adjacent to bony trabeculae; associated with bone abnormalities
2. perivascular: blood vessels surrounded by mast cell lesions
3. parafollicular: targetoid lesion with central core of mast cells surrounded by rim of lymphocytes or vice versa
4. diffuse: extensive infiltrates diffusely replacing hematopoietic elements; associated with mast cell leukemia; prominent bony changes common

Associated clonal hematopoietic non-mast cell lineage disorder (myeloid or lymphoid) may be present

Associated clonal hematopoietic non-mast cell disorder may mask concurrent systemic mastocytosis

Frequent fibrosis within mast cell lesions

With prolonged disease may find sclerotic lesions with decreased numbers of mast cells (burned out lesions)

Osteosclerosis common with more extensive diffuse disease

Identification of lesions required for the diagnosis; immunohistochemistry for tryptase may be particularly useful

Bone marrow aspirate	May see increased mast cells within and outside of particles
	Mast cells are atypical, exhibiting spindled morphology, decreased cytoplasmic granularity, increased nuclear lobation; degranulation common; variable blastic chromatin
	Mitoses very rare even in aggressive disease
	Mast cell numbers may be discordant with degree of bone marrow involvement; often attributable to decreased aspirability secondary to associated reticulin fibrosis

*Findings vary depending on degree of tumor burden and clinical variant type

References: [Horny 2008, 2009, Krokowski 2005, Parker 2000]

t14.32 Diagnostic Criteria for Various Bone Marrow Mastocytosis Entities

Entity	Criteria
SM:*	
Major	Multifocal, dense aggregates of mast cells
Minor	>25% of mast cells are morphologically atypical (eg, spindled, immature nuclear features)
	KIT D816V mutation detected
	Abnormal immunophenotypic expression of CD2 and/or CD25 on the mast cells
	Serum tryptase level ≥20 ng/mL
Indolent SM	Meets SM criteria
	No medullary or extramedullary disease dysfunction
	Often cutaneous disease
SM-AHNMD	Meets SM criteria
	AHNMD: meets criteria for another hematopoietic malignancy (eg, AML, MPN)
Aggressive SM	Meets SM criteria
	Evidence of bone marrow effacement, cytopenias
	Evidence of symptomatic extramedullary disease; bony disease/fractures, organomegaly with organ dysfunction, GI involvement
MCL	Meets SM criteria
	>20% mast cells in bone marrow
	Usually diffuse involvement of bone marrow
	May see circulating mast cells, but not required; aleukemic MCL has <10% circulating mast cells

*Diagnosis made with 1 major and 2 minor criteria *or* 3 minor criteria
AML = acute myeloid leukemia; GI = gastrointestinal; MCL = mast cell leukemia; MPN = myeloproliferative neoplasm; SM = systemic mastocytosis; SM-AHNMD = systemic mastocytosis with associated clonal hematological non-mast cell lineage disease

Reference: [Horny 2008]

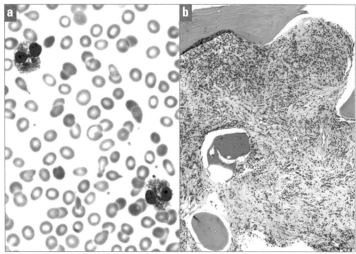

i14.107 *This composite shows the peripheral blood* **a** *and bone marrow core biopsy* **b** *in systemic mastocytosis with associated eosinophilia and teardrop erythrocytes in the peripheral blood, in conjunction with an effaced bone marrow showing osteosclerosis and marked fibrosis. (Wright and H&E)*

The remainder of the discussion will focus primarily on the peripheral blood and bone marrow manifestations of SM. Since the bone marrow and spleen are the most recognized sites of involvement by SM, an adequate bone marrow biopsy is currently regarded as essential for disease evaluation. The current WHO classification recognizes several bone marrow subtypes of SM **t14.29**. The clinical, physical, and radiologic findings are highly variable, and generally reflect the extent and activity of mast cell disease **t14.30** [Gotlib 2009] .

Similarly, hematologic and morphologic findings in systemic mastocytosis show a spectrum of pathologic abnormalities reflecting the degree of bone marrow impairment **t14.31**. The diagnostic criteria for the various systemic mastocytosis entities are detailed in **t14.32**. For the most part, mastocytosis is a morphologic diagnosis requiring confirmation with immunohistochemistry, genetic studies, and/or clinical information **t14.32**.

In the peripheral blood of patients with SM, anemia and eosinophilia (with variable dysplastic changes) are not uncommon **i14.107**. Circulating mast cells are distinctly unusual except in the rare cases of mast cell leukemia or end-stage mastocytosis. In patients with associated non-mast cell myeloid neoplasms, circulating blasts or dysplastic features may be noted.

In the bone marrow, aspirate smears may show a disproportionately low number of mast cells due to the fibrosis typically associated with the mast cell lesions **i14.107**. However, examination of aspirable bone marrow particles and surrounding cells may show increased mast cells with normal morphology or pathologic features, including spindled morphology, immature chromatin, multinucleation, and degranulation **i14.105**, **i14.108**, **i14.109**.

In bone marrow biopsy sections, mast cell lesions are distinctive and most often focal in nature, but are occasionally diffuse **i14.110**. The lesions may be paratrabecular, perivascular, or parafollicular in location **i14.110**. Both focal and diffuse lesions are often associated with increased fibrosis. In diffuse systemic mastocytosis, there is prominent osteosclerosis and the bone appears thickened with irregular remodeling of the trabeculae **i14.111**. The perivascular lesions may induce prominent medial hypertrophy. The mast cell lesions are composed of a variably polymorphic admixture of lymphocytes, eosinophils, and histocytes, in addition to the dense aggregates of mast cells **i14.110**, **i14.112**, **i14.113**. The lymphocytes may form the central focus of the lesion surrounded by mast cells or vice versa **i14.110**. The mast cells within these lesions may be round or spindled and have

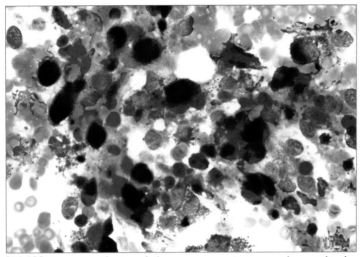

i14.108 *Low magnification of a bone marrow aspirate smear shows strikingly increased mast cells in systemic mastocytosis. (Wright)*

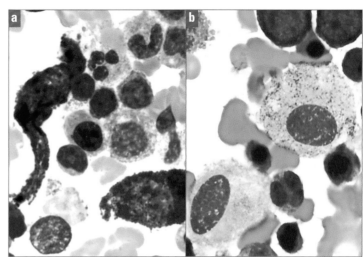

i14.109 *This composite from 2 cases of systemic mastocytosis shows well granulated and spindled mast cells in one case **a**, while the mast cells are predominately degranulated in the second case **b**. (Wright) (courtesy C Sever, MD)*

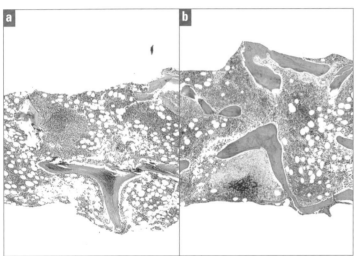

i14.110 *These bone marrow core biopsy sections from 2 patients with systemic mastocytosis show classic target lesions. (H&E) (**b** courtesy I Maric, MD)*

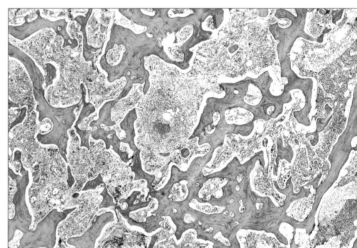

i14.111 *Low magnification of systemic mastocytosis shows extensive osteosclerosis in addition to a target lesion. (H&E) (courtesy D Canioni, MD)*

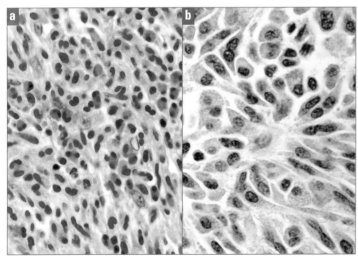

i14.112 *This composite shows the intermediate- and high-magnification features of systemic mastocytosis. Note spindled cell morphology and abundant admixture of eosinophils. (H&E) (courtesy I Maric, MD, and C Sever, MD)*

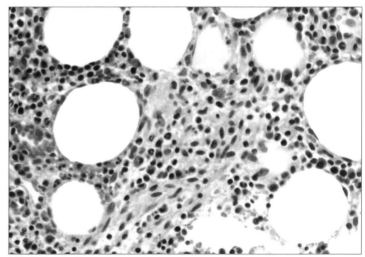

i14.113 *This bone marrow core biopsy section in systemic mastocytosis shows a subtle infiltrate of round mast cells with clear cytoplasm creating a discrete lesion. (H&E)*

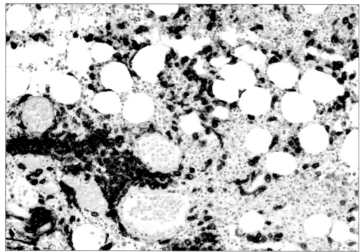

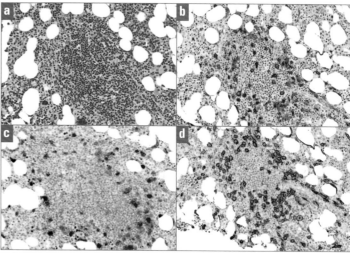

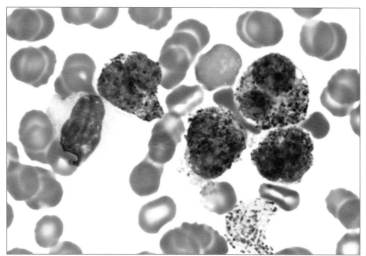

i14.114 *Immunoperoxidase staining for CD117 highlights both discrete mast cell lesions as well as a diffuse increase in mast cells in systemic mastocytosis. Note spindled morphology of some mast cells. (immunoperoxidase for CD117)*

i14.115 *This composite illustrates the morphological and immunohisto-chemical features of a target lesion in systemic mastocytosis. Morphologic features include a central core of lymphocytes* **a**, *while the mast cells surrounding the lymphocyte aggregate are positive for tryptase* **b**, *CD25* **c**, *and CD117* **d**. *(H&E and immunoperoxidase for tryptase, CD25, and CD117)*

moderate amounts of clear or eosinophilic cytoplasm i14.112, i14.113. The granules are often inconspicuous, as are mitotic figures. Immunohistochemical stains for CD117 and tryptase highlight the often subtle mast cell infiltrates i14.114. Tryptase is reportedly more specific but has been reported to be positive in basophils and some blast cells; therefore, use of CD34 for blasts and 2D7 or BB1 for basophils may be indicated [Samorapoomipichit 2001]. Expression of either CD25 or CD2 on mast cells is considered aberrant; CD25 coexpression is more frequent i14.115 [Hahn 2007, Horny 2008, Sotlar 2004].

Circulating mast cells are typical of mast cell leukemia i14.116. In mast cell leukemia, the bone marrow aspirates or core biopsy sections may show large numbers of mast cells, which are highlighted by toluidine blue staining i14.117, i14.118. The bone marrow biopsy is 100% cellular with sheets of mast cells i14.119. Tryptase immunohistochemistry reveals

i14.116 *This peripheral blood smear shows mast cell leukemia with striking leukocytosis. (Wright)*

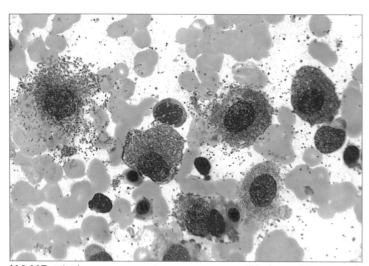

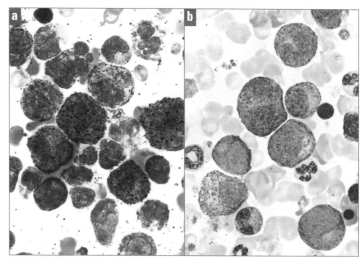

i14.117 *This bone marrow aspirate smear in mast cell leukemia. Note normal morphologic features of these leukemic mast cells. (Wright)*

i14.118 *This composite highlights the cytologic features of mast cell leukemia* **a** *as well as the toluidine blue positivity* **b** *from a patient with mast cell leukemia. (Wright and toluidine blue) (courtesy R McKenna, MD)*

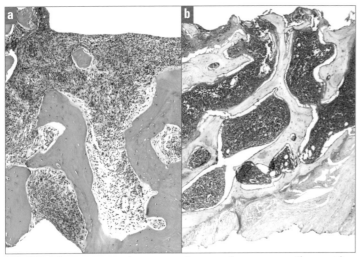

i14.119 *This composite is from a case of extensive bone marrow effacement by mast cell leukemia with associated marked osteosclerosis. (H&E and immunoperoxidase for tryptase)*

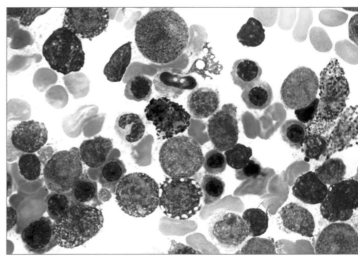

i14.120 *Concurrent systemic mastocytosis and acute erythroid leukemia is evident on this bone marrow aspirate smear. Note abundant abnormal mast cells, erythroblasts, and myeloblasts. (Wright)*

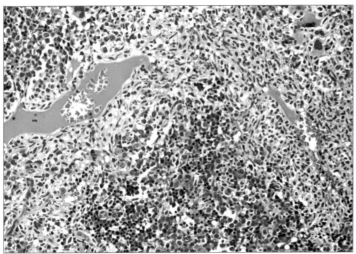

i14.121 *On this bone marrow core biopsy section, there is a distinct zoning of the abnormal mast cell infiltrates surrounding blood vessels and the dark blue areas, which are comprised of erythroblasts and myeloblasts, of this case of concurrent systemic mastocytosis and acute erythroid leukemia. (H&E)*

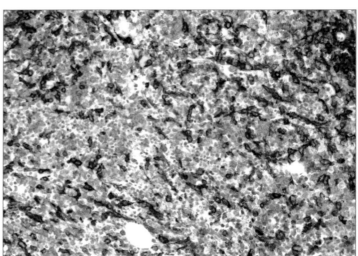

i14.122 *Numerous strongly CD117 positive spindled mast cells are evident on this bone marrow core biopsy section in conjunction with more weakly CD117 positive erythroblasts and myeloblasts in concurrent systemic mastocytosis and acute erythroid leukemia. (immunoperoxidase for CD117)*

the numerous atypical mast cells **i14.119**. In cases of prolonged disease, the bone marrow lesions may take on a "burned out" appearance, in which the entire lesion becomes sclerotic and mast cells virtually absent.

In some cases of systemic mastocytosis, an associated clonal hematopoietic non-mast-cell lineage disease (AHNMD) may be present. Thus, it is critical to assess the background marrow constituents carefully in all cases that would otherwise be diagnosed as SM. AHNMD may range most commonly from another myeloproliferative neoplasm or acute myeloid leukemia to less common lymphoid or plasma cell disorders. In such instances, the morphologic features typical of these associated neoplasms are evident simultaneously with the mastocytosis **i14.120, i14.121, i14.122, i14.123, i14.124**. In some instances of SM, increased granulocytic and

megakaryocytic lineages suggest a concurrent AHNMD, but clear-cut features of an MPN are not present. Clinical follow-up and/or assessment for a genetic aberration that would be diagnostic of MPN (*JAK2, BCR-ABL1*) is warranted.

In some cases of SM with AHNMD, the underlying mastocytosis is initially missed as it is obscured by a dominant bone marrow infiltrative disorder **i14.125**. This so-called "occult" SM is identified after treatment for the initial lesion reveals the classic underlying focal, compact/dense aggregates of mastocytosis **i14.126**. The disease is appropriately termed SM-AHNMD and has been most often seen in AML with t(8;21); a clonal relationship between the 2 neoplasms suggests a common neoplastic progenitor cell [Bernd 2004, Nagai 2007, Pullarkat 2007, 2009].

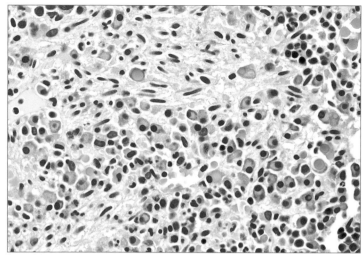

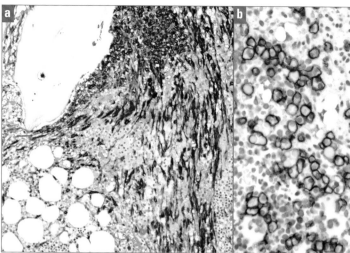

i14.123 *Concurrent spindled systemic mastocytosis is evident in conjunction with myeloma in this bone marrow core biopsy section (H&E) (courtesy C Ross, MD)*

i14.124 *This immunohistochemical composite of systemic mastocytosis with concurrent myeloma shows the striking paratrabecular tryptase positive mast cell infiltrates* **a**, *while the myeloma cells are highlighted by CD138* **b**. *(immunoperoxidase for tryptase and CD138) (courtesy C Ross, MD)*

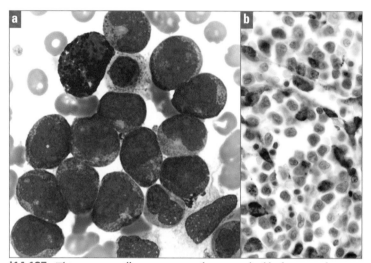

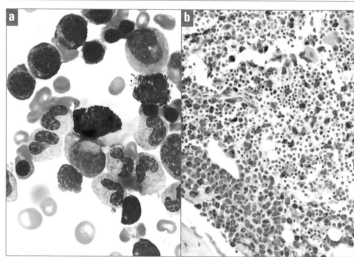

i14.125 *This composite illustrates a case of acute myeloid leukemia with t(8;21) with an associated but occult systemic mastocytosis, which is highlighted by tryptase staining* **b**. *(Wright and immunoperoxidase for tryptase)*

i14.126 *Following AML therapy, the acute myeloid leukemia with t(8;21) was in morphologic remission* **a**, *while concurrently the proportion of mast cells increased tremendously* **b**. *(Wright and immunoperoxidase for tryptase)*

It is now well known that mastocytosis is almost always accompanied by an underlying D816V activating mutation in the *KIT* gene (rare variant mutations reported) [Bodemer 2010]. Not only does this mutation meet one of the minor diagnostic criteria **t14.32**, it also indicates a general resistance to treatment by the tyrosine kinase inhibitor imatinib mesylate. Rare cases of familial *KIT* mutations are reported.

Survival in mastocytosis is highly variable and depends mainly on the disease subtype [Valent 2003]. Indolent SM shows a near-normal life expectancy, while mast cell leukemia is highly aggressive [Horny 2008, Pardanani 2010]. In SM-AHNMD, the prognosis is generally driven by the type of associated hematologic malignancy [Horny 2004, Pardanani 2009]. Other poor prognostic factors identified in mastocytosis include advanced age, weight loss, anemia, and thrombocytopenia [Lim 2009].

The differential diagnosis of mastocytosis is broad and includes mast cell hyperplasia, cells with "clear" morphology, focal bone marrow lesions with a polymorphous cellular infiltrate and/or fibrosis, metastatic disease, and disorders of bone. For the most part, careful morphologic review and/ or generous use of immunohistochemistry will reveal the nature of the bone marrow pathology. Recognition that SM can coexist with another potentially much more overt lesion should be remembered. In addition, the diagnostician must be aware that most cases of SM are diagnosed initially in bone marrow; therefore, a high index of suspicion and generous use of immunohistochemistry is essential.

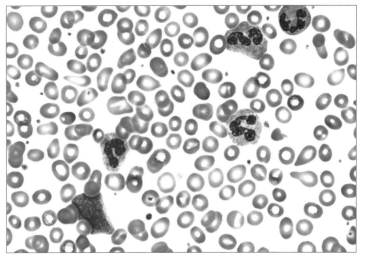

i14.127 *This peripheral blood smear is from a child with longstanding blood abnormalities thought to have a familial myeloproliferative neoplasm. JAK2 testing and conventional cytogenetics were normal. The peripheral blood shows rare circulating blasts, leukocytosis, and thrombocytosis. (Wright)*

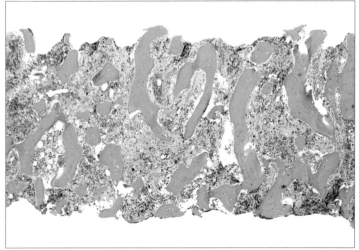

i14.128 *This bone marrow core biopsy section from a child with longstanding hematologic abnormalities suggestive of a familial myeloproliferative neoplasm shows osteosclerosis and marked myelofibrosis. (H&E)*

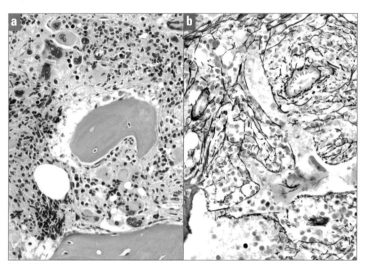

i14.129 *This high-magnification composite of a child with a possible familial myeloproliferative neoplasm shows increased and atypical megakaryocytes **a** in conjunction with marked myelofibrosis **b**. (H&E and reticulin)*

t14.33 Familial MPNs: ET, PV, PMF

Definition: 2 relatives in the same pedigree have the same MPN; ET, PV, or PMF

Major distinction from acquired MPN is that the genetic defect is constitutional

Familial MPN is distinct from familial erythrocytosis and/or thrombocytosis for at least 3 reasons: multilineage myeloproliferation, monoclonal hematopoiesis, and complex inheritance patterns

There is a genetic predisposition to acquiring the *JAK2* mutation

The *JAK2* V617F mutation rates in familial PV (55%-78%), ET (50%-69%), and PMF (75%-90%) differ from sporadic MPN

The clinical and hematologic features appear to be similar to sporadic MPN

Prevalence is at least 7% of all MPNs

ET= essential thrombocythemia; MPN = myeloproliferative neoplasm; PMF = primary myelofibrosis; PV = polycythemia vera

References: [Bellanne-Chantelot 2006, Cario 2005, Percy 2009, Rumi 2006, 2008]

[14.6] Familial MPNs

Familial MPNs have been described and require distinction from familial erythrocytosis and/or thrombocytosis that often arise from a constitutional single genetic defect [Percy 2009]. The general features of familial MPNs are listed in t14.33 [Landgren 2008, Skoda 2005, Rumi 2008, Teofili 2007a]. Familial MPN shows similar hematologic and bone marrow morphology to sporadic MPN. The peripheral blood shows variable cytoses, basophilia, leukoerythroblastosis, and atypical platelets i14.127. The core biopsy features are heterogeneous with abnormal megakaryocyte morphology, clustering, variably patchy residual hematopoiesis, and frequent fibrosis and osteosclerosis i14.128, i14.129.

[14.7] Leukemic Transformation of MPNs

The morphologic transformation of MPNs to myelofibrosis and/or acute leukemia is well known. Fibrotic transformations (so-called "spent phase of PV," fibrotic phase of PMF, and fibrotic accelerated phase in CML) are discussed in the individual disease sections.

In addition to bone marrow fibrosis and relentless enlarging organomegaly, leukemic transformation occurs in a subset of MPNs [Bacher 2007, Beer 2009a, Chim 2005, Ding 2009b, Finazzi 2005, Gangat 2007b, Hultdin 2007, Mesa 2005, Tam 2008, Yin 2006]. While less common in the *BCR-ABL1–* MPNs, blastic transformation is associated with a poor prognosis [Bacher 2007]. The mechanism of leukemic transformation may be the result of the natural disease course or prior treatment with certain chemotherapeutic agents (eg, alkylating agents, hydroxycarbamide, radioactive phosphorus, etc.) [Beer 2009a, Chim 2005, Ding 2009b, Finazzi 2005, Gangat 2007b,

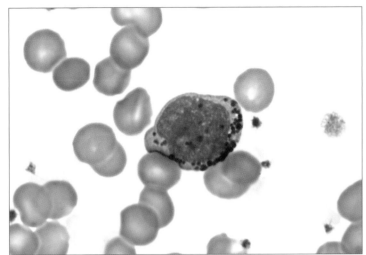

i14.130 *This peripheral blood smear is from a 79-year-old male who developed acute myeloid leukemia following hydroxyurea therapy for a myeloproliferative neoplasm. Note the immature basophil precursor in conjunction with profound anemia, while platelets are increased. (Wright)*

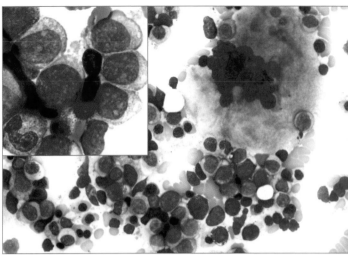

i14.131 *This bone marrow aspirate smear composite is from a patient who developed likely therapy-related acute myeloid leukemia following chemotherapy for a myeloproliferative neoplasm. Note markedly hyperlobated megakaryocyte in conjunction with markedly increased myeloblasts. (Wright)*

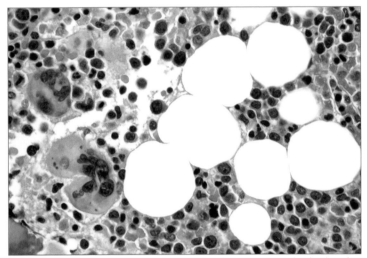

i14.132 *This bone marrow core biopsy section from a patient who developed acute myeloid leukemia following treatment for a myeloproliferative neoplasm shows persistent increased and hyperlobated megakaryocytes in conjunction with markedly increased myeloblasts. (H&E)*

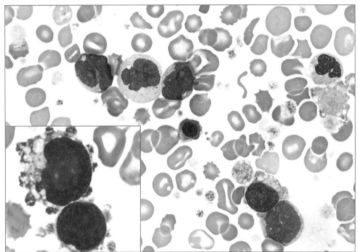

i14.133 *This peripheral blood smear composite is from a patient who developed a myeloid neoplasm following long-term chemotherapy for polycythemia vera. Note the tremendous immature megakaryocytic component to the myeloid neoplasm. (Wright)*

Mesa 2005, Tam 2008]. In some cases, the acquisition of a *RUNX1* mutation may promote leukemic transformation [Ding 2009b].

The non-CML MPN-acute leukemia transformations are most often of myeloid origin; very rare cases of lymphoblastic leukemia are described [Camos 1999, Woronzoff-Dashkoff 1996]. The peripheral blood findings often show progressive/worsening cytopenias with an increasing blast count and possible dysplasia **i14.130**. The bone marrow/peripheral blood shows ≥20% blasts. Those leukemias related to prior therapy exhibit multilineage dysplasia and often have complex cytogenetic abnormalities, including abnormalities of chromosomes 5 and 7. Megakaryocyte features of the primary MPN may persist **i14.131, i14.132**. A megakaryocytic component in acute leukemia transformation may be seen **i14.133**. Leukemic

blasts in transformed *JAK2* V617F+ MPN are often *JAK2* V617F– [Theocharides 2007].

[14.8] **Differential Diagnosis**

Many neoplastic and non-neoplastic disorders show morphologic features that may overlap with MPN. Although the differential diagnostic considerations for each of the myeloproliferative neoplasms have been discussed in the individual disease sections, an attempt to broadly categorize some of these considerations is presented in **t14.34**. This table is by no means all-inclusive, and the reader is also referred to the individual disease sections for further discussion. In general, the myeloid neoplasms that exhibit the greatest

t14.34 Differential Diagnosis of MPNs

Entity	Comments
Cytosis(es) with hypercellular bone marrow and blasts <20%	
Colony-stimulating factor effect	(see Chapter 10)
Paraneoplastic, cytokine-mediated phenomenon due to underlying neoplasm	Manifests as neutrophilia
Severe infection or inflammatory condition	History
Low blast count AML	Detection of inv(16), t(8;21), or t(15;17) (see Chapter 18)
MDS/MPN	Usually cytopenias, myelodysplastic features, and/or monocytosis (see Chapter 17)
Viral infection	Examples include EBV, CMV
Variably cellular BM with minimal/mild fibrosis, abnormal megakaryocytes, and blasts <20%	
Regenerative BM after toxic chemo-therapy, radiation, or other insult	History
Gray platelet syndrome	Thrombocytopenia
Autoimmune myelofibrosis	Usually peripheral cytopenias, history of autoimmunity
Valproic acid	History of drug ingestion
Human immunodeficiency virus-1	(see Chapter 33)
Immune thrombocytopenia (ITP)	(see Chapter 12)
MDS with fibrosis	Myelodysplastic features
Focal or diffuse fibrotic lesions in BM possibly with abnormal/ entrapped megakaryocytes (see t14.22)	
Osteosclerosis (see t14.23)	

AML = acute myeloid leukemia; BM = bone marrow; CMV = cytomegalovirus; EBV = Epstein-Barr virus; MDS = myelodysplastic syndrome; MPN = myeloproliferative neoplasm

References: [Moritake 2009, Oluwole 2009, Pich 2009, Pullarkat 2003, Sakka 2006]

overlap with MPN are the MDS/MPNs i14.134, i14.135. Key features useful in distinguishing MPN from MDS/MPN are the cytopenia(s), dysplasia, variably increased blasts, and small dysplastic megakaryocytes characteristic of MDS/ MPN. Collagen vascular disorders can also closely mimic MPN (as detailed in [14.5] "Classification," p 272) i14.136. Finally, anaplastic lymphoma cells can mimic the atypical enlarged megakaryocytes of MPN i14.137. Recognition of these and other diagnostic pitfalls is essential as is integration of all available clinical, hematologic, immunophenotypic, and genetic data.

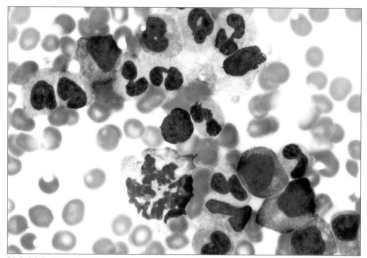

i14.134 *This bone marrow aspirate smear is from a patient with neutrophilia, basophilia, and mild monocytosis in the peripheral blood with associated thrombocytopenia. This bone marrow aspirate smear shows increased and dysplastic neutrophils with a slight increase in myeloblasts compatible with a myelodysplastic/myeloproliferative neoplasm. (Wright) (courtesy C Sever, MD)*

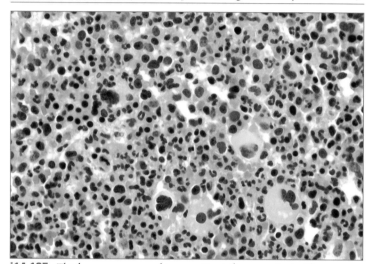

i14.135 *This bone marrow core biopsy section is from a patient with a myelodysplastic/myeloproliferative neoplasm. Note hypercellularity in conjunction with increased megakaryocytes,s which show nuclear hypolobation more characteristic of a myelodysplastic than a myeloproliferative process. (H&E) (courtesy C Sever, MD)*

[14.9] Components of the Diagnostic Interpretation of MPNs

Key to the work-up and diagnosis of a myeloproliferative neoplasm is the integration of morphologic features with clinical, hematologic, and genetic data. This is a systematic process that methodically excludes known non-neoplastic and neoplastic mimickers and subclassifies the MPN as is feasible t14.35. Often the accompanying clinical information is not available; however, such data should be subsequently incorporated into the individual case rather than rendering a less specific or "unclassifiable" MPN diagnosis. As needed, specific clinical, laboratory and/or genetic testing should be suggested in the final bone marrow report.

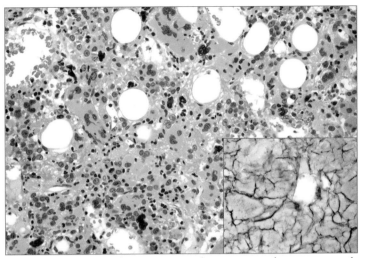

i14.136 *This composite bone marrow core biopsy section is from a patient with severe rheumatoid arthritis who developed a myeloproliferative-appearing bone marrow picture characterized by hypercellularity, increased megakaryocytes, and reticulin fibrosis (inset). (H&E and reticulin) (courtesy C Sever, MD)*

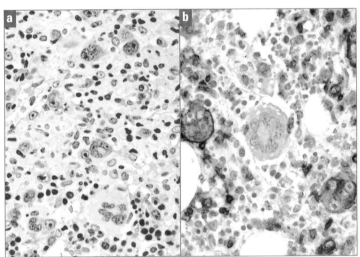

i14.137 *This composite from a patient with bone marrow involvement by anaplastic large cell lymphoma shows morphologic overlap with primary myelofibrosis. Note the enlarged and multi-nucleated lymphoma cells that mimic megakaryocytes morphologically **a**, while immunoperoxidase staining for CD30 clearly distinguishes the anaplastic large cell lymphoma cells from the negative megakaryocytes **b**. (H&E and immunoperoxidase for CD30) (courtesy R Macaulay, MD)*

t14.35 Components of the Diagnostic Interpretation

Discriminate benign/reactive disorder from true MPN; provide rationale for diagnosis

In early/prodromal stages of disease, be precise about the diagnosis and adhere to WHO 2008 criteria

Delineate specific subtype of MPN as possible

Integrate genetics as needed (eg, *BCR-ABL1*+, *KIT* D816V mutation positive)

Since MPN, unclassifiable, is a diagnosis of exclusion, provide a list of needed additional tests/data that would potentially resolve diagnostic uncertainty

MPN = myeloproliferative neoplasm

[14.10] Clues and Caveats

1. A systematic approach is essential in the successful diagnosis of myeloproliferative neoplasms, with integration of clinical, hematologic, morphologic, and genetic information.

2. Myeloproliferative neoplasms are characterized by autonomous proliferation of 1 or more hematopoietic lineages, with intact maturation and increased cell counts in the blood (ie, effective hematopoiesis) showing a predominance of mature cells.

3. In addition to elevated cell count(s), other blood clues to a myeloproliferative neoplasm include basophilia, leukoerythroblastic features, and circulating megakaryocytes.

4. Megakaryocyte morphology is key in the subclassification of myeloproliferative neoplasms:

   a. Small, uniform hypolobated megakaryocytes are typical for chronic myelogenous leukemia.

   b. Markedly enlarged, uniformly hyperlobated megakaryocytes typify essential thrombocythemia.

   c. Highly pleomorphic megakaryocytes with variably dark, bulbous nuclei are characteristic of primary myelofibrosis.

5. Genetic assessment is essential in all myeloproliferative neoplasms:

   a. *BCR-ABL1* defines chronic myelogenous leukemia.

   b. *JAK2* mutations are common in polycythemia vera, essential thrombocythemia, and primary myelofibrosis, but are especially frequent in polycythemia vera.

   c. *KIT* mutations are recurrent in systemic mastocytosis.

   d. Other cytogenetic abnormalities can be used to exclude non-neoplastic disorders or to confirm transformation of an established myeloproliferative neoplasm.

6. Utility of flow cytometric immunophenotyping is limited in the diagnosis of myeloproliferative neoplasms, but is useful in blast transformation.

7. Idiopathic cytosis of uncertain significance should be applied to cases that do not fulfill criteria for myeloproliferative neoplasms in which non-neoplastic causes have been reasonably excluded.

8. Of all the myeloproliferative neoplasms, only the natural history of chronic myelogenous leukemia is characterized by predictable clonal evolution to first accelerated then blast phase.

9. Imatinib therapy, although not curative, greatly reduces the incidence of transformation in chronic myelogenous leukemia.

10. Any hematolymphoid lineage can comprise the blast phase of chronic myelogenous leukemia; myeloid blast phase predominates.

11. The "neutrophilic" variant of chronic myelogenous leukemia is characterized by p230 BCR-ABL1 fusion product, marked neutrophilia with very limited left shift, and enlarged megakaryocytes closely mimicking chronic neutrophilic leukemia.

12. Criteria for the diagnosis of non-chronic myelogenous leukemia myeloproliferative neoplasms are complex, encompassing clinical, hematologic, laboratory, and genetic parameters.

13. Myeloproliferative neoplasms such as chronic eosinophilic leukemia, not otherwise specified, and chronic neutrophilic leukemia are diagnoses of exclusion.

14. Eosinophil dysplasia is not useful in distinguishing a primary from a secondary eosinophilia.

15. Clonal eosinophilias driven by *PDGFRA*, *PDGFRB*, and *FGFR1* mutations are excluded from chronic eosinophilic leukemia, not otherwise specified.

16. Concurrent iron deficiency can confound the classic hematologic profile of polycythemia vera.

17. Polycythemia vera can transform to a post-polycythemic myelofibrotic (so-called "spent") phase, which can be indistinguishable from advanced primary myelofibrosis.

18. The bone marrow in essential thrombocythemia can be normocellular, while hypercellularity characterizes all other myeloproliferative neoplasms, including chronic myelogenous leukemia.

19. Cellular phase primary myelofibrosis can be associated with marked thrombocytosis; these cases may be indistinguishable from essential thrombocythemia.

20. Similar to the clinically occult causes of physiologically inappropriate secondary erythrocytosis, the causes of sustained secondary eosinophilias may be obscure.

21. Osteosclerosis may be evident in cellular-phase primary myelofibrosis and is also common in post-polycythemic myelofibrosis and in systemic mastocytosis.

22. Dilated sinuses with prominent intrasinusoidal hematopoiesis are most prominent in primary myelofibrosis.

23. Myeloma can be associated with a blood and bone marrow picture indistinguishable from chronic neutrophilic leukemia.

24. The associated clonal hematopoietic disorder in cases of systemic mastocytosis can obscure the occult mast cell infiltrates. This is especially true when the associated hematolymphoid neoplasm is acute myeloid leukemia.

25. Even without a confounding associated hematolymphoid disorder, bone marrow lesions in systemic mastocytosis may be subtle and are easily overlooked, especially since systemic mastocytosis is often initially diagnosed in bone marrow.

[14.11] Acknowledgments

The authors acknowledge the photographic contributions of D Canioni, MD, M Irani, MD, J Jones, MD, R Macaulay, MD, I Maric, MD, R McKenna, MD, J Mo, MD, B Nelson, MD, C Ross, MD, J Said, MD, C Sever, MD, D Williams, MD, W Williams, MD, and C Wilson, MD.

[14.12] References

Abdel-Wahab OI, Levine RL [2009] Primary myelofibrosis: update on definition, pathogenesis, and treatment. *Annu Rev Med* 60:233-245.

Aboudola S, Murugesan G, Szpurka H, et al [2007] Bone marrow phospho-STAT5 expression in non-CML chronic myeloproliferative disorders correlates with *JAK2* V617F mutation and provides evidence of in vivo *JAK2* activation. *Am J Surg Pathol* 31:233-239.

Agis H, Fureder W, Bankl HC, et al [1996] Comparative immunophenotypic analysis of human mast cells, blood basophils and monocytes. *Immunology* 87:535-543.

Agis H, Krauth MT, Bohm A, et al [2006] Identification of basogranulin (BB1) as a novel immunohistochemical marker of basophils in normal bone marrow and patients with myeloproliferative disorders. *Am J Clin Pathol* 125:273-281.

Ahmed A, Chang CC [2006] Chronic idiopathic myelofibrosis: clinico-pathologic features, pathogenesis, and prognosis. *Arch Pathol Lab Med* 130:1133-1143.

Akin C [2006] Molecular diagnosis of mast cell disorders: a paper from the 2005 William Beaumont Hospital Symposium on Molecular Pathology. *J Mol Diagn* 8:412-419.

Altura RA, Head DR, Wang WC [2000] Long-term survival of infants with idiopathic myelofibrosis. *Br J Haematol* 109:459-462.

Alvarez-Larran A, Bellosillo B, Martinez-Aviles L, et al [2009] Postpolycythaemic myelofibrosis: frequency and risk factors for this complication in 116 patients. *Br J Haematol* 146:504-509.

Amato D, Memon S, Wang C [2008] Myeloblastic transformation of chronic neutrophilic leukaemia. *Br J Haematol* 142:148.

Anand M, Kumar R, Singh S [2004] Megakaryoblastic lineage of peripheral blood blasts of CML blast crisis identified by budding dysplastic platelets. *Am J Hematol* 75:239-240.

Anastasi J, Musvee T, Roulston D, et al [1998] Pseudo-Gaucher histiocytes identified up to 1 year after transplantation for CML are BCR/ABL-positive. *Leukemia* 12:233-237.

Baccarani M, Cortes J, Pane F, et al [2009] Chronic myeloid leukemia: an update of concepts and management recommendations of European LeukemiaNet. *J Clin Oncol* 27:6041-6051.

Bacher U, Haferlach T, Kern W, et al [2007] A case of chronic myeloproliferative syndrome followed by precursor T-cell acute lymphoblastic leukemia. *Cancer Genet Cytogenet* 175:52-56.

Bain B, Brunning R, Vardiman J, Thiele J [2008a] Chronic neutrophilic leukaemia. In: Swerdlow S, Campo E, Harris N, et al, eds. *WHO Classification of Tumours of Haematopoietic and Lymphoid Tissues.* 4th ed. Lyon, France: IARC Press; 38-39.

Bain B, Gilliland D, Vardiman J, Horney H-P [2008b] Chronic eosinophilic leukaemia, not otherwise specified. In: Swerdlow S, Campo E, Harris N, et al, eds. *WHO Classification of Tumours of Haematopoietic and Lymphoid Tissues.* 4th ed. Lyon, France: IARC Press; 51-53.

Bain BJ [2004] Relationship between idiopathic hypereosinophilic syndrome, eosinophilic leukemia, and systemic mastocytosis. *Am J Hematol* 77:82-85.

Bain BJ, Fletcher SH [2007] Chronic eosinophilic leukemias and the myeloproliferative variant of the hypereosinophilic syndrome. *Immunol Allergy Clin North Am* 27:377-388.

Barbui T, Carobbio A, Rambaldi A, Finazzi G [2009] Perspectives on thrombosis in essential thrombocythemia and polycythemia vera: is leukocytosis a causative factor? *Blood* 114:759-763.

Barbui T, Carobbio A, Cervantes F, et al [2010] Thrombosis in primary myelofibrosis: incidence and risk factors. *Blood* 115:778-782.

Barni S, Mandala M, Cazzaniga M, et al [2006] Bisphosphonates and metastatic bone disease. *Ann Oncol* 17Suppl2:ii91-95.

Barosi G, Bergamaschi G, Marchetti M, et al [2007] JAK2 V617F mutational status predicts progression to large splenomegaly and leukemic transformation in primary myelofibrosis. *Blood* 110:4030-4036.

Bartram CR, de Klein A, Hagemeijer A, et al [1983] Translocation of c-ab1 oncogene correlates with the presence of a Philadelphia chromosome in chronic myelocytic leukaemia. *Nature* 306:277-280.

Basquiera AL, Soria NW, Ryser R, et al [2009] Clinical significance of V617F mutation of the JAK2 gene in patients with chronic myeloproliferative disorders. *Hematology* 14:323-330.

Bass RD, Pullarkat V, Feinstein DI, et al [2001] Pathology of autoimmune myelofibrosis. *Am J Clin Pathol* 116:211-216.

Baxter EJ, Scott LM, Campbell PJ, et al [2005] Acquired mutation of the tyrosine kinase JAK2 in human myeloproliferative disorders. *Lancet* 365:1054-1061.

Beer PA, Delhommeau F, Le Couedic JP, et al [2009a] Two routes to leukemic transformation following a JAK2 mutation-positive myeloproliferative neoplasm. *Blood* epub ahead of print December 11, 2009; DOI 10.1182/blood-2009-08-236596.

Beer PA, Green AR [2009b] Pathogenesis and management of essential thrombocythemia. *Hematology Am Soc Hematol Educ Program* 621-628.

Bellanne-Chantelot C, Chaumarel I, Labopin M, et al [2006] Genetic and clinical implications of the Val617Phe JAK2 mutation in 72 families with myeloproliferative disorders. *Blood* 108:346-352.

Bennett J [1845] Case of hypertrophy of the spleen and liver in which death took place from suppuration of the blood. *Edinburgh Med Surg J* 64:413-423.

Bernd HW, Sotlar K, Lorenzen J, et al [2004] Acute myeloid leukaemia with t(8;21) associated with "occult" mastocytosis. Report of an unusual case and review of the literature. *J Clin Pathol* 57:324-328.

Bizzozero OJ, Jr, Johnson KG, Ciocco A [1966] Radiation-related leukemia in Hiroshima and Nagasaki, 1946-1964. I. Distribution, incidence, and appearance time. *N Engl J Med* 274:1095-1101.

Bock O, Hoftmann J, Theophile K, et al [2008] Bone morphogenetic proteins are overexpressed in the bone marrow of primary myelofibrosis and are apparently induced by fibrogenic cytokines. *Am J Pathol* 172:951-960.

Bock O, Loch G, Schade U, et al [2005] Osteosclerosis in advanced chronic idiopathic myelofibrosis is associated with endothelial overexpression of osteoprotegerin. *Br J Haematol* 130:76-82.

Bock O, Schlue J, Mengel M, et al [2004] Thrombopoietin receptor (Mpl) expression by megakaryocytes in myeloproliferative disorders. *J Pathol* 203:609-615.

Bodemer C, Hermine O, Palmerini F, et al [2010] Pediatric mastocytosis is a clonal disease associated with D(816)V and other activating *c-KIT* mutations. *J Invest Dermatol* 130:804-815.

Bohm J, Schaefer HE [2002] Chronic neutrophilic leukaemia: 14 new cases of an uncommon myeloproliferative disease. *J Clin Pathol* 55:862-864.

Boruchov AM [2009] Thrombocytopenia in myelodysplastic syndromes and myelofibrosis. *Semin Hematol* 46:S37-43.

Boveri E, Passamonti F, Rumi E, et al [2008] Bone marrow microvessel density in chronic myeloproliferative disorders: a study of 115 patients with clinico-pathological and molecular correlations. *Br J Haematol* 140:162-168.

Branford S, Seymour JF, Grigg A, et al [2007] BCR-ABL messenger RNA levels continue to decline in patients with chronic phase chronic myeloid leukemia treated with imatinib for >5 years and approximately half of all first-line treated patients have stable undetectable BCR-ABL using strict sensitivity criteria. *Clin Cancer Res* 13:7080-7085.

Buesche G, Ganser A, Schlegelberger B, et al [2007] Marrow fibrosis and its relevance during imatinib treatment of chronic myeloid leukemia. *Leukemia* 21:2420-2427.

Buesche G, Hehlmann R, Hecker H, et al [2003] Marrow fibrosis, indicator of therapy failure in chronic myeloid leukemia—prospective long-term results from a randomized-controlled trial. *Leukemia* 17:2444-2453.

Buhr T, Busche G, Choritz H, et al [2003] Evolution of myelofibrosis in chronic idiopathic myelofibrosis as evidenced in sequential bone marrow biopsy specimens. *Am J Clin Pathol* 119:152-158.

Buschle M, Janssen JW, Drexler H, et al [1988] Evidence for pluripotent stem cell origin of idiopathic myelofibrosis: clonal analysis of a case characterized by a N-ras gene mutation. *Leukemia* 2:658-660.

Cacace E, Salis G, Ruggiero V, Perpignano G [2006] Systemic mast cell disease: a rare cause of osteoporosis. *Clin Exp Rheumatol* 24:210.

Camos M, Cervantes F, Montoto S, et al [1999] Acute lymphoid leukemia following polycythemia vera. *Leuk Lymphoma* 32:395-398.

Campbell PJ, Bareford D, Erber WN, et al [2009] Reticulin accumulation in essential thrombocythemia: prognostic significance and relationship to therapy. *J Clin Oncol* 27:2991-2999.

Campiotti L, Grandi AM, Biotti MG, et al [2007] Megakaryocytic blast crisis as first presentation of chronic myeloid leukemia. *Am J Hematol* 82:231-233.

Caramazza D, Hussein K, Siragusa S, et al [2010] Chromosome 1 abnormalities in myeloid malignancies: a literature survey and karyotype-phenotype associations. *Eur J Haematol* 84:191-200.

Cario H, Goerttler PS, Steimle C, et al [2005] The JAK2 V617F mutation is acquired secondary to the predisposing alteration in familial polycythaemia vera. *Br J Haematol* 130:800-801.

Cario H, McMullin MF, Pahl HL [2009] Clinical and hematological presentation of children and adolescents with polycythemia vera. *Ann Hematol* 88:713-719.

Carobbio A, Finazzi G, Guerini V, et al [2007] Leukocytosis is a risk factor for thrombosis in essential thrombocythemia: interaction with treatment, standard risk factors, and Jak2 mutation status. *Blood* 109:2310-2313.

Cervantes F, Dupriez B, Pereira A, et al [2009] New prognostic scoring system for primary myelofibrosis based on a study of the International Working Group for Myelofibrosis Research and Treatment. *Blood* 113:2895-2901.

Cervantes F, Passamonti F, Barosi G [2008] Life expectancy and prognostic factors in the classic BCR/ABL-negative myeloproliferative disorders. *Leukemia* 22:905-914.

Chim CS, Kwong YL, Lie AK, et al [2005] Long-term outcome of 231 patients with essential thrombocythemia: prognostic factors for thrombosis, bleeding, myelofibrosis, and leukemia. *Arch Intern Med* 165:2651-2658.

Chung HJ, Chi HS, Cho YU, et al [2008] Promyelocytic blast crisis of chronic myeloid leukemia during imatinib treatment. *Ann Clin Lab Sci* 38:283-286.

Chung HJ, Chi HS, Seo EJ, et al [2006] [Erythroleukemic blast crisis of chronic myeloid leukemia.]. *Korean J Lab Med* 26:255-262.

Corso A, Lazzarino M, Morra E, et al [1995] Chronic myelogenous leukemia and exposure to ionizing radiation—a retrospective study of 443 patients. *Ann Hematol* 70:79-82.

Crivellato E, Ribatti D [2009] The mast cell: an evolutionary perspective. *Biol Rev Camb Philos Soc* epub ahead of print November 24, 2009.

Cross NC, Daley GQ, Green AR, et al [2008] BCR-ABL1-positive CML and BCR-ABL1-negative chronic myeloproliferative disorders: some common and contrasting features. *Leukemia* 22:1975-1989.

Dameshek W [1951] Some speculations on the myeloproliferative syndromes. *Blood* 6:372-375.

De Stefano V, Za T, Rossi E, et al [2008] Recurrent thrombosis in patients with polycythemia vera and essential thrombocythemia: incidence, risk factors, and effect of treatments. *Haematologica* 93:372-380.

Delhommeau F, Dupont S, Della Valle V, et al [2009] Mutation in TET2 in myeloid cancers. *N Engl J Med* 360:2289-2301.

Delhommeau F, Dupont S, Tonetti C, et al [2007] Evidence that the *JAK2* G1849T (V617F) mutation occurs in a lymphomyeloid progenitor in polycythemia vera and idiopathic myelofibrosis. *Blood* 109:71-77.

Diamond T, Depczynski B [1996] Acquired osteosclerosis associated with intravenous drug use and hepatitis C infection. *Bone* 19:679-683.

Diez-Martin JL, Graham DL, Petitt RM, Dewald GW [1991] Chromosome studies in 104 patients with polycythemia vera. *Mayo Clin Proc* 66:287-299.

Dincol G, Nalcaci M, Dogan O, et al [2002] Coexistence of chronic neutrophilic leukemia with multiple myeloma. *Leuk Lymphoma* 43:649-651.

Ding J, Komatsu H, Iida S, et al [2009a] The Asn505 mutation of the *c-MPL* gene, which causes familial essential thrombocythemia, induces autonomous homodimerization of the c-Mpl protein due to strong amino acid polarity. *Blood* 114:3325-3328.

Ding J, Komatsu H, Wakita A, et al [2004] Familial essential thrombocythemia associated with a dominant-positive activating mutation of the *c-MPL* gene, which encodes for the receptor for thrombopoietin. *Blood* 103:4198-4200.

Ding Y, Harada Y, Imagawa J, et al [2009b] AML1/RUNX1 point mutation possibly promotes leukemic transformation in myeloproliferative neoplasms. *Blood* 114:5201-5205.

Dobson JT, Seibert J, Teh EM, et al [2008] Carboxypeptidase A5 identifies a novel mast cell lineage in the zebrafish providing new insight into mast cell fate determination. *Blood* 112:2969-2972.

Dorfman DM, Longtine JA, Fox EA, et al [1997] T-cell blast crisis in chronic myelogenous leukemia. Immunophenotypic and molecular biologic findings. *Am J Clin Pathol* 107:168-176.

Druker BJ, Guilhot F, O'Brien SG, et al [2006] Five-year follow-up of patients receiving imatinib for chronic myeloid leukemia. *N Engl J Med* 355:2408-2417.

Druker BJ, Tamura S, Buchdunger E, et al [1996] Effects of a selective inhibitor of the Abl tyrosine kinase on the growth of Bcr-Abl positive cells. *Nat Med* 2:561-566.

Elliott MA, Hanson CA, Dewald GW, et al [2005] WHO-defined chronic neutrophilic leukemia: a long-term analysis of 12 cases and a critical review of the literature. *Leukemia* 19:313-317.

Feng B, Verstovsek S, Jorgensen JL, Lin P [2010] Aberrant myeloid maturation identified by flow cytometry in primary myelofibrosis. *Am J Clin Pathol* 133:314-320.

Finazzi G, Caruso V, Marchioli R, et al [2005] Acute leukemia in polycythemia vera: an analysis of 1638 patients enrolled in a prospective observational study. *Blood* 105:2664-2670.

Fletcher S, Bain B [2007] Diagnosis and treatment of hypereosinophilic syndromes. *Curr Opin Hematol* 14:37-42.

Florena AM, Tripodo C, Di Bernardo A, et al [2009] Different immunophenotypical apoptotic profiles characterise megakaryocytes of essential thrombocythaemia and primary myelofibrosis. *J Clin Pathol* 62:331-338.

Frater JL, Tallman MS, Variakojis D, et al [2003] Chronic myeloid leukemia following therapy with imatinib mesylate (Gleevec). Bone marrow histopathology and correlation with genetic status. *Am J Clin Pathol* 119:833-841.

Galli SJ, Kalesnikoff J, Grimbaldeston MA, et al [2005] Mast cells as "tunable" effector and immunoregulatory cells: recent advances. *Annu Rev Immunol* 23:749-786.

Gangat N, Strand J, Lasho TL, et al [2008] Cytogenetic studies at diagnosis in polycythemia vera: clinical and *JAK2* V617F allele burden correlates. *Eur J Haematol* 80:197-200.

Gangat N, Strand J, Li CY, et al [2007a] Leucocytosis in polycythaemia vera predicts both inferior survival and leukaemic transformation. *Br J Haematol* 138:354-358.

Gangat N, Tefferi A, Thanarajasingam G, et al [2009] Cytogenetic abnormalities in essential thrombocythemia: prevalence and prognostic significance. *Eur J Haematol* 83:17-21.

Gangat N, Wolanskyj AP, McClure RF, et al [2007b] Risk stratification for survival and leukemic transformation in essential thrombocythemia: a single institutional study of 605 patients. *Leukemia* 21:270-276.

Ganly P, Hanrahan V, Baker B, Romeril K [2007] Identification of *JAK2* V617F in patients with polycythemia is highly correlated with conventional criteria for diagnosis of polycythemia vera. *Am J Hematol* 82:80-82.

Gianelli U, Iurlo A, Vener C, et al [2008] The significance of bone marrow biopsy and *JAK2* V617F mutation in the differential diagnosis between the "early" prepolycythemic phase of polycythemia vera and essential thrombocythemia. *Am J Clin Pathol* 130:336-342.

Gianelli U, Vener C, Raviele PR, et al [2007] VEGF expression correlates with microvessel density in Philadelphia chromosome-negative chronic myeloproliferative disorders. *Am J Clin Pathol* 128:966-973.

Gibson SE, Schade AE, Szpurka H, et al [2008] Phospho-STAT5 expression pattern with the MPL W515L mutation is similar to that seen in chronic myeloproliferative disorders with *JAK2* V617F. *Hum Pathol* 39:1111-1114.

Girodon F, Bonicelli G, Schaeffer C, et al [2009] Significant increase in the apparent incidence of essential thrombocythemia related to new WHO diagnostic criteria: a population-based study. *Haematologica* 94:865-869.

Gleich GJ, Leiferman KM [2009] The hypereosinophilic syndromes: current concepts and treatments. *Br J Haematol* 145:271-285.

Gotlib J [2009] On being metachromatic: mystique and misunderstanding in mastocytosis. *Am J Hematol* 84:779-781.

Gotlib J [2010] Eosinophilic myeloid disorders: new classification and novel therapeutic strategies. *Curr Opin Hematol* 17:117-124.

Grimwade LF, Happerfield L, Tristram C, et al [2009] Phospho-STAT5 and phospho-Akt expression in chronic myeloproliferative neoplasms. *Br J Haematol* 147:495-506.

Gruner BA, DeNapoli TS, Elshihabi S, et al [2003] Anemia and hepatosplenomegaly as presenting features in a child with rickets and secondary myelofibrosis. *J Pediatr Hematol Oncol* 25:813-815.

Guglielmelli P, Barosi G, Specchia G, et al [2009] Identification of patients with poorer survival in primary myelofibrosis based on the burden of *JAK2* V617F mutated allele. *Blood* 114:1477-1483.

Haas B [2009] Autoimmune thyroiditis associated with marrow fibrosis and pancytopenia. *Leuk Lymphoma* 50:2086-2088.

Haferlach T, Bacher U, Kern W, et al [2008] The diagnosis of BCR/ABL-negative chronic myeloproliferative diseases (CMPD): a comprehensive approach based on morphology, cytogenetics, and molecular markers. *Ann Hematol* 87:1-10.

Hahn HP, Hornick JL [2007] Immunoreactivity for CD25 in gastrointestinal mucosal mast cells is specific for systemic mastocytosis. *Am J Surg Pathol* 31:1669-1676.

Hallanger Johnson JE, Kearns AE, Doran PM, et al [2007] Fluoride-related bone disease associated with habitual tea consumption. *Mayo Clin Proc* 82:719-724.

Hasserjian RP, Boecklin F, Parker S, et al [2002] ST1571 (imatinib mesylate) reduces bone marrow cellularity and normalizes morphologic features irrespective of cytogenetic response. *Am J Clin Pathol* 117:360-367.

Helbig G, Wieczorkiewicz A, Dziaczkowska-Suszek J, et al [2009] T-cell abnormalities are present at high frequencies in patients with hypereosinophilic syndrome. *Haematologica* 94:1236-1241.

Higgs JR, Sadek I, Neumann PE, et al [2008] Familial essential thrombocythemia with spontaneous megakaryocyte colony formation and acquired *JAK2* mutations. *Leukemia* 22:1551-1556.

Hochhaus A, O'Brien SG, Guilhot F, et al [2009] Six-year follow-up of patients receiving imatinib for the first-line treatment of chronic myeloid leukemia. *Leukemia* 23:1054-1061.

Horny HP [2009] Mastocytosis: an unusual clonal disorder of bone marrow-derived hematopoietic progenitor cells. *Am J Clin Pathol* 132:438-447.

Horny HP, Metcalfe D, Bennett J, et al [2008] Mastocytosis. In: Swerdlow S, Campo E, Harris N, et al, eds. *WHO Classification of Tumours of Haematopoietic and Lymphoid Tissues.* 4th ed. Lyon, France: IARC Press; 54-63.

Horny HP, Sotlar K, Sperr WR, Valent P [2004] Systemic mastocytosis with associated clonal haematological non-mast cell lineage diseases: a histopathological challenge. *J Clin Pathol* 57:604-608.

Huang Q, Wu Y, Snyder DS, et al [2007] Clinical and pathologic analysis of 16 cases of relapsed chronic myeloid leukemia after stem cell transplantation. *Am J Clin Pathol* 128:565-570.

Hultdin M, Sundstrom G, Wahlin A, et al [2007] Progression of bone marrow fibrosis in patients with essential thrombocythemia and polycythemia vera during anagrelide treatment. *Med Oncol* 24:63-70.

Hussein K, Bock O, Theophile K, et al [2009a] *JAK2* V617F) allele burden discriminates essential thrombocythemia from a subset of prefibrotic-stage primary myelofibrosis. *Exp Hematol* 37:1186-1193 e1187.

Hussein K, Huang J, Lasho T, et al [2009b] Karyotype complements the International Prognostic Scoring System for primary myelofibrosis. *Eur J Haematol* 82:255-259.

Hussein K, Van Dyke DL, Tefferi A [2009c] Conventional cytogenetics in myelofibrosis: literature review and discussion. *Eur J Haematol* 82:329-338.

Hussein K, Pandanani AD, Van Dyke DL, et al [2010] International Prognostic Scoring System—independent cytogenetic risk categorization in primary myelofibrosis. *Blood* 115:496-499.

Irvine DA, Heaney NB, Holyoake TL [2010] Optomising chronic myeloid leukaemia therapy in the face of resistance to tyrosine-kinase inhibitors—a synthesis of clinical and laboratory data. *Blood Rev* 24:1-9.

Ishii T, Wang J, Zhang W, et al [2009] Pivotal role of mast cells in pruritogenesis in patients with myeloproliferative disorders. *Blood* 113:5942-5950.

James C, Ugo V, Le Couedic JP, et al [2005] A unique clonal *JAK2* mutation leading to constitutive signalling causes polycythaemia vera. *Nature* 434:1144-1148.

Johansson P [2006] Epidemiology of the myeloproliferative disorders polycythemia vera and essential thrombocythemia. *Semin Thromb Hemost* 32:171-173.

Kako S, Kanda Y, Sato T, et al [2007] Early relapse of *JAK2* V617F-positive chronic neutrophilic leukemia with central nervous system infiltration after unrelated bone marrow transplantation. *Am J Hematol* 82:386-390.

Khalidi HS, Brynes RK, Medeiros LJ, et al [1998] The immunophenotype of blast transformation of chronic myelogenous leukemia: a high frequency of mixed lineage phenotype in "lymphoid" blasts and a comparison of morphologic, immunophenotypic, and molecular findings. *Mod Pathol* 11:1211-1221.

Kim AS, Goldstein SC, Luger S, et al [2008a] Sudden extramedullary T-lymphoblastic blast crisis in chronic myelogenous leukemia: a nonrandom event associated with imatinib? *Am J Clin Pathol* 129:639-648.

Kim M, Lee S, Jung CK, et al [2008b] Transient trisomy 8 abnormality in Philadelphia-negative cells during imatinib mesylate treatment of chronic myelogenous leukemia. *Int J Lab Hematol* 30:508-512.

Kirsch R, Geboes K, Shepherd NA, et al [2008] Systemic mastocytosis involving the gastrointestinal tract: clinicopathologic and molecular study of 5 cases. *Mod Pathol* 21:1508-1516.

Kneilling M, Rocken M [2009] Mast cells: novel clinical perspectives from recent insights. *Exp Dermatol* 18:488-496.

Kobayashi S, Yamashita K, Takeoka T, et al [2002] Calpain-mediated X-linked inhibitor of apoptosis degradation in neutrophil apoptosis and its impairment in chronic neutrophilic leukemia. *J Biol Chem* 277:33968-33977.

Kovanen PT [2009] Mast cells in atherogenesis: actions and reactions. *Curr Atheroscler Rep* 11:214-219.

Kralovics R [2008] Genetic complexity of myeloproliferative neoplasms. *Leukemia* 22:1841-1848.

Kralovics R, Passamonti F, Buser AS, et al [2005] A gain-of-function mutation of *JAK2* in myeloproliferative disorders. *N Engl J Med* 352:1779-1790.

Kralovics R, Stockton DW, Prchal JT [2003] Clonal hematopoiesis in familial polycythemia vera suggests the involvement of multiple mutational events in the early pathogenesis of the disease. *Blood* 102:3793-3796.

Krokowski M, Sotlar K, Krauth MT, et al [2005] Delineation of patterns of bone marrow mast cell infiltration in systemic mastocytosis: value of CD25, correlation with subvariants of the disease, and separation from mast cell hyperplasia. *Am J Clin Pathol* 124:560-568.

Kurosawa H, Okuya M, Matsushita T, et al [2009] *JAK2* V617F mutation-positive childhood essential thrombocythemia associated with cerebral venous sinus thrombosis. *J Pediatr Hematol Oncol* 31:678-680.

Kuter DJ, Bain B, Mufti G, et al [2007] Bone marrow fibrosis: pathophysiology and clinical significance of increased bone marrow stromal fibres. *Br J Haematol* 139:351-362.

Kvasnicka H, BJ, Brunning R, Thiele J, et al [2008] Myeloproliferative neoplasm, unclassifiable. In: Swerdlow S, Campo E, Harris N, et al, eds. *WHO Classification of Tumours of Haematopoietic and Lymphoid Tissues.* 4th ed. Lyon, France: IARC Press; 64-65.

Kvasnicka HM, Thiele J [2007] Classification of Ph-negative chronic myeloproliferative disorders—morphology as the yardstick of classification. *Pathobiology* 74:63-71.

Kvasnicka HM, Thiele J [2010] Prodromal myeloproliferative neoplasms: the 2008 WHO classification. *Am J Hematol* 85:62-69.

Landgren O, Goldin LR, Kristinsson SY, et al [2008] Increased risks of polycythemia vera, essential thrombocythemia, and myelofibrosis among 24,577 first-degree relatives of 11,039 patients with myeloproliferative neoplasms in Sweden. *Blood* 112:2199-2204.

Larsen TS, Christensen JH, Hasselbalch HC, Pallisgaard N [2007] The *JAK2* V617F mutation involves B- and T-lymphocyte lineages in a subgroup of patients with Philadelphia-chromosome negative chronic myeloproliferative disorders. *Br J Haematol* 136:745-751.

Larsen TS, Pallisgaard N, Moller MB, Hasselbalch HC [2008] High prevalence of arterial thrombosis in *JAK2* mutated essential thrombocythaemia: independence of the V617F allele burden. *Hematology* 13:71-76.

Lee JK, Whittaker SJ, Enns RA, Zetler P [2008] Gastrointestinal manifestations of systemic mastocytosis. *World J Gastroenterol* 14:7005-7008.

Levine RL, Pardanani A, Tefferi A, Gilliland DG [2007] Role of *JAK2* in the pathogenesis and therapy of myeloproliferative disorders. *Nat Rev Cancer* 7:673-683.

Levine RL, Wadleigh M, Cools J, et al [2005] Activating mutation in the tyrosine kinase *JAK2* in polycythemia vera, essential thrombocythemia, and myeloid metaplasia with myelofibrosis. *Cancer Cell* 7:387-397.

Lierman E, Cools J [2009] Recent breakthroughs in the understanding and management of chronic eosinophilic leukemia. *Expert Rev Anticancer Ther* 9:1295-1304.

Lim DJ, Oh EJ, Park CW, et al [2007] Pancytopenia and secondary myelofibrosis could be induced by primary hyperparathyroidism. *Int J Lab Hematol* 29:464-468.

Lim KH, Tefferi A, Lasho TL, et al [2009] Systemic mastocytosis in 342 consecutive adults: survival studies and prognostic factors. *Blood* 113:5727-5736.

Ma X, Vanasse G, Cartmel B, et al [2008] Prevalence of polycythemia vera and essential thrombocythemia. *Am J Hematol* 83:359-362.

Marchetti M, Falanga A [2008] Leukocytosis, JAK2 V617F mutation, and hemostasis in myeloproliferative disorders. *Pathophysiol Haemost Thromb* 36:148-159.

Marchioli R, Finazzi G, Landolfi R, et al [2005] Vascular and neoplastic risk in a large cohort of patients with polycythemia vera. *J Clin Oncol* 23:2224-2232.

Martinelli G, Rondoni M, Ottaviani E, et al [2007] Hypereosinophilic syndrome and molecularly targeted therapy. *Semin Hematol* 44:S4-S16.

Mauro MJ, Loriaux M, Deininger MW [2004] Ph-positive and -negative myeloproliferative syndromes may co-exist. *Leukemia* 18:1305-1307.

McLornan DP, Percy MJ, Jones AV, et al [2005] Chronic neutrophilic leukemia with an associated V617F JAK2 tyrosine kinase mutation. *Haematologica* 90:1696-1697.

McNamara C, Grigg A, Szer J, et al [2003] Morphological effects of imatinib mesylate (STI571) on the bone marrow and blood of patients with Philadelphia chromosome (Ph) positive chronic myeloid leukaemia. *Clin Lab Haematol* 25:119-125.

Melillo L, Tieghi A, Candoni A, et al [2009] Outcome of 122 pregnancies in essential thrombocythemia patients: a report from the Italian registry. *Am J Hematol* 84:636-640.

Melo JV [1996] The diversity of BCR-ABL fusion proteins and their relationship to leukemia phenotype. *Blood* 88:2375-2384.

Melo JV, Myint H, Galton DA, Goldman JM [1994] P190BCR-ABL chronic myeloid leukaemia: the missing link with chronic myelomonocytic leukaemia? *Leukemia* 8:208-211.

Merluzzi S, Frossi B, Gri G, et al [2010] Mast cells enhance proliferation of B lymphocytes and drive their differentiation towards IgA-secreting plasma cells. *Blood* epub ahead of print January 25, 2010; DOI 10.1182/blood-2009-10-250126.

Merzianu M, Medeiros LJ, Cortes J, et al [2005] inv(16)(p13q22) in chronic myelogenous leukemia in blast phase: a clinicopathologic, cytogenetic, and molecular study of 5 cases. *Am J Clin Pathol* 124:807-814.

Mesa RA, Hanson CA, Li CY, et al [2002] Diagnostic and prognostic value of bone marrow angiogenesis and megakaryocyte *c-Mpl* expression in essential thrombocythemia. *Blood* 99:4131-4137.

Mesa RA, Li CY, Ketterling RP, et al [2005] Leukemic transformation in myelofibrosis with myeloid metaplasia: a single-institution experience with 91 cases. *Blood* 105:973-977.

Metcalfe DD [2008] Mast cells and mastocytosis. *Blood* 112:946-956.

Michiels JJ [2004] Bone marrow histopathology and biological markers as specific clues to the differential diagnosis of essential thrombocythemia, polycythemia vera and prefibrotic or fibrotic agnogenic myeloid metaplasia. *Hematol J* 5:93-102.

Michiels JJ, Thiele J [2002] Clinical and pathological criteria for the diagnosis of essential thrombocythemia, polycythemia vera, and idiopathic myelofibrosis (agnogenic myeloid metaplasia). *Int J Hematol* 76:133-145.

Millot F, Traore P, Guilhot J, et al [2005] Clinical and biological features at diagnosis in 40 children with chronic myeloid leukemia. *Pediatrics* 116:140-143.

Morel P, Duhamel A [2010] Comparison of prognostic scoring systems in primary myelofibrosis. *Blood* 115:745; author reply 745-746.

Moritake H, Ikeda T, Manabe A, et al [2009] Cytomegalovirus infection mimicking juvenile myelomonocytic leukemia showing hypersensitivity to granulocyte-macrophage colony-stimulating factor. *Pediatr Blood Cancer* 53:1324-1326.

Nagai S, Ichikawa M, Takahashi T, et al [2007] The origin of neoplastic mast cells in systemic mastocytosis with AML1/ETO-positive acute myeloid leukemia. *Exp Hematol* 35:1747-1752.

Nakatani T, Imamura T, Ishida H, et al [2008] Frequency and clinical features of the JAK2 V617F mutation in pediatric patients with sporadic essential thrombocythemia. *Pediatr Blood Cancer* 51:802-805.

Neureiter D, Kemmerling R, Ocker M, et al [2008] Differential diagnostic challenge of chronic neutrophilic leukemia in a patient with prolonged leukocytosis. *J Hematop* 1:23-27.

Noguchi T, Ikeda K, Yamamoto K, et al [2001] Severe bleeding tendency caused by leukemic infiltration and destruction of vascular walls in chronic neutrophilic leukemia. *Int J Hematol* 74:437-441.

Nowell P, Hungerford D [1960] A minute chromosome in human chronic granulocytic leukemia. *Science* 132:1497-1500.

O'Malley DP, Sen J, Juliar BE, Orazi A [2005] Evaluation of stroma in human immunodeficiency virus/acquired immunodeficiency syndrome-affected bone marrows and correlation with CD4 counts. *Arch Pathol Lab Med* 129:1137-1140.

Oehler VG, Yeung KY, Choi YE, et al [2009] The derivation of diagnostic markers of chronic myeloid leukemia progression from microarray data. *Blood* 114:3292-3298.

Oh SH, Park TS, Kim HR, et al [2009] Chronic myelogenous leukemia showing biphenotypic blast crisis followed by lineage switch to B lymphoblastic leukemia. *Leuk Res* 33:e195-198.

Ohyashiki JH, Ohyashiki K, Shimamoto T, et al [1995] Ecotropic virus integration site-1 gene preferentially expressed in post-myelodysplasia acute myeloid leukemia: possible association with GATA1, GATA2, and stem cell leukemia gene expression. *Blood* 85:3713-3718.

Oluwole O, Awujo A, Ivonye C, Sanders L [2009] Myelodysplastic/myeloproliferative disorder with severe leukocytosis: a case report. *Am J Clin Oncol* 32:326-327.

Oren H, Duzovali O, Yuksel E, et al [1999] Development of acute promyelocytic leukemia with isochromosome 17q after BCR/ABL positive chronic myeloid leukemia. *Cancer Genet Cytogenet* 109:141-143.

Pane F, Frigeri F, Sindona M, et al [1996] Neutrophilic-chronic myeloid leukemia: a distinct disease with a specific molecular marker (BCR/ABL with C3/A2 junction). *Blood* 88:2410-2414.

Pardanani A, Lim KH, Lasho TL, et al [2009] Prognostically relevant breakdown of 123 patients with systemic mastocytosis associated with other myeloid malignancies. *Blood* 114:3769-3772.

Pardanani A, Tefferi A [2010] Systemic mastocytosis in adults: a review on prognosis and treatment based on 342 Mayo Clinic patients and current literature. *Curr Opin Hematol* epub ahead of print January 13, 2010.

Pardanani AD, Levine RL, Lasho T, et al [2006] MPL515 mutations in myeloproliferative and other myeloid disorders: a study of 1182 patients. *Blood* 108:3472-3476.

Parker R [2000] Hematologic aspects of systemic mastocytosis. *Hematol Oncol Clin North Am* 14:557-568.

Passamonti F, Rumi E, Arcaini L, et al [2009] Blast phase of essential thrombocythemia: a single center study. *Am J Hematol* 84:641-644.

Passamonti F, Rumi E, Arcaini L, et al [2008a] Prognostic factors for thrombosis, myelofibrosis, and leukemia in essential thrombocythemia: a study of 605 patients. *Haematologica* 93:1645-1651.

Passamonti F, Rumi E, Caramella M, et al [2008b] A dynamic prognostic model to predict survival in post-polycythemia vera myelofibrosis. *Blood* 111:3383-3387.

Passamonti F, Rumi E, Pungolino E, et al [2004] Life expectancy and prognostic factors for survival in patients with polycythemia vera and essential thrombocythemia. *Am J Med* 117:755-761.

Patel BB, Mohamed AN, Schiffer CA [2006] "Acute myelogenous leukemia like" translocations in CML blast crisis: 2 new cases of inv(16)/t(16;16) and a review of the literature. *Leuk Res* 30:225-232.

Patnaik MM, Tefferi A [2009a] The complete evaluation of erythrocytosis: congenital and acquired. *Leukemia* 23:834-844.

Patnaik MM, Tefferi A [2009b] Molecular diagnosis of myeloproliferative neoplasms. *Expert Rev Mol Diagn* 9:481-492.

Percy MJ, Rumi E [2009] Genetic origins and clinical phenotype of familial and acquired erythrocytosis and thrombocytosis. *Am J Hematol* 84:46-54.

Peterson L [2008] Prefibrotic myelofibrosis: is this diagnosis valid? *Blood* 111:1-2.

Pettigrew HD, Teuber SS, Kong JS, Gershwin ME [2009] Contemporary challenges in mastocytosis. *Clin Rev Allergy Immunol* epub ahead of print 29 July 2009.

Piaggio G, Rosti V, Corselli M, et al [2009] Endothelial colony-forming cells from patients with chronic myeloproliferative disorders lack the disease-specific molecular clonality marker. *Blood* 114:3127-3130.

Pich A, Riera L, Sismondi F, et al [2009] *JAK2* V617F activating mutation is associated with the myeloproliferative type of chronic myelomonocytic leukaemia. *J Clin Pathol* 62:798-801.

Policitemia GIs [1995] Polycythemia vera: the natural history of 1213 patients followed for 20 years. *Ann Intern Med* 123:656-664.

Ponzoni M, Savage DG, Ferreri AJ, et al [2004] Chronic idiopathic myelofibrosis: independent prognostic importance of bone marrow microvascular density evaluated by CD105 (endoglin) immunostaining. *Mod Pathol* 17:1513-1520.

Pullarkat ST, Pullarkat V, Kroft SH, et al [2009] Systemic mastocytosis associated with t(8;21)(q22;q22) acute myeloid leukemia. *J Hematop* 2:27-33.

Pullarkat ST, Vardiman JW, Slovak ML, et al [2008] Megakaryocytic blast crisis as a presenting manifestation of chronic myeloid leukemia. *Leuk Res* 32:1770-1775.

Pullarkat V, Bass RD, Gong JZ, et al [2003] Primary autoimmune myelofibrosis: definition of a distinct clinicopathologic syndrome. *Am J Hematol* 72:8-12.

Pullarkat V, Bedell V, Kim Y, et al [2007] Neoplastic mast cells in systemic mastocytosis associated with t(8;21) acute myeloid leukemia are derived from the leukemic clone. *Leuk Res* 31:261-265.

Quintas-Cardama A, Cortes J [2008] Therapeutic options against *BCR-ABL1* T315I-positive chronic myelogenous leukemia. *Clin Cancer Res* 14:4392-4399.

Rameshwar P, Chang VT, Thacker UF, Gascon P [1998] Systemic transforming growth factor-β in patients with bone marrow fibrosis—pathophysiological implications. *Am J Hematol* 59:133-142.

Randi ML, Putti MC, Scapin M, et al [2006] Pediatric patients with essential thrombocythemia are mostly polyclonal and V617F*JAK2* negative. *Blood* 108:3600-3602.

Reeder TL, Bailey RJ, Dewald GW, Tefferi A [2003] Both B and T lymphocytes may be clonally involved in myelofibrosis with myeloid metaplasia. *Blood* 101:1981-1983.

Reid AG, De Melo VA, Elderfield K, et al [2009] Phenotype of blasts in chronic myeloid leukemia in blastic phase-analysis of bone marrow trephine biopsies and correlation with cytogenetics. *Leuk Res* 33:418-425.

Reilly JT [2002] Chronic neutrophilic leukaemia: a distinct clinical entity? *Br J Haematol* 116:10-18.

Reilly JT [1997] Idiopathic myelofibrosis: pathogenesis, natural history and management. *Blood Rev* 11:233-242.

Reilly JT [2008] Pathogenetic insight and prognostic information from standard and molecular cytogenetic studies in the BCR-ABL-negative myeloproliferative neoplasms (MPNs). *Leukemia* 22:1818-1827.

Rizzi R, Pastore D, Liso A, et al [2004] Autoimmune myelofibrosis: report of 3 cases and review of the literature. *Leuk Lymphoma* 45:561-566.

Rohrbacher M, Hasford J [2009] Epidemiology of chronic myeloid leukaemia (CML). *Best Pract Res Clin Haematol* 22:295-302.

Rollison DE, Howlader N, Smith MT, et al [2008] Epidemiology of myelodysplastic syndromes and chronic myeloproliferative disorders in the United States, 2001-2004, using data from the NAACCR and SEER programs. *Blood* 112:45-52.

Rothenberg ME, Klion AD, Roufosse FE, et al [2008] Treatment of patients with the hypereosinophilic syndrome with mepolizumab. *N Engl J Med* 358:1215-1228.

Rowe JM, Lichtman MA [1984] Hyperleukocytosis and leukostasis: common features of childhood chronic myelogenous leukemia. *Blood* 63:1230-1234.

Rowley JD [1973] Letter: a new consistent chromosomal abnormality in chronic myelogenous leukaemia identified by quinacrine fluorescence and Giemsa staining. *Nature* 243:290-293.

Rumi E [2008] Familial chronic myeloproliferative disorders: the state of the art. *Hematol Oncol* 26:131-138.

Rumi E, Passamonti F, Della Porta MG, et al [2007] Familial chronic myeloproliferative disorders: clinical phenotype and evidence of disease anticipation. *J Clin Oncol* 25:5630-5635.

Rumi E, Passamonti F, Pietra D, et al [2006] *JAK2* (V617F) as an acquired somatic mutation and a secondary genetic event associated with disease progression in familial myeloproliferative disorders. *Cancer* 107:2206-2211.

Saint-Martin C, Leroy G, Delhommeau F, et al [2009] Analysis of the 10-eleven translocation 2 (TET2) gene in familial myeloproliferative neoplasms. *Blood* 114:1628-1632.

Sakka V, Tsiodras S, Giamarellos-Bourboulis EJ, Giamarellou H [2006] An update on the etiology and diagnostic evaluation of a leukemoid reaction. *Eur J Intern Med* 17:394-398.

Salgado C, Feliu E, Blade J, et al [1992] A second bone marrow biopsy as a cause of a false diagnosis of myelofibrosis. *Br J Haematol* 80:407-409.

Samorapoomipichit P, Kiener HP, Schernthaner G-H, et al [2001] Detection of tryptase in cytoplasmic granules of basophils in patients with chronic myeloid leukemia and other myeloid neoplasms. *Blood* 98:2580-2583.

Sanchez CP [2008] Mineral metabolism and bone abnormalities in children with chronic renal failure. *Rev Endocr Metab Disord* 9:131-137.

Sanchez S, Ewton A [2006] Essential thrombocythemia: a review of diagnostic and pathologic features. *Arch Pathol Lab Med* 130:1144-1150.

Schaub FX, Looser R, Li S, et al [2010] Clonal analysis of *TET2* and *JAK2* mutations suggests that *TET2* can be a late event in the progression of myeloproliferative neoplasms. *Blood* 115:2003-2007.

Schwartz KM, Skinner JA [2008] Hepatitis C-associated osteosclerosis: a case report. *Skeletal Radiol* 37:679-681.

Scolnik MP, Palacios MF, Acevedo SH, et al [1998] Promyelocytic blast crisis of chronic myelogenous leukaemia with translocations (9;22) and (15;17). *Leuk Lymphoma* 31:231-236.

Sheikha A [2004] Fatal familial infantile myelofibrosis. *J Pediatr Hematol Oncol* 26:164-168.

Shigekiyo T, Miyagi J, Chohraku M, et al [2008] Bleeding tendency in chronic neutrophilic leukemia. *Int J Hematol* 88:240-242.

Skoda R, Prchal JT [2005] Lessons from familial myeloproliferative disorders. *Semin Hematol* 42:266-273.

Sotlar K, Horny HP, Simonitsch I, et al [2004] CD25 indicates the neoplastic phenotype of mast cells: a novel immunohistochemical marker for the diagnosis of systemic mastocytosis (SM) in routinely processed bone marrow biopsy specimens. *Am J Surg Pathol* 28:1319-1325.

Soupir CP, Vergilio JA, Dal Cin P, et al [2007] Philadelphia chromosome-positive acute myeloid leukemia: a rare aggressive leukemia with clinicopathologic features distinct from chronic myeloid leukemia in myeloid blast crisis. *Am J Clin Pathol* 127:642-650.

Sperr WR, El-Samahi A, Kundi M, et al [2009] Elevated tryptase levels selectively cluster in myeloid neoplasms: a novel diagnostic approach and screen marker in clinical haematology. *Eur J Clin Invest* 39:914-923.

Steensma DP, Dewald GW, Lasho TL, et al [2005] The *JAK2* V617F activating tyrosine kinase mutation is an infrequent event in both "atypical" myeloproliferative disorders and myelodysplastic syndromes. *Blood* 106:1207-1209.

Steurer M, Zoller H, Augustin F, et al [2007] Increased angiogenesis in chronic idiopathic myelofibrosis: vascular endothelial growth factor as a prominent angiogenic factor. *Hum Pathol* 38:1057-1064.

Swolin B, Weinfeld A, Westin J [1988] A prospective long-term cytogenetic study in polycythemia vera in relation to treatment and clinical course. *Blood* 72:386-395.

Szpurka H, Tiu R, Murugesan G, et al [2006] Refractory anemia with ringed sideroblasts associated with marked thrombocytosis (RARS-T), another myeloproliferative condition characterized by *JAK2* V617F mutation. *Blood* 108:2173-2181.

Tagariello G, Di Gaetano R, Sartori R, et al [2009] The *JAK2* V617F) tyrosine kinase mutation in blood donors with upper-limit haematocrit levels. *Blood Transfus* 7:111-116.

Tam CS, Nussenzveig RM, Popat U, et al [2008] The natural history and treatment outcome of blast phase BCR-ABL-myeloproliferative neoplasms. *Blood* 112:1628-1637.

Tefferi A [2008a] The history of myeloproliferative disorders: before and after Dameshek. *Leukemia* 22:3-13.

Tefferi A [2009a] Molecular drug targets in myeloproliferative neoplasms: mutant *ABL1, JAK2, MPL, KIT, PDGFRA, PDGFRB* and *FGFR1. J Cell Mol Med* 13:215-237.

Tefferi A, Gilliland G [2006a] Classification of chronic myeloid disorders: from Dameshek towards a semi-molecular system. *Best Pract Res Clin Haematol* 19:365-385.

Tefferi A, Gotlib J, Pardanani A [2010] Hypereosinophilic syndrome and clonal eosinophilia: point-of-care diagnostic algorithm and treatment update. *Mayo Clin Proc* 85:158-164.

Tefferi A, Pardanani A [2007a] Evaluation of "increased" hemoglobin in the *JAK2* mutations era: a diagnostic algorithm based on genetic tests. *Mayo Clin Proc* 82:599-604.

Tefferi A, Pardanani A, Lim KH, et al [2009b] TET2 mutations and their clinical correlates in polycythemia vera, essential thrombocythemia and myelofibrosis. *Leukemia* 23:905-911.

Tefferi A, Patnaik MM, Pardanani A [2006b] Eosinophilia: secondary, clonal and idiopathic. *Br J Haematol* 133:468-492.

Tefferi A, Schad CR, Pruthi RK, et al [1995a] Fluorescent in situ hybridization studies of lymphocytes and neutrophils in chronic granulocytic leukemia. *Cancer Genet Cytogenet* 83:61-64.

Tefferi A, Silverstein MN, Noel P [1995b] Agnogenic myeloid metaplasia. *Semin Oncol* 22:327-333.

Tefferi A, Skoda R, Vardiman JW [2009c] Myeloproliferative neoplasms: contemporary diagnosis using histology and genetics. *Nat Rev Clin Oncol* 6:627-637.

Tefferi A, Thiele J, Orazi A, et al [2007b] Proposals and rationale for revision of the World Health Organization diagnostic criteria for polycythemia vera, essential thrombocythemia, and primary myelofibrosis: recommendations from an ad hoc international expert panel. *Blood* 110:1092-1097.

Tefferi A, Vardiman JW [2008b] Classification and diagnosis of myeloproliferative neoplasms: the 2008 World Health Organization criteria and point-of-care diagnostic algorithms. *Leukemia* 22:14-22.

Teofili L, Cenci T, Martini M, et al [2009] The mutant *JAK2* allele burden in children with essential thrombocythemia. *Br J Haematol* 145:430-432.

Teofili L, Giona F, Martini M, et al [2007a] Markers of myeloproliferative diseases in childhood polycythemia vera and essential thrombocythemia. *J Clin Oncol* 25:1048-1053.

Teofili L, Giona F, Martini M, et al [2007b] The revised WHO diagnostic criteria for Ph-negative myeloproliferative diseases are not appropriate for the diagnostic screening of childhood polycythemia vera and essential thrombocythemia. *Blood* 110:3384-3386.

Teofili L, Martini M, Cenci T, et al [2007c] Different STAT-3 and STAT-5 phosphorylation discriminates among Ph-negative chronic myeloproliferative diseases and is independent of the V617F JAK-2 mutation. *Blood* 110:354-359.

Theocharides A, Boissinot M, Girodon F, et al [2007] Leukemic blasts in transformed *JAK2* V617F-positive myeloproliferative disorders are frequently negative for the *JAK2* V617F mutation. *Blood* 110:375-379.

Thiele J, Kvasnicka H, Orazi A, et al [2008a] Polycythaemia vera. In: Swerdlow S, Campo E, Harris N, et al, eds. *WHO Classification of Tumours: Pathology and Genetics: Tumours of Haematopoietic and Lymphoid Tissues.* Lyon, France: IARC Press; 40-43.

Thiele J, Kvasnicka H, Orazi A, et al [2008b] Essential thrombocythemia. In: Swerdlow S, Campo E, Harris N, et al, eds. *WHO Classification of Tumours: Pathology and Genetics: Tumours of Haematopoietic and Lymphoid Tissues.* Lyon, France: IARC Press; 48-50.

Thiele J, Kvasnicka H, Tefferi A, et al [2008c] Primary myelofibrosis. In: Swerdlow S, Campo E, Harris N, et al, eds. *WHO Classification of Tumours: Pathology and Genetics: Tumours of Haematopoietic and Lymphoid Tissues.* Lyon, France: IARC Press; 44-47.

Thiele J, Kvasnicka HM [2003a] Chronic myeloproliferative disorders with thrombocythemia: a comparative study of 2 classification systems (PVSG, WHO) on 839 patients. *Ann Hematol* 82:148-152.

Thiele J, Kvasnicka HM [2005a] Hematopathologic findings in chronic idiopathic myelofibrosis. *Semin Oncol* 32:380-394.

Thiele J, Kvasnicka HM [2006a] Myelofibrosis in chronic myeloproliferative disorders—dynamics and clinical impact. *Histol Histopathol* 21:1367-1378.

Thiele J, Kvasnicka HM, Diehl V [2005b] Initial (latent) polycythemia vera with thrombocytosis mimicking essential thrombocythemia. *Acta Haematol* 113:213-219.

Thiele J, Kvasnicka HM, Fischer R [1999] Histochemistry and morphometry on bone marrow biopsies in chronic myeloproliferative disorders—aids to diagnosis and classification. *Ann Hematol* 78:495-506.

Thiele J, Kvasnicka HM, Fischer R, Diehl V [1997] Clinicopathological impact of the interaction between megakaryocytes and myeloid stroma in chronic myeloproliferative disorders: a concise update. *Leuk Lymphoma* 24:463-481.

Thiele J, Kvasnicka HM, Schmitt-Graeff A, et al [2005c] Bone marrow changes in chronic myelogenous leukaemia after long-term treatment with the tyrosine kinase inhibitor STI571: an immunohistochemical study on 75 patients. *Histopathology* 46:540-550.

Thiele J, Kvasnicka HM, Schmitt-Graeff A, et al [2000] Bone marrow features and clinical findings in chronic myeloid leukemia—a comparative, multicenter, immunohistological and morphometric study on 614 patients. *Leukemia and Lymphoma* 36:295-308.

Thiele J, Kvasnicka HM, Schmitt-Graeff A, et al [2002] Follow-up examinations including sequential bone marrow biopsies in essential thrombocythemia (ET): a retrospective clinicopathological study of 120 patients. *Am J Hematol* 70:283-291.

Thiele J, Kvasnicka HM, Schmitt-Graeff A, Diehl V [2003b] Bone marrow histopathology following cytoreductive therapy in chronic idiopathic myelofibrosis. *Histopathology* 43:470-479.

Thiele J, Kvasnicka HM, Vardiman J [2006b] Bone marrow histopathology in the diagnosis of chronic myeloproliferative disorders: a forgotten pearl. *Best Pract Res Clin Haematol* 19:413-437.

Thiele J, Kvasnicka HM, Zankovich R, Diehl V [2001] Clinical and morphological criteria for the diagnosis of prefibrotic idiopathic (primary) myelofibrosis. *Ann Hematol* 80:160-165.

Tilak V, Rai M, Singh VP, et al [2007] Hepatocellular carcinoma presenting as neutrophilic leukaemoid reaction—a rare entity. *J Indian Med Assoc* 105:462, 464-465.

Tolar J, Teitelbaum SL, Orchard PJ [2004] Osteopetrosis. *N Engl J Med* 351:2839-2849.

Uemura Y, Taguchi T, Kubota T, et al [2009] Neutrophil function and cytokine-specific signaling in chronic neutrophilic leukemia. *Int J Lab Hematol* 31:36-47.

Vaidya R, Siragusa S, Huang J, et al [2009] Mature survival data for 176 patients younger than 60 years with primary myelofibrosis diagnosed between 1976 and 2005: evidence for survival gains in recent years. *Mayo Clin Proc* 84:1114-1119.

Valent P [2009] Pathogenesis, classification, and therapy of eosinophilia and eosinophil disorders. *Blood Rev* 23:157-165.

Valent P, Akin C, Sperr WR, et al [2003] Diagnosis and treatment of systemic mastocytosis: state of the art. *Br J Haematol* 122:695-717.

Valent P, Dahinden CA [2010] Role of interleukins in the regulation of basophil development and secretion. *Curr Opin Hematol* 17:60-66.

van Daele PL, Beukenkamp BS, Geertsma-Kleinekoort WM, et al [2009] Immunophenotyping of mast cells: a sensitive and specific diagnostic tool for systemic mastocytosis. *Neth J Med* 67:142-146.

van Rhee F, Hochhaus A, Lin F, et al [1996] p190 *BCR-ABL* mRNA is expressed at low levels in p210-positive chronic myeloid and acute lymphoblastic leukemias. *Blood* 87:5213-5217.

Vardiman J, Brunning R, Arber D, et al [2008a] Introduction and overview of the classification of the myeloid neoplasms. In: Swerdlow S, Campo E, Harris N, et al, eds. *WHO Classification of Tumours: Pathology and Genetics: Tumours of Haematopoietic and Lymphoid Tissues.* Lyon, France: IARC Press; 18-30.

Vardiman J, Melo J, Baccarani M, Thiele J [2008b] Chronic myelogenous leukaemia, *BCR-ABL1* positive. In: Swerdlow S, Campo E, Harris N, et al, eds. *WHO Classification of Tumours: Pathology and Genetics: Tumours of Haematopoietic and Lymphoid Tissues.* Lyon, France: IARC Press; 32-37.

Vardiman JW [2009a] Chronic myelogenous leukemia, *BCR-ABL1+. Am J Clin Pathol* 132:250-260.

Vardiman JW, Thiele J, Arber DA, et al [2009b] The 2008 revision of the WHO classification of myeloid neoplasms and acute leukemia: rationale and important changes. *Blood* 114:937-951.

Vega F, Medeiros LJ, Lang WH, et al [2002] The stromal composition of malignant lymphoid aggregates in bone marrow: variations in architecture and phenotype in different B-cell tumours. *Br J Haematol* 117:569-576.

Verma D, Kantarjian HM, Jones D, et al [2009] Chronic myeloid leukemia (CML) with P190 *BCR-ABL*: analysis of characteristics, outcomes, and prognostic significance. *Blood* 114:2232-2235.

Virchow R [1845] Weisses Blut. *N Notiz Geb Natur-u Heilk* 36:151-156.

Wang SA, Pozdnyakova O, Jorgensen JL, et al [2009] Detection of paroxysmal nocturnal hemoglobinuria clones in patients with myelodysplastic syndromes and related bone marrow diseases, with emphasis on diagnostic pitfalls and caveats. *Haematologica* 94:29-37.

Wenstrup RJ, Roca-Espiau M, Weinreb NJ, Bembi B [2002] Skeletal aspects of Gaucher disease: a review. *Br J Radiol* 75Suppl1:A2-12.

Wilkins BS, Erber WN, Bareford D, et al [2008] Bone marrow pathology in essential thrombocythemia: interobserver reliability and utility for identifying disease subtypes. *Blood* 111:60-70.

Woronzoff-Dashkoff KK, Litz CE [1996] Acute lymphoblastic leukemia in a case of essential thrombocythemia. *Am J Clin Pathol* 106:206-208.

Wu Y, Slovak ML, Snyder DS, Arber DA [2006] Coexistence of inversion 16 and the Philadelphia chromosome in acute and chronic myeloid leukemias : report of 6 cases and review of literature. *Am J Clin Pathol* 125:260-266.

Xu Y, Dolan MM, Nguyen PL [2003] Diagnostic significance of detecting dysgranulopoiesis in chronic myeloid leukemia. *Am J Clin Pathol* 120:778-784.

Yanagisawa K, Ohminami H, Sato M, et al [1998] Neoplastic involvement of granulocytic lineage, not granulocytic-monocytic, monocytic, or erythrocytic lineage, in a patient with chronic neutrophilic leukemia. *Am J Hematol* 57:221-224.

Yin CC, Cortes J, Barkoh B, et al [2006] t(3;21)(q26;q22) in myeloid leukemia: an aggressive syndrome of blast transformation associated with hydroxyurea or antimetabolite therapy. *Cancer* 106:1730-1738.

Yin CC, Medeiros LJ, Glassman AB, Lin P [2004] t(8;21)(q22;q22) in blast phase of chronic myelogenous leukemia. *Am J Clin Pathol* 121:836-842.

Yoon SY, Li CY, Tefferi A [2000] Megakaryocyte *c-Mpl* expression in chronic myeloproliferative disorders and the myelodysplastic syndrome: immuno-peroxidase staining patterns and clinical correlates. *Eur J Haematol* 65:170-174.

Yoshida M, Nishikawa Y, Yamamoto Y, et al [2009] Mast cell leukemia with rapidly progressing portal hypertension. *Pathol Int* 59:817-822.

Myeloid and Lymphoid Neoplasms with Eosinophilia (MLNE) and Abnormalities of *PDGFRA, PDGFRB,* or *FGFR1*

David Czuchlewski, MD

The myeloid and lymphoid neoplasms with eosino-philia ("MLNE" seems the best abbreviation of this unwieldy name) and abnormalities of *PDGFRA*, *PDGFRB*, or *FGFR1* are among the entities recently promoted to the status of distinct diagnostic entities in the 2008 WHO classification [Bain 2008]. Since the presence of key alterations involving the 3 indicated genes provides a relatively simple route to definitive diagnosis, the main challenge with these entities lies in the initial recognition of their highly variable manifestations. The most important unifying element in these disorders is the consistent (although not universal) presence of eosinophilia. As such, in this chapter we will first consider MLNE in the context in which they are most likely to figure prominently: the clinical and diagnostic workup of unexplained eosinophilia.

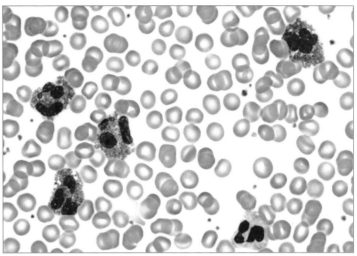

i15.1 *A T-cell clone was detected in this patient with unexplained eosinophilia. Note marked mature eosinophilia on this blood smear. The occurrence of chronic eosinophilia should prompt examination for T-cell lymphoma or populations of T cells with aberrant immunophentoype, both of which may produce a reactive eosinophilia, presumably due to abnormal cytokine production. (Wright)*

[15.1] Eosinophilia

Persistent eosinophilia presents to the clinician and hemato-pathologist a broad differential diagnosis. Eosinophilia may be either clonal/neoplastic or nonclonal/reactive. The distinction is sometimes difficult to make and usually involves extensive clinical and laboratory analysis. The approach to the diagnosis of eosinophilia may be broken down into several successive steps:

1. Establish the presence of significant eosinophilia
2. Investigate reactive causes of eosinophilia
3. Investigate neoplasms in which clonal eosinophilia may be seen
4. In the absence of positive findings in steps 2 or 3, establish 1 of 3 possible diagnoses:
   a. chronic eosinophilic leukemia, not otherwise specified
   b. idiopathic hypereosinophilic syndrome
   c. idiopathic hypereosinophilia

The recognition of MLNE has to some degree simplified the situation, in that there are now additional diagnostic entities to which patients may be definitively assigned. The detection of MLNE in a patient with eosinophilia takes place in step 3 of this algorithm. It should be noted that although we separate the consideration of reactive and neoplastic processes into distinct steps for the purpose of clarity, in practice these investigations would likely be carried out simultaneously. This is particularly true when patients present with very high eosinophil counts and/or tissue destruction (most frequently cardiac) from eosinophilic cytokine-mediated damage, a clinically urgent situation in which diagnosis should not be delayed. Cardiac damage often takes the form of endomyocardial fibrosis, which produces a restrictive cardiomyopathy, or valvular damage. Eosinophilia may also produce pulmonary fibrosis and gastrointestinal and central nervous system symptoms.

When the clinical situation allows, it is prudent to establish the characteristics of the eosinophilia before committing to an exhaustive investigation (step 1). In general, a threshold of $1.5 \times 10^3/\mu L$ ($1.5 \times 10^9/L$) is used to designate eosino-philia deserving further clinical attention. Similarly, eosino-philia present at such a level for longer than 6 months clearly necessitates further workup and is indeed necessary for establishing a diagnosis of hypereosinophilic syndrome or hypereosinophilia. However, clinical investigation of significant eosinophilia should rarely, if ever, be delayed to demonstrate chronicity, especially if tissue damage is present or suspected.

The second step in the aforementioned algorithm involves the exclusion of reactive causes of eosinophilia (see **t10.12**, p 195). Non-neoplastic processes to be considered include allergy, drug reaction, parasitic disease, Kimura disease, and pulmonary diseases such as hypersensitivity pneumonitis and Loeffler pneumonia. In addition, eosinophilia may arise in the setting of cytokine production by malignancies, including T-cell lymphoma and classical Hodgkin lymphoma. Eosinophilia has also been described in the presence of circulating T-cell subsets with abnormal immunophe-notype, though the precise relationship between such populations and current or subsequent T-cell lymphoma is not entirely clear **i15.1**. B lymphoblastic leukemia with t(5;14) (q31;32) is characterized by an *IL3-IGH@* fusion which leads to upregulation of interleukin (IL) 3 production and consequent eosinophilia **i15.2** [Meeker 1990]. In all of these cases, the eosinophils are not themselves clonal, but are simply

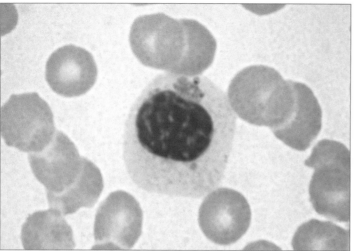

i15.2 *Abnormal eosinophilic morphology in a case of B-cell lymphoblastic leukemia with t(5;14). This rearrangement involves the IL3 gene and is thought to drive a reactive eosinophilia by altering cytokine production. Note that abnormal morphology (hypolobation and hypogranularity) may be present in reactive eosinophilia as seen on this blood smear. (Wright)*

i15.3 *Reactive eosinophils in a patient receiving exogenous interleukin (IL) 2 and IL-4 for therapeutic reasons. Note the mild hypersegmentation; eosinophil morphology is an unreliable guide to clonality, since benign processes can show abnormalities as seen in this blood smear. (Wright)*

responding to the altered environment produced by the unrelated tumor cells.

In contrast, step 3 involves the detection of a set of neoplasms in which eosinophils are *part* of clonal myelopoiesis. Acute myeloid leukemia (AML), myeloproliferative neoplasms, myelodysplastic disorders, and myelodysplastic/myeloproliferative neoplasms must all be ruled out using standard techniques as detailed throughout this book. In particular, since chronic myelogenous leukemia (CML) often demonstrates clonal eosinophilia, morphologic and molecular consideration must be given to this diagnosis. AML with inv(16)(p13.1q22) or t(16;16)(p13.1;q22) should also receive special consideration in this setting. Eosinophilic morphology is of little help in these investigations, because reactive cases often show altered morphology (including abnormal granulation and lobation) and clonal cases may show unremarkable eosinophilic morphology **i15.3**.

It is at this point that evidence of *PDGFRA*, *PDGFRB*, or *FGFR1* abnormalities should be sought. Molecular rearrangement of these genes is associated with clonal eosinophilia, sometimes in a background characteristic of other myeloid and lymphoid malignancies. However, as these genetic lesions may also present as isolated chronic eosinophilia, testing should not be reserved for situations in which features of other myeloid or lymphoid malignancies are present. Conventional karyotype of adequate resolution suffices to exclude *PDGFRB* and *FGFR1* rearrangements, but a specific fluorescence in situ hybridization (FISH) assay must be performed to detect the presence of the most common *PDGFRA* rearrangement [Bain 2007].

If all of these investigations are nondiagnostic, then the algorithm concludes with 3 possible diagnoses (step 4).

Chronic eosinophilic leukemia, not otherwise specified, is the diagnosis if, having excluded all of the above:

1. there is a clonal cytogenetic or molecular abnormality, or
2. blasts comprise >2% of the peripheral blood cellularity, or
3. blasts comprise >5% of the bone marrow cellularity [Bain 2008].

If these criteria are not fulfilled, but there is evidence of tissue damage from the eosinophilia, the diagnosis is idiopathic hypereosinophilic syndrome. In the absence of tissue damage, some prefer the term *idiopathic hypereosinophilia* [Gotlib 2008].

[15.2] Myeloid and Lymphoid Neoplasms with *PDGFRB* Rearrangement

Having established a baseline approach to general eosinophilia, we now turn to the specific eosinophilic disorders produced by the genetic rearrangements encompassed within MLNE.

Two of these entities involve genes encoding receptors for platelet-derived growth factor (PDGF). PDGF is a dimer of 2 disulfide-linked polypeptide chains that acts as a paracrine growth factor important in embryonic development [Betsholtz 1995]. PDGF binds the cell surface receptor tyrosine kinases PDGFRα and PDGFRβ, which dimerize and activate signaling pathways important to growth [Andrae 2008, Kelly 1991]. This system facilitates the development of many organ systems, and plays a specific role in the survival and migration of embryonic hematopoietic precursors [Andrae 2008, Cho 2002, Finzsch 2008]. Comparatively little is known about the function of PDGF after embryogenesis, but autocrine or paracrine stimulation by PDGF stimulates growth in a number of tumor types [Andrae 2008].

t15.1 Reported Cytogenetic Abnormalities Involving PDGFRB*

Cytogenetic Abnormality	Genes
t(5;12)(q31~33;p12~13)	ETV6-PDGFRB
t(1;3;5)(p36;p21;q33)	WDR48-PDGFRB
der(1)t(1;5)(p34;q33), der(5)t(1;5)(p34;q15), der(11)ins(11;5)(p12;q15q33)	GPIAP1-PDGFRB
t(1;5)(q21;q33)	TPM3-PDGFRB
t(1;5)(q23;q33)	PDE4DIP-PDGFRB
t(2;5)(p21;q33)	SPTBN1-PDGFRB
t(4;5)(q21;q33), t(4;5;5)(q23;q31;q33)	PRKG2-PDGFRB
t(3;5)(p21-25;q31-35)	GOLGA4-PDGFRB
t(5;7)(q33;q11.2)	HIP1-PDGFRB
t(5;10)(q33;q21)	CCDC6-PDGFRB
t(5;10)(q33;q22)	H4-PDGFRB
t(5;12)(q31-33;q24)	GIT2-PDGFRB
t(5;14)(q33;q24)	NIN-PDGFRB
t(5;14)(q33;q22)	KIAA1509-PDGFRB
t(5;14)(q33;q32)	CEV14-PDGFRB
t(5;15)(q33;q22)	TP53BP1-PDGFRB
t(5;16)(q33;p13)	NDE1-PDGFRB
t(5;17)(q33-34;q11.2)	MYO18A-PDGFRB
t(5;17)(q33;p13)	RABEP1-PDGFRB
t(5;17)(q33;p11.2)	SPECC1-PDGFRB

*Red indicates most common

References: [Bain 2007, Gallagher 2008, Tefferi 2007, Walz 2009a]

Translocation involving PDGFB was identified in 1994 in a case of apparent chronic myelomonocytic leukemia [Golub 1994]. The t(5;12) fused ETV6 to PDGFRB. Soon thereafter the transforming potential of this fusion protein was demonstrated [Carroll 1996]. Many additional PDGFRB translocation partners have been described t15.1, but the t(5;12) is the most common rearrangement. Clinical interest in PDGFRB rearrangement soared with the realization that treatment with imatinib resulted in prompt and durable remission in the vast majority of rearranged cases [Apperley 2002, David 2007, Walz 2007].

The majority of PDGFRB rearrangements occur in cases with 2 features:

1. Presentation as apparent chronic myelomonocytic leukemia
2. The presence of significant eosinophilia

However, it is crucial to bear in mind that some cases give rise to phenotypes more consistent with chronic eosinophilic leukemia, atypical CML, and very rarely AML, juvenile myelomonocytic leukemia, and even chronic basophilic leukemia. In addition, some cases lack eosinophilia. Thus, PDGFRB rearranged cases illustrate 2 important principles that we will also stress in the discussion of the other MLNE entities:

1. The presentation of MLNE can be highly variable and (despite the presence of "with eosinophilia" in the name) cases may occasionally even lack eosinophilia
2. If the characteristic genetic abnormality is detected, MLNE should be diagnosed regardless of the phenotype; thus, both chronic myelomonocytic leukemia (CMML)-like and AML-like cases are subsumed into the category "myeloid neoplasms with PDGFRB rearrangement"

All cases described thus far have carried 5q rearrangements visible by conventional cytogenetics. Of note, although 5q33 is the band most often cited in the literature as affected, the breakpoint may be assigned variably from 5q31-5q33. Thus, particular attention should be paid to this entire region when examining the karyogram, especially from a case of apparent CMML. Unfortunately, ETV6 and PDGFRB are not the only genes in this area that are translocated in hematopoietic malignancies [Cools 2002], and 5q translocations not directly involving PDGFRB fusion may not respond to imatinib. Indeed, the IL3 gene is also located at 5q31, and rearrangement of IL3 can upregulate production of this cytokine and thereby drive a reactive eosinophilia. While the direct participation of PDGFRB may be demonstrated by FISH or molecular analysis, FISH may be falsely negative in some cases of documented PDGFRB rearrangement, and molecular detection requires the use of specific primers for the translocation partner, which may differ from the usual ETV6 [Steer 2002]. Therefore, in cases with a 5q31-33 breakpoint, a trial of imatinib may be the simplest and most cost-effective way of interrogating for the presence of the PDGFRB fusion. If this therapy does not result in the expected response, further clarification of the precise molecular topography would be justified.

[15.3] Myeloid and Lymphoid Neoplasms with PDGFRA Rearrangement

The myeloid and lymphoid neoplasms with PDGFRA rearrangement are similar in etiology to those with PDGFRB rearrangement in that the receptor tyrosine kinase involved in the translocation normally binds PDGF, and in that the disease is imatinib-responsive. Also, the phenotype of the resulting malignancy may be variable as is the case for PDGFRB. PDGFRA rearrangements typically present with chronic eosinophilia (and often neutrophilia), but may also feature AML or T-cell lymphoblastic leukemia as the main hematologic manifestation [Metzgeroth 2007]. Rare cases present as CMML with eosinophilia [Zota 2008]. Eosinophilia is described as

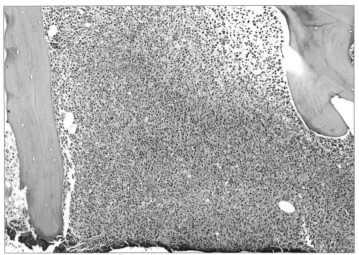

i15.4 *Low-power magnification of bone marrow section from a patient with rearrangement of* PDGFRA. *Note marked hypercellularity with increased eosinophils among the granulocytic cells. (H&E) (courtesy W Finn, MD)*

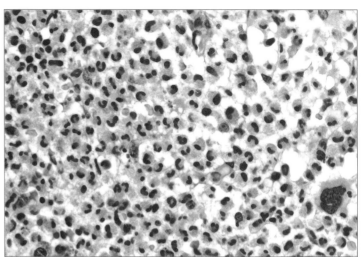

i15.5 *High-power magnification of bone marrow core biopsy specimen from a patient with chronic eosinophilic leukemia due to rearrangement of* PDGFRA *(see* i15.4*). (H&E) (courtesy W Finn, MD)*

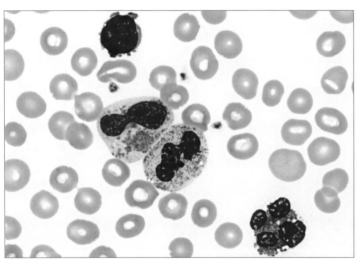

i15.6 *Eosinophilic abnormalities in the blood sample of a patient with rearrangement of* PDGFRA. *The eosinophil on the left shows abnormal granulation, and the eosinophil on the lower right has abnormal lobation. Morphologic abnormalities are neither sensitive nor specific for MLNE, but if present, should raise the possibility of these entities (see* i15.4*,* i15.5*). (Wright) (courtesy W Finn, MD)*

t15.2 Reported Cytogenetic Abnormalities Involving PDGFRA*

Cytogenetic Abnormality	Genes
del(14q12)	FIP1L1-PDGFRA†
t(2;4)(p24;q12)	STRN-PDGFRA
t(4;10)(q12;p11)	KIF5B-PDGFRA
t(4;12)(q2?3;p1?2)	ETV6-PDGFRA
t(4;22)(q12;q11)	BCR-PDGFRA
ins(9;4)(q33;q12q25)	CDK5RAP2-PDGFRA

*Red indicates most common
†Fluorescence in situ hybridization (FISH) is necessary to detect this small interstitial deletion; conventional karyotype of sufficient resolution, or FISH probes designed to detect *PDGFRA* break-apart, are appropriate to detect the remainder of rearrangements in this table

References: [Curtis 2007, Fink 2009, Tefferi 2007]

a generally invariant feature in *PDGFRA* rearrangements i15.4, i15.5, i15.6.

Laboratory testing for *PDGFRA* rearrangements differs significantly from the strategy for the other 2 MLNE disorders. Whereas *PDGFRB* and *FGFR1* rearrangements are detectable by routine high-resolution karyotype, the most common *PDGFRA* rearrangement arises via a microdeletion at 4q12 that fuses *PDGFRA* to its neighbor *FIP1L1*. This microdeletion is invisible on routine cytogenetics, but can be detected with FISH. Often the target of the FISH probe is the gene *CHIC2*, which lies within the small 800-kb deleted region [Fink 2009, Pardanani 2003]. As with *PDGFRB*, other fusion partners have been described t15.2. One particularly noteworthy translocation is the t(4;22)(q12;q11), which

joins *BCR* and *PDGFRA*. The resulting myeloproliferative disorder has features intermediate between CML and eosinophilic leukemia [Bain 2007]. In some cases eosinophilia is not a prominent finding; therefore, this unusual translocation may be a rare cause of myeloproliferative disorders that appear to represent CML but lack the necessary t(9;22). Importantly, variant *PDGFRA* translocations are detectable using 3-color FISH probes that not only reveal the *CHIC2* deletion, but also allow the deduction of a translocation involving the region [Fink 2009]. It is important to clarify the specific layout and discriminatory power of the probe set used by the cytogenetic laboratory in suspected cases of *PDGFRA* rearrangement. Many of the variant translocations will also be visible on routine karyotype [Curtis 2007, Tefferi 2007]. Detection of *PDGFRA* rearrangement is exceedingly important for patient care, since treatment with imatinib will induce sustained response (even

t15.3 Reported Cytogenetic Abnormalities Involving *FGFR1**

Cytogenetic Abnormality	Genes
t(8;13)(p11;q12)	*ZNF198-FGFR1*
t(8;9)(p11;q33)	*CEP110-FGFR1*
t(6;8)(q27;p11-12)	*FRFG10P1-FGFR1*
t(7;8)(q34;p11)	*TIF1-FGFR1*
t(8;11)(p11;p15)	*FGFR1-?*
t(8;22)(p11;q11)	*BCR-FGFR1*
t(8;12)(p11;q15)	*CPSF6-FGFR1*
t(8;17)(p11;q23)	*MYO18A-FGFR1*
t(8;19)(p12;q13.3)	*HERVK-FGFR1*
ins(12;8)(p11;p11p22)	*FGFR10P2-FGFR1*

*Red indicates most common

References: [Bain 2007, Hidalgo-Curtis 2008, Tefferi 2007]

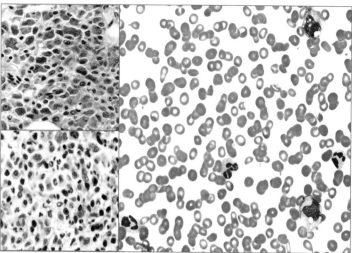

i15.7 *This composite illustrates blood and bone marrow core biopsy features from a 39-year-old male with a history of T-ALL and t(8;13) involving* FGFR1 *in which the blood showed a CMML-like picture, while the bone marrow core biopsy shows increased eosinophils, immature myeloid cels, and increased TdT+ blasts. Consequently, a diagnosis of "myeloid and lymphoid neoplasm with* FGFR1 *abnormality" is appropriate. (Wright, H&E, immunoperoxidase for TdT) (courtesy D Cornfield, MD)*

in cases presenting as T-cell lymphoblastic leukemia), barring resistance mutations in the fusion protein [Helbig 2008, Simon 2008].

Close analysis of the *FIP1L1-PDGFRA* breakpoints suggests that this recurrent rearrangement occurs through illegitimate nonhomologous end joining (a type of DNA repair) following double-strand breaks, the location of which may be constrained by local chromatin structure [Walz 2009b]. Some data suggest that the severity of MLNE with *FIP1L1-PDGFRA* rearrangement may be influenced by the presence of a single nucleotide polymorphism (SNP) in the gene encoding a subunit of the receptor for IL-5, a key cytokine mediating eosinophilic proliferation [Burgstaller 2007].

[15.4] Myeloid and Lymphoid Neoplasms with *FGFR1* Rearrangement

As is the case with *PDGFRA* and *PDGFRB*, *FGFR1* signaling is critical in embryogenesis. Mutations in *FGFR1* cause some syndromic forms of craniosynostosis [Passos-Bueno 2008]. Aberrant activation of *FGFR1* tyrosine kinase is seen in various neoplasms and characterizes a specific subset of MLNE cases [Acevedo 2009].

MLNE with *FGFR1* rearrangement presents in an even more heterogeneous manner than do cases with *PDGFR* rearrangements. Indeed, an earlier diagnostic descriptor for such cases was "8p11 stem cell syndrome," underscoring that an early precursor cell, with several lineage pathways available for differentiation, was affected. MLNE with *FGFR1* presents variously as chronic eosinophilic leukemia, AML, T- or B-cell lymphoblastic leukemia, or acute leukemia of ambiguous lineage i15.7. Eosinophilia is present in approximately 90% of cases, providing an important diagnostic clue but again illustrating the concept that lack of eosinophilia does not exclude the possibility

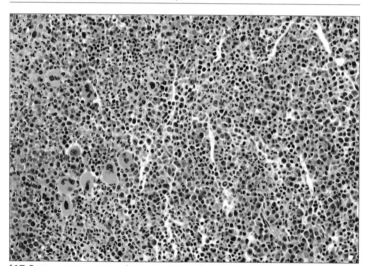

i15.8 *Bone marrow core biopsy specimen from a patient who presented with unexplained chronic eosinophilia. Conventional cytogenetics disclosed a t(8;9), one of the reported* FGFR1 *translocations, which is diagnostic of MLNE. (H&E) (courtesy S Gheith, MD)*

of MLNE. Detection of the *FGFR1* rearrangement, with a number of different translocation partners t15.3, is accomplished by high-resolution karyotype i15.8.

[15.5] The Problem of Overlap between Systemic Mastocytosis and Myeloid and Lymphoid Neoplasms with *PDGFR* Rearrangements

Mast cells are increased in some cases with either *PDGFRA* or *PDGFRB* rearrangements; these mast cells may be spindled in shape and can show aberrant expression of CD2 and/or CD25. Serum tryptase may also be somewhat elevated. These findings,

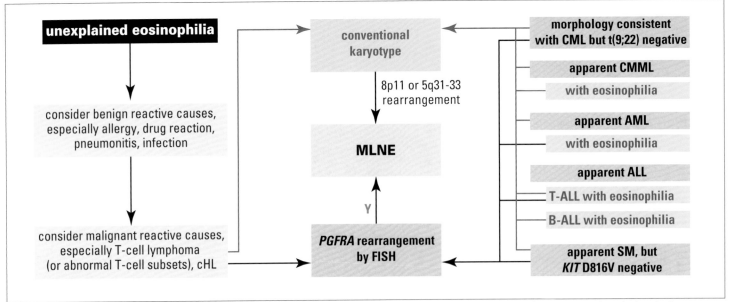

f15.1 *Diagnostic synthesis of cases in which MLNE should be suspected and addressed via conventional cytogenetics and/or FISH. In the right-hand column, conventional cytogenetics would usually be performed on a routine basis when these diagnoses are made, even without eosinophilia or the possibility of MLNE. In these cases, the routine study should detect the 8p11 or 5q31-33 rearrangement, and all that is necessary is to recognize these breakpoints as consistent with MLNE. In contrast, FISH for PDGFRA rearrangement is not routinely performed, and specific findings, as listed in the right-hand column, should prompt such testing.*

cHL = classical Hodgkin lymphoma; FISH = fluorescence in situ hybridization; MLNE = myeloid and lymphoid neoplasms with eosinophilia and abnormalities of PDGFRA, PDGFRB, or FGFR1; SM = systemic mastocytosis

in combination, may fulfill the diagnostic criteria for systemic mastocytosis. Indeed, the early literature reports some *PDGFR* rearrangements as occurring in systemic mastocytosis with eosinophilia. (These cases usually lack the *KIT* D816V mutation.)

This overlap presents an interesting challenge to the diagnostician. Mastocytosis may be diagnosed in conjunction with an "associated clonal hematological non-mast cell lineage disease" (SM-AHNMD). One might be tempted to render such a diagnosis in cases of *PDGFR* rearrangement with mastocytosis: systemic mastocytosis via the fulfillment of the relevant criteria, and a clonal myeloid neoplasm via the *PDGFR* rearrangement. However, it is preferable to diagnose such cases as MLNE, without a separate diagnosis of systemic mastocytosis, for 2 reasons. First, as we note above, the specific lineage that proliferates in MLNE does not generally influence the diagnosis. Thus, the diagnosis of MLNE is made whether the *PDGFRA* rearrangement presents as chronic eosinophilic leukemia or T-cell lymphoblastic leukemia. The involvement of the mast cell lineage, while dramatic, should not necessarily lead one to contradict this principle. Second, the most critical piece of diagnostic information in cases of apparent systemic mastocytosis in the setting of *PDGFR* rearrangement is, in fact, the presence of this genetic lesion, since these cases will respond to imatinib, while cases of systemic mastocytosis with *KIT* D816V mutations will be resistant. Top-line diagnosis of such cases as MLNE facilitates the communication of this critical point. The World Health Organization 2008 classification also follows this scheme of division, noting that mast cell infiltrates in MLNE tend to be less dense than in unambiguous systemic mastocytosis [Bain 2008].

[15.6] ### Diagnostic Synthesis of Myeloid and Lymphoid Neoplasms with Eosinophilia and Abnormalities of *PDGFRA*, *PDGFRB*, or *FGFR1*

Throughout this chapter, we have stressed that MLNE represents a hematologically heterogeneous group of disorders. The main barrier to their diagnosis is not the laboratory-based detection of the genetic lesions, but rather the index of suspicion of the clinician and hematopathologist. In order not to miss a case of MLNE, the diagnostician must keep a sharp look-out for cytogenetic abnormalities involving the critical regions (5q31-33, 4q12, and 8p11) in all cases of myeloproliferative neoplasms, myelodysplastic/myeloproliferative neoplasms, and acute leukemias. We conclude with a figure that summarizes the complex morphologic and clinical clues to the presence of MLNE, separating the workup into 2 main categories in which MLNE should be suspected:

1. Cases of unexplained eosinophilia
2. Specific clinical presentations of hematologic malignances that may suggest the presence of the pathognomonic rearrangements, especially when eosinophilia is also present **f15.1**

[15.7] ### Clues and Caveats

1. Myeloid and lymphoid neoplasms with eosinophilia and abnormalities of *PDGFRA*, *PDGFRB*, or *FGFR1* (MLNE) were first recognized as diagnostic entities in the World Health Organization 2008 classification. All feature rearrangement of genes encoding receptor tyrosine kinases.

2. MLNE frequently presents as unexplained chronic eosinophilia or possible "chronic eosinophilic leukemia."

3. MLNE may present with the phenotype of other hematologic malignancies, including CMML, CML, AML, acute lymphoblastic leukemia, and systemic mastocytosis. In these cases eosinophilia is typically (but not always) present.

4. Testing for MLNE often figures in the workup of chronic or unexplained eosinophilia.

5. In the absence of a MLNE rearrangement, unexplained eosinophilia may fulfill criteria for "chronic eosinophilic leukemia, not otherwise specified," if clonality is detected or the blast count is sufficiently high.

6. Conventional karyotype is adequate to detect rearrangements involving PDGFRB and FGFR1.

7. 5q31-33 or 8p11 rearrangements in *any* myeloid neoplasm or lymphoblastic leukemia should trigger consideration of a possible PDGFRB and FGFR1 rearrangement, respectively.

8. *PDGFRA* rearrangement is often a cryptic deletion at 4q12 requiring FISH or molecular techniques for detection. Since this deletion is not visible on routine karyotype, this FISH assay is usually indicated in the workup of unexplained eosinophilia.

9. Imatinib is highly effective in treating cases with PDGFRA and PDGFRB rearrangements. It is not effective in cases with FGFR1 rearrangement.

[15.8] Acknowledgments
The author thanks D Cornfield, MD, W Finn, MD, and S Gheith, MD, for providing illustrations.

[15.9] References

Acevedo VD, Ittmann M, Spencer DM [2009] Paths of FGFR-driven tumorigenesis. *Cell Cycle* 8:580-588.

Andrae J, Gallini R, Betsholtz C [2008] Role of platelet-derived growth factors in physiology and medicine. *Genes Dev* 22:1276-1312.

Apperley JF, Gardembas M, Melo JV, et al [2002] Response to imatinib mesylate in patients with chronic myeloproliferative diseases with rearrangements of the platelet-derived growth factor receptor beta. *N Engl J Med* 347:481-487.

Bain B, Gilliland D, Horny H-P, Vardiman J [2008] Myeloid and lymphoid neoplasms with eosinophilia and abnormalities of *PDGFRA, PDGFRB,* or *FGFR1.* In: Swerdlow S, Campo E, Harris N, et al, eds. *WHO Classification of Tumours of Haematopoietic and Lymphoid Tissues.* 4th ed. Lyon, France: IARC Press; 68-73.

Bain BJ, Fletcher SH [2007] Chronic eosinophilic leukemias and the myeloproliferative variant of the hypereosinophilic syndrome. *Immunol Allergy Clin North Am* 27:377-388.

Betsholtz C [1995] Role of platelet-derived growth factors in mouse development. *Int J Dev Biol* 39:817-825.

Burgstaller S, Kreil S, Waghorn K, et al [2007] The severity of *FIP1L1-PDGFRA*-positive chronic eosinophilic leukaemia is associated with polymorphic variation at the IL5RA locus. *Leukemia* 21:2428-2432.

Carroll M, Tomasson MH, Barker GF, et al [1996] The TEL/platelet-derived growth factor beta receptor (*PDGF* beta R) fusion in chronic myelomonocytic leukemia is a transforming protein that self-associates and activates *PDGF* beta R kinase-dependent signaling pathways. *Proc Natl Acad Sci USA* 93:14845-14850.

Cho NK, Keyes L, Johnson E, et al [2002] Developmental control of blood cell migration by the *Drosophila* VEGF pathway. *Cell* 108:865-876.

Cools J, Mentens N, Odero MD, et al [2002] Evidence for position effects as a variant ETV6-mediated leukemogenic mechanism in myeloid leukemias with a t(4;12)(q11-q12;p13) or t(5;12)(q31;p13). *Blood* 99:1776-1784.

Curtis CE, Grand FH, Musto P, et al [2007] Two novel imatinib-responsive *PDGFRA* fusion genes in chronic eosinophilic leukaemia. *Br J Haematol* 138:77-81.

David M, Cross NC, Burgstaller S, et al [2007] Durable responses to imatinib in patients with *PDGFRB* fusion gene-positive and *BCR-ABL*-negative chronic myeloproliferative disorders. *Blood* 109:61-64.

Fink SR, Belongie KJ, Paternoster SF, et al [2009] Validation of a new three-color fluorescence in situ hybridization (FISH) method to detect *CHIC2* deletion, *FIP1L1/PDGFRA* fusion and *PDGFRA* translocations. *Leuk Res* 33:843-846.

Finzsch M, Stolt CC, Lommes P, Wegner M [2008] Sox9 and Sox10 influence survival and migration of oligodendrocyte precursors in the spinal cord by regulating PDGF receptor alpha expression. *Development* 135:637-646.

Gallagher G, Horsman DE, Tsang P, Forrest DL [2008] Fusion of *PRKG2* and *SPTBN1* to the platelet-derived growth factor receptor beta gene (*PDGFRB*) in imatinib-responsive atypical myeloproliferative disorders. *Cancer Genet Cytogenet* 181:46-51.

Golub TR, Barker GF, Lovett M, Gilliland DG 1994 Fusion of *PDGF* receptor beta to a novel ets-like gene, *tel,* in chronic myelomonocytic leukemia with t(5;12) chromosomal translocation. *Cell* 77:307-316.

Gotlib J, Cools J [2008] Five years since the discovery of *FIP1L1-PDGFRA*: what we have learned about the fusion and other molecularly defined eosinophilias. *Leukemia* 22:1999-2010.

Helbig G, Stella-Holowiecka B, Majewski M, et al [2008] A single weekly dose of imatinib is sufficient to induce and maintain remission of chronic eosinophilic leukaemia in *FIP1L1-PDGFRA*-expressing patients. *Br J Haematol* 141:200-204.

Hidalgo-Curtis C, Chase A, Drachenberg M, et al [2008] The t(1;9)(p34;q34) and t(8;12)(p11;q15) fuse pre-mRNA processing proteins SFPQ (PSF) and CPSF6 to ABL and FGFR1. *Genes Chromosomes Cancer* 47:379-385.

Kelly JD, Haldeman BA, Grant FJ, et al [1991] Platelet-derived growth factor (PDGF) stimulates PDGF receptor subunit dimerization and intersubunit trans-phosphorylation. *J Biol Chem* 266:8987-8992.

Meeker TC, Hardy D, Willman C, et al [1990] Activation of the interleukin-3 gene by chromosome translocation in acute lymphocytic leukemia with eosinophilia. *Blood* 76:285-289.

Metzgeroth G, Walz C, Score J, et al [2007] Recurrent finding of the *FIP1L1-PDGFRA* fusion gene in eosinophilia-associated acute myeloid leukemia and lymphoblastic T-cell lymphoma. *Leukemia* 21:1183-1188.

Pardanani A, Ketterling RP, Brockman SR, et al [2003] *CHIC2* deletion, a surrogate for *FIP1L1-PDGFRA* fusion, occurs in systemic mastocytosis associated with eosinophilia and predicts response to imatinib mesylate therapy. *Blood* 102:3093-3096.

Passos-Bueno MR, Serti Eacute AE, Jehee FS, et al [2008] Genetics of craniosynostosis: genes, syndromes, mutations and genotype-phenotype correlations. *Front Oral Biol* 12:107-143.

Simon D, Salemi S, Yousefi S, Simon HU [2008] Primary resistance to imatinib in Fip1-like 1-platelet-derived growth factor receptor alpha-positive eosinophilic leukemia. *J Allergy Clin Immunol* 121:1054-1056.

Steer EJ, Cross NC [2002] Myeloproliferative disorders with translocations of chromosome 5q31-35: Role of the platelet-derived growth factor receptor Beta. *Acta Haematol* 107:113-122.

Tefferi A, Gilliland DG [2007] Oncogenes in myeloproliferative disorders. *Cell Cycle* 6:550-566.

Walz C, Metzgeroth G, Haferlach C, et al [2007] Characterization of three new imatinib-responsive fusion genes in chronic myeloproliferative disorders generated by disruption of the platelet-derived growth factor receptor beta gene. *Haematologica* 92:163-169.

Walz C, Haferlach C, Hanel A, et al [2009a] Identification of a *MYO18A-PDGFRB* fusion gene in an eosinophilia-associated atypical myeloproliferative neoplasm with a t(5;17)(q33-34;q11.2). *Genes Chromosomes Cancer* 48:179-183.

Walz C, Score J, Mix J, et al [2009b] The molecular anatomy of the *FIP1L1-PDGFRA* fusion gene. *Leukemia* 23:271-278.

Zota V, Miron PM, Woda BA, et al [2008] Eosinophilia with *FIP1L1-PDGFRA* fusion in a patient with chronic myelomonocytic leukemia. *J Clin Oncol* 26:2040-2041.

CHAPTER

Myelodysplastic Syndromes

Kathryn Foucar, MD

The successful diagnosis of a myelodysplastic syndrome (MDS) requires the integration of clinical, hematologic, morphologic, and genetic features. In some cases, especially low-grade disorders, MDS is a diagnosis of exclusion that can be made only after a thorough assessment to exclude non-neoplastic disorders. In contrast, the challenge in high-grade MDS is often the distinction between MDS and low blast count acute myeloid leukemia (AML). This chapter will focus on guiding the diagnostician by providing clues to recognize and subclassify MDS, warnings about diagnostic traps, and strategies to effectively evaluate specimens received to assess for possible MDS. The reader is referred to Chapter 13 for comparisons of the prototypic hematologic, morphologic, and bone marrow features among all myeloid neoplasms. As delineated in Chapter 13, each category of myeloid neoplasm exhibits prototypic hemogram, blood and bone marrow morphology, and core biopsy features.

There are 4 primary components in the definition of MDS. This clonal hematopoietic (HP) stem cell disorder is characterized by:

1. Unexplained and persistent cytopenia(s)
2. Dysplasia in at least 1 hematopoietic lineage
3. Ineffective hematopoiesis with bone marrow hypercellularity (increased apoptosis)
4. Risk of transformation to AML [Brunning 2008c, Orazi 2009, Vardiman 2008b]

The designation *idiopathic cytopenia of undetermined significance* (ICUS) has been proposed for cytopenia cases without dysplasia, reserving a diagnosis of MDS for cases with morphologic dysplasia [Valent 2007, Wimazal 2007]. Similarly, cases with persistent cytopenias *without* dysplasia but with an MDS-type cytogenetic abnormality can be called presumptive, but not definitive, MDS [Valent 2007].

The clinician plays the pivotal role in excluding other causes of persistent cytopenias, while the pathologist should interpret and oversee the routine and specialized testing performed on blood and bone marrow specimens **t16.1**. Primary tasks for the diagnostician include the enumeration of blasts in blood and bone marrow and the determination of type and extent of dysplasia and architectural abnormalities in erythroid, granulocytic, and megakaryocytic lineages. Flow cytometric immunophenotyping, although not required, can provide information about aberrant antigen expression to supplement the morphologic assessment for dysplasia. In contrast, conventional karyotyping should be considered in all cases, because this is the crucial method used to establish clonality, definitively excluding non-neoplastic disorders. Cytogenetic studies also contribute significant prognostic information. Other specialized tests, including flow cytometry for paroxysmal nocturnal hemoglobinuria (PNH), fluorescence in situ hybridization (FISH), and various molecular tests, should be considered on a case-by-case

t16.1 Approach to the Diagnosis of MDS

Clinical and hematologic features	Comprehensive clinical evaluation
	Document persistent cytopenia(s)
	Exclude non-MDS causes for cytopenias
Blood and bone marrow	Morphologic assessment for type and degree of MDS-related dysplastic features of individual cells on good quality specimens
	Assessment of BM architecture/topobiology to determine normal vs abnormal localizations and distribution of HP lineages and immature cells
	Blast enumeration
Conventional cytogenetics	Essential diagnostic test; requires adequate BM aspirate specimen
Flow cytometry	Not required for either blast enumeration (may be problematic) or assessment of lineage dysplasia based on aberrant antigen expression profile (complex interpretations)
	May provide useful ancillary information
Diagnostic interpretation	Requires integration of clinical, hematologic, morphologic, and genetic findings
	Provide WHO 2008 subtype:
	refractory anemia or refractory cytopenia with unilineage dysplasia
	myelodysplasia with isolated del(5q)
	refractory anemia with ring sideroblasts
	refractory cytopenia with multilineage dysplasia (with/without ring sideroblasts)
	refractory anemia with excess blasts-1, -2
	myelodysplastic syndrome, unclassifiable

BM = bone marrow; HP = hematopoietic; MDS = myelodysplastic syndrome; WHO = World Health Organization

basis. The results of all routine and specialized tests should be integrated into the diagnosis.

[16.1] Incidence, Epidemiology, and Pathogenesis

The prototypic patient with MDS is elderly (median age, 72 years). Incidence rates can approach 50 per 100,000 in this age group [Hofmann 2005, Steensma 2006, Strom 2008]. Only about 10% of MDS patients are <50 years old. MDS is exceedingly uncommon in children, in whom the incidence rate is below 0.01 per 100,000 [Bernasconi 2007, Strom 2008]. The development of MDS in younger patients is often linked to either underlying constitutional disorders or prior therapy. In recent years the incidence of therapy-related MDS (t-MDS) has been steadily increasing because of improved outcomes for patients treated with chemotherapy with or without autologous stem cell transplantation [Steensma 2006, Strom 2008].

The pathophysiology of MDS is complex, with a wide array of potential genetic changes, multiple clinical and biologic subtypes, and progression of many cases from early to high-grade processes. However, at the most general level, MDS represents a clonal proliferation (thus accounting for the hypercellularity seen in most cases) combined with increased apoptosis (thus resulting in ineffective hematopoiesis and cytopenias). The progression toward high-grade MDS and the transformation to AML involve the acquisition of additional molecular alterations that increase cell survival [Bernasconi 2008].

Because genetic changes vary by case and by subtype, we will use the del(5q), one of the best understood MDS-associated molecular abnormalities, as an illustrative example. Though at least 41 genes are contained within the minimal region of deletion in patients with the isolated del(5q), only 1 of these genes has been shown both to induce an MDS phenotype when experimentally inhibited *and* to correct the MDS phenotype when experimentally resupplied to cells harboring the del(5q) [Itzykson 2008]. This gene, *RPS14*, codes for a ribosomal subunit. Although the specific role of *RPS14* in hematopoiesis is not entirely clear, many other bone marrow failure syndromes, including Diamond-Blackfan anemia and Shwachman-Diamond syndrome, also involve abnormalities in ribosomal assembly. The del(5q) occurs in only a portion of MDS cases, and other cytogenetic abnormalities likely carry their own specific cellular consequences. High-resolution analysis has uncovered submicroscopic copy number changes throughout the genome, both in cases with normal karyotype and in cases with other visible karyotypic abnormalities [Paulsson 2006, Starczynowski 2008]. Thus, nonuniform but recurrent genetic changes, whether visible on the karyogram or not, are characteristic of MDS and likely serve as initiating or pivotal events in the development of MDS.

Clonal genetic changes alone do not account for the characteristic hematopoietic failure of MDS, which is associated with increased apoptosis and very often mediated by an immune response [Rosenfeld 2000, Sloand 2008]. CD8+ T cells from some MDS patients suppress colony formation in vivo, and are often clonal or oligoclonal, indicating a cellular immune response directed toward the marrow elements [Baumann 2002, Epling-Burnette 2007, Epperson 2001, Huh 2009, Melenhorst 2002]. In at least some cases, these T cells specifically destroy the malignant cells, perhaps upon recognizing novel or upregulated proteins generated by mutations [Sloand 2005, 2008]. However, apoptosis is increased in *both* the clonal and the background nonclonal marrow cells in MDS [Li 2004]. The apoptosis in the normal marrow elements may be due to an "innocent bystander" effect, in which they succumb to cytokines generated by the immune response. Indeed, increased levels of inflammatory cytokines and factors that suppress hematopoiesis, including tumor necrosis factor-α (TNF-α), interferon-γ (IFN-γ), Fas ligand, and TNF-related apoptosis-inducing ligand, are increased in the serum of MDS patients [Kerbauy 2007, Kitagawa 1997]. The progression to high-grade

MDS and AML occurs as additional genetic changes render the malignant cells insensitive to apoptotic stimuli and enhance their proliferative capacity [Bernasconi 2008, Rosenfeld 2000] (see **sidebar 16.1** for further discussion of MDS pathophysiology.)

[sidebar 16.1] **From Pathophysiology to Treatment (and Back Again) in MDS**

While we have considered therapeutic options to be generally beyond the scope of this book, in certain cases (eg, all-trans-retinoic acid [ATRA] in acute promyelocytic leukemia, imatinib in chronic myelogenous leukemia) a therapy directly targets a causative abnormality and thus becomes of interest to the student of pathology. Certain recent advances in the treatment of MDS belong to this category.

The immune system directly promotes apoptosis in many MDS bone marrows, especially via activation of CD8+ cytotoxic T cells [Baumann 2002, Epling-Burnette 2007, Epperson 2001, Huh 2009, Melenhorst 2002]. This response is further tied to changes in the T-cell regulatory population (Treg) and similar disturbances of immune regulation [Alfinito 2010, Kiladjian 2007, Kordasti 2007, Wu 2008]. These observations prompted the introduction of immunosuppression as a treatment for MDS. Though results have varied, a subset of cases (ranging from 15%-90%) clinically respond to immunosuppression [Kasner 2009]. Among the criteria that best predict response are age younger than 60 years, limited transfusion dependence, and HLA-DR15 [Melchert 2008, Saunthararajah 2002, 2003]. Interestingly, this HLA type is also significantly overrepresented in aplastic anemia, highlighting the importance of aberrant immune activity in this entity as well [Sugimori 2007].

The accumulation of additional genetic changes accompanies the evolution to high-grade MDS or AML. Loss of expression of tumor suppressor genes is central to this process and, as in all tumors, chromosomal deletion is one of the key mechanisms. In MDS, however, inactivation of these genes by aberrant hypermethylation plays an unusually important role (attachment of methyl groups to so-called CpG islands, often in the promoter regions of genes, silences expression). Pharmacologic reversal of this process would be expected to "reactivate" some of these tumor suppressor genes and ameliorate the MDS phenotype. In fact, 2 drugs, 5-azacitidine and its derivative, decitabine, achieve this goal. Both are cytidine analogues that are incorporated into DNA, where they irreversibly bind DNA methyltransferases responsible for maintaining stable methylation [Christman 2002]. By occupying and depleting methyltransferases, the drugs decrease the global degree of methylation throughout the genome. In the context of MDS, this leads to hematologic improvement, transfusion independence, and/or increased interval to the development of AML [Kasner 2009].

If the success of immunosuppressive and hypomethylating regimens makes logical sense based on the underlying pathophysiology, there is 1 new MDS treatment that does not fit this mold. Lenalidomide, an analogue of the drug thalidomide, has shown great success, especially in the treatment of patients with MDS with isolated del(5q) [List 2006]. It is far from clear, however, which of lenalidomide's wide array of documented effects is responsible for this karyotypic specificity. Among the candidates are immunomodulation, antiangiogenesis, antiadhesion, inhibition of tumor necrosis factor-α (TNF-α) production, and direct induction of apoptosis [Jadersten 2009]. Haploinsufficiency for the *RPS14* gene is thought to play a crucial role in MDS with isolated del(5q) [Itzykson 2008]. However, the direct connection between *RPS14*, which codes for a ribosomal subunit, and hematopoietic failure remains to be established. Indeed, recent data suggest that the interaction of lenalidomide with cell-cycle control phosphatases encoded by genes on 5q may be the crucial pharmacologic mechanism [Wei 2009]. The remarkable efficacy of lenalidomide in patients with isolated del(5q) may yet provide a key insight into the exact mechanism by which deletion of the region contributes to the development of MDS.

[16.2] Prognostic Factors in MDS

Because of the association with both overall survival and progression rate over time to AML, significant emphasis has been placed on delineating prognostic factors in MDS t16.2 [Alessandrino 2008, Bernasconi 2007, Greenberg 1997, Haase 2007, Kao 2008, Malcovati 2005b, 2007, Verburgh 2007]. Several systems have been devised to incorporate key prognostic factors; the International Prognostic Scoring System (IPSS) was proposed in 1997, while the World Health Organization (WHO) classification-based prognostic scoring system (WPSS) was proposed in 2007 t16.3 [Greenberg 1997, Malcovati 2007]. Overall median survival time ranges from 141 months for very-low-risk MDS patients to 9 months for very-high-risk patients, while cumulative probability of transformation to AML at 5 years ranges from 0.03 for very-low-risk patients to 0.84 for high-risk patients [Malcovati 2007].

t16.2 Prognostic Factors in Myelodysplasia*

Factor	Comment
Age	Worse outcome linked to older age
Cytopenia(s)[†]	Severity of anemia most consistent hematologic factor linked to outcome
	Worst outcome for patients with hemoglobin <8 g/dL
	Number of cytopenias utilized in IPSS score
% blasts in BM	Generally categorized by progressively increasing ranges: <5, 5-10, 11-20
Karyotype	Good risk: normal, −Y, del(5q), del(20q)
	Poor risk: complex (≥3) abnormalities, −7, del(7q)
	Intermediate risk: other abnormalities (for IPSS and WPSS scores)
	Median survival 53 months for patients with normal karyotype; 9 months for patients with complex abnormal karyotype
WHO subtype	Lowest risk: RA, RARS, RA with del(5q)
	Intermediate risk (2 groups): RCMD (with/without RS); RAEB-1
	Highest risk: RAEB-2 (for WPSS score)
Multilineage dysplasia	Significant factor in some studies; linked to WPSS
Transfusion requirement	Significant factor in WPSS

*See t16.3 for IPSS and WPSS
[†]A recent study suggests that lymphopenia (≤1.2×10⁹/L) is linked to adverse outcomes [Jacobs 2010]
BM = bone marrow; IPSS = International Prognostic Scoring System; RA = refractory anemia; RAEB = refractory anemia with excess blasts; RARS = refractory anemia with ring sideroblasts; RCMD = refractory cytopenia with multilineage dysplasia; RS = ring sideroblasts; WHO = World Health Organization; WPSS = WHO-classification based prognostic scoring system

References: [Alessandrino 2008, Bernasconi 2007, Greenberg 1997, Haase 2007, Kao 2008, Malcovati 2005b,2007, Verburgh 2007]

t16.3 Prognostic Factor Scoring Systems in Myelodysplastic Syndromes

IPSS

Score	0	0.5	1	1.5	2
% BM blasts	<5	5-10		11-15	20-30*
Karyotype (see t16.2)	Good	Intermediate		Poor	
Number of cytopenias	0-1	2-3			

WPSS

Score	0	1	2	3
WHO category	RA, RARS, RA del(5q)	RCMD, RCMD-RS	RAEB-1	RAEB-2
Karyotype (see t16.2)	Good	Intermediate	Poor	
Transfusion requirement	No	Regular[†]		

Overall IPSS Score		Overall WPSS Score	
Total Score	**Comments[‡]**	**Total Score**	**Comments**
0	Low risk; median survival 5.7 years	0	Very low risk; 90% 5-year survival
0.5-1.0	Intermediate 1; median survival 3.5 years	1	Low risk; 70% 5-year survival
1.5-2.0	Intermediate 2; median survival 1.2 years	2	Intermediate risk; 50% 5-year survival
≥2.5	High risk ; median survival 0.4 years	3-4	High risk; 20% 5-year survival

*Cases classified as AML based on WHO 2001 and 2008
[†]Tranfusions at least every 8 weeks over a 4-month period
[‡]Cases with 20%-30% blasts included in IPSS; these cases now fulfill criteria for AML
AML = acute myeloid leukemia; BM = bone marrow; IPSS = International Prognostic Scoring System; RA = refractory anemia; RAEB = refractory anemia with excess blasts; RARS = refractory anemia with ring sideroblasts; RCMD = refractory cytopenia with multilineage dysplasia; RS = ring sideroblasts; WHO = World Health Organization; WPSS = WHO-classification-based prognostic scoring system

References: [Greenberg 1997, Malcovati 2007]

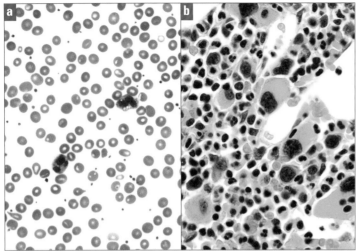

i16.1 *This composite from a patient with low-grade myelodysplasia shows moderate anemia with macrocytosis (note lack of polychromasia)* **a**, *while the bone marrow shows hypercellularity with increased and clustered hypolobated megakaryocytes* **b**. *(Wright, H&E)*

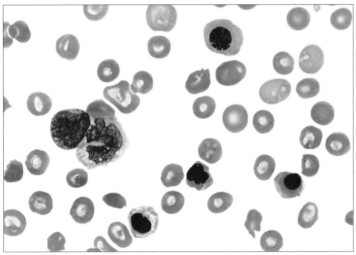

i16.2 *This peripheral blood smear is from a patient with refractory anemia with excess blasts-2 and shows severe cytopenias, circulating blasts, numerous nucleated red blood cells, and an enlarged, hypogranular platelets. (Wright)*

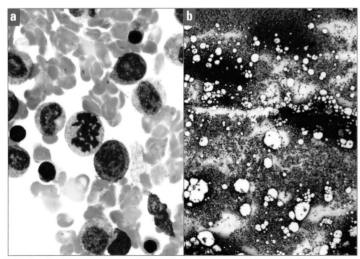

i16.3 *This bone marrow composite from a patient with high-grade myelodys-plasia shows increased blasts* **a** *and a markedly hypercellular bone marrow as evidenced on low magnification* **b**. *(Wright)*

[16.3] Hematologic Features and Minimal Diagnostic Criteria

Single or multilineage cytopenias are a hallmark of MDS, while hypercellularity, intact maturation, architectural abnormalities, variable percentage of blasts (<20%), and hematopoietic lineage dysplasia together comprise the prototypic profile of MDS in bone marrow i16.1, i16.2, i16.3, i16.4, t16.4 [Bernasconi 2007, Brunning 2008c, Steensma 2006, Vardiman 2008b].

t16.4 Prototypic Blood and Bone Marrow Features of MDS

Blood	
Anemia	85% of cases
	<10 g/dL in 60% of patients
	Often macrocytic (reduced polychromasia)
Neutropenia	40% of cases
	Functional defects common
	Dysplastic features common
Thrombocytopenia	30%-40% of cases
	Functional defects common
	May be dysplastic
Pancytopenia	15% of cases
	Dysplastic features common
Circulating blasts	Common in more high grade MDS
	Percentage critical for classification

Bone Marrow	
Cellularity	Typically hypercellular (90% of cases) with intact HP lineage maturation
Blast %, dysplasia	Blast %, individual cell dysplasia assessment critical for classification
Architecture/ topobiology	Abnormal localization of both immature myeloid cells (ALIP) and megakaryocytes common
	Abnormal localization of granulocytic and erythroid cells common
	Increased megakaryocytes with clustering and dysplasia (may be paratrabecular)
Bone marrow stroma and bone	Subset of cases (~10%) may show fibrosis or hypocellularity
	Bony trabeculae usually normal
	Sinuses usually normal
	Histiocytes increased
	Small vessel neoangiogenesis; larger vessels unremarkable

HP = hematopoietic ; MDS = myelodysplastic syndrome

References: [Bernasconi 2007, Brunning 2008c, Steensma 2006, Vardiman 2008b]

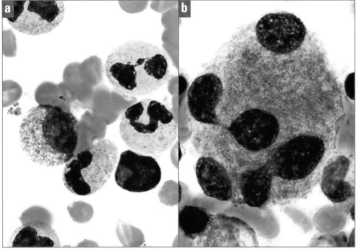

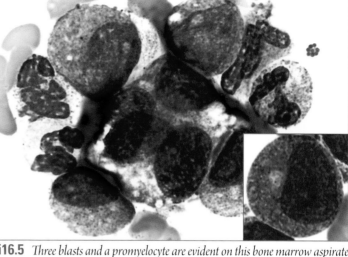

i16.4 *This composite highlights the prototypic dysplastic changes in a patient with high-grade myelodysplasia including numerous hypogranular and hypolobated neutrophils* **a** *in conjunction with a markedly abnormal megakaryocyte with separate nuclei* **b**. *(Wright)*

i16.5 *Three blasts and a promyelocyte are evident on this bone marrow aspirate smear, while the inset shows a classic promyelocyte with a prominent clear paranuclear hof (Golgi region). (Wright)*

[16.3.1] **Blast Enumeration**

The percentage of blasts in blood and bone marrow includes myeloblasts, monoblasts, promonocytes, and megakaryoblasts, but myeloblasts are by far the most frequent blast type in MDS **i16.5** [Vardiman 2008b]. Megakaryoblasts should be distinguished from maturing megakaryocytic cells **i16.6**. Blasts are counted as a percentage of total nucleated cells, but both lymphocytes and plasma cells should be excluded in patients with underlying lymphoid/plasma cell neoplasms [Vardiman 2008b]. Similarly, maturing megakaryocytic cells are not included in these differential cell counts. Because both chronic myelomonocytic leukemias and juvenile myelomonocytic leukemias are included among cases of MDS/MPN (myelodysplastic/myeloproliferative neoplasms), monoblasts and promonocytes are seldom a significant component of blasts in MDS.

Consequently, the main challenge in blast enumeration in MDS is the distinction between a myeloblast (agranular and granular subtypes) and a promyelocyte [Mufti 2008]. Although the nuclear chromatin shows progressive condensation with successive stages of maturation, the presence of an eccentric nucleus with a distinctly visible paranuclear Golgi zone (hof) is the primary feature used to identify early promyelocytes **i16.5** [Mufti 2008]. Cells with these features are not included in the blast percentage. The blast percentage is always <20% in MDS, and in many cases the blast count falls within the normal range (see **[16.5]** "Classification of MDS," p 343). Accurate blast enumeration may be problematic on suboptimal specimens; immunohistochemical assessment for CD34 may be helpful in these situations. Although the WHO 2008 criteria for MDS blast percentage is based on total nucleated cells, recent investigators suggest that outcomes may be better

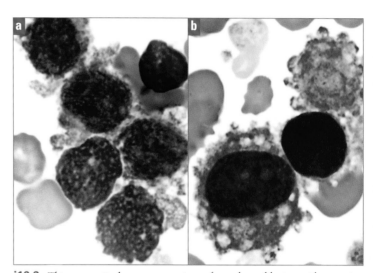

i16.6 *This composite shows a comparison of megakaryoblasts* **a** *with maturing megakaryocytic cells* **b**. *Only megakaryoblasts are included in the blast percentage. (Wright)*

predicted by basing the blast percentage on nonerythroid cells for erythroid-predominant (≥50%) cases, analogous to AML criteria [Wang 2008]. If the erythroid predominant case consists largely of erythroblasts, a diagnosis of acute erythroid leukemia should be considered (see Chapter 18).

[16.3.2] **Hematopoietic Lineage Dysplasia and Architectural Assessment**

The confirmation of dysplasia in erythroid, granulocytic, and megakaryocytic lineage cells is challenging for several reasons. First, at least 10% of cells in a given lineage must show dysplasia by WHO 2008 criteria, and the type of morphologic abnormality used to qualify as "dysplasia" must be of a "MDS" type **t16.5**. These dysplastic features involve nuclear and cytoplasmic abnormalities in erythroid,

t16.5 Dysplastic Features in Myelodysplasia

Lineage	Blood	Bone Marrow
Erythroid	No specific features required	Nuclei: budding, multinucleation, karyorrhexis, megaloblastic changes, internuclear bridging
	Often see anisopoikilocytosis, macrocytosis (both non-specific)*	Cytoplasm: ring sideroblasts, vacuolization, PAS positivity
		Biopsy: loss of colony formation
Granulocytic	Nuclei: hyposegmentation, hypersegmentation, myelokathexis-like thin interlobar strands	Nuclei: hyposegmentation, variable left shift, megaloblastic changes
	Cytoplasm: hypogranularity, often with Döhle body–like structures	Cytoplasm: hypogranularity, enlarged pseudo Chédiak-Higashi granules, Auer rods[†]
	Left shift, variable % myeloblasts	Biopsy: ALIP
Megakaryocytic[‡]	Large, hypogranular platelets	Nuclei: hypolobation, widely spaced nuclei (multinucleation), micromegakaryocytes
		Biopsy: increased numbers, small overall size, clustering, abnormal paratrabecular localization; CD34 positivity of megakaryocytes
Monocytic[§]	Immature, abnormal forms	Nuclei: dispersed chromatin, nucleoli
	If monocytosis present, should consider MDS/MPN	Cytoplasm: hypogranular

*Rare cases of MDS show striking anisopoikilocytosis with spherocytes mimicking microangiopathic hemolytic anemia; other rare cases exhibit an acquired α thalassemia picture (see t16.11)
[†]Auer rods very rare in MDS; consider low blast count acute myeloid leukemia
[‡]Dysplasia quantitated on core biopsy based on assessment of 30 megakaryocytes
[§]Monocytosis not compatible with diagnosis of MDS; consider MDS/MPN

ALIP = abnormal localization of immature precursors; MDS/MPN = myelodysplastic/myeloproliferative neoplasm; PAS = periodic acid-Schiff

References: [Brunning 2008c, Steensma 2006, Vardiman 2008b]

granulocytic, and megakaryocytic cells i16.7, i16.8, i16.9, i16.10, i16.11, i16.12, i16.13, i16.14, i16.15, i16.16, i16.17, i16.18, i16.19, i16.20, i16.21. Features on biopsy sections are also used to categorize dysplasia, especially for megakaryocytes, and immunohistochemistry can be used to assess the hemato-poietic architecture, which is frequently abnormal in MDS i16.17, i16.20, i16.21, i16.22, i16.23, i16.24, i16.25. In addition, the assessment for abnormal localization of immature

precursors (ALIP) is best done on core biopsy sections by integrating morphology and immunohistochemistry i16.26, i16.27, i16.28. Technically excellent blood smears, bone marrow aspirate smears, and core biopsy sections are essential for the assessment of dysplasia. The assessment of neutrophil cytoplasmic granularity is especially problematic on suboptimally stained smears.

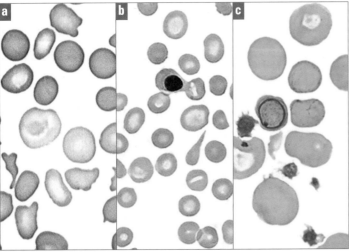

i16.7 *Peripheral blood smears from 3 patients with myelodysplasia illustrate the spectrum of RBC abnormalities. Note occasional hypochromic forms, moderate to marked anisopoikilocytosis, and rare Cabot rings. (Wright)*

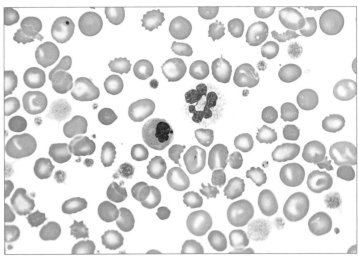

i16.8 *Marked anisopoikilocytosis including circulating normoblasts is evident on this peripheral blood smear from a patient with myelodysplasia. Note hypogranular neutrophil. (Wright)*

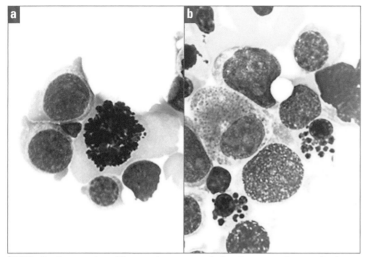

i16.9 *Striking erythroid karyorrhexis in myelodysplasia is evident on this bone marrow aspirate smear composite. (Wright)*

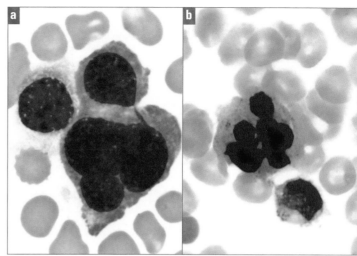

i16.10 *This composite illustrates pseudocongenital dyserythropoietic anemia-like multinucleation in a patient with myelodysplasia. (Wright)*

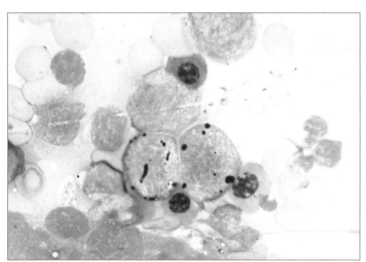

i16.11 *The various patterns of periodic acid-Schiff (PAS) reactivity in erythroid elements in myelodysplasia are illustrated on this bone marrow aspirate smear. Note distinctly globular (beaded) reaction pattern in immature erythroid cells, while maturing orthochromic normoblasts exhibit a diffuse cytoplasmic positivity. (PAS)*

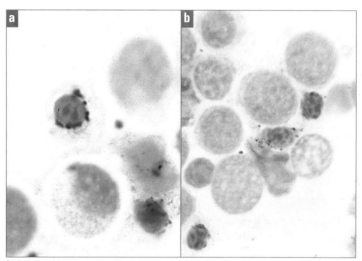

i16.12 *This composite illustrates multiple ring sideroblasts in 2 cases of myelodysplasia. (Prussian blue)*

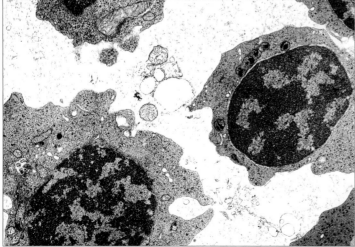

i16.13 *Electron micrograph illustrates iron within paranuclear mitochondria in a patient with myelodysplasia with ring sideroblasts. (electron microscopy)*

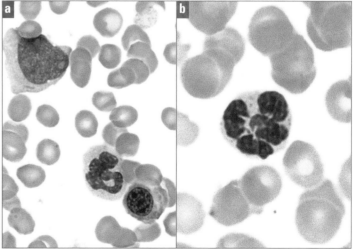

i16.14 *Composite of peripheral blood smears from a child **a** and an adult **b** with myelodysplasia illustrate circulating myeloblasts, hypogranular neutrophils, and hypersegmented neutrophils. (Wright)*

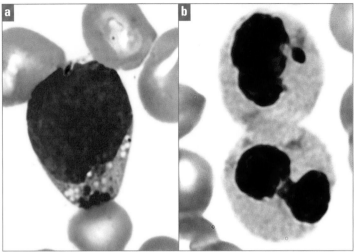

i16.15 *This composite illustrates granulocytic lineage abnormalities in 2 patients with myelodysplasia. A myeloblast with pseudo Chédiak-Higashi granules is evident in the peripheral blood **a**, while neutrophils which exhibit profoundly hypogranular cytoplasm and Döhle bodies in conjunction with nuclear hyposegmentation are evident **b**. (Wright)*

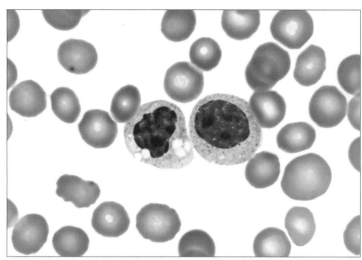

i16.16 *Hypercondensed chromatin is evident in 2 neutrophils from a patient with myelodysplasia. Note nuclear hyposegmentation. (Wright)*

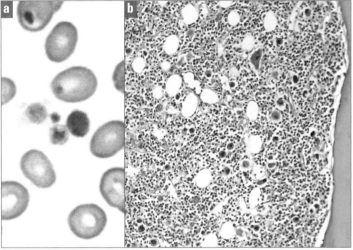

i16.17 *This composite shows peripheral blood **a** and a bone marrow core biopsy **b** specimens from a patient with myelodysplasia in which the circulating platelets are large and hypogranular; the bone marrow specimen shows hypercellularity with increased hypolobated megakaryocytes. (Wright, H&E)*

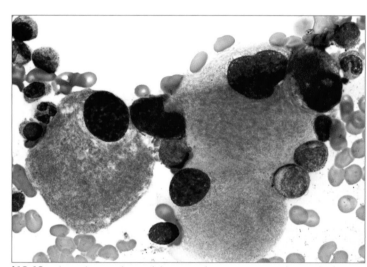

i16.18 *Three abnormal monolobate megakaryocytes are evident in this bone marrow aspirate smear from a patient with myelodysplasia. (Wright)*

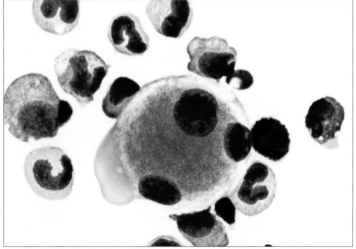

i16.19 *A megakaryocyte with 3 separate nuclei (so-called "pawn ball" megakaryocyte) is evident on this cytospin smear from a patient with myelodysplasia. (Wright)*

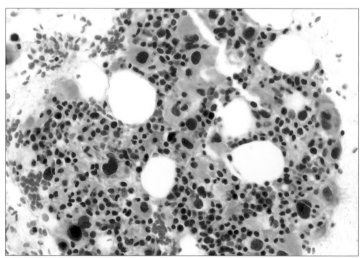

i16.20 *This bone marrow clot section is from a 76-year-old female with pancytopenia. Note overall hypercellular bone marrow with markedly increased megakaryocytes, which show clustering and nuclear hypolobation. (H&E)*

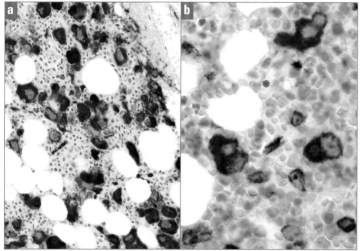

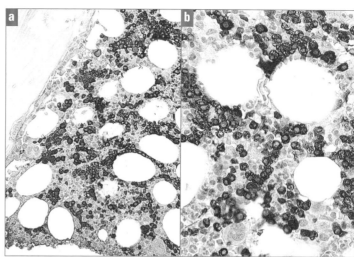

i16.21 *This composite of 2 patients with myelodysplasia demonstrates megakary-ocytes highlighted by immunoperoxidase staining for CD42b* **a**, *and increased and minimally clustered myeloblasts in conjunction with CD34+ megakaryocytes, a common feature in myelodysplasia, highlighted by CD34 immunohistochemical staining* **b** . *(immunoperoxidase for CD42b and CD34)*

i16.22 *This composite highlights normal erythroid colony formation at low* **a** *and intermediate* **b** *magnification. Note tendency for erythroid cells to show clustering, so-called colony formation. (immunoperoxidase for hemoglobin A)*

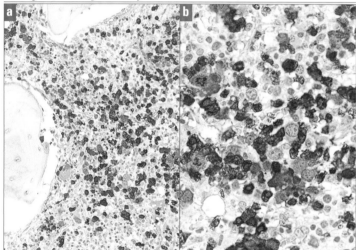

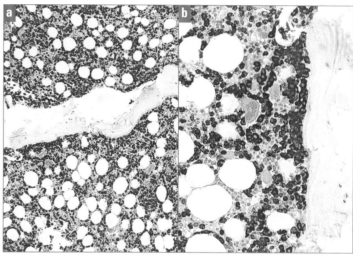

i16.23 *This composite shows the low- and intermediate-magnification appearance of disrupted red cell colonies, a typical feature in more high-grade myelodysplastic processes. Note loss of colony formation. (immunoperoxidase for hemoglobin A)*

i16.24 *This composite highlights normal myeloperoxidase staining at low* **a** *and intermediate* **b** *magnification. Note paratrabecular localization of brightly myeloperoxidase-positive immature granulocytic cells. (immunoperoxidase for myeloperoxidase)*

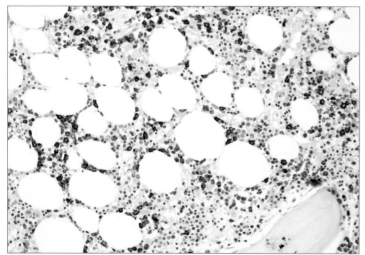

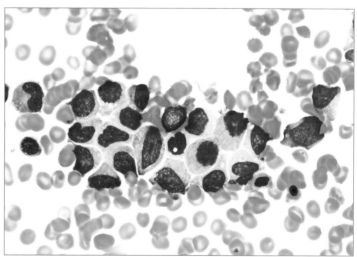

i16.25 *This bone marrow core biopsy section from a patient with myelodys-plasia illustrates abnormal localization of immature precursors (ALIP) in that the brightly myeloperoxidase positive cells are aggregated distally from their normal paratrabecular localization. (immunoperoxidase for myeloperoxidase)*

i16.26 *Abnormal localization of immature precursors is evident on this bone marrow aspirate smear in which immature granulocytic cells hold together in clusters. (Wright)*

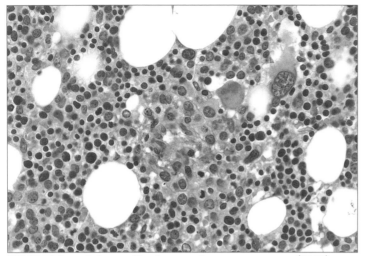

i16.27 *A focus of abnormal localization of immature precursors (ALIP) is evident in the center of this bone marrow core biopsy section. (H&E)*

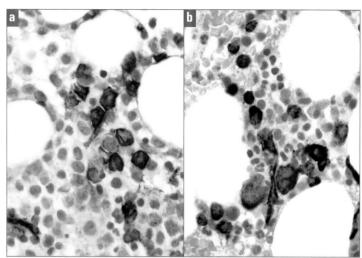

i16.28 *This composite illustrates the immunohistochemical features of abnormal localization of immature precursors (ALIP) in that a cluster of CD34+ cells is evident* **a***, while both clustering of CD34+ cells and CD34+ megakaryocytes are evident in another patient with ALIP* **b***. (immunoperoxidase for CD34)*

[16.3.3]   **Minimal Diagnostic Criteria**

Based on an integrative approach, definitive diagnosis of MDS is possible in many cases **t16.6** [Valent 2007, Wimazal 2007]. Once a diagnostic threshold has been achieved, the application of WHO criteria for subclassification is relatively straightforward (see **[16.6]** "Unique Types of MDS," p 350). However, many cases may exhibit some, but not all, features of MDS. In these cases, cytogenetic confirmation is essential (see **[16.5]** "Classification of MDS," p 343). Other specialized tests may provide strong support for a diagnosis of MDS, but the value of these tests in MDS is not as clear-cut as cytogenetics **t16.6** (see **[16.5]** "Classification of MDS," p 343).

[16.3.4]   **Idiopathic Cytopenia of Uncertain (Undetermined) Significance**

The designation ICUS has been proposed for cases in which unexplained prolonged cytopenia(s) is/are well-documented, blasts are not increased, dysplasia is absent, and cytogenetics are either normal or not performed [Valent 2007, Wimazal 2007]. Careful assessment is required to exclude other causes of cytopenia(s), and close clinical follow-up is essential. Subsequent bone marrow examinations may provide definitive evidence of MDS [Valent 2007].

[16.4]   **Specialized Studies in MDS**

[16.4.1]   **Conventional Cytogenetics**

Even though there are no MDS-defining cytogenetic abnormalities, conventional karyotyping is still by far the most important specialized test in the evaluation of a patient for possible MDS. A clonal abnormal conventional karyotype is detected in 40%-60% of all cases of MDS and in >85% of cases of t-MDS [Bernasconi 2007, Brunning 2008c, Haase 2007, Steensma 2006,

t16.6 Minimal Diagnostic Criteria in MDS

Definitive Diagnosis of MDS

Sustained cytopenia(s)
Other causes of cytopenia(s) excluded
Dysplasia ≥10% of cells in at least 1 hematopoietic lineage
5%-19% blasts in bone marrow
With/without clonal cytogenetic abnormality of MDS type (see **[16.4]**)

or

Same as above except blasts not increased
Other causes of cytopenias excluded
Dysplasia ≥10% of cells in at least 1 hematopoietic lineage
Clonal cytogenetic abnormality of MDS type (cytogenetic confirmation especially important in unilineage cytopenia/dysplasia cases)

Presumptive Diagnosis of MDS

Sustained cytopenia(s) without dysplasia
Other causes of cytopenia(s) excluded
Clonal cytogenetic abnormality of MDS type
Other presumptive criteria:
    abnormal flow cytometric immunophenotype compatible with MDS **t16.9**
    clonal hematopoiesis based on molecular assay (eg, HUMARA)
    RAS mutations based on molecular assay

Idiopathic Cytopenia of Uncertain (Undetermined) Significance (ICUS)

Sustained cytopenia(s) without dysplasia
All other causes of cytopenia(s) excluded
Normal blast percentage
Lack of any presumptive criteria
Subsequent bone marrow examination, special studies required for definitive diagnosis

HUMARA = human androgen receptor assay; MDS = myelodysplastic syndrome

References: [Valent 2007, Wimazal 2007]

t16.7 Cytogenetic Abnormalities in MDS*

Abnormality[†]	Frequency (%)		Comments in de novo MDS[‡]
	MDS	t-MDS	
del(5q)	10-25	40	Median survival 80 months
+8[§]	10-20		Median survival 25 months
−7, del(7q)	10-15	50	Median survival 14 months
del(20q)[§]	5-8		Median survival 70 months; macrocytosis, thrombocytopenia, minimal (if any) dysplasia
del(11q)	3-7		Median survival 16 months
del(17p)	1-3	25	Small neutrophils, pseudo Pelger-Huët nuclei, cytoplasmic vacuoles; often seen in t-MDS
+21	1-5		Median survival 100 months
−5	1-5		Median survival 15 months
−Y[§]	1-5		Most predictive of myeloid neoplasm when detected in all metaphases
Complex karyotype	15		Median survival 9 months
Balanced translocation	<1	2-3	Variety of translocations described

*Karyotype is a prognostically significant factor used in prognosis scoring systems (see **t16.3**)
[†]50% of all MDS cases have an abnormal conventional karyotype [Haase 2007]
[‡]Comments relate to de novo MDS unless specified
[§]The presence of +8, del(20q), or −Y as sole chomosomal abnormalities in the absence of morphologic dysplasia is *not* considered presumptive evidence of MDS when combined with idiopathic persistent cytopenia(s), in contrast to other abnormalities listed here
MDS = myelodysplastic syndrome; t-MDS = therapy-related MDS

References: [Bernasconi 2007, Brunning 2008c, Gupta 2007, Haase 2007, Hofmann 2005, Ogata 2006, Steensma 2006, Wong 2008]

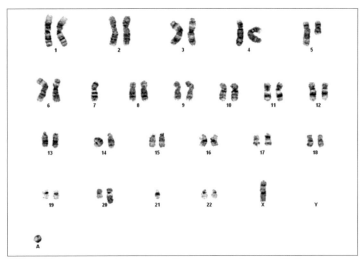

f16.1 *This conventional karyotype of bone marrow from an elderly patient with refractory cytopenia with multilineage dysplasia shows complex adverse risk cytogenetic abnormalities including del(5q) and monosomy 7.*

t16.8 Frequency of Cytogenetic Abnormalities Based on WHO Subtype of MDS

Subtype	% with Cytogenetic Abnormality	% with Unfavorable Karyotype
RA	30-40	15-20
MDS del(5q)	100*	0
RARS	10-25	0
RCMD[†]	40-50	10-20
RCMD-RS[†]	40-60	16-25
RAEB-1	55-70	15-25
RAEB-2	50-75	15-25
MDS-U	60	NA

*Defined by karyotype
[†]Same subtype in WHO 2008

MDS = myelodysplastic syndrome; NA = not available; RA = refractory anemia; RAEB = refractory anemia with excess blasts; RARS = refractory anemia with ring sideroblasts; RCMD = refractory cytopenia with multilineage dysplasia; WHO = World Health Organization

References: [Bernasconi 2007, Germing 2006b, Haase 2007]

Vardiman 2008b]. Although there are no cytogenetic abnormalities unique to MDS, certain abnormalities are quite characteristic of MDS and comprise the MDS-associated cytogenetic features that can be used to confirm this diagnosis **t16.7**. The most common cytogenetic abnormalities in MDS involve a gain or loss of chromosomal material, often involving chromosomes 5, 7, and 8 **f16.1**.

Karyotype is also an important prognostic factor used in both current prognostic scoring systems, IPSS and WPSS (see **t16.3**). Karyotype is also linked to specific WHO subtypes of MDS in that adverse prognostic types of karyotypic abnormalities are more frequently identified in more high-grade MDS **t16.8**. Median survival times range from 53 months for MDS patients with normal karyotypes to 9 months for patients with complex cytogenetic abnormalities [Haase 2007].

[16.4.2] **Fluorescence In Situ Hybridization (FISH)**
Conventional cytogenetics is the preferred mode of bone marrow assessment in patients with suspected MDS, but FISH studies also have a role in the assessment of cryptic

abnormalities and in situations in which conventional cytogenetic study is unsuccessful/unavailable [Bernasconi 2003, Cherry 2003, Pitchford 2010]. In addition, FISH testing may reveal clonal cytogenetic abnormalities in specimens with a normal karyotype, but a large probe set is required [Bernasconi 2003].

[16.4.3] **Other Molecular Genetic Tests in MDS**
Various molecular genetic tests have been applied to MDS specimens to detect single-nucleotide polymorphisms, *FLT3* mutations, *BMI1* expression, and for gene expression profiling of CD34+ cells [Boultwood 2007, Georgiou 2006, Gondek 2008, Mihara 2006, Mohamedali 2007]. These molecular tests provide information about the pathophysiology of MDS, potential targeted therapy options,

and enhance patient risk stratification for early therapeutic interventions. Further incorporation of molecular testing into routine MDS assessment is likely, especially as targeted therapy options expand.

[16.4.4] Immunophenotyping in MDS

Although the usefulness of immunohistochemical staining in MDS specimens for CD34, myeloperoxidase, and various megakaryocyte antigens is well-established, the role of flow cytometric immunophenotyping (FCI) in MDS diagnosis is more controversial t16.9 [Cherian 2005a,2005b, Della Porta 2006, Maftoun-Banankhah 2008, Malcovati 2005a, Matarraz 2008, Ogata 2006, Orazi 2009, Pirruccello 2006, Scott 2008, Sternberg 2005, Tsao 2007, Valent 2007, van de Loosdrecht 2008, Wang 2009]. While FCI is useful for the delineation of CD34+ cells, the usual caveats about hemodilution of the specimen, lysing of erythroid cells, and other factors artifactually skewing CD34 percentages apply [Loken 2008]. Furthermore, the assessment of CD34+ cells for aberrant antigen expression requires that numerous antibodies be used in a multicolor assessment [Ogata 2006, Pirruccello 2006]. Because the abnormal myeloid cells in MDS deviate from normal cells in terms of the pattern of antigen expression with maturation, assessment of these patterns of antigen expression by FCI has become common in MDS [Stetler-Stevenson 2009]. However, the FCI assessment of individual lineages or individual cell types such as granulocytes or monocytes also requires at least 4-color (usually 6- to 8-color) flow cytometry, numerous antibodies, specific gating strategies, and fairly subjective visual evaluation of complex patterns t16.9 [Cherian 2005a,2005b, Della Porta 2006, Loken 2008, Malcovati 2005a]. In addition, many specimen handling and technical factors can influence these complex patterns of antigen expression [Loken 2008]. In many cases, especially those cases of morphologically straightforward MDS, the extent of FCI aberrations generally parallels that seen on morphologic examination [Della Porta 2006, van de Loosdrecht 2008]. However, FCI may be particularly useful in morphologically indeterminate cases in which positive FCI may provide presumptive evidence of MDS [Stetler-Stevenson 2001, 2009, Truong 2009]. Because the interpretation of FCI data regarding maturation expression profiles is complex, the use of scoring systems to separate cases into normal, mild, moderate, and severe categories based on the number of immunophenotypic abnormalities is recommended [Cherian 2005a, 2005b, Loken 2008, Scott 2008, Stetler-Stevenson 2009, van de Loosdrecht 2008]. This FCI score may even predict outcome in MDS patients undergoing stem cell transplant [Scott 2008].

[16.4.5] Hematogones in Myelodysplasia

One distinctive finding by comprehensive FCI of bone marrow specimens from patients with MDS is that immunophenotypic hematogones are consistently reduced below levels detected in age-/sex-matched controls [Maftoun-Banankhah 2008, Matarraz 2008, Ogata 2006, Tsao 2007]. Because standardization of the FCI

t16.9 Flow Cytometric Immunophenotyping in MDS

Immunophenotypic Assessment	Aberrant Features/Comments
CD34+ myeloid cells	Coexpression of CD11c, CD15, CD4, CD7, CD10, CD19, CD56
	Abnormal patterns of CD34 and CD117 expression
	Decreased CD45 intensity
	Absent CD13, CD33, or HLA-DR
CD34+ lymphoid cells	Cells with immunophenotypic profile of hematogones significantly reduced
Granulocytes/ maturing myeloid cells	Reduced side scatter of granulocytes
	Coexpression of CD11a, CD66, CD56, CD34
	Reduced CD10, CD13, CD33 expression
Erythroid lineage cells	Synchronous expression of CD71 and glycophorin A (GlyA)
	Increased expression of CD105
	Coexpression of CD34, CD117, CD235a
Monocytic cells	Abnormal expression profile for HLA-DR, CD13, CD14, CD33, CD45, CD36
	Coexpression of CD56, CD7, CD19, CD34
Reduced hematogones	Immature B-cell population exhibiting spectrum of maturation
	Hematogones reduced in low-grade MDS compared with bone marrow specimens from age-matched controls
Paroxysmal nocturnal hemoglobinuria	Loss/reduced expression of GPI-associated antigens (eg, CD14 on monocytes, CD24 on granulocytes, CD55/CD59 on a subset of erythrocytes, granulocytes, or monocytes

References: [Cherian 2005a,2005b, Della Porta 2006, Maftoun-Banankhah 2008, Malcovati 2005a, Matarraz 2008, Ogata 2006, Orazi 2009, Pirruccello 2006, Scott 2008, Sternberg 2005, Tsao 2007, Valent 2007, van de Loosdrecht 2008, Wang 2009]

patterns of antigen expression in hematogone populations is good, a negative association with MDS may be a useful adjunct in the diagnosis of morphologically indeterminate cases, especially since reduced hematogones may be more evident in patients with "early" (low-risk) MDS [Sternberg 2005].

[16.4.6] Paroxysmal Nocturnal Hemoglobinuria Studies

There are several reasons why assessment for underlying paroxysmal nocturnal hemoglobinuria (PNH) is important in the evaluation of patients for possible MDS. First, PNH, especially the hypoproliferative variant, may mimic MDS by producing a chronic anemia without an adequate reticulocyte response [Orazi 2009]. Other cytopenias may also be present in these patients. Second, low-level PNH clones may be identified in patients with MDS [Wang 2009]. The best testing modality for PNH is FCI for reduced expression of GPI-associated antigens (see Chapters 6 and 11 for more details) [Orazi 2009, Wang 2009]. The detection of a prominent

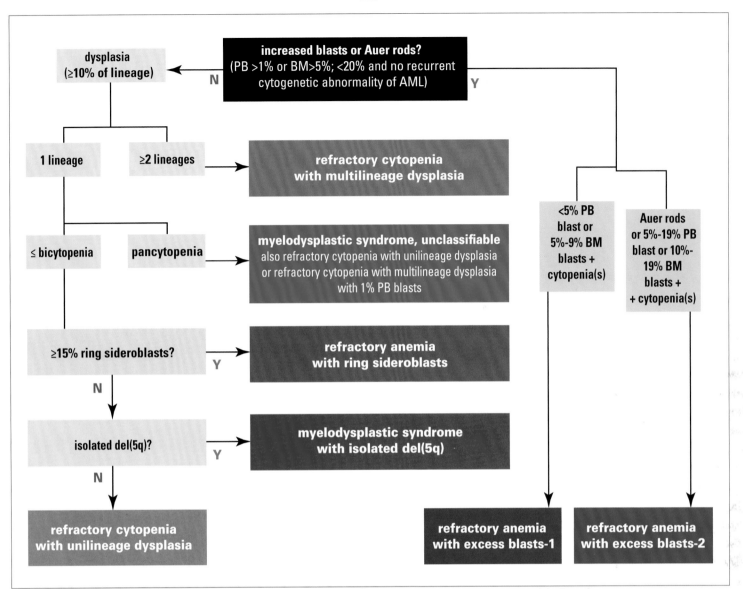

f16.2 *Myelodysplasia algorithm. BM = bone marrow; PB = peripheral blood (redrawn with permission, courtesy C Pitchford, MD)*

population of cells with reduced expression of GPI-associated antigens favors PNH, while finding a smaller subset of abnormal populations supports a diagnosis of MDS.

[16.5] Classification of MDS

The classification requirements and key features of the WHO 2008 subtypes of MDS are detailed in **f16.2** and **t16.10** [Bernasconi 2007, Brunning 2008a, 2008b, 2008c, Haase 2007, Hasserjian 2008a, Orazi 2008b, 2009, Steensma 2006, Vardiman 2008b]. The blood and bone marrow criteria are generally easy to apply in MDS provided that specimens are of good quality and that the diagnostician is adept at blast identification, blast enumeration, and the assessment of specific dysplastic features for all hematopoietic lineages as discussed earlier in this chapter **f16.2**. The number of MDS, unclassifiable cases is generally <5% in large series [Bernasconi 2007]. Iron stains should be performed routinely on bone marrow aspirate smears to assess for ring sideroblasts and dysplastic

coarse iron granules. Cytochemical stains, such as myeloperoxidase and nonspecific esterase, may be necessary in some cases for determination of blast lineage. As emphasized earlier, neither erythroblasts nor promyelocytes are included in the blast percentage.

[16.5.1] Refractory Cytopenias with Unilineage Dysplasia (RCUD)

Refractory anemia accounts for the clear-cut majority of cases of RCUD. Indeed both refractory neutropenia and refractory thrombocytopenia are sufficiently rare in adults to warrant strong consideration of other differential diagnostic possibilities [Brunning 2008b]. The complete blood count may show a single cytopenia or bicytopenia. Cases of pancytopenia with low blood/bone marrow blast counts and unilineage dysplasia should be classified as MDS, unclassifiable (MDS-U) [Brunning 2008b]. Aside from cytopenia(s), the blood smear may be unremarkable or

t16.10 WHO Classification of Myelodysplastic Syndromes (MDS)*

Subtype (% All MDS)	Blood Cytopenia (Other)	% Blots[†]	Dysplasia	Bone Marrow % Blasts[†]	Auer Rods	Dysplasia	Ring Sideroblasts	Median Survival (Months)	% 5 Year Survival Rate	% Evolution to AML at 5 Years
RCUD (RA, RN, RT) (10%-18%)	**Unicytopenia** (rarely **bicytopenia**) **No pancytopenia** No monocytosis	<1%	1 lineage ± macrocytosis	<5%	N	≥10% in 1 lineage	Absent or <15% erythroid cells	70-100	90%	2%-15%
MDS iso del(5q) (5%-10%)	**Anemia** (usually macrocytic) **Platelets normal to increased**	<1%	Usually absent	<5%	N	**Normal to increased hypolobated megakaryocytes**	Absent	145	88%	<10%-20%
RARS (4%-12%)	**Anemia** No monocytosis	<1% (usually absent)	Erythrocytes Macrocytosis common Dimorphic RBCs	<5%	N	≥10% dysplastic erythroid cells	≥15% erythroid cells	>100	>98%	2%
RCMD (30%-40%)	**Uni- or bicytopenia** **No monocytosis** **No pancytopenia**	<1%	>1 lineage	<5%	N	≥10% dysplastic cells in 2 or 3 lineages	±	30-60	60%	20%
RAEB-1 (15%-20%)	**Uni- to pancytopenia** **No monocytosis**	<5%	1-3 lineages	5%-9%	N	≥10% in 1-3 lineages	±	16-40	25%	25%
RAEB-2 (20%)	**Uni- to pancytopenia** **No monocytosis**	5%-19%	1-3 lineages	10%-19%	**Y (may be present)**	≥10% in 1-3 lineages	±	9-20	25%	35%-50%
MDS-U (<5%)	**Uni- to pancytopenia[‡]** No monocytosis	≤1%	1-3 lineages	<5%	N	**Dysplastic cells present, but <10% if clonal cytogenetic abnormality** ≥10% in 1-3 lineages[‡]	±	NA	NA	28%

*Bold indicates WHO 2008 requirement

[†]Recent authors suggest that, similar to AML, blast percentage should be based on nonerythroid cells for cases of MDS in which the erythroid lineage accounts for ≥50% of total cells [Wang 2008]

[‡]Note MDS-U criteria are complex; key blood feature is pancytopenia; in cases lacking pancytopenia, multilineage dysplasia must be present

MDS-U = myelodysplastic syndrome, unclassifiable; NA = not available; RA = refractory anemia; RAEB = refractory anemia with excess blasts; RARS = refractory anemia with ring sideroblasts; RCMD = refractory cytopenia with multilineage dysplasia; RCUD = refractory cytopenias with unilineage dysplasia; RN = refractory neutropenia; RT = refractory thrombocytopenia; WHO = World Health Organization

References: [Bernasconi 2007, Brunning 2008a, 2008b, 2008c, Germing 2006b, Haase 2007, Hasserjian 2008a, Malcovati 2005b, Orazi 2008b, 2009, Steensma 2006, Vardiman 2008b]

show nonspecific anisopoikilocytosis and/or macrocytosis i16.29. The bone marrow is typically hypercellular and the extent of dysplasia is best assessed by integrating features from aspirate smears, core biopsy sections, and iron stains.

[16.5.2] **Myelodysplasia with Isolated del(5q)**

This MDS subtype is defined by the presence of isolated del(5q) t16.10 [Hasserjian 2008b]. This distinctive subtype of MDS was recognized >30 years ago by the unique profile of elderly female patients with macrocytic anemia, thrombocytosis, and hypolobated megakaryocytes i16.30, i16.31,

i16.32, i16.33 [Hasserjian 2008b, Mohamedali 2009]. Although patients who match this profile have a good outcome and relatively low risk of evolution to AML, other MDS patients with isolated del(5q) have a more adverse outcome [Holtan 2008]. Therapy with lenalidomide can reduce the transfusion requirement and prolong survival in cases of MDS with isolated del(5q) [Ades 2009, List 2006].

[16.5.3] **Refractory Anemia with Ring Sideroblasts**

In refractory anemia with ring sideroblasts (RARS) dysplastic changes are restricted to the erythroid lineage

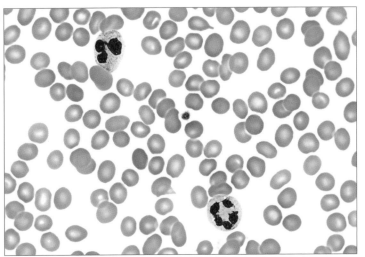

i16.29 *This peripheral blood smear is from a patient with refractory anemia who had a macrocytic anemia and thrombocytopenia in conjunction with a normal absolute neutrophil count. (Wright)*

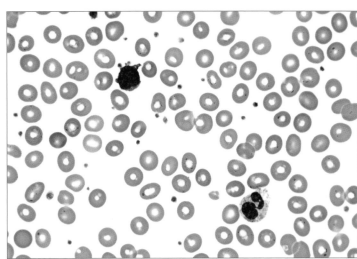

i16.30 *This peripheral blood smear is from a patient with myelodysplasia and isolated del(5q). The patient had a mild macrocytic anemia in conjunction with thrombocytosis and a normal absolute neutrophil count. (Wright)*

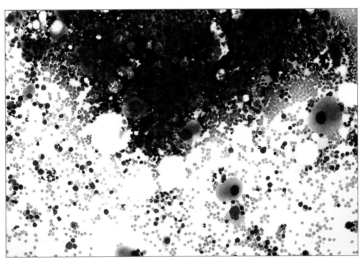

i16.31 *This bone marrow aspirate smear is from a patient with myelodysplasia with isolated del(5q) and shows a hypercellular bone marrow with increased hypolobated megakaryocytes. (Wright)*

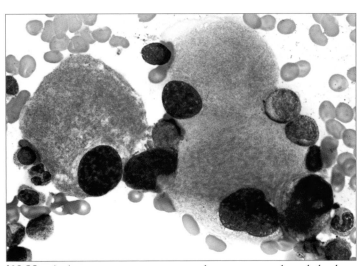

i16.32 *This bone marrow aspirate smear is from a patient with myelodysplasia and isolated del(5q) and shows multiple monolobate megakaryocytes, which characterize this distinctive subtype of low-grade myelodysplasia. (Wright)*

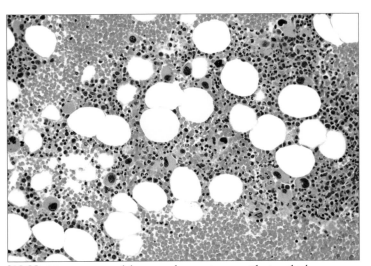

i16.33 *Numerous monolobate megakaryocytes are evident on this bone marrow clot section from a patient with myelodysplasia and isolated del(5q). (H&E)*

and ring sideroblasts (at least 5 paranuclear iron granules covering 1/3 of the diameter of the nucleus) must account for ≥15% of erythroid lineage cells in bone marrow **i16.34** (see **i16.12**). These ring sideroblasts are attributed to aberrant mitochondrial ferritin due to upregulation of *FTMT* and other genes involved in this process very early in erythropoiesis (see **i16.13**) [Tehranchi 2005]. Ring sideroblasts can be seen in other more high-grade types of MDS and in many non-neoplastic disorders (see **[16.8]** "Differential Diagnosis of MDS," p 352). Storage iron is often increased, either linked to chronic transfusion requirements or intrinsic defects in iron homeostasis [Chee 2008]. Investigators have identified hemochromatosis-associated gene mutations in patients with RARS with elevated ferritin levels not related to transfusion requirements **i16.35** [Nearman 2007].

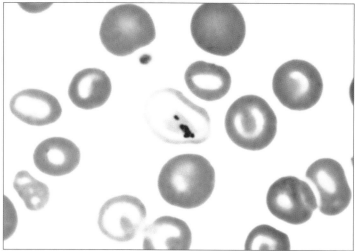

i16.34 *This peripheral blood smear is from a patient with refractory anemia and ring sideroblasts. Note dimorphic red bloods cells and prominent Pappenheimer bodies within erythrocytes. (Wright)*

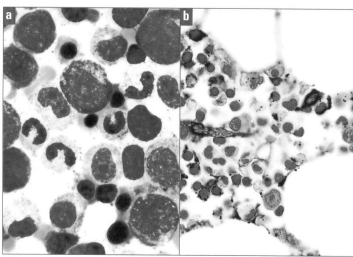

i16.35 *This composite illustrates abundant erythroid lineage cells without significant dysplasia on a bone marrow aspirate smear **a**, while markedly increased storage and erythroid iron is present on the core biopsy section. Note ring sideroblasts. See **i16.12** and **i16.13** for ring sideroblasts. (Wright and Prussian blue)*

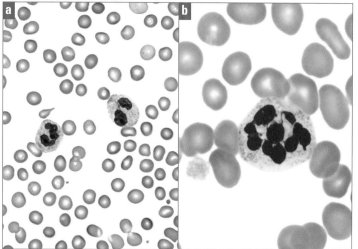

i16.36 *This composite is from 2 patients with refractory cytopenia with multilineage dysplasia. Note macrocytic anemia with thrombocytopenia and dysplastic neutrophil **a**, while the other blood smear shows a markedly hypersegmented and hypogranular neutrophil. Note large hypogranular platelet **b**. (Wright)*

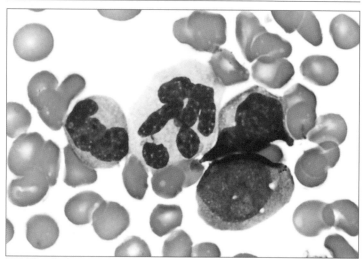

i16.37 *This bone marrow aspirate smear shows markedly abnormal mature neutrophils in conjunction with a granular blast in a patient with refractory cytopenia with multilineage dysplasia. (Wright)*

Circulating blasts are rarely, if ever seen, and bone marrow blast percentages are within normal range **i16.34**, **i16.35** [Hasserjian 2008a]. Erythroid lineage cells predominate in bone marrow, while granulocytic and megakaryocytic lineages are unremarkable or show very infrequent dysplastic features **i16.35**. Outcome is good, and transformations to AML are infrequent in patients with RARS **t16.10**.

[16.5.4] **Refractory Cytopenia with Multilineage Dysplasia**

By definition, cases of refractory cytopenia with multilineage dysplasia (RCMD) must show ≥10% dysplastic cells in ≥2 hematopoietic lineages **t16.10** [Brunning 2008a]. Blast counts are low in blood and bone marrow **i16.36**, **i16.37**. Megakaryocyte dysplasia is best assessed on core biopsy sections, and at least 30 megakaryocytes should be assessed,

although modifications to the megakaryocyte dysplasia requirements for RCMD have been proposed based on outcome studies **i16.38**, **i16.39** [Matsuda 2007]. The number of ring sideroblasts is quite variable but may exceed 15% of erythroid lineage cells in the bone marrow **i16.40**.

[16.5.5] **Refractory Anemia with Excess Blasts**

In refractory anemia with excess blasts (RAEB), the blast percentage in blood ranges from 2%-19%, while the bone marrow contains 5%-19% myeloblasts **i16.41**, **i16.42** [Orazi 2008b]. Based on these blood and bone marrow blast percentages, cases are classified as either RAEB-1 or RAEB-2 **t16.10**. In addition, the identification of Auer rods in a case of true MDS warrants the diagnosis of RAEB-2, but the diagnostician must exclude a diagnosis of low blast count AML **i16.43**. The dysplastic features noted in cases of RAEB-1 and RAEB-2, although similar to

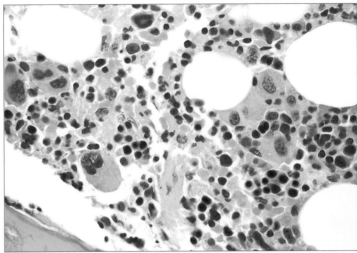

i16.38 *This bone marrow core biopsy section shows overall hypercellularity with clustered and hypolobated megakaryocytes in a patient with refractory cytopenia with multilineage dysplasia. (H&E)*

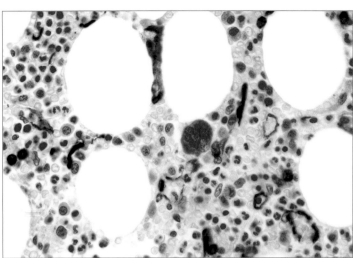

i16.39 *Immunohistochemical staining for CD34 shows increased and minimally clustered myeloblasts in conjunction with neoangiogenesis and CD34+ megakaryocytes in this bone marrow core biopsy from a patient with refractory cytopenia with multilineage dysplasia. (immunoperoxidase for CD34)*

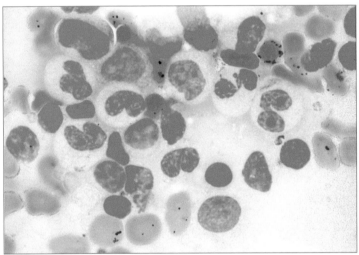

i16.40 *Occasional ring sideroblasts in conjunction with dysplastic coarse iron granules are evident in this bone marrow aspirate smear from a patient with refractory cytopenia with multilineage dysplasia. (Prussian blue)*

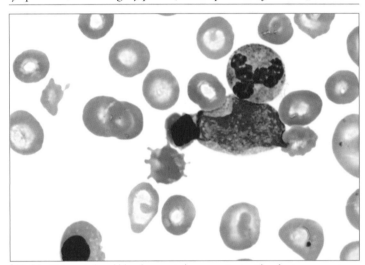

i16.41 *This peripheral blood smear is from a patient with refractory anemia with excess blasts-2 and shows marked pancytopenia, a circulating blast, and dysplastic erythroid and neutrophilic cells. (Wright)*

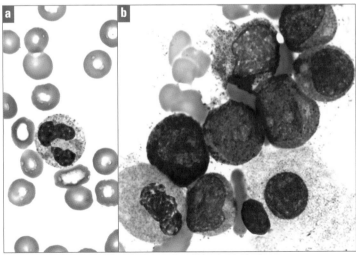

i16.42 *This composite illustrates peripheral blood **a** and a bone marrow aspirate smear **b** in a patient with refractory anemia with excess blasts. Note striking dysplasia of granulocytic cells in conjunction with increased myeloblasts. (Wright)*

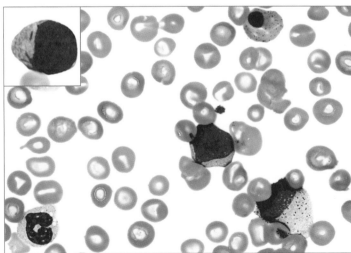

i16.43 *This peripheral blood smear is from a patient with refractory anemia with excess blasts-2 in which rare blasts containing Auer rods were identified (inset). Note circulating blasts in blood in conjunction with significant cytopenias, dysplastic neutrophils, and a circulating nucleated red blood cell. (Wright)*

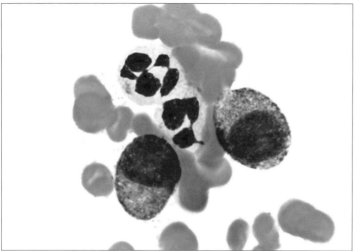

i16.44 *2 hypogranular dysplastic neutrophils adjacent to 2 granular blasts are evident in this bone marrow aspirate smear from a patient with refractory anemia with excess blasts-1. Note absence of hof in granular myeloblasts. (Wright)*

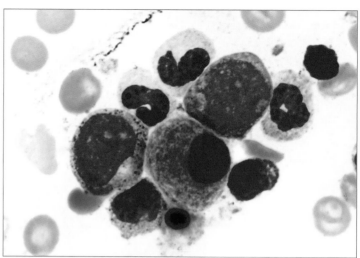

i16.45 *This bone marrow aspirate smear from a patient with refractory anemia with excess blasts shows multilineage dysplasia characterized by a myeloblast with pseudo-Chédiak-Higashi granules, hypogranular neutrophils, and a small monolobated megakaryocyte. (Wright)*

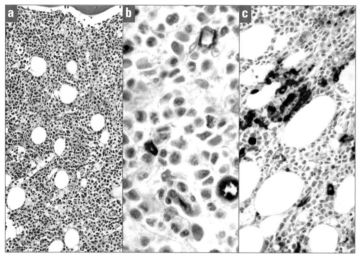

i16.46 *This composite illustrates the morphologic and immunohistochemical features of refractory anemia with excess blasts-2. Note hypercellular bone marrow* **a** *with increased neoangiogenesis and increased myeloblasts* **b**, *while megakaryocytes are increased, clustered, and hypolobated* **c**. *On bone marrow aspirate smears, 13% blasts were identified by differential counts. (H&E and immunoperoxidase for CD34 and CD42b)*

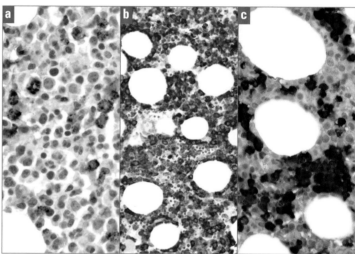

i16.47 *This composite illustrates the aberrant immunohistochemical features in a patient with refractory anemia with excess blasts. Increased and clustered CD34+ cells are evident* **a**, *while myeloperoxidase staining shows prominent non-paratrabecular myeloid aggregates (abnormal localization of immature precursors)* **b**, *and hemoglobin A stain shows disruption in colony formation* **c**. *(immunoperoxidase for CD34, myeloperoxidase, and hemoglobin A)*

other MDS subtypes, may be more pronounced **i16.44**, **i16.45** [Brunning 2008c, Orazi 2009]. However, cases with less overt dysplasia do occur, and immunohistochemical assessment of bone marrow core biopsy sections may be useful in that architectural abnormalities are common in RAEB **i16.46**, **i16.47**. The usefulness of the WHO classification in predicting outcome in RAEB has been confirmed in large studies [Germing 2006a].

[16.5.6] **Myelodysplastic Syndrome, Unclassifiable**

The designation of myelodysplasia, unclassifiable, is applied in several fairly distinct and complex situations **i16.48**, **i16.49** [Orazi 2008a]. First, cases demonstrating pancytopenia in which other features are compatible with RCUD are considered as unclassifiable. Second, cases in which 1% blasts are noted in

the blood, while other features are compatible with RCUD or RCMD are also considered unclassifiable. Finally, cases with prolonged cytopenias, ≤1% blood blasts, <5% bone marrow blasts, dysplasia (but <10%), and an MDS-associated clonal cytogenetic abnormality are considered unclassifiable [Orazi 2008a]. Close follow-up is warranted in these patients.

[16.5.7] **Childhood Myelodysplastic Syndrome**

Unlike MDS in adults, the incidence of MDS in children is very low. Childhood MDS is different from MDS in adults in many important respects [Baumann 2008, Strom 2008]. In children it is essential to distinguish de novo MDS from bone marrow disorders that develop in children with underlying diverse constitutional disorders (especially Down syndrome and

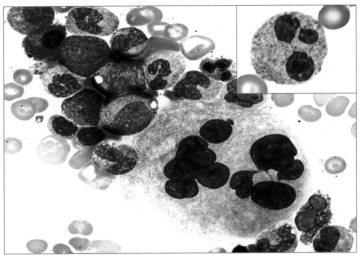

i16.48 *This composite shows the peripheral blood and bone marrow aspirate smear features from a patient with myelodysplastic syndrome, unclassifiable. This patient has severe pancytopenia, while the bone marrow aspirate smear (inset) shows markedly dysplastic megakaryocytes; other lineages are unremarkable. (Wright)*

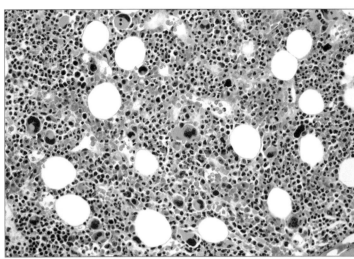

i16.49 *This bone marrow biopsy from a patient with myelodysplastic syndrome, unclassifiable, shows hypercellularity with increased atypical megakaryocytes (see **i16.48**). (H&E)*

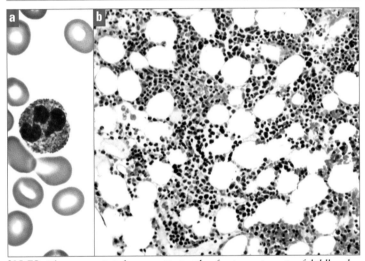

i16.50 *This composite is from a patient with refractory cytopenia of childhood type myelodysplasia. Note pancytopenia, most notably marked thrombocytopenia, in peripheral blood **a**, while the bone marrow core biopsy **b** shows marked hypocellularity with markedly reduced megakaryocytes. (Wright, H&E)*

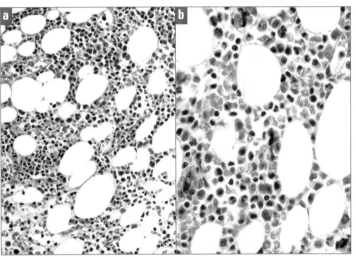

i16.51 *This composite of a bone marrow core biopsy from a patient with refractory cytopenia of childhood-type myelodysplasia shows virtual absence of megakaryocytes by CD42b staining **a**, while CD34 staining shows only scattered positive myeloblasts **b**. (immunoperoxidase for CD42b and CD34)*

bone marrow failure disorders) and from therapy-related MDS [Baumann 2008, Elghetany 2007, Niemeyer 2008, Strom 2008]. The distinction between childhood MDS and aplastic anemia is essential in patients with refractory cytopenia of childhood, while more high-grade MDS such as RAEB must be distinguished from low blast count AML.

The WHO 2008 subtypes of MDS do not apply well to pediatric cases, but children can occasionally develop RAEB, which shows general overlap with adult cases. The 20% myeloblast threshold for AML may not apply as well to pediatric cases, and the distinction between MDS and AML may be more problematic in children [Baumann 2008, Hasle 2003, Niemeyer 2008].

A provisional WHO 2008 category of refractory cytopenia of childhood (RCC) has been proposed. These children more often have sustained neutropenia and/or thrombocytopenia rather than, or in addition to, anemia; profound bone marrow hypocellularity is typical **i16.50** [Baumann 2008, Kardos 2003, Niemeyer 2008]. Distinction from aplastic anemia is based in part on the identification of dysplasia In general, detection of clonal cytogenetic abnormalities is not currently considered a reliable discriminator between aplastic anemia and MDS (Chapter 17). However, an exception is made in children specifically for monosomy 7, which, if present at presentation, should be treated as MDS [Marsh 2009]. The types of dysplastic features noted in RCC are generally similar to those seen in specimens from adults, but blasts are not increased and megakaryocytes are often markedly decreased. Step sectioning and immunohistochemical assessment may be required to detect these infrequent megakaryocytes and assess them for dysplasia **i16.51**. Identification of micromegakaryocytes is an important feature used to distinguish RCC from aplastic anemia [Baumann 2008, Niemeyer 2008].

[16.6]   Unique Types of MDS

There are many morphologic variants in MDS, ranging from hypocellular MDS to presumptive MDS in cases in which sustained, unexplained cytopenias are detected *without* dysplasia but with an MDS-associated clonal cytogenetic abnormality **t16.11** [Akiyama 2005, Barlogie 2008, Buesche 2008, Czader 2009, Haas 2009, Hanson 2008, Huang 2008, Jaen 1990, Lai 1995, Lim 2007, McClure 1999, Orazi 2009,

Pedersen-Bjergaard 2008, Singh 2007, Sloand 2009, Steensma 2003, 2005, Valent 2007, Vardiman 2008a, Willis 2005]. The salient features, key tips, and caveats for these diverse morphologic variants are listed in **t16.11**. In MDS with Auer rods, exclusion of low blast count AML is the top priority, while many neoplastic and non-neoplastic causes of hypocellularity must be excluded in hypocellular (h-) MDS (see **i16.43**) **i16.52**. In h-MDS, the detection of dysplasia,

t16.11   Unique Types of Myelodysplasia

Subtype	Comments/Clues/Tips/Caveats
MDS with Auer rods	Auer rods can be seen in RAEB-2, CMML-2, and AML
	Distinction between low blast count AML and RAEB-2 critical (cytogenetic assessment for AML-defining translocations)
	Rare reports in cases otherwise fulfilling criteria for RCMD, RARS, RAEB-1; rapid evolution to AML
Hypocellular MDS (h-MDS)	5%-10% of MDS cases
	Profound cytopenias; granulocytic and megakaryocytic dysplasia most useful
	More prevalent in pediatric MDS and in females
	Most cases RA (low IPSS score)
	Some cases respond to immunosuppressive therapy
	Cellularity <30% in younger patients; <20% in elderly
	Differential diagnosis includes AA, HCL, h-AML, T-LGL, PNH, toxic myelopathy
MDS with fibrosis	10% of MDS; 50% of t-MDS
	Associated with multilineage dysplasia, higher blast counts, clonal cytogenetic abnormalities, prior chemotherapy
	Adverse prognosis, decreased survival time
	Many myeloid neoplasms may show fibrosis (see **t16.12**)
MDS with del(17p)	Rare genetic subtype of MDS, MDS/MPN, or AML
	Increased frequency in t-MDS
	Excessive nuclear chromatin clumping, hyposegmentation of neutrophils
	Neutrophils small overall size, vacuolated
	Adverse outcome; high frequency of progression to AML
MDS with normal morphology and clonal MDS-type cytogenetic abnormality	Documentation of clonal cytogenetic abnormality of MDS type provides presumptive evidence of MDS in patients with sustained cytopenias with other causes excluded, even if dysplasia not present
	Rare patients with normal CBC, blood and bone marrow morphology may have clonal non-MDS type cytogenetic abnormality (+15) without subsequent development of a hematologic disorder
MDS with acquired α thalassemia	Linked to inactivating somatic mutations of *ATRX* which causes down-regulation in α-globin gene expression
	Acquired mutation in patients with MDS
	Male predominance
Therapy-related MDS (see Chapter 18)	WHO MDS subclassification not relevant
	Distinction between t-MDS and t-AML not relevant
	Complex cytogenetic abnormalities common
	Poor outcome
	Increasing incidence following chemotherapy with/without radiation and with/without autologous stem cell transplantation
	Similar to MDS and AML, Class I and II mutations identified
	Abnormal karyotype in 90%
	Multilineage dysplasia, variable blast percentage, fibrosis common

AML = acute myeloid leukemia; CBC = complete blood count; CMML = chronic myelomonocytic leukemia; IPSS = International Prognostic Scoring System; MDS = myelodysplastic syndrome; MPN = myeloproliferative neoplasm; RA = refractory anemia; RAEB - refractory anemia with excess blasts; RARS = refractory anemia with ring sideroblasts; RCMD = refractory anemia with multilineage dysplasia; t-AML = therapy-related AML; t-MDS = therapy-related MDS

References: [Akiyama 2005, Barlogie 2008, Buesche 2008, Czader 2009, Haas 2009, Hanson 2008, Huang 2008, Jaen 1990, Lai 1995, Lim 2007, McClure 1999, Orazi 2009, Pedersen-Bjergaard 2008, Singh 2007, Sloand 2009, Steensma 2003, 2005, Valent 2007, Vardiman 2008a, Willis 2005]

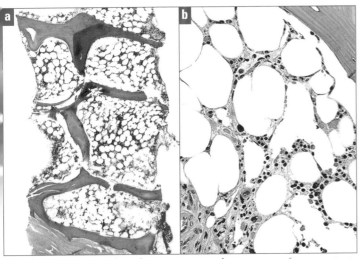

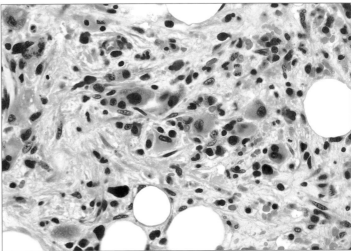

i16.52 *This composite shows bone marrow core biopsy sections from a patient with hypocellular myelodysplasia. Note overall hypocellularity at low magnification, while an atypical megakaryocyte is apparent on high magnification. (H&E)*

i16.53 *Clustered, small, hypolobated megakaryocytes in conjunction with marked fibrosis are evident in this bone marrow core biopsy section from a patient with myelodysplasia with fibrosis. (H&E)*

t16.12 Myeloid Neoplasms with Fibrosis*

Disorder	Key Tip(s)
Mastocytosis	Osteosclerosis, mast cell lesions
Primary myelofibrosis	Osteosclerosis, dilated sinuses, pleomorphic megakaryocytes
Spent phase of polycythemia vera	History of polycythemia vera
CML with fibrosis	Small megakaryocytes, basophilia, *BCR-ABL1*
MDS/MPN with fibrosis	Monocytosis
MDS with fibrosis	Multilineage dysplasia, pancytopenia
Acute megakaryocytic leukemia	Immature and abnormal mature megakaryocytes
Acute panmyelosis with fibrosis	Estimated 20%-25% myeloblasts by CD34, multilineage dysplasia
Acute myeloid leukemia with fibrosis	Blast percentage ≥20%, but can be markedly increased

*See Chapters 14, 17, 18 for more details; ranked by lowest to highest predicted CD34 positivity
CML = chronic myelogenous leukemia; MDS = myelodysplastic syndrome; MDS/MPN = myelodysplastic/myeloproliferative neoplasm

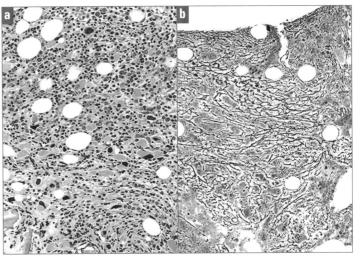

i16.54 *Bone marrow biopsy section composite illustrates atypical megakaryocytic proliferation* **a** *and marked reticulin fibrosis* **b** *in a patient with myelodysplasia with fibrosis. (H&E and reticulin)*

especially in granulocytic cells and megakaryocytes, is particularly valuable, since these abnormalities are unlikely to be present in aplastic anemia, hypocellular hairy cell leukemia, T-cell large granular lymphocytic leukemia, and paroxysmal nocturnal hemoglobinuria **i16.52** [Huang 2008, Orazi 2009, Sloand 2009]. The distinction between h-MDS and aplastic anemia can be especially problematic if clonal cytogenetic abnormalities are detected. The detection of an MDS-type cytogenetic abnormality does support a diagnosis of h-MDS, but some authors report similar cytogenetic abnormalities in aplastic anemia (see Chapter 7 for details). The blast percentage is key in distinguishing h-MDS from h-AML; CD34 immunohistochemical staining is useful in these cases.

MDS with fibrosis is uniquely challenging because the bone marrow is frequently inaspirable, compromising both morphologic assessment and the success of cytogenetics and flow cytometric immunophenotyping. Cases of MDS exhibiting fibrosis are generally of higher grade based on blast percentage and multilineage dysplasia **i16.53**, **i16.54**. Both morphologic findings and immunohistochemical staining on core biopsy sections for CD34, myeloperoxidase, CD61, and other megakaryocytic antigens are essential in distinguishing fibrotic MDS from the many other myeloid neoplasms that can exhibit fibrosis **t16.12**.

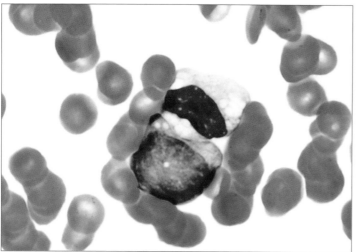

i16.55 *This peripheral blood smear shows a circulating blast in conjunction with a dysplastic mononuclear pseudo Pelger-Huët neutrophil in a patient with therapy-related myelodysplasia. (Wright)*

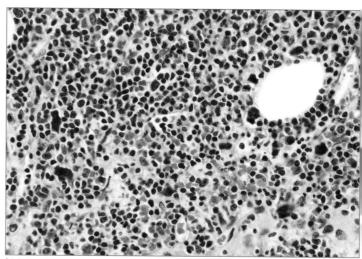

i16.56 *This bone marrow core biopsy from a patient with therapy-related myelodysplasia shows residual chronic lymphocytic leukemia (upper left) side by side with myelodysplasia characterized by hypercellularity and abnormal megakaryocytes (lower right). (H&E)*

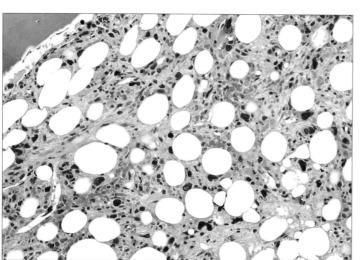

i16.57 *This bone marrow core biopsy shows hypocellularity, marked fibrosis, and increased atypical megakaryocytes in a patient who developed therapy-related myelodysplasia 7 years after autologous bone marrow transplantation. (H&E)*

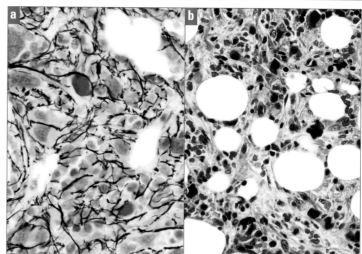

i16.58 *This composite illustrates markedly increased reticulin fibrosis **a** in conjunction with mild collagen fibrosis **b** in a patient with therapy-related myelodysplasia. Collagen fibrosis occurs only infrequently in this setting. (reticulin and trichrome)*

The incidence of therapy-related secondary myeloid neoplasms is increasing because of the prolonged survival of patients treated with chemotherapy. Although all therapy-related myeloid neoplasms are merged in WHO 2008, a fair number of cases will closely resemble either MDS or AML [Czader 2009, Singh 2007]. General features of t-MDS include pronounced multilineage dysplasia, variable blast percentage (≤20%), and fibrosis **i16.55, i16.56, i16.57, i16.58**.

transformation (<5%), while the predicted rate of leukemic transformation is 15% for RCUD (typically RA) and RCMD, 20% for MDS with isolated del(5q), 25% for RAEB-1, 30% for MDS-U, and >50% for RAEB-2 [Bernasconi 2007, Malcovati 2005b]. The morphologic features of MDS-associated AML are variable and some cases may show very limited differentiation **i16.59, i16.60, i16.61, i16.62**.

[16.8] Differential Diagnosis of MDS

Many neoplastic and non-neoplastic disorders show overlap with MDS in some respect. **t16.13** attempts to categorize differential diagnostic considerations based on several features, including disorders with ineffective hematopoiesis, cytopenias with dysplasia, macrocytosis, and ring

[16.7] Transformation to AML

Increased risk of AML is one of the defining parameters of MDS. The frequency of this transformation varies by MDS subtype (see **t16.10**) [Bernasconi 2007, Sridhar 2009]. Cases of RARS show the lowest incidence of acute leukemic

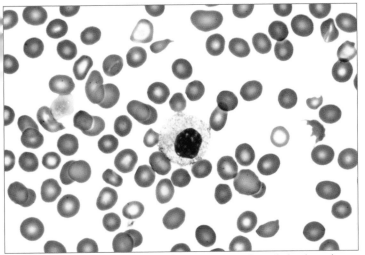

i16.59 *This peripheral blood smear from a patient with myelodysplasia that transformed to acute erythroid/myeloid leukemia shows profound pancytopenia with markedly dysplastic neutrophils, platelets, and red blood cells. (Wright)*

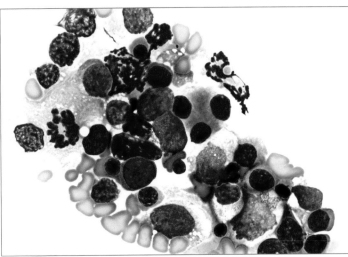

i16.60 *This bone marrow aspirate smear shows increased myeloblasts, a predominance of erythroid lineage cells, and a dysplastic pawn-ball-type megakaryocyte in this patient who developed acute erythroid/myeloid leukemia after myelodysplasia. (Wright)*

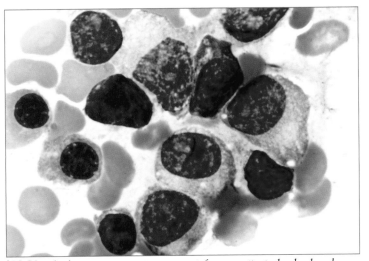

i16.61 *This bone marrow aspirate smear is from a patient who developed an acute undifferentiated leukemia after therapy for refractory cytopenia with multilineage dysplasia. Note blasts are agranular, and flow cytometric immunophenotyping showed a stem cell phenotype. (Wright)*

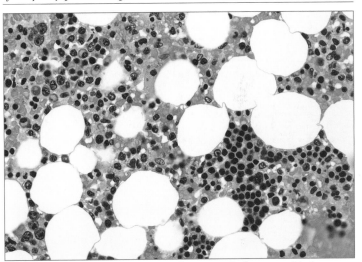

i16.62 *This bone marrow clot section shows partial effacement of the bone marrow core biopsy by an acute undifferentiated leukemia that developed after therapy for refractory cytopenia with multilineage dysplasia. (H&E)*

sideroblasts. Some disorders can manifest with several of these MDS-type features, thus exhibiting significant overlap with MDS i16.63, i16.64, i16.65 [Alcindor 2002, Brunning 2008c, Hasle 1994, Huff 2007, Orazi 2009, Ozbek 2004, Rezuke 1991, Yarali 2002]. All of these differential diagnostic considerations are discussed in more detail in other chapters.

Disorders categorized by circulating blasts are segregated by patient age in t16.14. As noted, MDS is one of many causes of circulating blasts, and a systematic approach in conjunction with generous use of bone marrow examination and specialized testing may be required for a definitive diagnosis. The challenging differential diagnosis between MDS and low blast count AML has been emphasized in this chapter. Both careful blast enumeration and cytogenetics for an AML-defining translocation may help in this distinction. Careful adherence to WHO criteria should allow distinction between MDS and other myeloid neoplasms (see Chapter 13 for strategies and tips in the approach to myeloid neoplasms). The diagnostician must have sufficient clinical information to know if a patient has received cytokine therapy, because recombinant granulocyte colony-stimulating factor is linked to circulating blasts and to an increase in bone marrow immaturity, especially early in therapy.

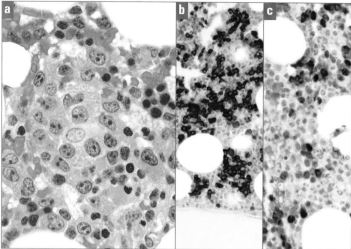

i16.63 *This composite is from a patient with a prolonged collagen vascular disease who developed abnormal localization of immature precursors evident by H&E **a** and myeloperoxidase staining **b**, while abnormal loss of erythroid colony formation is evident by hemoglobin A staining **c**. (H&E, immunoperoxidase for myeloperoxidase and hemoglobin A)*

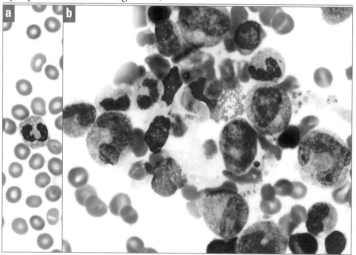

i16.64 *This case of megaloblastic anemia secondary to vitamin B$_{12}$ deficiency mimicked myelodysplasia; the patient presented with pancytopenia with hyposegmented neutrophils in the peripheral blood **a**, while the corresponding bone marrow aspirate smear showed hypercellularity with striking megaloblastic changes **b**. (Wright)*

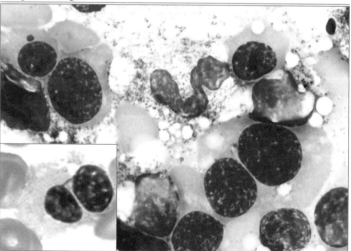

i16.65 *Dysplastic neutrophils and erythroid lineage cells are evident in this bone marrow and peripheral blood (inset) from a patient with human immunodeficiency virus 1. (Wright)*

t16.13 Differential Diagnosis of Myelodysplasia*

Cytopenias with Hypercellular Bone Marrow (ineffective hematopoiesis)

Collagen vascular disorders (ALIP may be present)‡

Chronic infections, HIV-1, EBV, parvovirus, leishmaniasis‡

Megaloblastic anemia

Cytokine therapy (early) (ALIP)

Copper deficiency (consider homeopathic/denture paste use)

Paroxysmal nocturnal hemoglobinuria‡

Acute leukemias/other myeloid neoplasms

Chronic lymphoid neoplasms (hairy cell leukemia)‡

Paraneoplastic phenomenon in solid tumors

Numerous constitutional disorders† (CDA, myelokathexis, congenital sideroblastic anemia)

Cytopenias with Dysplasia

Megaloblastic anemia

Autoimmune disorders/collagen vascular diseases

Copper deficiency (other essential element deficiency)

Chronic viral infections especially HIV-1; parvovirus in immunosuppressed patients

Heavy metal/toxic exposures (arsenic, alcohol)

Medications (valproic acid)/supplements (zinc)

Toxic myelopathy

Chemotherapy

Cytokine therapy

Numerous constitutional disorders† (CDA, congenital megaloblastic and sideroblastic anemias, myelokathexis, microdeletion 22q11.2)

Macrocytosis

Megaloblastic anemia

Copper deficiency (consider homeopathic/denture paste use)

Medications (zidovudine, valproic acid, hydroxyurea, folate antagonists)

Congenital sideroblastic anemia†

Alcohol

Ring Sideroblasts

Zinc toxicity/copper deficiency

Medications (isoniazide, cycloserine)

Alcohol abuse

Nutritional deficiency (copper deficiency)

Constitutional disorders (congenital sideroblastic anemia, Pearson syndrome)

Other myeloid neoplasms

*See other chapters for details about individual disorders
†Easily identifiable constitutional RBC disorders such as thalassemia, sickle cell anemia not included
‡Not all cases with this diagnosis exhibit a hypercellular bone marrow, but hypercellularity is present in a substantial proportion of cases
ALIP = abnormal localization of immature precursors; CDA = congenital dyserythropoietic anemia; EBV = Epstein-Barr virus; HIV = human immunodeficiency virus

References: [Alcindor 2002, Brunning 2008c, Hasle 1994, Huff 2007, Orazi 2009, Ozbek 2004, Rezuke 1991, Sibley 2009, Yarali 2002]

t16.14 Blasts in Blood: Key Age-Based Considerations

Newborn/Infant	Child/Teenager
Physiologic at birth	Down syndrome-related disorders
Infection	Infection/other severe systemic disorders*
Other severe stress	
Down syndrome-related disorders	Bone marrow metastasis
Other constitutional disorders (eg, osteopetrosis)	Other constitutional disorders
	Cytokine therapy
Juvenile myelomonocytic leukemia (JMML)	Acute leukemia
	Chronic leukemia (CML, JMML)
Congenital acute leukemia	MDS
Adult	**Elderly**
Cytokine therapy	Bone marrow metastasis
Severe systemic disorder	Cytokine therapy
Bone marrow metastasis	Chronic myeloid neoplasm (MDS, MDS/MPN, MPN, CML)
Chronic myeloid neoplasm (CML, MPN, MDS/MPN, MDS	
	Severe systemic disorder
Acute leukemia	Acute leukemia
Toxic insult/myelopathy	Toxic insult/myelopathy

*Includes autoimmune disorders, chronic infections

CML = chronic myelogenous leukemia; MDS = myelodysplastic syndrome; MPN = myeloproliferative neoplasm

t16.15 Components of the Diagnostic Interpretation in MDS

Provide justification for MDS diagnosis and give WHO subtype; include percent blasts in blood and bone marrow

Provide information regarding lineages with ≥10% dysplastic cells and cellularity

Comment on any other unique morphologic/cytochemical features

Comment on results and significance of any additional studies such as CD34, CD42b, CD61, myeloperoxidase, and hemoglobin A immunoperoxidase assessment of bone marrow architecture and immature cell localization

Integrate results of flow cytometric immunophenotyping

Integrate genotypic data and comment on prognostic significance (may require later integrated report)

Comment on an association, if any, with underlying genetic/immune disorders, antecedent chemotherapy, or toxic exposure

If MDS subtype is a "diagnosis of exclusion" (eg, refractory anemia), provide data used to refute other differential diagnostic considerations

Recommend additional tests/studies to potentially resolve "suspicious for MDS but not diagnostic" type cases

MDS = myelodysplastic syndrome; WHO = World Health Organization

[16.9] # Components of the Diagnostic Interpretation

Components of the diagnostic interpretation in MDS cases are listed in t16.15. The diagnostic report is of greatest use to clinicians and patients if the justification for the MDS diagnosis and WHO subtype are clearly stated. Unique features should be mentioned along with their significance, if known. The immunohistochemical architectural features help support individual lineage dysplasia assessment, and general myeloblast percentage estimates should correlate with differential cell counts. Results of specialized studies should be integrated; this may require a follow-up report once genetic testing is completed. Recommend additional testing as necessary to resolve inconclusive cases.

[16.10] ## Clues and Caveats

1. MDS is characterized by prolonged, unexplained cytopenias and ineffective hematopoiesis due to increased bone marrow apoptosis.
2. Poor specimen quality is a major factor in diagnostic errors and in low diagnostic concordance.
3. The diagnosis of MDS requires the integration of clinical, hematologic, morphologic, and cytogenetic features; non-neoplastic causes of cytopenias must be excluded.
4. Although myeloblasts comprise the majority of blasts in MDS, megakaryoblasts, monoblasts, and promonocytes are also included in the blast percentage. Erythroblasts and promyelocytes are not included in the blast percentage.
5. Myeloblasts may be agranular or granular; morphologic enumeration of blasts is essential; flow cytometric immunophenotyping is not a surrogate for morphologic enumeration.
6. The distinction between a myeloblast and a promyelocyte is based on the presence of a clear paranuclear golgi area in promyelocytes.
7. Myelodysplastic disorders with an associated monocytosis $\geq 1.0 \times 10^9/L$ are included in MDS/MPN and are not included in MDS.
8. Conventional cytogenetics is the most valuable specialized test in MDS and should be performed routinely.
9. Low-grade MDS must be distinguished from numerous non-neoplastic causes of cytopenia, dysplasias, and ineffective hematopoiesis. Disorders showing the most overlap with MDS include megaloblastic anemia, copper deficiency, chronic viral infections, collagen vascular disorders, arsenic exposure, and rare constitutional disorders.

10. MDS can occur at any age, but clearly predominates in the elderly; MDS in children and young adults is rare and may be linked to underlying constitutional disorders or prior chemotherapy.

11. MDS-type dysplasia must be evident in ≥10% of erythroid and granulocytic cells; at least 30 megakaryocytes should be assessed for dysplasia on core biopsy sections.

12. In addition to dysplastic features of individual cells, abnormal localization of hematopoietic lineages on core biopsy sections is a feature of MDS.

13. Cases of prolonged, unexplained cytopenia without either increased blasts or morphologic dysplasia and normal (or not performed) karyotype should be designated as ICUS.

14. No cytogenetic finding is unique to MDS, but MDS-associated cytogenetic abnormalities include gains or losses of chromosome material, especially involving chromosomes 5, 7, and 8.

15. The designation MDS, unclassifiable includes cases that otherwise fulfill criteria for RCUD but exhibit pancytopenia and cases that otherwise fulfill criteria for RCUD or RDMD but exhibit 1% blasts in blood.

16. The designation MDS, unclassifiable is also applied to cases with some, but not ≥10%, dysplastic cells, in conjunction with a clonal MDS-type cytogenetic abnormality.

17. A presumptive diagnosis of MDS can be made in cases of persistent cytopenias that lacks dysplasia if a clonal cytogenetic abnormality of MDS type is present.

18. Comprehensive flow cytometric immunophenotyping can be used to delineate aberrant patterns of antigen expression in mature and immature hematopoietic lineage cells in cases of MDS.

19. The severity of aberrant antigen expression by flow cytometry generally parallels the degree of morphologic dysplasia and the grade of the MDS.

20. Hematogones are often decreased in low-grade MDS.

21. PNH clones may be present in MDS, but they are usually detected on only a small subset of cells.

22. Both the IPSS and WPSS predict outcome in MDS. The IPSS is based on percentage of blasts in bone marrow, number of cytopenias, and karyotype. The WPSS is based on WHO category, karyotype, and transfusion requirement.

23. MDS in children differs from adults; children with refractory cytopenia(s) often have markedly hypocellular bone marrows mimicking aplastic anemia; assessment for neutrophil and megakaryocyte dysplasia is crucial.

24. About 10% of MDS in adults will be either hypocellular or fibrotic.

25. Although Auer rods may be present in RAEB-2, it is essential to exclude low blast count AML by cytogenetic assessment for AML-defining translocations.

26. Immunohistochemical staining, especially for CD34, is useful in assessing for the localization, overall number (estimated), and clustering of myeloblasts on bone marrow core biopsy sections; dysplastic megakaryocytes may be CD34 positive.

27. Transformation to AML varies by MDS subtype and is highest in RAEB-2.

28. The incidence of therapy-related myeloid neoplasms is increasing; t-MDS and t-AML are biologically similar and are merged for classification and treatment purposes.

[16.11] **Acknowledgements**

The author acknowledges the photographic contributions of R Brynes, MD, and C Sever, MD; Clovis Pitchford for f16.2.

[16.12] **References**

Ades L, Boehrer S, Prebet T, et al [2009] Efficacy and safety of lenalidomide in intermediate-2 or high-risk myelodysplastic syndromes with 5q deletion: results of a phase 2 study. *Blood* 113:3947-3952.

Akiyama T, Matsunaga T, Terui T, et al [2005] Involvement of transforming growth factor-β and thrombopoietin in the pathogenesis of myelodysplastic syndrome with myelofibrosis. *Leukemia* 19:1558-1566.

Alcindor T, Bridges KR [2002] Sideroblastic anaemias. *Br J Haematol* 116:733-743.

Alessandrino EP, Della Porta MG, Bacigalupo A, et al [2008] WHO classification and WPSS predict posttransplantation outcome in patients with myelodysplastic syndrome: a study from the Gruppo Italiano Trapianto di Midollo Osseo (GITMO). *Blood* 112:895-902.

Alfinito F, Sica M, Luciano L, et al [2010] Immune dysregulation and dyserythropoiesis in the myelodysplastic syndromes. *Br J Haematol* 148:90-98.

Barlogie B, Tricot G, Haessler J, et al [2008] Cytogenetically defined myelodysplasia after melphalan-based autotransplantation for multiple myeloma linked to poor hematopoietic stem-cell mobilization: the Arkansas experience in >3,000 patients treated since 1989. *Blood* 111:94-100.

Baumann I, Niemeyer C, Bennett J, Shannon K [2008] Childhood myelodysplastic syndrome. In: Swerdlow S, Campo E, Harris N, et al, eds. *WHO Classification of Tumours: Pathology and Genetics: Tumours of Haematopoietic and Lymphoid Tissues.* Lyon, France: IARC Press; 104-107.

Baumann I, Scheid C, Koref MS, et al [2002] Autologous lymphocytes inhibit hemopoiesis in long-term culture in patients with myelodysplastic syndrome. *Exp Hematol* 30:1405-1411.

Bernasconi P [2008] Molecular pathways in myelodysplastic syndromes and acute myeloid leukemia: relationships and distinctions—a review. *Br J Haematol* 142:695-708.

Bernasconi P, Cavigliano PM, Boni M, et al [2003] Is FISH a relevant prognostic tool in myelodysplastic syndromes with a normal chromosome pattern on conventional cytogenetics? a study on 57 patients. *Leukemia* 17:2107-2112.

Bernasconi P, Klersy C, Boni M, et al [2007] World Health Organization classification in combination with cytogenetic markers improves the prognostic stratification of patients with de novo primary myelodysplastic syndromes. *Br J Haematol* 137:193-205.

Boultwood J, Pellagatti A, Cattan H, et al [2007] Gene expression profiling of CD34+ cells in patients with the 5q– syndrome. *Br J Haematol* 139:578-589.

Brunning R, Bennett J, Matutes E, et al [2008a] Refractory cytopenia with multilineage dysplasia. In: Swerdlow S, Campo E, Harris N, et al, eds. *WHO Classification of Tumours: Pathology and Genetics: Tumours of Haematopoietic and Lymphoid Tissues.* Lyon, France: IARC Press; 98-99.

Brunning R, Hasserjian R, Porwit A, et al [2008b] Refractory cytopenia with unilineage dysplasia. In: Swerdlow S, Campo E, Harris N, et al, eds. *WHO Classification of Tumours: Pathology and Genetics: Tumours of Haematopoietic and Lymphoid Tissues.* Lyon, France: IARC Press; 94-95.

Brunning R, Orazi A, Germing U, et al [2008c] Myelodysplastic syndromes/ neoplasms, overview. In: Swerdlow S, Campo E, Harris N, et al, eds. *WHO Classification of Tumours: Pathology and Genetics: Tumours of Haematopoietic and Lymphoid Tissues.* Lyon, France: IARC Press; 88-93.

Buesche G, Teoman H, Wilczak W, et al [2008] Marrow fibrosis predicts early fatal marrow failure in patients with myelodysplastic syndromes. *Leukemia* 22:313-322.

Chee CE, Steensma DP, Wu W, et al [2008] Neither serum ferritin nor the number of red blood cell transfusions affect overall survival in refractory anemia with ringed sideroblasts. *Am J Hematol* 83:611-613.

Cherian S, Moore J, Bantly A, et al [2005a] Flow-cytometric analysis of peripheral blood neutrophils: a simple, objective, independent and potentially clinically useful assay to facilitate the diagnosis of myelodysplastic syndromes. *Am J Hematol* 79:243-245.

Cherian S, Moore J, Bantly A, et al [2005b] Peripheral blood MDS score: a new flow cytometric tool for the diagnosis of myelodysplastic syndromes. *Cytometry B Clin Cytom* 64:9-17.

Cherry AM, Brockman SR, Paternoster SF, et al [2003] Comparison of interphase FISH and metaphase cytogenetics to study myelodysplastic syndrome: an Eastern Cooperative Oncology Group (ECOG) study. *Leuk Res* 27:1085-1090.

Christman JK [2002] 5-Azacytidine and 5-aza-2'-deoxycytidine as inhibitors of DNA methylation: mechanistic studies and their implications for cancer therapy. *Oncogene* 21:5483-5495.

Czader M, Orazi A [2009] Therapy-related myeloid neoplasms. *Am J Clin Pathol* 132:410-425.

Della Porta MG, Malcovati L, Invernizzi R, et al [2006] Flow cytometry evaluation of erythroid dysplasia in patients with myelodysplastic syndrome. *Leukemia* 20:549-555.

Elghetany MT [2007] Myelodysplastic syndromes in children: a critical review of issues in the diagnosis and classification of 887 cases from 13 published series. *Arch Pathol Lab Med* 131:1110-1116.

Epling-Burnette PK, Painter JS, Rollison DE, et al [2007] Prevalence and clinical association of clonal T-cell expansions in myelodysplastic syndrome. *Leukemia* 21:659-667.

Epperson DE, Nakamura R, Saunthararajah Y, et al [2001] Oligoclonal T cell expansion in myelodysplastic syndrome: evidence for an autoimmune process. *Leuk Res* 25:1075-1083.

Georgiou G, Karali V, Zouvelou C, et al [2006] Serial determination of FLT3 mutations in myelodysplastic syndrome patients at diagnosis, follow up or acute myeloid leukaemia transformation: incidence and their prognostic significance. *Br J Haematol* 134:302-306.

Germing U, Strupp C, Kuendgen A, et al [2006a] Refractory anaemia with excess of blasts (RAEB): analysis of reclassification according to the WHO proposals. *Br J Haematol* 132:162-167.

Germing U, Strupp C, Kuendgen A, et al [2006b] Prospective validation of the WHO proposals for the classification of myelodysplastic syndromes. *Haematologica* 91:1596-1604.

Gondek LP, Tiu R, O'Keefe CL, et al [2008] Chromosomal lesions and uniparental disomy detected by SNP arrays in MDS, MDS/MPD, and MDS-derived AML. *Blood* 111:1534-1542.

Greenberg P, Cox C, LeBeau MM, et al [1997] International scoring system for evaluating prognosis in myelodysplastic syndromes. *Blood* 89:2079-2088.

Gupta R, Soupir CP, Johari V, Hasserjian RP [2007] Myelodysplastic syndrome with isolated deletion of chromosome 20q: an indolent disease with minimal morphological dysplasia and frequent thrombocytopenic presentation. *Br J Haematol* 139:265-268.

Haas PS, Roy NB, Gibbons RJ, et al [2009] The role of X-inactivation in the gender bias of patients with acquired α-thalassaemia and myelodysplastic syndrome (ATMDS). *Br J Haematol* 144:538-545.

Haase D, Germing U, Schanz J, et al [2007] New insights into the prognostic impact of the karyotype in MDS and correlation with subtypes: evidence from a core dataset of 2124 patients. *Blood* 110:4385-4395.

Hanson CA, Steensma DP, Hodnefield JM, et al [2008] Isolated trisomy 15: a clonal chromosome abnormality in bone marrow with doubtful hematologic significance. *Am J Clin Pathol* 129:478-485.

Hasle H, Kerndrup G, Jacobsen BB, et al [1994] Chronic parvovirus infection mimicking myelodysplastic syndrome in a child with subclinical immuno-deficiency. *Am J Pediatr Hematol Oncol* 16:329-333.

Hasle H, Niemeyer CM, Chessells JM, et al [2003] A pediatric approach to the WHO classification of myelodysplastic and myeloproliferative diseases. *Leukemia* 17:277-282.

Hasserjian R, Gattermann N, Bennett J, et al [2008a] Refractory anemia with ring sideroblasts. In: Swerdlow S, Campo E, Harris N, et al, eds. *WHO Classification of Tumours: Pathology and Genetics: Tumours of Haematopoietic and Lymphoid Tissues.* Lyon, France: IARC Press; 96-97.

Hasserjian R, Le Beau M, List A, et al [2008b] Myelodysplastic syndrome with isolated del(5q). In: Swerdlow S, Campo E, Harris N, et al, eds. *WHO Classification of Tumours: Pathology and Genetics: Tumours of Haematopoietic and Lymphoid Tissues.* Lyon, France: IARC Press; 102.

Hofmann WK, Koeffler HP [2005] Myelodysplastic syndrome. *Annu Rev Med* 56:1-16.

Holtan SG, Santana-Davila R, Dewald GW, et al [2008] Myelodysplastic syndromes associated with interstitial deletion of chromosome 5q: clinico-pathologic correlations and new insights from the pre-lenalidomide era. *Am J Hematol* 83:708-713.

Huang TC, Ko BS, Tang JL, et al [2008] Comparison of hypoplastic myelodys-plastic syndrome (MDS) with normo-/hypercellular MDS by International Prognostic Scoring System, cytogenetic and genetic studies. *Leukemia* 22:544-550.

Huff JD, Keung YK, Thakuri M, et al [2007] Copper deficiency causes reversible myelodysplasia. *Am J Hematol* 82:625-630.

Huh YO, Medeiros LJ, Ravandi F, et al [2009] T-cell large granular lymphocyte leukemia associated with myelodysplastic syndrome: a clinicopathologic study of 9 cases. *Am J Clin Pathol* 131:347-356.

Itzykson R, Gardin C, Fenaux P [2008] Meeting report: myelodysplastic syndromes at ASH 2007. *Leukemia* 22:893-897.

Jacobs NL, Holtan SG, Porrata LF, et al [2010] Host immunity affects survival in myelodysplastic syndromes: independent prognostic value of the absolute lymphocyte count. *Am J Hematol* 85:160-163.

Jadersten M, Hellstrom-Lindberg E [2009] Myelodysplastic syndromes: biology and treatment. *J Intern Med* 265:307-328.

Jaen A, Irriguible D, Milla F, et al [1990] Abnormal chromatin clumping in leucocytes: a clue to a new subtype of myelodysplastic syndrome. *Eur J Haematol* 45:209-214.

Kao JM, McMillan A, Greenberg PL [2008] International MDS risk analysis workshop (IMRAW)/IPSS reanalyzed: impact of cytopenias on clinical outcomes in myelodysplastic syndromes. *Am J Hematol* 83:765-770.

Kardos G, Baumann I, Passmore SJ, et al [2003] Refractory anemia in childhood: a retrospective analysis of 67 patients with particular reference to monosomy 7. *Blood* 102:1997-2003.

Kasner MT, Luger SM [2009] Update on the therapy for myelodysplastic syndrome. *Am J Hematol* 84:177-186.

Kerbauy DB, Deeg HJ [2007] Apoptosis and antiapoptotic mechanisms in the progression of myelodysplastic syndrome. *Exp Hematol* 35:1739-1746.

Kiladjian JJ, Fenaux P, Caignard A [2007] Defects of immune surveillance offer new insights into the pathophysiology and therapy of myelodysplastic syndromes. *Leukemia* 21:2237-2239.

Kitagawa M, Saito I, Kuwata T, et al [1997] Overexpression of tumor necrosis factor (TNF)-α and interferon (IFN)-γ by bone marrow cells from patients with myelodysplastic syndromes. *Leukemia* 11:2049-2054.

Kordasti SY, Ingram W, Hayden J, et al [2007] CD4+CD25high Foxp3+ regulatory T cells in myelodysplastic syndrome (MDS). *Blood* 110:847-850.

Lai JL, Preudhomme C, Zandecki M, et al [1995] Myelodysplastic syndromes and acute myeloid leukemia with 17p deletion. An entity characterized by specific dysgranulopoiesis and a high incidence of P53 mutations. *Leukemia* 9:370-381.

Li X, Bryant CE, Deeg HJ [2004] Simultaneous demonstration of clonal chromosome abnormalities and apoptosis in individual marrow cells in myelodysplastic syndrome. *Int J Hematol* 80:140-145.

Lim ZY, Killick S, Germing U, et al [2007] Low IPSS score and bone marrow hypocellularity in MDS patients predict hematological responses to antithymocyte globulin. *Leukemia* 21:1436-1441.

List A, Dewald G, Bennett J, et al [2006] Lenalidomide in the myelodysplastic syndrome with chromosome 5q deletion. *N Engl J Med* 355:1456-1465.

Loken MR, van de Loosdrecht A, Ogata K, et al [2008] Flow cytometry in myelodysplastic syndromes: report from a working conference. *Leuk Res* 32:5-17.

Maftoun-Banankhah S, Maleki A, Karandikar NJ, et al [2008] Multiparameter flow cytometric analysis reveals low percentage of bone marrow hematogones in myelodysplastic syndromes. *Am J Clin Pathol* 129:300-308.

Malcovati L, Della Porta MG, Lunghi M, et al [2005a] Flow cytometry evaluation of erythroid and myeloid dysplasia in patients with myelodysplastic syndrome. *Leukemia* 19:776-783.

Malcovati L, Germing U, Kuendgen A, et al [2007] Time-dependent prognostic scoring system for predicting survival and leukemic evolution in myelodysplastic syndromes. *J Clin Oncol* 25:3503-3510.

Malcovati L, Porta MG, Pascutto C, et al [2005b] Prognostic factors and life expectancy in myelodysplastic syndromes classified according to WHO criteria: a basis for clinical decision making. *J Clin Oncol* 23:7594-7603.

Marsh JC, Ball SE, Cavenagh J, et al [2009] Guidelines for the diagnosis and management of aplastic anemia. *Br J Haematol* 147:43-70.

Matarraz S, Lopez A, Barrena S, et al [2008] The immunophenotype of different immature, myeloid, and B-cell lineage-committed CD34+ hematopoietic cells allows discrimination between normal/reactive and myelodysplastic syndrome precursors. *Leukemia* 22:1175-1183.

Matsuda A, Germing U, Jinnai I, et al [2007] Improvement of criteria for refractory cytopenia with multilineage dysplasia according to the WHO classification based on prognostic significance of morphological features in patients with refractory anemia according to the FAB classification. *Leukemia* 21:678-686.

McClure RF, Dewald GW, Hoyer JD, Hanson CA [1999] Isolated isochromosome 17q: a distinct type of mixed myeloproliferative disorder/myelodysplastic syndrome with an aggressive clinical course. *Br J Haematol* 106:445-454.

Melchert M, List A [2008] Targeted therapies in myelodysplastic syndrome. *Semin Hematol* 45:31-38.

Melenhorst JJ, Eniafe R, Follmann D, et al [2002] Molecular and flow cytometric characterization of the CD4 and CD8 T-cell repertoire in patients with myelodysplastic syndrome. *Br J Haematol* 119:97-105.

Mihara K, Chowdhury M, Nakaju N, et al [2006] Bmi-1 is useful as a novel molecular marker for predicting progression of myelodysplastic syndrome and patient prognosis. *Blood* 107:305-308.

Mohamedali A, Gaken J, Twine NA, et al [2007] Prevalence and prognostic significance of allelic imbalance by single-nucleotide polymorphism analysis in low-risk myelodysplastic syndromes. *Blood* 110:3365-3373.

Mohamedali A, Mufti GJ [2009] Van-den Berghe's 5q– syndrome in 2008. *Br J Haematol* 144:157-168.

Mufti GJ, Bennett JM, Goasguen J, et al [2008] Diagnosis and classification of myelodysplastic syndrome: International Working Group on Morphology of Myelodysplastic Syndrome (IWGM-MDS) consensus proposals for the definition and enumeration of myeloblasts and ring sideroblasts. *Haematologica* 93:1712-1717.

Nearman ZP, Szpurka H, Serio B, et al [2007] Hemochromatosis-associated gene mutations in patients with myelodysplastic syndromes with refractory anemia with ringed sideroblasts. *Am J Hematol* 82:1076-1079.

Niemeyer CM, Baumann I [2008] Myelodysplastic syndrome in children and adolescents. *Semin Hematol* 45:60-70.

Ogata K, Kishikawa Y, Satoh C, et al [2006] Diagnostic application of flow cytometric characteristics of CD34+ cells in low-grade myelodysplastic syndromes. *Blood* 108:1037-1044.

Orazi A, Brunning R, Baumann I, Hasserjian R [2008a] Myelodysplastic syndrome, unclassifiable. In: Swerdlow S, Campo E, Harris N, et al, eds. *WHO Classification of Tumours: Pathology and Genetics: Tumours of Haematopoietic and Lymphoid Tissues.* Lyon, France: IARC ; 103.

Orazi A, Brunning R, Hasserjian R, et al [2008b] Refractory anemia with excess blasts. In: Swerdlow S, Campo E, Harris N, et al, eds. *WHO Classification of Tumours: Pathology and Genetics: Tumours of Haematopoietic and Lymphoid Tissues.* Lyon, France: IARC Press; 100-101.

Orazi A, Czader MB [2009] Myelodysplastic syndromes. *Am J Clin Pathol* 132:290-305.

Ozbek N, Derbent M, Olcay L, et al [2004] Dysplastic changes in the peripheral blood of children with microdeletion 22q11.2. *Am J Hematol* 77:126-131.

Paulsson K, Heidenblad M, Strombeck B, et al [2006] High-resolution genome-wide array-based comparative genome hybridization reveals cryptic chromosome changes in AML and MDS cases with trisomy 8 as the sole cytogenetic aberration. *Leukemia* 20:840-846.

Pedersen-Bjergaard J, Andersen MK, Andersen MT, Christiansen DH [2008] Genetics of therapy-related myelodysplasia and acute myeloid leukemia. *Leukemia* 22:240-248.

Pirruccello SJ, Young KH, Aoun P [2006] Myeloblast phenotypic changes in myelodysplasia. CD34 and CD117 expression abnormalities are common. *Am J Clin Pathol* 125:884-894.

Pitchford C, Hettinga A, Reichard K [2010] Fluorescence in situ hybridization testing for –5/5q, –7/7q, +8, and del(20q) in primary myelodysplastic syndrome correlates with conventional cytogenetics in the setting of an adequate study. *Am J Clin Pathol* 133:240-264.

Rezuke WN, Anderson C, Pastuszak WT, et al [1991] Arsenic intoxication presenting as a myelodysplastic syndrome: a case report. *Am J Hematol* 36:291-293.

Rosenfeld C, List A [2000] A hypothesis for the pathogenesis of myelodysplastic syndromes: implications for new therapies. *Leukemia* 14:2-8.

Saunthararajah Y, Nakamura R, Nam JM, et al [2002] HLA-DR15 (DR2) is overrepresented in myelodysplastic syndrome and aplastic anemia and predicts a response to immunosuppression in myelodysplastic syndrome. *Blood* 100:1570-1574.

Saunthararajah Y, Nakamura R, Wesley R, et al [2003] A simple method to predict response to immunosuppressive therapy in patients with myelodysplastic syndrome. *Blood* 102:3025-3027.

Scott BL, Wells DA, Loken MR, et al [2008] Validation of a flow cytometric scoring system as a prognostic indicator for posttransplantation outcome in patients with myelodysplastic syndrome. *Blood* 112:2681-2686.

Sibley A, Maddox AM [2009] Myelodysplasia and copper deficiency induced by denture paste. *Am J Hematol* 84:612.

Singh ZN, Huo D, Anastasi J, et al [2007] Therapy-related myelodysplastic syndrome: morphologic subclassification may not be clinically relevant. *Am J Clin Pathol* 127:197-205.

Sloand EM [2009] Hypocellular myelodysplasia. *Hematol Oncol Clin North Am* 23:347-360.

Sloand EM, Mainwaring L, Fuhrer M, et al [2005] Preferential suppression of trisomy 8 compared with normal hematopoietic cell growth by autologous lymphocytes in patients with trisomy 8 myelodysplastic syndrome. *Blood* 106:841-851.

Sloand EM, Rezvani K [2008] The role of the immune system in myelodysplasia: implications for therapy. *Semin Hematol* 45:39-48.

Sridhar K, Ross DT, Tibshirani R, et al [2009] Relationship of differential gene expression profiles in CD34+ myelodysplastic syndrome marrow cells to disease subtype and progression. *Blood* 114:4847-4858.

Starczynowski DT, Vercauteren S, Telenius A, et al [2008] High-resolution whole genome tiling path array CGH analysis of CD34+ cells from patients with low-risk myelodysplastic syndromes reveals cryptic copy number alterations and predicts overall and leukemia-free survival. *Blood* 112:3412-3424.

Steensma DP, Bennett JM [2006] The myelodysplastic syndromes: diagnosis and treatment. *Mayo Clin Proc* 81:104-130.

Steensma DP, Dewald GW, Hodnefield JM, et al [2003] Clonal cytogenetic abnormalities in bone marrow specimens without clear morphologic evidence of dysplasia: a form fruste of myelodysplasia? *Leuk Res* 27:235-242.

Steensma DP, Gibbons RJ, Higgs DR [2005] Acquired α-thalassemia in association with myelodysplastic syndrome and other hematologic malignancies. *Blood* 105:443-452.

Sternberg A, Killick S, Littlewood T, et al [2005] Evidence for reduced B-cell progenitors in early (low-risk) myelodysplastic syndrome. *Blood* 106:2982-2991.

Stetler-Stevenson M, Arthur DC, Jabbour N, et al [2001] Diagnostic utility of flow cytometric immunophenotyping in myelodysplastic syndrome. *Blood* 98:979-987.

Stetler-Stevenson M, Yuan CM [2009] Myelodysplastic syndromes: the role of flow cytometry in diagnosis and prognosis. *Int J Lab Hematol* 31:479-483.

Strom SS, Velez-Bravo V, Estey EH [2008] Epidemiology of myelodysplastic syndromes. *Semin Hematol* 45:8-13.

Sugimori C, Yamazaki H, Feng X, et al [2007] Roles of DRB1 *1501 and DRB1 *1502 in the pathogenesis of aplastic anemia. *Exp Hematol* 35:13-20.

Tehranchi R, Invernizzi R, Grandien A, et al [2005] Aberrant mitochondrial iron distribution and maturation arrest characterize early erythroid precursors in low-risk myelodysplastic syndromes. *Blood* 106:247-253.

Truong F, Smith BR, Stachurski D, et al [2009] The utility of flow cytometric immunophenotyping in cytopenic patients with a non-diagnostic bone marrow: a prospective study. *Leuk Res* 33:1039-1046.

Tsao L, Reichard K, Foucar K [2007] Diagnostic utility of flow cytometlric enumeration of hematogones in MDS bone marrows. *Mod Pathol* 20(Suppl 2):262A.

Valent P, Horny HP, Bennett JM, et al [2007] Definitions and standards in the diagnosis and treatment of the myelodysplastic syndromes: consensus statements and report from a working conference. *Leuk Res* 31:727-736.

van de Loosdrecht AA, Westers TM, Westra AH, et al [2008] Identification of distinct prognostic subgroups in low- and intermediate-1-risk myelodysplastic syndromes by flow cytometry. *Blood* 111:1067-1077.

Vardiman J, Arber D, Brunning R, et al [2008a] Therapy-related myeloid neoplasms. In: Swerdlow S, Campo E, Harris N, et al, eds. *WHO Classification of Tumours: Pathology and Genetics: Tumours of Haematopoietic and Lymphoid Tissues.* Lyon, France: IARC Press; 127-129.

Vardiman J, Brunning R, Arber D, et al [2008b] Introduction and overview of the classification of the myeloid neoplasms. In: Swerdlow S, Campo E, Harris N, et al, eds. *WHO Classification of Tumours: Pathology and Genetics: Tumours of Haematopoietic and Lymphoid Tissues.* Lyon, France: IARC Press; 18-30.

Verburgh E, Achten R, Louw VJ, et al [2007] A new disease categorization of low-grade myelodysplastic syndromes based on the expression of cytopenia and dysplasia in one vs more than one lineage improves on the WHO classification. *Leukemia* 21:668-677.

Wang SA, Pozdnyakova O, Jorgensen JL, et al [2009] Detection of paroxysmal nocturnal hemoglobinuria clones in patients with myelodysplastic syndromes and related bone marrow diseases, with emphasis on diagnostic pitfalls and caveats. *Haematologica* 94:29-37.

Wang SA, Tang G, Fadare O, et al [2008] Erythroid-predominant myelodysplastic syndromes: enumeration of blasts from nonerythroid rather than total marrow cells provides superior risk stratification. *Mod Pathol* 21:1394-1402.

Wei S, Chen X, Rocha K, et al [2009] A critical role for phosphatase haplodeficiency in the selective suppression of deletion 5q MDS by lenalidomide. *Proc Natl Acad Sci USA* 106:12974-12979.

Willis MS, McKenna RW, Peterson LC, et al [2005] Low blast count myeloid disorders with Auer rods: a clinicopathologic analysis of 9 cases. *Am J Clin Pathol* 124:191-198.

Wimazal F, Fonatsch C, Thalhammer R, et al [2007] Idiopathic cytopenia of undetermined significance (ICUS) vs low-risk MDS: the diagnostic interface. *Leuk Res* 31:1461-1468.

Wong AK, Fang B, Zhang L, et al [2008] Loss of the Y chromosome: an age-related or clonal phenomenon in acute myelogenous leukemia/myelodysplastic syndrome? *Arch Pathol Lab Med* 132:1329-1332.

Wu L, Li X, Chang C, et al [2008] Deviation of type I and type II T cells and its negative effect on hematopoiesis in myelodysplastic syndrome. *Int J Lab Hematol* 30:390-399.

Yarali N, Fisgin T, Duru F, Kara A [2002] Myelodysplastic features in visceral leishmaniasis. *Am J Hematol* 71:191-195.

Myelodysplastic/ Myeloproliferative Neoplasms

Kathryn Foucar, MD

The 4 disorders included as subtypes of myelodysplastic/myeloproliferative neoplasms (MDS/MPNs) t17.1 are unique among the myeloid neoplasms in that both dysplastic and proliferative features are evident simultaneously at initial presentation. Consequently, MDS/MPNs exhibit both effective and ineffective hematopoiesis [Vardiman 2008c].

A multiparameter approach is required for diagnosis. Key clinical information includes patient symptoms and physical examination findings such as splenomegaly, lymphadenopathy, or other sites of extramedullary disease. Other clinical information such as duration of complete blood count (CBC) abnormalities, careful history for previous hematologic disorders, and (especially in children) family history and evidence for constitutional disorders are all relevant to the diagnosis of MDS/MPN. Importantly, a diagnosis of MDS/MPN should not be rendered in patients with an established diagnosis of antecedent MDS or MPN. Instead, transformation of the antecedent myeloid neoplasm is a more appropriate consideration [Orazi 2008b, Vardiman 2008c].

Once it is determined that a de novo disorder is present, critical blood and bone marrow parameters need to be assessed t17.2. The prototypic complete blood count (CBC) from a patient with MDS/MPN shows at least one "cytosis" and at least one "cytopenia" i17.1 [Foucar 2009, Orazi 2008b, Vardiman 2008c]. Attention must also be paid to both the absolute monocyte count and the percentage of monocytes, because these parameters are critical for subclassification. Similarly, accurate delineation of myeloblasts, monoblasts, and promonocytes is essential to determine the percent blasts/blast equivalents i17.2. Promonocytes (blast equivalents) are distinguished from monocytes based on dispersed chromatin, delicately folded nuclei, and cytoplasmic basophilia as compared

t17.1 Myelodysplastic/Myeloproliferative Neoplasms

Chronic myelomonocytic leukemia

Atypical chronic myeloid leukemia, *BCR-ABL1*–

Juvenile myelomonocytic leukemia

Myelodysplastic/myeloproliferative neoplasm, unclassifiable

Reference: [Swerdlow 2008]

t17.2 Diagnostic Approach to Myelodysplastic/Myeloproliferative Neoplasms

Blood Requirements

At least 1 lineage "cytosis" (effective hematopoiesis)

At least 1 lineage "cytopenia" (ineffective hematopoiesis)

Numeral requirements for "cytosis"	WBC ≥13 × 10³/µL (≥13 × 10⁹/L)
	Platelet count ≥450 × 10³/µL (≥450 × 10⁹/L)
	Absolute monocyte count >1.0 × 10³/µL (>1.0 × 10⁹/L)

Cytopenias defined as below age/sex-related normal ranges

Dysplasia of at least one hematopoietic lineage

Blasts and blast equivalents <20%

Bone Marrow Requirements

Hypercellularity

Proliferation of 1 or more hematopoietic lineage(s)

Dysplasia of at least 1 or more hematopoietic lineage(s)

Assess monocytic component by cyto- or immunohistochemistry

Blasts and blast equivalents <20%

WBC = white blood cell

References: [Orazi 2006, 2008a, 2008b, Vardiman 2008c]

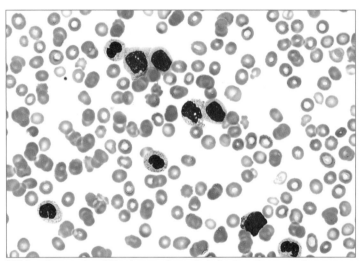

i17.1 *This peripheral blood smear shows the hybrid combination of leukocytosis in conjunction with significant anemia and thrombocytopenia in this patient with myelodysplastic/myeloproliferative neoplasm. (Wright)*

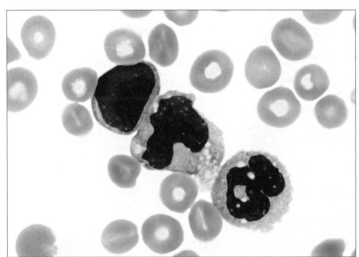

i17.2 *This peripheral blood smear shows a myeloblast (top), promonocyte (center), and a mature monocyte (bottom) from a patient with myelodysplastic/myeloproliferative neoplasm. Note significant anemia and thrombocytopenia. (Wright)*

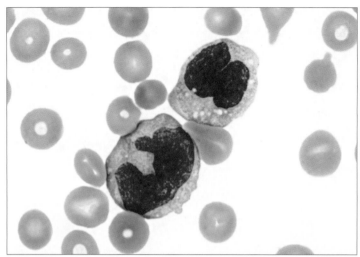

i17.3 *This peripheral blood smear shows a promonocyte with an adjacent atypical monocyte. The promonocyte (bottom) shows finer nuclear chromatin, clearly visible nucleoli, and moderate amounts of basophilic cytoplasm. The atypical monocyte shows greater nuclear maturity and a more slate gray appearance to the cytoplasm. (Wright)*

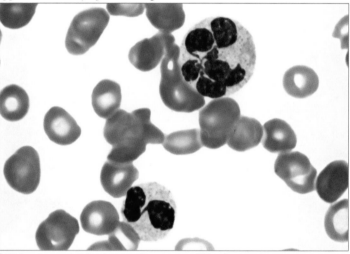

i17.4 *Neutrophil dysplasia in this peripheral blood smear from a patient with myelodysplastic/myeloproliferative neoplasm consists of both hypo- and hypersegmentation of the nuclei in conjunction with hypogranular cytoplasm. (Wright)*

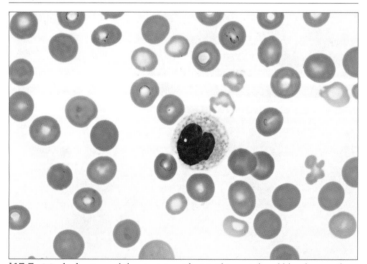

i17.5 *Marked anisopoikilocytosis is evident in this peripheral blood smear from a patient with myelodysplastic/myeloproliferative neoplasm. Note dysplastic neutrophil as well. (Wright)*

t17.3 Criteria for Dysplasia

Neutrophil Lineage

Hypogranular cytoplasm with/without Döhle bodies

Nuclear segmentation defects (hyposegmentation most common)

Hypercondensed nuclear chromatin

Megaloblastic changes

Functional defects of neutrophils

Abnormal localization of immature precursors on core biopsy (IHC for CD34 and MPO)

Megakaryocyte Lineage

Large, hypogranular platelets

Functional defects of platelets

Broad size range of megakaryocytes

Nuclear lobulation defects (hypo- or hyperlobulated)

Megakaryocyte clustering on core biopsy

Erythroid Lineage

Anisopoikilocytosis

Defects in hemoglobinization

Nuclear lobulation, budding, karyorrhexis

Megaloblastic changes

Loss of colony formation by IHC on core biopsy

Ring sideroblasts/increased dysplastic coarse iron granules

IHC = immunohistochemistry; MPO = myeloperoxidase

---

with the more grayish cytoplasm and more condensed chromatin of maturing monocytes **i17.2, i17.3**. Recent reports suggest that factors secreted by the clonal dysplastic neutrophilic cells inhibit monocyte differentiation, producing atypical monocytosis [Droin 2010].

The next key step in both blood and bone marrow evaluation is the documentation of dysplasia in at least one hematopoietic (HP) lineage using specific criteria **t17.3**. Blood smears are optimal for assessing neutrophil, platelet, and erythrocyte dysplasia, while the entire spectrum of hematopoietic lineage morphology is best assessed on bone marrow aspirate smears and core biopsy sections **i17.4, i17.5, i17.6, i17.7**. Immunohistochemical stains and iron stains can be used to document dysplasia **i17.8**.

Genetic assessment is essential to exclude other myeloid neoplasms that may exhibit some features of MDS/MPN. Thus, conventional cytogenetics or molecular testing must be performed to *exclude BCR-ABL1*, and mutations of *PDGFRA*, *PDGFRB*, *FGFR1*, isolated del(5q), and inv(3). The detection of any of these genetic abnormalities should prompt consideration of alternate World Health Organization (WHO) 2008 myeloid neoplasms [Vardiman 2008c].

Although there are no defining cytogenetic abnormalities in MDS/MPN, *RAS* mutations are common at the molecular level, especially in juvenile myelomonocytic leukemia (JMML), but

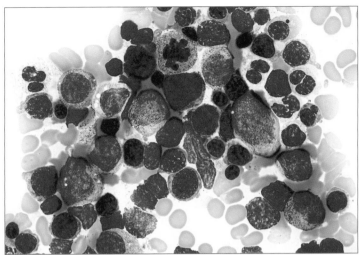

i17.6 *This bone marrow aspirate smear is hypercellular with a left shift of the granulocytic lineage. Note that mature neutrophils have hypogranular cytoplasm and nuclear hyposegmentation. (Wright)*

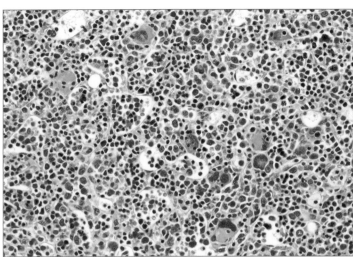

i17.7 *This bone marrow core biopsy section from a patient with myelodysplastic/ myeloproliferative neoplasm is virtually 100% cellular and shows increased numbers of abnormal megakaryocytes. (H&E)*

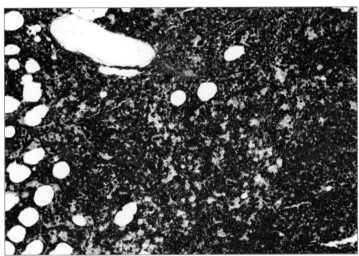

i17.8 *Intense myeloperoxidase positivity of this bone marrow core biopsy section from a patient with atypical chronic myelogenous leukemia is reflective of the striking granulocytic proliferation in the bone marrow. (immunoperoxidase for myeloperoxidase)*

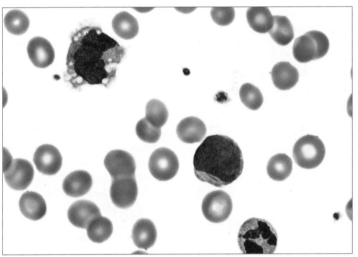

i17.9 *This peripheral blood smear is from a patient with chronic myelomonocytic leukemia-2, in which an Auer rod is evident in the blast located near the center. (Wright)*

also in other MDS/MPNs. Similarly, monosomy 7 is relatively common in JMML; the detection of monosomy 7 supports a diagnosis of JMML but it is not required for diagnosis. Recent studies document *TET2* mutations in a significant proportion of cases of MDS/MPN; the pathogenic role of this mutation has not been delineated [Jankowska 2009]. As with all myeloid neoplasms, the detection of a clonal cytogenetic abnormality excludes non-neoplastic differential diagnostic considerations.

[17.1] Chronic Myelomonocytic Leukemia (CMML)

Chronic myelomonocytic leukemia is the most common type of MDS/MPN encountered in clinical practice. Patients are elderly, there is a male predominance, and many patients have splenomegaly and extramedullary disease at other sites [Orazi 2008a]. Once alternate myeloid neoplasms have been excluded

by genetic testing for *BCR-ABL1*, *PDGFRA*, and *PDGFRB*, the salient blood and bone marrow features of CMML include:

1. Persistent monocytosis of $>1.0 \times 10^3/\mu L$ ($>1.0 \times 10^9/L$)
2. <20% blasts/blast equivalents in blood and bone marrow
3. Dysplasia of at least one myeloid lineage

If dysplasia cannot be documented, a diagnosis of CMML can still be rendered if the monocytosis persists for at least 3 months, a clonal cytogenetic abnormality is detected, and causes of secondary monocytosis have been excluded [Orazi 2008a].

Chronic myelomonocytic leukemia is further subdivided into CMML-1 with blasts/blast equivalents <5% in blood and <10% in bone marrow. Criteria for CMML-2 include 5%-19% in blood, 10%-19% blasts/blast equivalents in bone marrow *or* detection of Auer rods irrespective of blast percentage **i17.9** [Orazi 2008a, Vardiman 2008c].

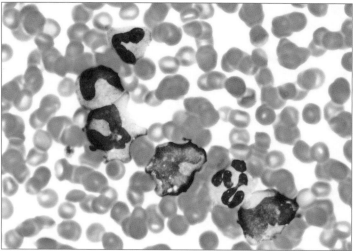

i17.10 *This peripheral blood smear from a patient with chronic myelomonocytic leukemia shows a marked increase in both neutrophils and monocytes. Note hypogranular cytoplasm of neutrophils and immaturity of the monocytic cells. (Wright) (courtesy C Sever, MD)*

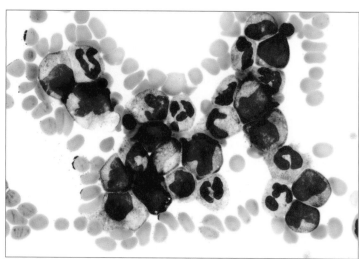

i17.11 *This bone marrow aspirate smear from a patient with chronic myelomonocytic leukemia shows increased overall cellularity with a significant increase in granulocytic cells. Monocytes are present, but less conspicuous. (Wright) (courtesy C Sever, MD)*

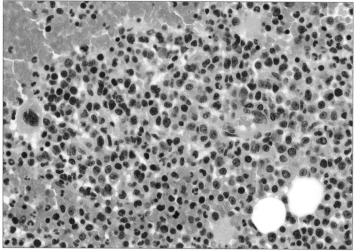

i17.12 *This bone marrow clot section shows virtually 100% cellularity and a marked expansion of granulocytic cells in this patient with chronic myelomonocytic leukemia. (H&E) (courtesy C Sever, MD)*

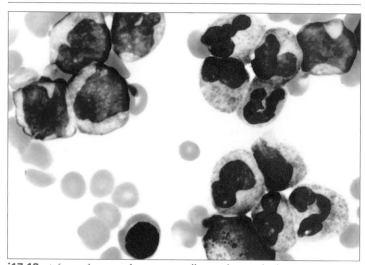

i17.13 *A focus of increased monocytic cells is evident on this bone marrow aspirate smear from a patient with chronic myelomonocytic leukemia. Note immaturity of monocytic cells. (Wright) (courtesy C Sever, MD)*

The white blood cell (WBC) count is highly variable in CMML, but usually elevated. Generally, a neutrophilia accompanies the required absolute monocytosis, but some cases show neutropenia i17.10. Dysplasia is typically evident in the neutrophil lineage, while monocyte immaturity may also be evident i17.10. Careful distinction between atypical monocytes and promonocytes (blast equivalents) on technically adequate specimens is essential (see i17.3). Either basophilia or eosinophilia may be present, but neither is typically prominent, especially if disorders with abnormalities of *PDGFRA* and *B* and systemic mastocytosis have been appropriately excluded.

As is characteristic of all MDS/MPNs, the bone marrow is typically hypercellular in CMML. Both aspirate smears and biopsy sections exhibit a granulocytic proliferation with monocytosis i17.11. The myeloid to erythroid (M:E) ratio may

exceed 10:1 i17.12. The monocytic component within the bone marrow is typically less conspicuous than in the blood i17.13. Often either cytochemical staining for nonspecific esterase (NSE) or immunohistochemical staining for CD163, lysozyme, CD68R, and/or CD68 may help highlight the monocytic cells, especially if granulocytic markers are used to distinguish this alternate lineage i17.14 [Ngo 2008, Orazi 2006]. Abnormal localization of immature precursors (ALIP) can also be assessed on core biopsy sections with CD34 and myeloperoxidase histochemical stains. CD34 immunohistochemical staining is also useful in highlighting the differences in the percentages of blasts in CMML 1 (<10% blasts) and CMML 2 (10%-19% blasts), but morphologic blast percentage determination is essential [Ngo 2008, Orazi 2006].

Both dyserythropoiesis and dysmegakaryopoiesis are common in CMML. Erythroid dysplasia is best appreciated

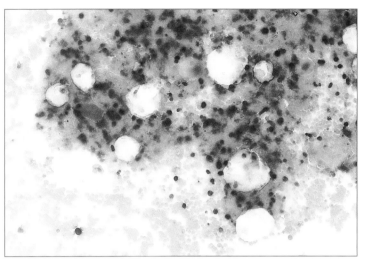

i17.14 *The monocytic component of chronic myelomonocytic leukemia is highlighted by nonspecific esterase staining of this bone marrow aspirate smear. (Nonspecific esterase)*

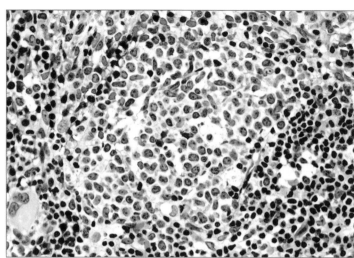

i17.15 *This bone marrow core biopsy shows a lymphoid aggregate (right) adjacent to a nodule of plasmacytoid dendritic cells (so-called monocytic nodule, center) in this patient with chronic myelomonocytic leukemia. (H&E)*

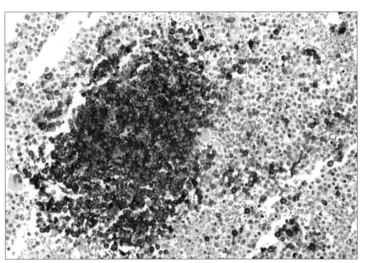

i17.16 *Immunoperoxidase for CD123 can be used to highlight these nodules of plasmacytoid dendritic cells in bone marrow core biopsy sections (as well as sections from other sites) in patients with chronic myelomonocytic leukemia. (immunoperoxidase for CD123)*

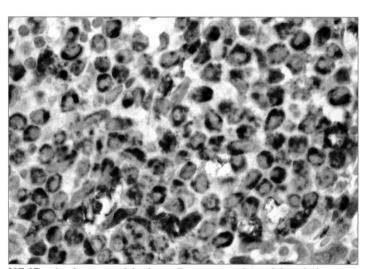

i17.17 *The plasmacytoid dendritic cells comprising this nodule in the bone marrow are CD68+ in this patient with chronic myelomonocytic leukemia. (immunoperoxidase for CD68)*

on Wright and Prussian blue stained bone marrow aspirate smears, while both aspirate smears and core biopsies are useful for highlighting megakaryocyte dysplasia. On both H&E and immunohistochemical staining for CD42b or CD31, abnormal megakaryocyte size and clustering can be appreciated. Often smaller, dysplastic megakaryocytes predominate (see **i17.7**) [Orazi 2006, 2008a, 2008b].

One distinctive feature of CMML is the identification of nodules of plasmacytoid dendritic cells highlighted with CD123 staining **i17.15, i17.16, i17.17, i17.18**. These discrete nodules contain cells with round nuclei, dispersed chromatin, and eosinophilic cytoplasm with distinct cell membranes **i17.19, i17.20**. Often cell turnover is brisk, and tingible body macrophages may be present [Chen 2003, Mongkonsritragoon 1998, Orazi 2006, 2008b]. These monocytic nodules are highly associated with CMML and may be present within extramedullary sites of

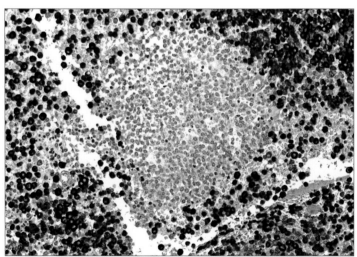

i17.18 *Myeloperoxidase highlights numerous positive cells in chronic myelomonocytic leukemia in this bone marrow core biopsy section, while the plasmacytoid dendritic cell nodule is negative. (immunoperoxidase for myeloperoxidase)*

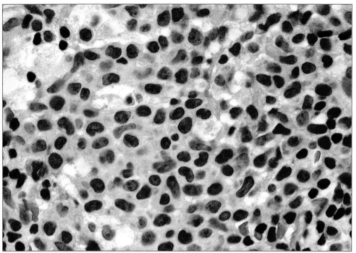

i17.19 *High-power magnification of a plasmacytoid nodule from a bone marrow core biopsy section shows some immaturity and cytologic atypia. (H&E)*

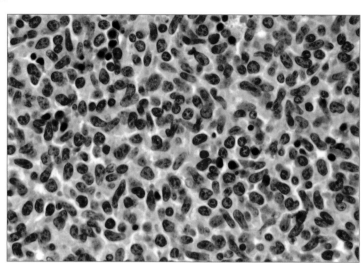

i17.20 *The cytologic features of another example of a plasmacytoid dendritic nodule on a bone marrow core biopsy are illustrated. Note relatively finely dispersed nuclear chromatin. (H&E)*

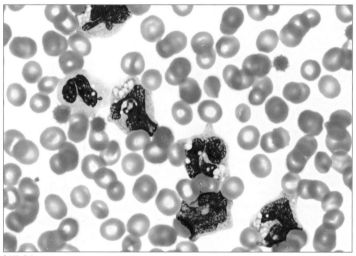

i17.21 *This peripheral blood smear shows a striking monocytosis. Although there is some nuclear immaturity, atypical monocytes predominate (see **i17.22**). (Wright)*

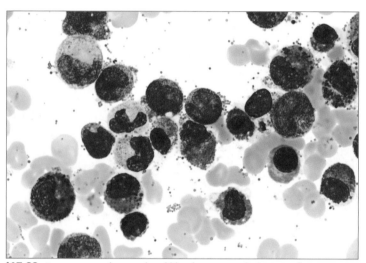

i17.22 *In contrast to the peripheral blood smear in which atypical, yet mature, monocytes predominate **i17.21**, this bone marrow aspirate smear shows a striking left shift with numerous blasts and abnormal eosinophils in a case confirmed to be acute myeloid leukemia with inv(16), despite the resemblance of the peripheral blood to chronic myelomonocytic leukemia. (Wright)*

disease. At least some studies confirm a clonal relationship between the plasmacytoid dendritic cells and the underlying CMML [Orazi 2008b].

Currently, flow cytometric immunophenotyping does not play a major role in the diagnosis of CMML. However, many aberrant patterns of antigen expression have been described, which may be useful in distinguishing CMML from non-neoplastic disorders [Lacronique-Gazaille 2007, Xu 2005]. The expression profile of monocytic antigens such as CD64, CD36, and CD14 can help document the monocytic lineage derivation of the neoplastic cells, but reduced expression of these antigens has been described in CMML [Lacronique-Gazaille 2007, Xu 2005]. Expression of CD56 is more prevalent in CMML than in non-neoplastic monocytic disorders [Lacronique-Gazaille 2007, Xu 2005].

Cytogenetic abnormalities are common in CMML, but none is specific. The most frequently described findings

include trisomy 8, monosomy 7, del(7q), and structural abnormalities of 12p [Orazi 2008a]. Although no genetic features are recurrent in CMML, these studies provide definitive exclusionary information. As described earlier, the detection of *BCR-ABL1* gene rearrangement or rearrangements of *PDGFRA*, *PDGFRB*, or *FGFR1* all define other distinctive biologic entities; the diagnosis of CMML is not appropriate for these cases. Similarly, the detection of either 11q23 translocations or isolated del(5q) should prompt careful consideration of other myeloid neoplasms.

Although transformation to acute myeloid leukemia (AML) may occur, a more significant issue at the time of diagnosis of CMML is to document that the bone marrow blast/blast equivalent percentage is <20%. Cases in which the blood findings are compatible with CMML may actually

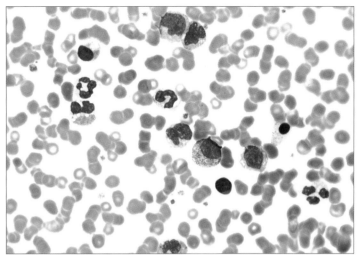

i17.23 *In addition to numerous neutrophils and monocytes, this peripheral blood smear also shows a marked eosinophilia. Although the blood picture is compatible with chronic myelomonocytic leukemia with eosinophilia, the bone marrow showed extensive systemic mastocytosis. (Wright)*

t17.4 WHO Criteria for Juvenile Myelomonocytic Leukemia

Blood	Absolute monocytosis >1.0 × 10³/µL (>1.0 × 10⁹/L)
	<20% blasts/blast equivalents (promonocytes)
Bone marrow	<20% blasts/blast equivalents (promonocytes)
Genetics	Absent *BCR-ABL1*
	Absent t(9;22)(q34;q11.2)
Additional criteria (≥2 required)	Increased hemoglobin F level for age
	Immature granulocytic cells in blood
	WBC >10 × 10³/µL (>10 × 10⁹/L)
	Clonal cytogenetic abnormality including monosomy 7
	In vitro GM-CSF hypersensitivity of myeloid progenitor cells

GM-CSF = granulocyte monocyte colony-stimulating factor; WBC = white blood cell; WHO = World Health Organization

References: [Baumann 2008]

demonstrate acute myelomonocytic leukemia (AMML) in the bone marrow **i17.21, i17.22**. Consequently, a diagnosis of CMML based solely on blood assessment should be interpreted with caution. In these situations, a strong recommendation should be made to confirm the diagnosis of CMML in bone marrow.

Transformation of CMML to AML can be manifested by progressive increases in the percentage of blood or bone marrow blasts/blast equivalents, progressive dysplasia, and cytopenias, and an increased size of CD34+ collections on clot or core biopsy sections. Recent studies suggest an association between *RUNX1* mutations and progression to AML in CMML patients [Kuo 2009].

As emphasized, the differential diagnosis of CMML is broad and includes neoplastic and non-neoplastic disorders. Furthermore, cases of CMML-like disorders with eosinophilia have been placed in a new WHO category if specific genetic mutations are present (see Chapter 15). In addition, cases of systemic mastocytosis can exhibit a blood picture that fulfills the criteria for CMML with eosinophilia **i17.23**.

[17.2] Juvenile Myelomonocytic Leukemia (JMML)

The WHO 2008 diagnostic criteria for juvenile myelomonocytic leukemia are listed on **t17.4**. JMML is unique among the MDS/MPNs in that the vast majority of cases occur in young children, usually 3 years of age or younger, and the pathogenesis is relatively well delineated **sidebar 17.1** [Emanuel 2008, Koike 2008, Niemeyer 2008, Tartaglia 2003]. Dysregulation of the granulocyte monocyte colony-stimulating factor (GM-CSF)/RAS signal transduction pathway via multiple different activating mutations is considered to be the key pathophysiologic mechanism in JMML [Baumann 2008, Loh 2009]. A germline mutation of *NRAS* has been identified in one case of JMML [De Filippi 2009]. Increased sensitivity to GM-CSF in cell culture studies is a reflection of these molecular/genetic events [Emanuel 2008, Koike 2008].

Although there are many clinical clues to the diagnosis of JMML, including young age, association with neurofibromatosis 1, hepatosplenomegaly, lymphadenopathy, and skin lesions, examination of the peripheral blood is essential [Baumann 2008]. The peripheral blood in patients with JMML exhibits a profile of prototypic features including sustained monocytosis (often with some evidence of nuclear atypia and immaturity), leukocytosis, thrombocytopenia, and often anemia **i17.24, i17.25, i17.26** [Baumann 2008]. The morphologic delineation of monoblasts, promonocytes, and mature atypical monocytes is essential in distinguishing JMML from AMML. Blasts and promonocytes (blast equivalents) must comprise <20% of cells; promonocytes are typically <5% **i17.26** [Baumann 2008].

The bone marrow is typically hypercellular **i17.27**. Again, blasts and blast equivalents must account for <20% of total nucleated cells. There is usually a marked predominance of granulocytic lineage cells, while the monocytic component is often less conspicuous than that noted in the blood. Cytochemical and/or immunohistochemical stains may be useful in highlighting monocytic cells, but the specificity of many immunohistochemical stains is not as optimal as cytochemical nonspecific esterase (NSE) staining **i17.28, i17.29, i17.30**. Dysplasia is generally not prominent. Other less common findings include erythroid lineage proliferation and reticulin fibrosis. The identification of definitive Auer rods excludes a diagnosis of JMML and favors acute myeloid leukemia (AML).

[sidebar 17.1] Genetics of Syndromic and Nonsyndromic Juvenile Myelomonocytic Leukemia

If the constitutional bone marrow failure syndromes are caused by inherited mutations resulting in *ineffective* hematopoiesis, then the syndromic presentation of JMML could be thought of as a corollary: an MDS/MPN resulting from inherited mutations. JMML is particularly noted to occur in conjunction with neurofibromatosis 1 (NF1) and Noonan syndrome (NS). While not all cases of JMML occur in the setting of congenital syndromes, the subset of syndromic cases has provided key mechanistic insights that have proven applicable to sporadic JMML as well.

NF1 is an autosomal dominant disorder with high penetrance but variable expressivity, meaning that different patients may develop differing manifestations of the disease. Most commonly, patients demonstrate café au lait spots, Lisch nodules, axillary and/or inguinal freckling, and multiple cutaneous neurofibromas. While there is a low risk of malignant transformation of the cutaneous neurofibromas, deeper plexiform neurofibromas may undergo transformation to malignant peripheral nerve sheath tumors; patients with NF1 are also at increased risk for diverse other malignancies, including glioma, pheochromocytoma, medulloblastoma and, as noted earlier, JMML. NF1 is caused by germline mutation of *NF1*, the gene product of which, neurofibromin, hydrolyzes GTP bound to active RAS, thus converting RAS to an inactive state. In the absence of neurofibromin, RAS remains active and exerts proliferative effects. JMML and other NF1-associated malignancies arise in part when acquired loss of the second, unmutated allele leads to total eradication of neurofibromin-mediated control of the RAS pathway. Clinically, NF1 is diagnosed in 11% of all cases of JMML [Niemeyer 2008]. However, when sporadic cases of JMML (ie, cases occurring in patients without clinical evidence of NF1) are assessed, approximately 15% show *NF1* mutations [Side 1998].

The coexistence of *NF1* mutations and JMML demonstrates the importance of the RAS/MAPK pathway in the development of JMML, as does the consideration of JMML in light of NS, an autosomal dominant disorder characterized by short stature, congenital heart defects and developmental delays.

Additional features include characteristic facies, webbed neck, pectus defects, coagulopathy, and cryptorchidism. Children with NS present with an unusual MPN that may vary in aggressiveness; this process often fulfils the criteria for diagnosis of JMML [Niemeyer 2008]. The first gene found to be mutated in NS was *PTPN11*, which encodes the tyrosine phosphatase SHP2. A direct analogy to NF1-associated JMML was soon apparent: SHP2 relays growth signals to RAS, and the NS mutations produce constitutive activation of the protein and the pathway. Moreover, acquired mutations to *PTPN11* are found in 34% of sporadic JMML cases [Tartaglia 2003]. Subsequently, inherited mutations of a second gene, *KRAS*, were found in some patients with NS [Schubbert 2006], and acquired *RAS* gene mutations were identified in 20% of sporadic JMML [Koike 2008]. The implication was clear: NF1, NS, and JMML can all be produced by overactive RAS signaling, thus explaining the clinical overlap. If the mutations are germline, then NF1 or NS occur and the patient is at increased risk for JMML; if the mutations are acquired in a hematopoietic progenitor cell, then JMML may arise.

This neat story has been somewhat complicated by the discovery of an additional gene mutated in NS: *SOS1*, the protein product of which is recruited to the plasma membrane in the process of RAS activation. While this gene often harbors the causative mutation in NS, *SOS1* mutations are not described in JMML [Emanuel 2008, Kratz 2007, Roberts 2007]. Interestingly, *SOS1* mutations are also exceedingly rare across a broad range of malignancies [Swanson 2008]. Similarly, *RAF1* mutations may cause NS, but do not seem to be associated with JMML. It remains unclear why these alterations are sufficient to cause NS but depart from the pattern established above in their oncogenic potential. Conversely, mutations in *CBL* are present in some cases of JMML but have not yet been observed in NS.

A summary table presenting the frequencies of mutations in NF1, NS and JMML is provided below **tS17.1**. The success in pinpointing much of the molecular basis of JMML via NF1 and NS demonstrates the power of studying hematopoietic malignancies in the setting of inherited cancer susceptibility syndromes.

tS17.1 Frequency of Mutations in Neurofibromatosis Type 1 (NF1), Noonan Syndrome (NS), and Juvenile Myelomonocytic Leukemia (JMML)

Gene	NF-1	NS	JMML
PTPN11	—	50%	~35%
*KRAS**	—	<5%	20%-25%
SOS1	—	10%-13%	—
RAF1	—	3%-17%	—
NF1	>95%[†]	—	~25%
CBL	—	—	15%

NRAS may also be mutated in JMML; recent reports of germline mutation of *NRAS* in JMML patients
[†] Detection of *NF1* mutations may be limited by assay type and somatic mosaicism, explaining the slightly <100% detection rate

References: [Allanson 1997, De Felippi 2009, Emanuel 2008, Friedman 1997, Kratz 2007, Loh 2009, Side 1998, Tartaglia 2003]

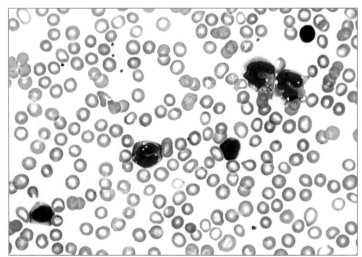

i17.24 *This peripheral blood smear is from a 5-year-old male with neurofibromatosis 1 and juvenile myelomonocytic leukemia. Note marked leukocytosis, anemia, and thrombocytopenia. (Wright) (courtesy W Finn, MD)*

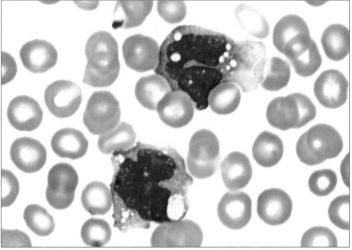

i17.25 *Although some nuclear immaturity is evident in the peripheral blood of this 5-year-old male with juvenile myelomonocytic leukemia, atypical monocytes predominate. (Wright) (courtesy W Finn, MD)*

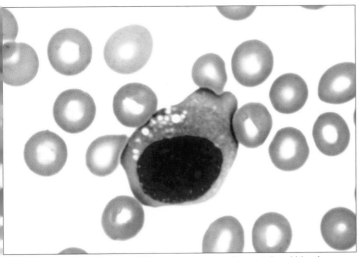

i17.26 *Rare circulating monoblasts are evident in this peripheral blood smear from a 5-year-old male with neurofibromatosis 1 and juvenile myelomonocytic leukemia. (Wright) (courtesy W Finn, MD)*

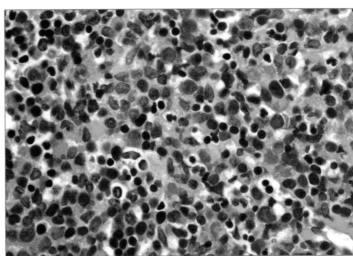

i17.27 *The bone marrow is virtually 100% cellular in this bone marrow core biopsy section from an infant with juvenile myelomonocytic leukemia associated with monosomy 7. (H&E)*

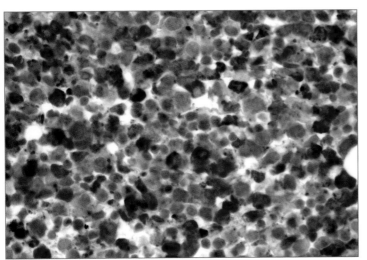

i17.28 *Immunoperoxidase staining for CD68 on this bone marrow core biopsy section shows numerous positive cells in this infant with juvenile myelomonocytic leukemia. (immunoperoxidase for CD68)*

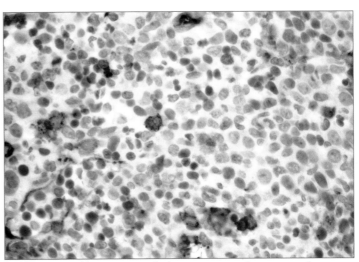

i17.29 *CD34+ blasts are rare in this bone marrow core biopsy section from an infant with juvenile myelomonocytic leukemia. (immunoperoxidase for CD34)*

Flow cytometric immunophenotyping is useful in documenting a monocytic component, but a distinctive flow "profile" has not been delineated. The detection of a substantial CD34+ population by flow cytometric immunophenotyping favors a diagnosis of AML.

By conventional karyotyping, monosomy 7 is detected in 25% of cases, while mutations in genes involved in the RAS signaling pathway are detected in >75% of cases [Loh 2009, Niemeyer 2008]. The detection of a translocation involving 11q23 supports a diagnosis of AML even in cases with a predominance of mature cells in blood **i17.31**.

The differential diagnosis of JMML includes both neoplastic and non-neoplastic disorders. The careful application of 2008 WHO classification criteria generally allows the distinction among JMML, chronic myelogenous leukemia (CML), AML, and other myeloid neoplasms.

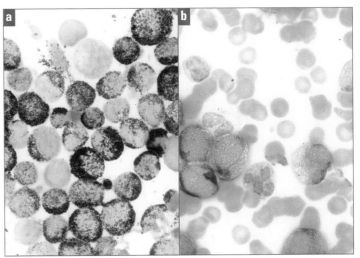

i17.30 *This composite of myeloperoxidase **a** and nonspecific esterase **b** is from a bone marrow aspirate smear from a 1-year-old patient with juvenile myelomonocytic leukemia. (Cytochemistry for myeloperoxidase, nonspecific esterase) (courtesy R Brynes, MD)*

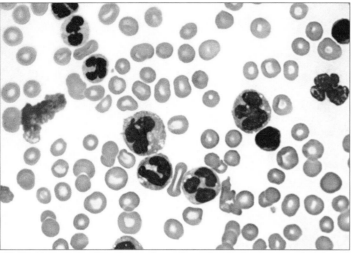

i17.31 *This peripheral blood smear from a 5-month-old infant shows a striking resemblance to juvenile myelomonocytic leukemia, yet 11q23 was detected with cytogenetic evaluation, which confirmed a diagnosis of acute myeloid leukemia. (Wright)*

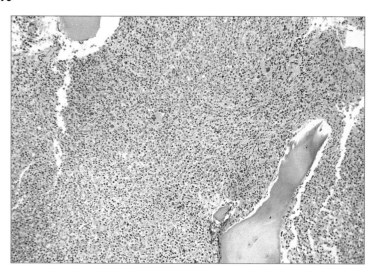

i17.32 *Bone marrow biopsy section from a patient with chronic Epstein-Barr virus infection shows striking hypercellularity mimicking myelodysplastic/myeloproliferative neoplasm. (H&E)*

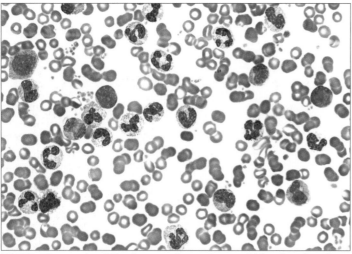

i17.33 *This peripheral blood smear is from a 69-year-old female with a white blood cell count of 161 × 10³/μL (161 × 10⁹/L) and morphologic features compatible with atypical chronic myelogenous leukemia. BCR-ABL1 was negative. Note hypogranular neutrophils, left shift, and anemia. (Wright)*

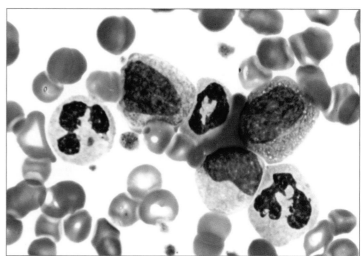

i17.34 *On high magnification, both left shift and dysplastic neutrophils are evident in this peripheral blood smear from a 69-year-old female with atypical chronic myelogenous leukemia. (Wright)*

Both genetic studies and careful delineation of blasts, promonocytes, and more mature forms facilitate these differential diagnostic distinctions i17.31. In addition to these neoplastic differential diagnostic considerations, chronic viral infections can be associated with splenomegaly and sustained monocytosis. In particular, chronic Epstein-Barr virus, cytomegalovirus, and human herpesvirus 6 can all mimic JMML i17.32 [Herrod 1983, Kirby 1990, Lorenzana 2002, Manabe 2004, Niemeyer 1998, Pinkel 1998, Toyoda 2004].

[17.3] Atypical Chronic Myelogenous Leukemia (aCML), *BCR-ABL1*– (aCML)

The 2008 WHO criteria for the diagnosis of aCML include genetic exclusions as well as fairly complex blood and bone marrow features t17.5 [Orazi 2008b, Vardiman 2008b]. As these complex criteria suggest, aCML is a diagnosis of exclusion, requiring comprehensive genetic testing and methodical evaluation of leukocytes in blood and bone marrow i17.33, i17.34, i17.35. One morphologic hallmark of aCML is striking dysgranulopoiesis. These dysplastic neutrophilic cells often exhibit hypogranular cytoplasm and nuclear segmentation defects i17.35. Pronounced nuclear clumping of neutrophils is also a feature [Orazi 2008b].

The bone marrow is typically hypercellular with a pronounced granulocytic lineage proliferation i17.36. Megakaryocytes may be increased and hypolobulated, mimicking *BCR-ABL1*+ CML i17.37. However, the degree of dysgranulopoiesis is much more dramatic in aCML. Dyserythropoiesis is also fairly common. The percent of

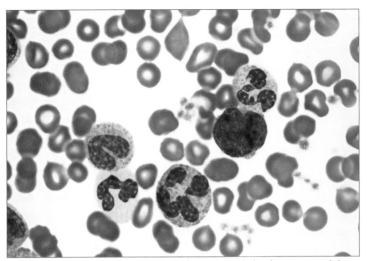

i17.35 *Anisopoikilocytosis, anemia, leukocytosis with dysplastic neutrophils, and left shift are all evident in this peripheral blood smear from a patient with atypical chronic myelogenous leukemia. (Wright)*

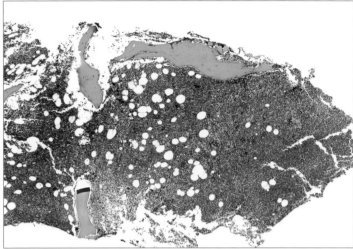

i17.36 *This bone marrow core biopsy section is markedly hypercellular for the patient's age in a case of atypical chronic myelogenous leukemia. Note increase in megakaryocytes. (H&E)*

t17.5 WHO Criteria for Atypical Chronic Myelogenous Leukemia, *BCR-ABL1*–

Blood	WBC ≥13 × 10³/μL (≥13.0 × 10⁹/L)
	Neutrophilia
	Left shift (promyelocytes, myelocytes, metamyelocytes) ≥10%
	Prominent dysgranulopoiesis
	Minimal to moderate basophilia (<2%)
	Absent to minimal monocytosis (<10%)
	<20% blasts/blast equivalents
Bone marrow	<20% blasts/blast equivalents
	Hypercellular with granulocytic proliferation
	Granulocytic lineage dysplasia
Genetics	Absence of *BCR-ABL1* or t(9;22)(q34;q11.2)
	Absence of *PDGFRA/B* rearrangements

References: [Vardiman 2008b]

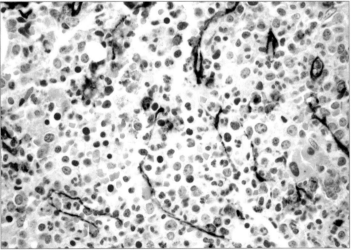

i17.37 *On higher magnification, the increase in atypical megakaryocytes is striking in this bone marrow core biopsy section from a patient with atypical chronic myelogenous leukemia. Note small megakaryocyte size and reduced megakaryocyte nuclear lobulation. (H&E)*

blasts must be <20% by definition **i17.38**. Neither flow cytometric immunophenotyping nor conventional cytogenetics provides definitive "proof" of aCML, but nonrecurrent clonal cytogenetic abnormalities are present in most cases [Vardiman 2008b]. *JAK2* mutations have not been appreciated in this disorder [Fend 2008].

[17.4] Myelodysplastic/Myeloproliferative Neoplasms, Unclassified (MDS/MPN-U)

Similar to other MDS/MPN, cases of MDS/MPN-U must first exhibit the requisite hybrid myelodysplastic and myeloproliferative features and represent a de novo disorder

i17.38 *This bone marrow core biopsy section shows mildly increased CD34+ blasts with some clustering in this patient with atypical chronic myelogenous leukemia. Note neoangiogenesis. (immunoperoxidase for CD34)*

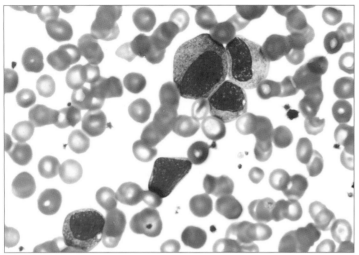

i17.39 *A diagnosis of myelodysplastic/myeloproliferative neoplasm, unclassified was made on this peripheral blood smear from a 54-year-old male with a white blood cell count of 15.5 × 10³/μL (15.5 × 10⁹/L), moderate anemia, and a normal platelet count. Although left shift of the granulocytic series is evident, striking neutrophil dysplasia is not a feature. (Wright)*

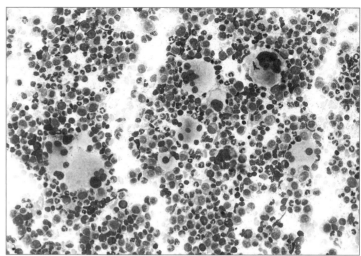

i17.40 *This bone marrow aspirate smear from a patient with myelodysplastic/myeloproliferative neoplasm, unclassified shows marked hypercellularity in conjunction with increased megakaryocytes showing a range of nuclear features. (Wright)*

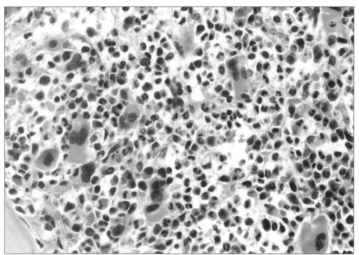

i17.41 *This bone marrow core biopsy section from an elderly patient with myelodysplastic/myeloproliferative neoplasm, unclassified shows marked hypercellularity and a marked increase in dysplastic, small megakaryocytes with nuclear hypolobulation. (H&E)*

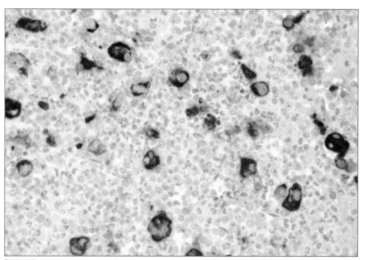

i17.42 *Immunoperoxidase staining for CD42b on this bone marrow core biopsy section from a patient with myelodysplastic/myeloproliferative neoplasm, unclassified shows markedly increased megakaryocytes, many of which are small and have reduced nuclear lobulation. (immunoperoxidase for CD42b)*

[Vardiman 2008a]. In addition, the diagnosis of MDS/MPN-U is to be used in cases that cannot be classified into any other MDS, MPN, or MDS/MPN category. Similar to other subtypes of MDS/MPN, multiple genetic subtypes are exclusionary, including *BCR-ABL1*, t(9;22)(q34;q11.2), rearrangements of *PDGFRA*, *PDGFRB*, *FGFR1*, isolated del(5q), t(3;3)(q21;q26), and inv3(q21q26) [Vardiman 2008a]. Furthermore, a diagnosis of MDS/MPN should *not* be rendered in patients with a recent history of either cytotoxic or growth factor therapy unless a clonal cytogenetic abnormality is detected. Instead, these patients should be re-evaluated after the cessation of these therapies to determine if the blood and bone marrow abnormalities, including blast percentages, are transient or sustained.

Once all of these exclusionary criteria are removed from consideration, the actual hematologic and morphologic features consist of documentation of *effective* hematopoiesis in one or more lineages based on WBC of 13.0 × 10³/μL (13.0 × 10⁹/L) or more and/or platelet count of ≥450 × 10³/μL (≥450 × 10⁹/L). Simultaneous *ineffective* hematopoiesis, usually anemia, must also be confirmed **i17.39** [Vardiman 2008a].

The bone marrow is typically hypercellular with proliferation of any or all hematopoietic lineages, but at least one lineage must show dysplastic features **t17.3, i17.40, i17.41, i17.42**. Blasts in the blood and bone marrow must be <20%.

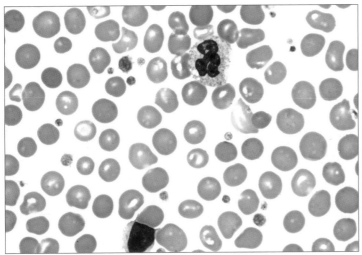

i17.43 *This peripheral blood smear from a 78-year-old female with a normal white blood cell count, a mild macrocytic anemia, and platelet count >1,000 × 10³/µL (>1.0 × 10⁹/L) is compatible with refractory anemia with ring sideroblasts associated with marked thrombocytosis. (Wright) (courtesy C Sever, MD)*

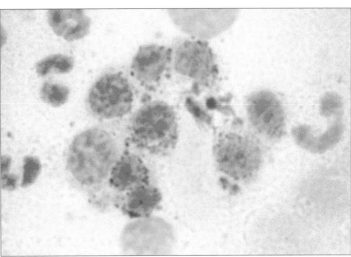

i17.44 *Numerous ring sideroblasts are evident in this iron stain of a bone marrow aspirate smear from a 78-year-old female with a diagnosis of refractory anemia with ring sideroblasts associated with marked thrombocytosis. (Prussian blue)*

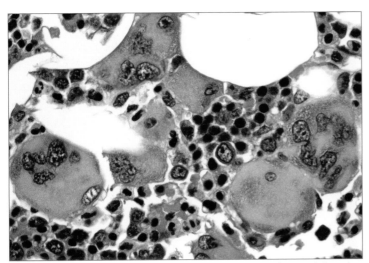

i17.45 *Huge hyperlobulated megakaryocytes reminiscent of essential thrombocythemia are evident on the bone marrow core biopsy section from a 78-year-old female with a diagnosis of presumed refractory anemia with ring sideroblasts associated with marked thrombocytosis (H&E) (courtesy C Sever, MD)*

more favorable outcome. The compelling overlap with ET has prompted recent authors to suggest that this category should be eliminated [Wardrop 2009]. Other investigators report molecular overlap between RARS-T and RAS, which, in conjunction with frequent *JAK2* mutations, does support a hybrid MDS/MPN molecular profile [Malcovati 2009]. Furthermore, other authors report survival differences between RARS-T and conventional ET, providing some evidence to support retention of this provisional category [Atallah 2008].

The constellation of features in RARS-T include anemia, often macrocytic, marked thrombocytosis, bone marrow hypercellularity with erythroid and megakaryocytic proliferation, 15% or more ring sideroblasts, <20% blasts, and hyperlobated megakaryocytes that are increased, often clustered, and indistinguishable from ET i17.43, i17.44, i17.45 [Orazi 2008b, Vardiman 2008a].

[17.4.1] **Provisional Category: Refractory Anemia with Ring Sideroblasts Associated with Marked Thrombocytosis (RARS-T)**

One 2001 WHO provisional entity, RARS-T, has been retained in the provisional category due to lack of generally accepted evidence that RARS-T is a distinctive entity [Wardrop 2009]. More than other cases of MDS/MPN, RARS-T closely overlaps with MPN in many key respects. Both the sustained thrombocytosis and the hyperlobated megakaryocytes overlap with essential thrombocythemia (ET) i17.43, i17.44, i17.45. Similarly, either *JAK2* or *MPL* mutations are detected in about 60% of cases of RARS-T, identical to the frequency of these mutations in ET and primary myelofibrosis [Gattermann 2007, Szpurka 2006, Vardiman 2008a, Wardrop 2009]. *JAK2* mutations in RARS-T are linked to a

[17.5] **Differential Diagnosis of MDS/MPN**

Although some key differential diagnostic considerations are included in the discussion of individual MDS/MPN subtypes, a broad list of neoplastic and non-neoplastic differential diagnostic considerations is presented in t17.6.

[17.6] **Components of the Diagnostic Interpretation**

As predicted from the complex and multifaceted diagnostic requirements, the successful diagnosis of a MDS/MPN requires clinical information, comprehensive morphologic and hematologic assessment of blood and bone marrow, as well as thorough cytogenetic/molecular analyses

t17.6 Differential Diagnosis of Myelodysplastic/Myeloproliferative Neoplasms

Non-Neoplastic Considerations

Chronic viral infections	EBV, CMV, HHV6
Collagen vascular disorders	Often more MPN-like, but may have concurrent anemia
Cytokine/growth factor therapy	rhG-CSF/GM-CSF Cytokine producing neoplasms
Other non-neoplastic causes of monocytosis	Many types of infection Inflammatory disorders

Neoplastic, Nonhematopoietic

Chemokine or cytokine producing carcinomas/sarcomas

Cytokine-producing lymphomas

Neoplastic, Hematopoietic

Myelodysplastic syndromes

Myeloproliferative neoplasms, including CML

Myeloid neoplasms with eosinophilia and abnormalities of *PDGFRA, PDGFRB, FGFR1*

Acute myeloid leukemias, including AMML

AMML = acute myelomonocytic leukemia; CML = chronic myelogenous leukemia; CMV = cytomegalovirus; EBV = Epstein-Barr virus; GM-CSF = granulocyte macrophage colony-stimulating factor; HHV6 = human herpesvirus 6; rhG-CSF = recombinant human granulocyte colony-stimulating factor

t17.7 Components of the Diagnostic Interpretation

Establish hybrid effective and ineffective lineage hematopoiesis

Exclude non-neoplastic causes of hematologic abnormalities, including underlying infection and/or cytokine therapy

Confirm dysplasia in at least one hematopoietic lineage

Quantify blasts and blast equivalents in blood and bone marrow

Confirm that disorder is de novo

Exclude transformation of previously diagnosed myeloid neoplasm

Use cytochemical stains (NSE) to confirm monocytic component as needed

Assess for ring sideroblasts with iron stain on bone marrow aspirate smear

Perform conventional cytogenetics and/or molecular studies for both exclusionary and inclusionary purposes

Exclude cases with *BCR-ABL1, PDGFRA, PDGFRB, FGFR1,* isolated del(5q), inv(3)/t(3;3) mutations

Assess for *JAK2* mutations, which are common in MDS/MPN-U, RARS-T

Assess for RAS pathway mutations in MDS/MPN, especially children with suspected JMML

JMML = juvenile myelomonocytic leukemia; MDS/MPN = myelodysplastic/myeloproliferative neoplasms; NSE = nonspecific esterase; RARS-T = refractory anemia with ring sideroblasts with thrombocytosis; RAS = *rat* sarcoma gene

t17.7. The decision to perform a bone marrow examination in these cases hinges on whether or not the hematologic and morphologic abnormalities in the blood can be attributed to underlying infection, cytokine therapy, or other causes. If abnormalities are "unexplained," bone marrow examination with cytogenetics/fluorescence in situ hybridization or molecular testing is warranted. These molecular genetic tests can be performed on blood samples if bone marrow examination is not an option. The contribution of flow cytometric immunophenotyping in the diagnosis of MDS/MPN is less clear cut, but flow cytometry is a good modality to determine lineage of blasts, as needed.

[17.7] Clues and Caveats

1. To be considered as a possible MDS/MPN, a case must exhibit both proliferative and dysplastic features at presentation.
2. The CBC should demonstrate both cytoses and cytopenia(s).
3. Dysplasia of at least one hematopoietic lineage must be present (rare exceptions).
4. Strict criteria for defining dysplasia in all hematopoietic lineages must be followed.
5. The diagnostician must be able to identify promonocytes (blast equivalents) and monoblasts/myeloblasts.
6. Delineation of promonocytes is key to the distinction between CMML or JMML and AMML.
7. Cytochemical NSE and/or immunohistochemistry may be essential in highlighting the monocytic component in bone marrow aspirate smears.
8. Nodules of CD123+ plasmacytoid dendritic cells (so-called monocytic nodules) may be evident on core biopsies or clot sections in CMML.
9. Blood findings may be compatible with CMML in some cases in which the bone marrow shows AMML.
10. JMML is the only MDS/MPN that primarily affects children usually younger than 3 years of age; associations with neurofibromatosis and other constitutional disorders have been established.
11. JMML must be distinguished from AML.
12. The detection of Auer rods in JMML-like processes supports AML.
13. The detection of 11q23 translocations supports AML, not MDS/MPN.
14. Some cases of myeloid malignancy with iso(17q) fulfill criteria for MDS/MPN.
15. Chronic viral infections can produce a blood and bone marrow picture that mimics JMML.
16. Diagnostic criteria for aCML are complex. Key features include marked leukocytosis, prominent dysplastic neutrophilia, cytopenias, and absence of cytogenetic/molecular features of CML and other genetically defined neoplasms.
17. The provisional category of RARS-T may represent cases of essential thrombocythemia that have ring sideroblasts.

[17.8] References

Allanson J [1997] Noonan syndrome. In: *GeneReviews at GeneTests: Medical Genetics Information Resource* (database online). URL: http://www.genetests.org. Updated October 2008.

Atallah E, Nussenzveig R, Yin CC, et al [2008] Prognostic interaction between thrombocytosis and JAK2 V617F mutation in the WHO subcategories of myelodysplastic/myeloproliferative disease-unclassifiable and refractory anemia with ringed sideroblasts and marked thrombocytosis. *Leukemia* 22:1295-1298.

Baumann I, Bennett J, Niemeyer C, et al [2008] Juvenile myelomonocytic leukaemia. In: Swerdlow S, Campo E, Harris N, et al, eds. *WHO Classification of Tumours: Pathology & Genetics: Tumours of Haematopoietic and Lymphoid Tissues.* Lyon, France: IARC Press; 82-84.

Chen YC, Chou JM, Ketterling RP, et al [2003] Histologic and immunohistochemical study of bone marrow monocytic nodules in 21 cases with myelodysplasia. *Am J Clin Pathol* 120:874-881.

Chen YC, Chou JM, Letendre L, Li CY [2005] Clinical importance of bone marrow monocytic nodules in patients with myelodysplasia: retrospective analysis of 21 cases. *Am J Hematol* 79:329-331.

De Filippi P, Zecca M, Lisini D, et al [2009] Germ-line mutation of the *NRAS* gene may be responsible for the development of juvenile myelomonocytic leukaemia. *Br J Haematol* 147:706-709.

Droin N, Jacquel A, Hendra JB, et al [2010] Alpha-defensins secreted by dysplastic granulocytes inhibit the differentiation of monocytes in chronic myelomonocytic leukemia. *Blood* 115:78-88.

Emanuel PD [2008] Juvenile myelomonocytic leukemia and chronic myelomonocytic leukemia. *Leukemia* 22:1335-1342.

Fend F, Horn T, Koch I, et al [2008] Atypical chronic myeloid leukemia as defined in the WHO classification is a JAK2 V617F negative neoplasm. *Leuk Res* 32:1931-1935.

Foucar K [2009] Myeloproliferative/myelodysplastic neoplasms. *Am J Clin Pathol* 132:281-289.

Friedman J [1997] Neurofibromatosis 1. In: *GeneReviews at GeneTests: Medical Genetics Information Resource* (database online). URL: http://www.genetests.org. Updated June 2009.

Gattermann N, Billiet J, Kronenwett R, et al [2007] High frequency of the JAK2 V617F mutation in patients with thrombocytosis (platelet count>600 × 10⁹/L) and ringed sideroblasts >15% considered as MDS/MPD, unclassifiable. *Blood* 109:1334-1335.

Herrod HG, Dow LW, Sullivan JL [1983] Persistent Epstein-Barr virus infection mimicking juvenile chronic myelogenous leukemia: immunologic and hematologic studies. *Blood* 61:1098-1104.

Jankowska AM, Szpurka H, Tiu RV, et al [2009] Loss of heterozygosity 4q24 and TET2 mutations associated with myelodysplastic/myeloproliferative neoplasms. *Blood* 113:6403-6410.

Kirby MA, Weitzman S, Freedman MH [1990] Juvenile chronic myelogenous leukemia: differentiation from infantile cytomegalovirus infection. *Am J Pediatr Hematol Oncol* 12:292-296.

Koike K, Matsuda K [2008] Recent advances in the pathogenesis and management of juvenile myelomonocytic leukaemia. *Br J Haematol* 141:567-575.

Kratz CP, Niemeyer CM, Thomas C, et al [2007] Mutation analysis of Son of Sevenless in juvenile myelomonocytic leukemia. *Leukemia* 21:1108-1109.

Kuo MC, Liang DC, Huang CF, et al [2009] RUNX1 mutations are frequent in chronic myelomonocytic leukemia and mutations of the C-terminal region might predict acute myeloid leukemia transformation. *Leukemia* 23:1426-1431.

Lacronique-Gazaille C, Chaury MP, Le Guyader A, et al [2007] A simple method for detection of major phenotypic abnormalities in myelodysplastic syndromes: expression of CD56 in CMML. *Haematologica* 92:859-860.

Loh ML, Sakai DS, Flotho C, et al [2009] Mutations in CBL occur frequently in juvenile myelomonocytic leukemia. *Blood* 114:1859-1863.

Lorenzana A, Lyons H, Sawaf H, et al [2002] Human herpesvirus 6 infection mimicking juvenile myelomonocytic leukemia in an infant. *J Pediatr Hematol Oncol* 24:136-141.

Malcovati L, Della Porta MS, Pietra D, et al [2009] Molecular and clinical features of refractory anemia with ringed sideroblasts associated with marked thrombocytosis. *Blood* 114:3538-3545.

Manabe A, Yoshimasu T, Ebihara Y, et al [2004] Viral infections in juvenile myelomonocytic leukemia: prevalence and clinical implications. *J Pediatr Hematol Oncol* 26:636-641.

Mongkonsritragoon W, Letendre L, Qian J, Li CY [1998] Nodular lesions of monocytic component in myelodysplastic syndrome. *Am J Clin Pathol* 110:154-162.

Ngo NT, Lampert IA, Naresh KN [2008] Bone marrow trephine morphology and immunohistochemical findings in chronic myelomonocytic leukaemia. *Br J Haematol* 141:771-781.

Niemeyer C, Fenu S, Hasle H, et al [1998] Response: Differentiating juvenile myelomonocytic leukemia from infectious disease. *Blood* 91:365-367.

Niemeyer CM, Kratz CP [2008] Paediatric myelodysplastic syndromes and juvenile myelomonocytic leukaemia: molecular classification and treatment options. *Br J Haematol* 140:610-624.

Orazi A, Bennett J, Germing U, et al [2008a] Chronic myelomonocytic leukaemia. In: Swerdlow S, Campo E, Harris N, et al, eds. *WHO Classification of Tumours: Pathology & Genetics: Tumours of Haematopoietic and Lymphoid Tissues.* Lyon, France: IARC Press; 76-79.

Orazi A, Chiu R, O'Malley DP, et al [2006] Chronic myelomonocytic leukemia: the role of bone marrow biopsy immunohistology. *Mod Pathol* 19:1536-1545.

Orazi A, Germing U [2008b] The myelodysplastic/myeloproliferative neoplasms: myeloproliferative diseases with dysplastic features. *Leukemia* 22:1308-1319.

Pinkel D [1998] Differentiating juvenile myelomonocytic leukemia from infectious disease. *Blood* 91:365.

Roberts AE, Araki T, Swanson KD, et al [2007] Germline gain-of-function mutations in SOS1 cause Noonan syndrome. *Nat Genet* 39:70-74.

Schubbert S, Zenker M, Rowe SL, et al [2006] Germline KRAS mutations cause Noonan syndrome. *Nat Genet* 38:331-336.

Side LE, Emanuel PD, Taylor B, et al [1998] Mutations of the NF1 gene in children with juvenile myelomonocytic leukemia without clinical evidence of neurofibromatosis, type 1. *Blood* 92:267-272.

Swanson KD, Winter JM, Reis M, et al [2008] SOS1 mutations are rare in human malignancies: implications for Noonan Syndrome patients. *Genes Chromosomes Cancer* 47:253-259.

Swerdlow S [2008] Myelodysplastic/myeloproliferative diseases. In: Swerdlow S, Campo E, Harris N, et al, eds. *WHO Classification of Tumours: Pathology & Genetics: Tumours of Haematopoietic and Lymphoid Tissues.* Lyon, France: IARC Press; 75-86.

Szpurka H, Tiu R, Murugesan G, et al [2006] Refractory anemia with ringed sideroblasts associated with marked thrombocytosis (RARS-T), another myeloproliferative condition characterized by JAK2 V617F mutation. *Blood* 108:2173-2181.

Tartaglia M, Niemeyer CM, Fragale A, et al [2003] Somatic mutations in PTPN11 in juvenile myelomonocytic leukemia, myelodysplastic syndromes and acute myeloid leukemia. *Nat Genet* 34:148-150.

Toyoda H, Ido M, Hori H, et al [2004] A case of juvenile myelomonocytic leukemia with concomitant cytomegalovirus infection. *J Pediatr Hematol Oncol* 26:606-608.

Vardiman J, Bennett J, Bain B, et al [2008a] Myelodysplastic/myeloproliferative neoplasm, unclassifiable. In: Swerdlow S, Campo E, Harris N, et al, eds. *WHO Classification of Tumours: Pathology & Genetics: Tumours of Haematopoietic and Lymphoid Tissues.* Lyon, France: IARC Press; 85-86.

Vardiman J, Bennett J, Bain B, et al [2008b] Atypical chronic myeloid leukaemia, BCR-ABL1 negative. In: Swerdlow S, Campo E, Harris N, et al, eds. *WHO Classification of Tumours: Pathology & Genetics: Tumours of Haematopoietic and Lymphoid Tissues.* Lyon, France: IARC Press; 80-81.

Vardiman J, Brunning R, Arber D, et al [2008c] Introduction and overview of the classification of the myeloid neoplasms. In: Swerdlow S, Campo E, Harris N, et al, eds. *WHO Classification of Tumours: Pathology & Genetics: Tumours of Haematopoietic and Lymphoid Tissues.* Lyon, France: IARC Press; 18-30.

Wardrop D, Steensma DP [2009] Is refractory anaemia with ring sideroblasts and thrombocytosis (RARS-T) a necessary or useful diagnostic category? *Br J Haematol* 144:809-817.

Xu Y, McKenna RW, Karandikar NJ, et al [2005] Flow cytometric analysis of monocytes as a tool for distinguishing chronic myelomonocytic leukemia from reactive monocytosis. *Am J Clin Pathol* 124:799-806.

CHAPTER 18

Acute Myeloid Leukemia

Kathryn Foucar, MD

Kaaren Reichard, MD

David Czuchlewski, MD

The successful diagnosis of acute myeloid leukemia (AML) has never been an easy task for the practicing pathologist, and the stakes have always been high. Not only are the morphologic features of a case often challenging, but major, urgent, potentially life-threatening treatment decisions hinge on this diagnosis. In acute promyelocytic leukemia (APL), the challenge is even greater, because any delay, even a few hours, will postpone notification of the clinician that the patient is at high risk for a potentially catastrophic hemorrhage. Consequently, the pathologist is faced with the expectation of providing a "correct" diagnosis as rapidly as possible.

Recent biologic insights in AML have even more dramatically expanded expectations of pathologists, with the advance from traditional morphologic and immunophenotypic evaluations to a biologic assessment of AML. This transition requires that the pathologist understand pathogenetic features of AML, since these mechanistic parameters are directly linked to prognosis, "curability," many distinctive clinical and morphologic features, optimal therapy, and appropriate minimal residual disease monitoring. The 2008 WHO classification of AML has set a new diagnostic standard in AML diagnosis by utilizing a recurrent genetic abnormality as the defining feature for many types of AML [Vardiman 2008b]. Thus, the state-of-the-art diagnosis of AML requires an integration of clinical, hematologic, morphologic, immunophenotypic, and genetic features. This process must occur in a systematic fashion and must be logical and cost effective.

[18.1] Definition

Acute myeloid leukemia is a clonal hematopoietic disorder that may be derived from either a hematopoietic stem cell or a lineage-specific progenitor cell. AML is characterized both by a predominance of immature forms (with variable, but incomplete, maturation) and loss of normal hematopoiesis. Single or multiple hematopoietic lineages may comprise the leukemic clone. The requisite blast/blast equivalent percentage is 20% in the peripheral blood and bone marrow; a lower percentage is acceptable in cases with AML-defining translocations and in acute erythroid leukemia (see [18.4] "Blasts and Blast Equivalents," p 380 for discussion of blasts/blast equivalents) [Vardiman 2008b].

The blast percentage is derived from counting all nucleated cells for AML diagnosis with the exception of acute erythroid leukemias in which the blast percentage is based on non-erythroid cells. In extramedullary sites, a diagnosis of myeloid sarcoma is equivalent to AML regardless of blood and bone marrow findings. Finally,

in 2 clinical situations (1. prior cytotoxic chemotherapy and/or radiation therapy and 2. Down syndrome), cases with features of myelodysplastic syndrome and those with features of AML are lumped together as "myeloid neoplasms" without regard to blast count, as there are no significant clinical or biologic differences in behavior tied to exceeding the 20% threshold. These basic definitional considerations are summarized in f18.1.

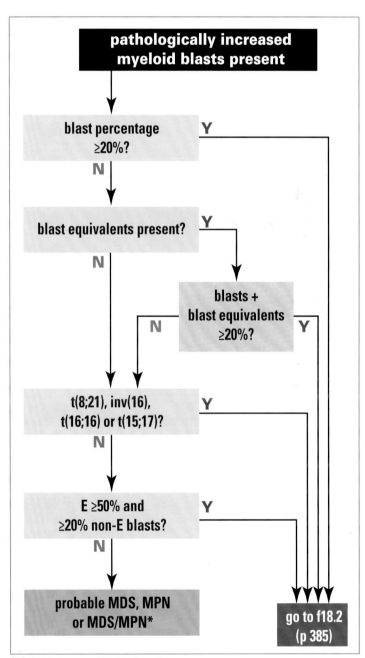

f18.1 *Definition of AML algorithm.*

Note that the MDS-like state in patients with Down syndrome <5 years of age or in patients with a prior cytotoxic therapy behaves biologically as AML regardless of blast count; see Chapters 16 & 17 for further assessment

AML= acute myeloid leukemia; E = erythroid cells; MDS = myelodysplastic syndrome; MPN = myeloproliferative neoplasm

t18.1 Selected Risk Factors for AML

Risk Factor	Comments
Inherited Genetic Disorders*	
Down syndrome	Acute leukemia 10-20 times that of individuals without trisomy 21
	Elevated risk of acute megakaryoblastic leukemia (~600 times normal)
	Transient abnormal myelopoiesis is a spontaneously remitting "leukemia-equivalent" unique to Down syndrome patients
Severe congenital neutropenia	Cumulative incidence of MDS and AML after 15 years of G-CSF therapy is 34%; risk is 11% at age 20
	Transformation is particularly associated with the acquisition of secondary mutations to the gene encoding the G-CSF receptor
	Cyclic neutropenia does not appear to share a significant risk of progression to MDS or AML
Shwachman-Diamond syndrome	Estimated incidence of MDS/AML is 19% at 20 years of age and 36% at 30 years, perhaps due to mitotic spindle destabilization in the absence of SBDS protein and consequent chromosomal instability
Dyskeratosis congenita	Head and neck squamous cell carcinomas dominate the cancer risk; however, the ratio of observed to expected cases of AML is 195:1 [Alter 2009]
Fanconi anemia	Ratio of observed to expected incidence of AML is 868:1
	Risk of early transformation is increased in D1 complementation group and in the Ashkenazi Jewish population
Environmental Exposures	
Ionizing radiation	Linked to the risk of secondary AML
Benzene exposure	Strong dose-response relationship with the development of AML
	Benzene-related cases may be reminiscent of therapy-related AML, a finding that recalls the use of benzene as an early form of chemotherapy
Cigarette smoking	Slightly increased risk of AML (average relative risk = 1.6); positive dose-response relationship with the number of cigarettes smoked; cigarette smoke contains benzene, which may be responsible for the increased risk
Pesticides/herbicides	Slightly increased risk of AML (meta-relative risk: 1.55)
Chemotherapy	
Topoisomerase II inhibitors	Agents include etoposide and teniposide
	Developing t-AML after such epipodophyllotoxins ~2%-12%, depending on regimen-related factors (see **t18.6**)
Alkylating chemotherapy	Agents include: melphalan, cyclophosphamide, nitrogen mustard, chlorambucil, busulfan, carboplatin, cisplatin, dacarbazine, procarbazine, carmustine, mitomycin C, thiotepa, and lomustine
	Early regimens: relative risks for secondary AML exceed 300
	Less toxic regimens (eg, ABVD): somewhat decreased the risk (see **t18.6**)
Anthracyclines and anthracenediones	Agents include daunorubicin, doxorubicin, and mitoxantrone (intercalating agents, but also act as topoisomerase II inhibitors)
	Increased risk of AML may be attributable to the latter mechanism of action
	Risk of secondary AML with these agents is less than with strong topoisomerase II inhibitors such as the epipodophyllotoxins, but incidence still substantial (1 study found relative risk with anthracycline therapy to be on the order of 2.7)
Anti-tubulin agents	Agents include taxanes, vincristine, and vinblastine (frequently administered with other classes of chemotherapeutic agents)
	Some anecdotal reports suggest an increased risk with taxanes, but other studies show no increase in incidence when taxanes are added to an anthracycline-based regimen
	WHO 2008 classification endorses these drugs as cytotoxic agents implicated in therapy-related hematologic neoplasms

*Many other inherited disorders are more weakly associated with increased risk for AML, including Li-Fraumeni syndrome, neurofibromatosis, Noonan syndrome and Klinefelter syndrome; patients with congenital amegakaryocytic thrombocytopenia are also at some increased risk of developing AML
~1/2 reported cancers associated with Diamond-Blackfan anemia are AML; the rarity of these bone marrow failure syndromes somewhat hinders precise risk quantification
ABVD = adriamycin (doxorubicin), bleomycin, vinblastine, and dacarbazine; AML = acute myeloid leukemia; G-CSF = granulocyte colony-stimulating factor; MDS = myelodysplastic syndrome

References: [Alter 2009, Belson 2007, Bhatia 1996, Burroughs 2009, Cimino 1991, Dale 2003, Donadieu 2005, Felix 1998, Freedman 2002, Geddis 2009, Green 2009, Hijiya 2009, Le Deley 2007, Leone 2007, Lipton 2006, Natelson 2007, Patt 2007, Rosenberg 2008a, 2008b, Van Maele-Fabry 2007, Vineis 2004, Xavier 2009, Yeasmin 2008]

[18.2] Epidemiology and Pathogenesis

The age-adjusted incidence of AML in the United States is 3.4 cases per 100,000 persons [Deschler 2006]. AML can occur in patients of any age, but in general, both the overall incidence and the proportion of total acute leukemias that are myeloid increase with age. Thus, acute lymphoblastic leukemia (ALL) predominates in children, with only one case of AML diagnosed for every 5 cases of ALL [Belson 2007]. For childhood AML, peak incidence occurs in the first year of life, then decreases until age 4, and thereafter remains relatively constant until adulthood [Gurney 1995]. The incidence of AML then increases through adulthood, during which period 70%-80% of acute leukemias are AML, with a marked spike in incidence in the elderly. Much of this increased incidence is attributable to AML with myelodysplasia-related changes, which becomes more common with age, while the incidence of de novo AML remains approximately constant across all adult age groups [Deschler 2006].

One of the central themes in this chapter will be that "AML" may best be considered an umbrella term for a heterogeneous group of myeloid leukemias that differ substantially in cause, age of onset, clinical features, and prognosis. For example, AML with t(1;22)(p13;q13); *RBM15-MKL1* is a de novo megakaryoblastic AML arising in infants and very young children, while megakaryoblastic leukemia *without* the t(1;22) often arises in children in the setting of Down syndrome. Epidemiologic and pathogenetic heterogeneity is the necessary consequence of the increasingly fine distinctions among subtypes of AML. Despite this heterogeneity, we can make some general observations about the disease states and environmental exposures that appear to increase an individual's risk for developing AML of various subtypes. These are listed and discussed in **t18.1**. The risk of AML is also substantially increased in patients with other hematopoietic disorders, including myelodysplastic syndrome (MDS), some myeloproliferative neoplasms (MPNs), MDS/MPN overlap syndromes, aplastic anemia, and paroxysmal nocturnal hemoglobinuria, in which case the development of AML may be due to progression of the underlying disease.

In general, AML arises following the accumulation (through inherited genetic mechanisms, environmental influences, sheer random chance, or some combination of these) of specific translocations, mutations, and other genetic alterations. Crucially, leukemogenesis often requires the acquisition of several cooperating genetic lesions. For example, the introduction of the fusion protein *RUNX1-RUNX1T1*, formed by the t(8;21)(q22;q22), into mice is insufficient to cause leukemia [Mrozek 2008b]. Similarly, introduction of an abnormally activated tyrosine kinase, which provides a pro-proliferative signal, results in a

t18.2 Class I and Class II Mutations in AML

Class I Mutations (Proliferation)	Class II Mutations (Impaired Differentiation)
FLT3	PML-RARA
KIT	RUNX1-RUNX1T1
RAS	CBFB-MYH11
PTPN11	MLL fusions
JAK2	CEBPA

*The mechanism of leukemogenesis for *NPM1* mutations remains somewhat unclear

Reference: [Vardiman 2008b]

myeloproliferative process rather than outright leukemia. However, leukemia supervenes when *both* abnormalities are present in the mice simultaneously [Grisolano 2003]. This and similar observations have given rise to the designation of AML-associated molecular genetic changes as either Class I or Class II, with the former conferring increased proliferation and the latter contributing to arrested hematopoietic differentiation **t18.2**. This distinction is largely irrelevant for diagnostic purposes, but it does underscore the important idea that cooperating alterations in multiple pathways are usually present in AML.

[18.3] Key Steps in the Diagnosis of AML

An attempt to outline key steps in the diagnosis of AML is made in **t18.3** (general approach strategies to all myeloid neoplasms are presented in Chapter 13). Although some of these steps are performed simultaneously or are overlapping, it is important for the diagnostician to understand the importance of basic CBC information in determining the likelihood that a patient has AML. This is especially important for rapid diagnosis of AML and appropriate utilization of specialized tests. Although the WBC is highly variable in AML, it is essential for the diagnostician to assess for hematopoietic failure (ie, neutropenia, anemia, and thrombocytopenia). Although preservation of a single hematopoietic lineage may be observed rarely, hematopoietic failure is an expected finding in AML.

If hematopoiesis is preserved (normal absolute neutrophil count, RBC parameters, and platelet count), a diagnosis of AML is very unlikely, and other diagnostic possibilities should be considered. In our experience, the rare examples of exceptions to this general rule have occurred in circumstances in which the blood and bone marrow examinations were performed for reasons unrelated to hematologic dysfunction, and early/partial involvement by acute leukemia was detected.

t18.3 Acute Myeloid Leukemia: Diagnostic Steps*

1. Evaluation of an abnormal CBC for possible AML (usually step 1 for the pathologist)

   Confirm HP failures, assess for blasts/blast equivalents (see step 2), and dysplasia
   WBC: non-specific; in AML can be low, normal, or high
   ANC: severe neutropenia characteristic of HP failure; typical in AML, but exceptions occur
   Circulating blasts: variable number and percent in AML, but key feature to assess in blood
   RBC features: severe anemia characteristic of HP failure, an expected feature of AML
      Polychromasia: reduced, since anemia is result of bone marrow production failure
      Other RBC pathology: non-specific
   Platelets: severe thrombocytopenia characteristic of HP failure

2. Identify morphologic blasts and blast equivalents in blood (and subsequent bone marrow, if performed)

   Morphologic assessment of nuclear features key for "blast" designation
   Distinguish from blast look-alikes and other immature hematopoietic cells
   Consider APL specifically; alert clinician if suspected based on morphology of immature cells and CBC data
   Cytochemistry, flow cytometric immunophenotyping, genetics can all be performed on blood as needed

3. Bone marrow examination often performed to address differential diagnoses from blood assessment or for protocol requirements

4. Determine lineage of blasts/blast equivalents (can be performed on blood or bone marrow)

   Morphology (nucleus and cytoplasm)
   Cytochemistry
   Immunophenotype
   Consider APL specifically and alert clinician if suspected

5. Enumeration of blasts/blast equivalents by morphology and differential cell count

   Blood (percentage; threshold ≥20%)
   Bone marrow (percentage; threshold ≥20%): blast count <20%, but Auer rods or other distinctive morphology suggests AML
   Unique situations compromising blast count:
      Fibrosis and/or necrosis
      Predominance (≥50%) of erythroid lineage
      Marked hypocellularity
      Technically poor specimen

6. Assess all lineages for dysplasia (core biopsy better for megakaryocyte assessment)

7. Identify biologic subtypes of AML based on:

   Distinctive morphologic features (eg, multilineage dysplasia)
   Recurrent cytogenetic subtypes
   Molecular assessment for *NPM1*, *CEBPA*, and *FLT3*
   Prior chemotherapy/radiation
   Antecedent hematologic disorder
   Constitutional disorder (eg, Down syndrome or other constitutional disorders)

8. For cases lacking diagnostic biologic features, exclude other differential diagnostic possibilities

9. Lineage-based classification for AML, NOS cases lacking identifiable biologic features

*Some diagnostic steps overlapping and/or simultaneous
ANC = absolute neutrophil count; APL = acute promyelocytic leukemia; CBC = complete blood count; HP = hematopoietic; NOS = not otherwise specified; RBC = red blood cell; WBC = white blood cell

Simultaneously with CBC assessment, the blood smear should be reviewed systematically for blasts, blast equivalents, other abnormal cells, and dysplasia (all hematopoietic lineages).

The identification, lineage determination, and enumeration of blasts/blast equivalents is also an integrative process that encompasses routine morphology, cytochemical staining, and flow cytometric immunophenotyping on blood or bone marrow (see [18.4] "Blasts and Blast Equivalents"). Throughout this diagnostic process, the pathologist must remain aware of both the urgency in rapid diagnosis of APL and the numerous diagnostic pitfalls/key problem areas in AML diagnosis (see [18.9] "Diagnostic Pitfalls in AML Diagnosis," p 419).

The molecular genetic data essential for the diagnosis of cases of AML with recurrent genetic abnormalities is often delayed compared to rapid morphology, cytochemical, and immunophenotypic assessment. Consequently, a final integrated report may not be generated for several days to several weeks. However, fluorescence in situ hybridization (FISH) testing offers a more rapid turnaround for assessment of specific genetic abnormalities depending upon probe availability. FISH testing is ideal for rapid assessment of AML-defining translocations, including t(15;17)(q22;q21)* in APL, which results in the fusion of *PML-RARA*.

A lineage-based classification can be used for an initial diagnosis if data supporting a specific biologic subtype is not available. However for the most part, with the exception of APL, lineage-based classification alone is not predictive of genotype. In addition, in the absence of a diagnostic biologic parameter, the diagnostician must exclude many differential diagnostic considerations. This can be especially problematic when specimens are suboptimal, fibrotic, necrotic, or show a blast percentage approximating 20%.

Frequent discussions with the clinical team are essential throughout the diagnostic process. Particular attention must be paid to rapid communication about possible APL, including recommendations for coagulation assessment. This dialogue with the clinical team is also essential to determining factors that can potentially influence the pathologist's interpretation, such as antecedent hematologic disorders, prior cytotoxic therapy, and recent granulocyte colony-stimulating factor (G-CSF) therapy.

[18.4] Blasts and Blast Equivalents

Blasts, blast equivalents, and other immature hematopoietic cells must be identified and distinguished from various blast look-alikes t18.4. For AML diagnosis, blasts include myeloblasts, monoblasts, and megakaryoblasts, while promonocytes are blast equivalents in all types of AML and promyelocytes are blast equivalents exclusively in acute promyelocytic leukemia.

*The t(15;17) *PML-RARA* translocation has been historically denoted as both t(15;17)(q22;q21) and t(15;17)(q22;q12). Currently the most accurate description is actually thought to be t(15;17)(q24;q21). For the sake of simplicity and consistency, we have chosen to use the t(15;17)(q22;q21) designation.

t18.4 Blasts, Blast Equivalents, Other Immature Cells in Blood and Bone Marrow

Cell Type	Key Morphologic Features	Cytochemistry	Immunophenotype/Comments*
Myeloblast	Large nucleus with finely dispersed chromatin and variably prominent nucleoli Relatively high nuclear/cytoplasmic ratio Variable number of cytoplasmic granules, may be concentrated in limited portion of cytoplasm	MPO+	CD34+, CD13+[†], CD33+[†], MPO+, HLA-DR+, vCD11c+, wCD45+, CD117 usually +
Promyelocyte	Nuclear chromatin slightly condensed; nucleoli variably prominent; nucleus often eccentric, and Golgi zone may be apparent Numerous cytoplasmic granules that may be more dispersed throughout cytoplasm Blast equivalent in APL *only* In APL, intense cytoplasmic granularity usually present Nuclear configuration variable, but nuclear folding and lobulation characteristic of microgranular variant of APL	Strong, uniform MPO+	CD13+, CD33+, MPO+, wCD45+, **CD34–, HLA-DR–** Loss of HLA-DR and acquisition of strong CD15 and CD11c associated with maturation Gradual loss of CD33 also characterizes successive maturation stages CD34 usually negative in hypergranular variant; often positive in microgranular variant
Monoblast	Moderate to low nuclear to cytoplasmic ratio, nuclear chromatin finely dispersed with variably prominent nucleoli; nuclei round to folded Abundant, slightly basophilic cytoplasm containing fine granulation and occasional vacuoles	NSE+	**CD34–**, HLA-DR+, CD13+, **CD33 bright +, CD36/CD64 coexpression**, vCD4+, CD11c+, wCD45+ Usually CD34– Occasional cases moderate CD45+
Promonocyte	Slightly condensed nuclear chromatin; variably prominent nucleoli Abundant finely granular blue/gray cytoplasm that may be vacuolated Very monocytic appearance with nuclear immaturity Consistent blast equivalent in AML	NSE+	**CD36/CD64 coexpression**, HLA-DR+, CD13+, **CD33 bright +**, vCD14+, CD4+, CD11c+, CD45+
Erythroblast	Relatively high nuclear/cytoplasmic ratio Nucleus round with slightly condensed chromatin; nucleoli variably prominent Moderate amounts of deeply basophilic cytoplasm that may be vacuolated Included in blast percentage *only* in acute erythroid leukemia	PAS+	**Glycophorin A+, hemoglobin A+**, CD71+, CD34–, CD45–, MPO–, myeloid antigens negative CD117 often positive
Megakaryoblast	Highly variable morphologic features; often not recognizable without special studies May be lymphoid-appearing with high nuclear to cytoplasmic ratio Nuclear chromatin fine to variably condensed Cytoplasm may be scant to moderate, is usually agranular or contains a few granules; blebbing or budding of cytoplasm may be evident Blasts may form cohesive clumps	NA	**CD34–, CD41+, CD61+**, CD33 bright +, CD13–, HLA-DR– (or dim) Progressive maturation characterized by loss of CD34 and acquisition of CD42 and von Willebrand factor
Blastic plasmacy-toid dendritic cell[§]	Variable morphology; not identified in either normal bone marrow or AML Often not recognizable without immunophenotyping May be lymphoid-appearing May show cytoplasmic tadpoles	MPO– NSE–	**CD4+, CD56+, CD123+**, CD43+, CD45+, HLA-DR+, vTdT+ CD123 not specific; seen in subset of AMLs (Discussed in detail in Chapter 19)

*Key flow cytometric clues to lineage assignment in boldface

[†]Rare AML lacks surface CD13 and CD33

[‡]False positive CD41 expression by flow cytometry may be secondary to platelet adherence to blasts

[§]See Chapter 19

AML = acute myeloid leukemia; APL = acute promyelocytic leukemia; MPO = myeloperoxidase; NSE = non-specific esterase; PAS = periodic acid-Schiff; v = variable antigen expression; w = weak antigen expression

References: [Dohner 2010, Vardiman 2008b]

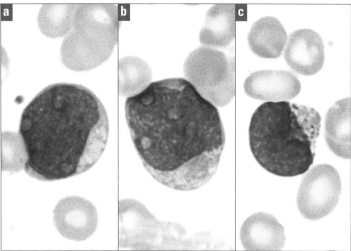

i18.1 *This bone marrow aspirate composite illustrates the spectrum of cytoplasmic granulation ranging from agranular **a** to granular (**b** and **c**) blast. Myeloblasts with granules lack other features of promyelocytes such as a prominent paranuclear hof. (Wright)*

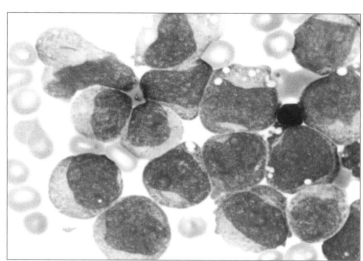

i18.2 *Bone marrow aspirate smear from a patient with acute myeloid leukemia includes both granular and agranular blasts. Note Auer rod (upper left cell). (Wright)*

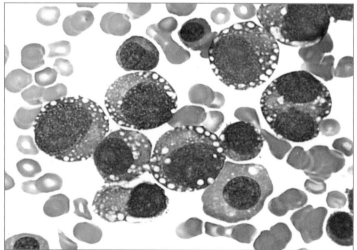

i18.3 *Megakaryoblasts show prominent cytoplasmic blebbing in a peripheral blood smear. (Wright)*

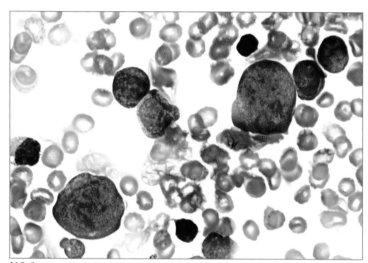

i18.4 *Several erythroblasts with deeply basophilic cytoplasm are present on this bone marrow aspirate smear. (Wright)*

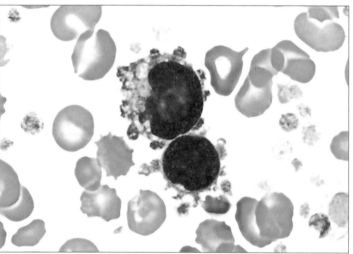

i18.5 *The erythroblasts in this case of acute pure erythroid leukemia account for ≥80% of cells. These erythroblasts show deeply basophilic cytoplasm with prominent vacuolization. (Wright)*

Erythroblasts are included in the blast percentage only in acute "pure" erythroid leukemia. Nuclear morphologic features are most critical in the decision that a cell is a blast exhibiting finely dispersed rather than condensed nuclear chromatin. Other useful nuclear features of blasts to assess include overall size, nucleoli, and nuclear configuration. Cytoplasmic features are very helpful in lineage determination, ie, sparse fine granules and Auer rods in myeloblasts, cytoplasmic blebbing in megakaryoblasts, and deeply basophilic, vacuolated cytoplasm in erythroblasts **t18.4, i18.1, i18.2, i18.3, i18.4, i18.5**. As their name implies, blastic plasmacytoid dendritic cell neoplasms can be derived from cells with morphologic features of blasts. These cells are not evident in normal bone marrow and are not generally included in the discussion of immature cell populations that need to be identified in cases of possible AML. However, for completeness, blastic plasmacytoid dendritic cells

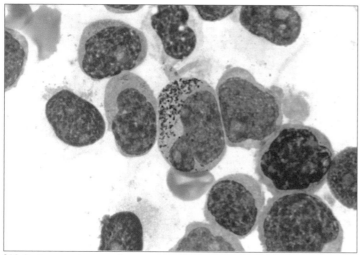

i18.6 *A promyelocyte with an eccentric nucleus, a paranuclear hof, and abundant cytoplasmic granules is present in the center of this bone marrow aspirate smear from a patient with acute myeloid leukemia with maturation. Promyelocytes are not included within the blast percentage for this type of AML. (Wright)*

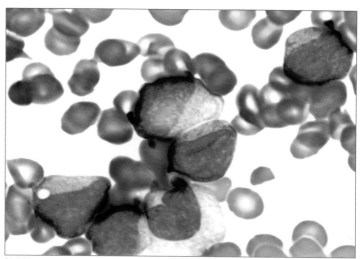

i18.7 *A spectrum of myeloblasts is present in this bone marrow aspirate smear including 2 blasts with Auer rods. (Wright)*

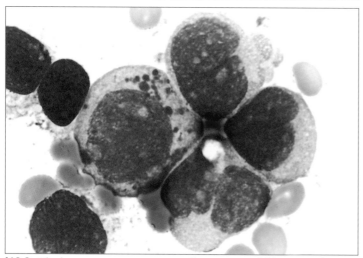

i18.8 *This bone marrow aspirate smear illustrates 4 myeloblasts, one of which contains pseudo Chédiak-Higashi granules. This granular blast is not a promyelocyte, because it lacks a prominent paranuclear hof. (Wright)*

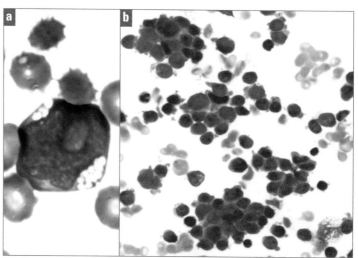

i18.9 *This composite shows a spectrum of unique features of myeloblasts, including a myeloblast with deeply basophilic and sharply vacuolated cytoplasm resembling Burkitt lymphoma **a**, while distinct clumping of myeloblasts mimics a metastatic tumor **b**. (Wright)*

are highlighted in **t18.4**, but the reader is referred to Chapter 19 for comprehensive discussion and illustrations.

Myeloblasts can be morphologically diverse, and the distinction between a granular blast and a promyelocyte with a distinct paranuclear hof (Golgi zone) is key **i18.1, i18.2, i18.6**. Auer rods are a key cytologic feature of myeloblasts, although Auer rods can be seen in promyelocytes in APL and even rarely in mature cells **i18.7**. Other unique features of myeloblasts include pseudo Chédiak-Higashi granules, nuclear indentation, deeply basophilic cytoplasm with vacuoles, and, rarely, clumping on aspirate smears mimicking a metastatic process **i18.8, i18.9**. Associations of some of these unusual morphologic features with immunophenotypic and molecular genetic properties have been reported [Chang 2006, Kussick 2004]. Cytochemical staining for myeloperoxidase is important in establishing the lineage of myeloblasts **i18.10**. Features of AML on bone

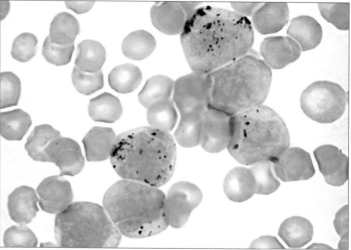

i18.10 *Cytochemical staining for myeloperoxidase illustrates a spectrum of scant to moderate positivity, which is characteristic of early granulocytic maturation in cases of acute myeloid leukemia. (myeloperoxidase cytochemical stain)*

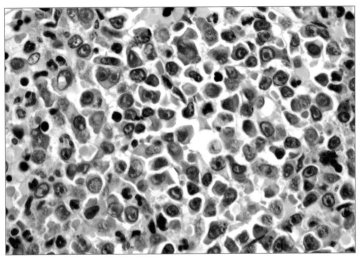

i18.11 *This bone marrow core biopsy section is effaced by a homogeneous infiltrate of acute myeloid leukemia cells. Note the large nuclear size, variably prominent nucleoli, and moderately abundant amounts of cytoplasm. (H&E)*

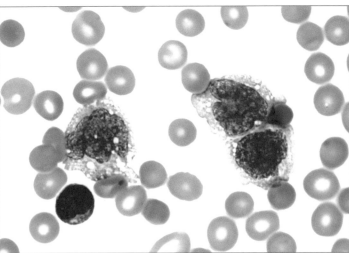

i18.12 *Monoblasts (right lower) and promonocytes (upper right and upper left) are evident in this peripheral blood smear from a patient with acute monocytic leukemia. Promonocytes are blast equivalents. (Wright)*

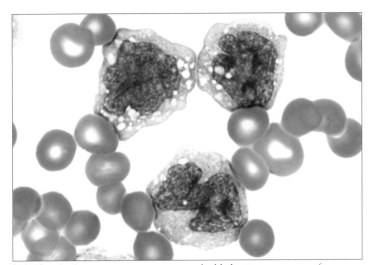

i18.13 *This bone marrow aspirate smear highlights 2 promonocytes (upper cells) and an immature, atypical monocyte (lower cell) in a case of acute monocytic leukemia. Promonocytes are blast equivalents. (Wright)*

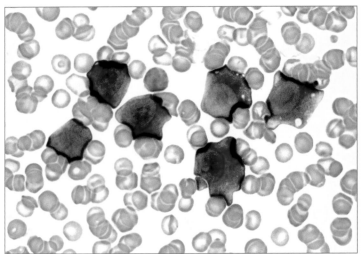

i18.14 *Intense reddish brown cytoplasmic nonspecific esterase positivity is evident in this acute monocytic leukemia. (cytochemical stain for nonspecific esterase)*

marrow core biopsy sections are also heterogeneous, but prototypic findings include a predominance of immature cells with dispersed chromatin, variably prominent nucleoli, and moderate amounts of eosinophilic cytoplasm i18.11. Monoblasts and promonocytes (blast equivalents) must also be successfully identified based on morphologic and cytochemical features i18.12, i18.13, i18.14.

Flow cytometric immunophenotyping (and to a lesser extent immunohistochemical staining) is a mainstay in assessing immaturity (weak CD45, CD34, CD117) and lineage in AML t18.4. Integration of morphology, limited cytochemistry, and immunophenotype is optimal in AML diagnosis t18.4, t18.5. However, the actual blast percentage is best assessed by morphology, and the percentage of CD34+ cells should not substitute for the morphologic percentage. Keep in mind that flow cytometry specimens

may show falsely low blast percentages due to hemodilution or falsely elevated blast percentages due to lysis of erythroid cells. Furthermore, many types of blasts (erythroblasts, monoblasts, megakaryoblasts) and blast equivalents (promyelocytes, promonocytes) typically lack CD34 expression.

Based on morphologic differential cell counts, the blast threshold in blood and bone marrow for AML diagnosis is 20% [Vardiman 2008b]. However, as noted earlier, there are exceptions to this general rule f18.1, and the blast/blast equivalent percentage must always be assessed in the overall context of a given case. Determining an accurate blast/blast equivalent percentage can be especially challenging in technically suboptimal, necrotic, or fibrotic specimens (see [18.9] "Diagnostic Pitfalls in AML Diagnosis," p 419). In these situations, immunohistochemical techniques may be helpful in determining lineage and immature cell populations on tissue sections. Similarly, cases with a marked expansion of the erythroid lineage can be difficult to diagnose (see [18.9] "Diagnostic Pitfalls in AML Diagnosis," p 419). Key features to assess include the overall percentage of erythroid lineage cells, the degree of maturation/differentiation of the erythroid lineage, the percentage of myeloid blasts among non-erythroid cells, and the extent of dysplasia.

[18.5] Classification of AML

In most cases, the integration of traditional clinical, hematologic, morphologic, cytochemical, and immuno-phenotypic data results in a confident diagnosis of AML. If a patient has Down syndrome, has a known history of antecedent myelodysplasia, or has had prior chemotherapy/radiation therapy, additional biologic information can be provided at the time of traditional assessment. However, the biologic classification of AML will often hinge upon molecular genetic studies. If a positive molecular genetic result is obtained, the AML will be subcategorized among the 9 molecular genetic subtypes in the 2008 WHO classification t18.5. If non-contributory molecular genetic and clinical results are obtained, the case will be subclassified based on traditional lineage-based criteria (see [18.7] "AML, Not Otherwise Specified (NOS)," p 408).

[18.6] Biologic Subtypes of AML

As illustrated in f18.2 and t18.5, there are essentially 2 ways to categorize specific biologic subtypes of AML: genetic findings and clinical setting. Many details pertaining to these subtypes are listed in t18.5, which serves as a quick reference guide for this section. In this section we will describe in some detail those cases of AML categorizable by clinical setting, as well as the genetically defined subtypes of AML.

[18.6.1]   **Molecular Genetic Biologic Subtypes of AML**

Core Binding Factor Acute Myeloid Leukemias

Core binding factor (CBF) AML includes AML with t(8;21) and AML with inv(16)/t(16;16). These 2 AML cytogenetic groups are often grouped together based on involvement of related CBF machinery and relatively overall favorable prognosis [Marcucci 2005]. The CBF genes are *RUNX1* (21q22, aka *AML1, CBFA2*) and *CBFB* (16q22). As part of the CBF heterodimer transcription factor complex, RUNX1 binds to DNA promoter sequences of genes needed for hematopoiesis, while CBFB protects the complex from proteolysis [Okumura 2008, Paschka 2008a, Speck 2002]. The chimeric proteins, produced as a result of the chromosomal rearrangements,

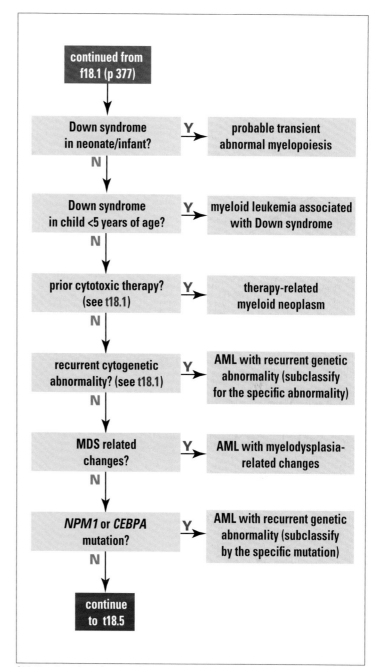

f18.2 *Flow chart for classification of AML by biologic subtypes.*

AML= acute myeloid leukemia; MDS = myelodysplastic syndrome

contribute to leukemogenesis by dysregulating the normal CBF transcriptional activity [Downing 2003, Helbling 2005].

AML with t(8;21)(q22;q22); RUNX1-RUNX1T1

AML with t(8;21)(q22;q22) is defined by the presence of this translocation, a variant translocation, or molecular *RUNX1-RUNX1T1* fusion, regardless of blast count f18.3 [Arber 2008a]. Clues and confirmatory tests for this distinct type of AML are listed in t18.5.

The peripheral blood findings are variable, but circulating blasts accompanied by cytopenias are common i18.15. Circulating mature granulocytes including neutrophils are a

t18.5 Clues and Confirmatory Tests for Biologic Types of AML (continued on next spread)

AML Subtype	Clinical Features	CBC/Blood Morphology	BM Aspirate
Recurrent Abnormalities			
AML t(8;21) (q22;q22); *(RUNX1-RUNX1T1)*	Young adults, myeloid sarcomas 10%-15% of pediatric AML 7% of adult AML	Cytopenias, circulating blasts with evidence of neutrophilic maturation	Blasts may be <20% Long tapered Auer rods Salmon-colored cytoplasm, rim of basophilia Manifests as AML with maturation
AML inv(16) (p13.1;q22) t(16;16) (p13.1;q22) *CBFB-MYH11*	Young adults Extramedullary disease 6%-12% pediatric AML 8% adult AML	Although variable, higher WBC and blast counts vs t(8;21) Monocytic cells, myeloid blasts predominate Cytopenias	Blasts may be <20% Abnormal eosinophils with admixed eosinophil/ basophil granules Variable monocytic component
AML t(15;17) (q22;q21); *PML-RARA**	Young adults DIC major complication 8%-15% pediatric AML 5%-12% adult AML	Leukocytosis—microgranular variant Leukopenia—hypergranular variant Profound thrombocytopenia Rare hyperbasophilic variant	Abnormal promyelocytes predominate (blasts may be <20%) Hypergranular variant (majority of cases): packed with granules, numerous Auer rods in single cell Microgranular variant (20% of cases): reniform, bilobed nuclei with scant to inconspicuous granules Strong uniform cytochemical MPO positivity
AML t(9;11) (p22;q23); *MLLT3-MLL*	More common in children Extramedullary disease (gingival, skin), DIC 5%-20% pediatric AML 4%-5% adult AML	Anemia, thrombocytopenia Variable WBC count and blasts	Monocytic blasts/blast equivalents
AML t(6;9) (p23;q34); *DEK-NUP214*	Young adults (median age 30 years) 1% of pediatric and adult AMLs	Basophilia (≥2%) in 50% of cases WBC may be lower than typical AML	Background myelodysplasia May see monocytic features, occasional ring sideroblasts
AML inv(3) (q21;q26.2) or t(3;3) (q21;q26.2) *RPN1-EVI1*	Possible hepatosplenomegaly	Normal or increased platelets Giant, hypogranular platelets; circulating, bare megakaryocytic nuclei	Many small, hypolobated megakaryocytes Multilineage dysplasia
AML t(1;22) (p13;q13); *RBM15-MKL1*	Restricted to infants or young children (<3 years of age) without Down syndrome Marked organomegaly	Megakaryoblasts with basophilic cytoplasm and cytoplasmic blebbing; smaller blasts may show a more lymphoblastic appearance	Megakaryoblasts with basophilic cytoplasm and cytoplasmic blebbing; smaller blasts may show a more lymphoblastic appearance Micromegakaryocytes are present Granulocytic and erythroid dysplasia not prominent
AML with mutated *NPM1*	Typically, de novo acute leukemia in older adult	WBC may be relatively high	Many, but not all cases show monocytic differentiation 80%-90% of acute monocytic leukemias have mutated *NPM1* High blast percentage
AML with mutated *CEBPA*	Occurs in 6%-15% of de novo AML; no age or sex predilection	Relatively high hemoglobin and blood blast count Relatively low platelet count	Most cases show features of AML with or without maturation; no specific morphologic features

*The t(15;17) PML-RARA translocation has been historically denoted as both t(15;17)(q22;q21) and t(15;17)(q22;q12); currently the most accurate description is actually thought to be t(15;17)(q24;q21); for the sake of simplicity and consistency, we have chosen to use the t(15;17)(q22;q21) designation

AML = acute myeloid leukemia; APL = acute promyelocytic leukemia; ATRA = all trans retinoic acid; BM = bone marrow; CBC = complete blood count; DIC = disseminated intravascular coagulation; HP = hematopoiesis; IHC = immunohistochemistry; MDS = myelodysplastic syndrome; MPN = myeloproliferative neoplasm; MPO = myeloperoxidase; MRD = minimal residual disease; PML = promyelocytic leukemia; WBC = while blood cell count

BM Biopsy	Flow Cytometry	Confirmatory Tests/Other
Hypercellular Increased blasts with evidence of granulocytic maturation Megakaryopoiesis and erythropoiesis decreased IHC: PAX5+, CD10+	Blasts: CD34+, CD117+, CD13+, CD33+, CD19+, CD79a+, TdT+ or CD56+ Frequent subpopulations reflecting granulocytic maturation in background	Favorable subtype Cytogenetics KIT activating mutations (12%-47%) may confer worse overall survival Molecular monitoring of RUNX1/RUNX1T1 for MRD
Hypercellular; admixture of immature and mature monocytic and granulocytic components	2 distinct populations: blasts (CD34+, CD117+, weak CD45+, myeloid antigens +) monocytic cells (CD45+, bright CD36/CD64 coexpression, CD33 bright+, CD34–, CD117–, HLA-DR+)	Favorable subtype Cytogenetics Molecular or FISH for CBFB-MYH11 if suspect cryptic fusion Trisomy 22 often also seen If +22 identified, may need FISH/molecular if karyotype otherwise normal KIT mutations (25%); significance unclear Molecular negativity may be associated with long-term remission
Hypercellular, dominated by cells with obvious granules in hypergranular variant Antibodies against PML show a nuclear granular pattern vs a speckled pattern in non-APL promyelocytes	Classically CD34–, HLA-DR–, CD33 bright+ CD2 and CD34 expression common in microgranular variant CD56 in 20% of cases; associated with worse outcome	Favorable subtype Cytogenetics Molecular for PML-RARA needed in rare cases with negative cytogenetics and FISH MRD monitoring (see Chapter 36) ATRA overcomes maturation block; used in combination with chemotherapy Arsenic trioxide also used in therapy of APL FLT3 mutations (~30%-40%); likely adverse effect
Hypercellular, monoblasts and promonocytes IHC: CD68+, lysozyme+, CD163+	Coexpression of CD36/CD64, HLA-DR+, CD33 bright+, CD4 weak+, CD56+, CD45+ CD34–, CD117– CD14 variable, often negative/dim	Intermediate risk Cytogenetics FISH for MLL
Background myelodysplasia (>60% of cases)	Typical myeloid phenotype: CD45 weak+, CD34+, CD117+, CD13+, CD33+	Poor prognosis Cytogenetics (abnormality may be overlooked) FLT3-ITD+ in ~70%-80%
Small, hypolobated megakaryocytes Cellularity and fibrosis variable	Blasts typically express CD34, CD13, CD33; may express CD7, CD41 and CD61	Poor risk Cytogenetics
Micromegakaryocytes are present There is usually collagen and/or reticular fibrosis Overall appearance may suggest metastatic tumor	Blasts typically express CD41 and CD61; CD42b more variable. CD36 may be positive. CD34, MPO, CD45 frequently negative, somewhat complicating lineage identification.	Cytogenetics Patients may respond to intensive chemotherapy
Usually markedly hypercellular	Blasts typically CD34 negative, with expression of CD14, CD11b and CD68 Monocytic antigens typically expressed (CD36/CD64)	Molecular (typically sizing via capillary electrophoresis for exon 12 mutations; "type A" mutation, a 4 base pair TCTG insertion most common); favorable outcome IHC for abnormal cytoplasmic NPM1 protein endorsed by WHO; some studies suggest molecular analysis may be preferred
Most cases show features of AML with or without maturation; no specific morphologic features assist in identifying CEBPA mutated cases	Blasts express typical myeloid antigens: usually CD34+, express CD7 in the majority of cases	Molecular (mutations described throughout gene, with 2 "hot-spots" at N-terminal and C-terminal) Favorable outcome

AML = acute myeloid leukemia; APL = acute promyelocytic leukemia; ATRA = all trans retinoic acid; BM = bone marrow; CBC = complete blood count; HP = hematopoiesis; IHC = immunohistochemistry; DIC = disseminated intravascular coagulation; MDS = myelodysplastic syndrome; MPN = myeloproliferative neoplasm; MPO = myeloperoxidase; MRD = minimal residual disease; PML = promyelocytic leukemia; WBC = while blood cell count

t18.5 Clues and Confirmatory Tests for Biologic Types of AML (continued from previous spread)

AML Subtype	Clinical Features	CBC/Blood Morphology	BM Aspirate
Other Biologic Subtypes			
AML with MDS-related changes (3 criteria; only 1 required)	Elderly; patient may have antecedent MDS, MDS/MPN (#1 criterion)	Cytopenias Single or multilineage dysplasia	Dysplasia of ≥50% of erythroid and/or granulocytic cells (#2 criterion)
Therapy-related myeloid neoplasm	History of chemotherapy and/or radiation therapy	Cytopenias Single or multilineage dysplasia common	Cases may meet criteria for AML, MDS, or MDS/MPN (see t18.8)
Down syndrome (DS)-related myeloid proliferation:			
Transient abnormal myelopoiesis (TAM)	Diagnosis of DS (including mosaic cases) Neonate/fetus Possible co-morbidities include cardiopulmonary failure, hyperviscosity, and hepatic fibrosis Spontaneous remission	Blasts are morphologically indistinguishable from those in myeloid leukemia associated with DS Basophilia may be present Possible thrombocytopenia with leukocytosis	Blasts are morphologically indistinguishable from those in myeloid leukemia associated with DS Erythroid and megakaryocytic dysplasia typically present
Myeloid leukemia associated with DS	Diagnosis of DS (including mosaic cases) Infant/young child (usually <4-5 yrs of age)	Blasts have megakaryoblastic features, with basophilic cytoplasm, coarse granules, and cytoplasmic blebbing Erythroid precursors, marked anisopoikilocytosis, and giant platelets may be seen Often cytopenias	Myeloid neoplasms falling into this category may show <20% blasts, as MDS and AML in this clinical setting are not clinically or biologically distinct Dyserythropoiesis and dysgranulopoiesis

AML = acute myeloid leukemia; APL = acute promyelocytic leukemia; ATRA = all trans retinoic acid; BM = bone marrow; CBC = complete blood count; DIC = disseminated intravascular coagulation; HP = hematopoiesis; IHC = immunohistochemistry; MDS = myelodysplastic syndrome; MPN = myeloproliferative neoplasm; MPO = myeloperoxidase; MRD = minimal residual disease; PML = promyelocytic leukemia; WBC = while blood cell count

References by subtype

8;21   [Boissel 2006, Cairoli 2006, Care 2003, Chen 2008, De 2007, Gamerdinger 2003, Huang 2006, Khoury 2003, Kozlov 2005, Leroy 2005, Marcucci 2003, 2005, Miyoshi 1993, Mrozek 2001, Paschka 2006, Rowe 2000, Schlenk 2004, Schnittger 2006, Tiacci 2004, Valbuena 2006, Weisser 2007]

inv(16)   [Boissel 2006, Cairoli 2006, Care 2003, Hung 2007, Marcucci 2003, 2005, Mrozek 2001, Paschka 2006, Rowe 2000, Schlenk 2004, Spencer 2007, Xu 2008]

15;17   [Ades 2005, Arber 2008a, Arbuthnot 2006, Bennett 2000, de Botton 2004, Doyle 2009, Foley 2001, Gomis 2004, Ito 2004, Kaito 2005, Kelaidi 2009, Lee 2003, Leu 2009, Mohamedbhai 2008, Mueller 2006, Ravandi 2009, Sanz 2009b, Stankova 2006, Tallman 2009, Wang 2008]

9;11   [Arber 2008a, Balgobind 2009, Dunphy 2007, Krasinskas 1998, Mrozek 1997, Xu 2006b]

6;9   [Alsabeh 1997, Chi 2008, Oyarzo 2004, Parcells 2006, Slovak 2006, Thiede 2002]

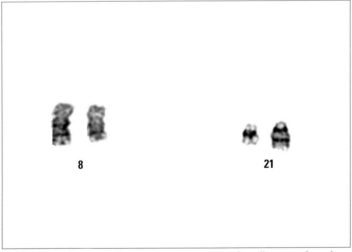

f18.3 *Partial karyotype showing chromosomes 8 and 21 illustrates t(8;21) (q22;q22). The abnormal chromosome of each pair is each on the right. (Giemsa trypsin Wright)*

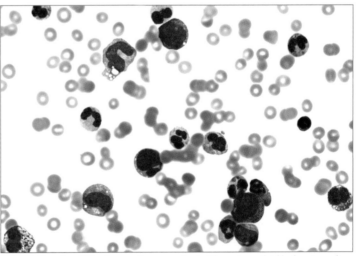

i18.15 *Peripheral blood smear from a patient with acute myeloid leukemia and t(8;21) shows prominent myeloid and monocytic maturation. Blasts are present, but maturation is prominent. Note profound anemia and thrombocytopenia. (Wright)*

BM Biopsy	Flow Cytometry	Confirmatory Tests/Other
Abnormal megakaryocytes	Aberrant antigen maturation profile variable; myeloid blasts (CD34+)	MDS-associated cytogenetic abnormalities (#3 criteria), not all cases (see t18.7)
Cases may meet criteria for AML, MDS, or MDS/MPN (see t18.8)	Variable; often aberrant	Two common subtypes: chromosomal losses/gains or 11q23 (*MLL*) translocation
Blast % may be lower than blood blast count Cellularity and blast % variable (in some cases explained by presence of blasts at sites of fetal HP)	Positive for CD34, CD56, CD13, CD33, CD7, CD4, CD41, CD61, CD42b.	*GATA1* mutation
Very dense fibrosis may be present Highly atypical megakaryocytes	In contrast to TAM, blasts are CD34- in ~50% of cases. CD56 and CD41 also more likely to be negative	*GATA1* mutation; cases of MDS or AML occurring in patients with DS who are older than age 5 *and* lack *GATA1* mutation are considered "conventional" MDS or AML

AML = acute myeloid leukemia; APL = acute promyelocytic leukemia; ATRA = all trans retinoic acid; BM = bone marrow; CBC = complete blood count; HP = hematopoiesis; IHC = immunohistochemistry; DIC = disseminated intravascular coagulation; MDS = myelodysplastic syndrome; MPN = myeloproliferative neoplasm; MPO = myeloperoxidase; MRD = minimal residual disease; PML = promyelocytic leukemia; WBC = while blood cell count

inv(3)	[Jotterand Bellomo 1992, Martinelli 2003, Nucifora 1997, Raza 2004, Testoni 1999]
t(1;22)	[Duchayne 2003, Mercher 2001, Niu 2009, Paredes-Aguilera 2003, Ribeiro 1993]
NPM1	[Becker 2010, Falini 2005, 2007, Konoplev 2009, Schnittger 2005, Tsou 2006, Yu 2006, Yun 2003]
CEBPA	[Baldus 2007, Bienz 2005, Dufour 2010, Frohling 2004, Koschmieder 2009, Pabst 2009, Schlenk 2008, Wouters 2009]
MDS-related changes	[Arber 2008b, Wandt 2008]
Therapy-related changes	[Czader 2009, Knight 2009, Pedersen-Bjergaard 2008, Rund 2005, Seedhouse 2007, Vardiman 2008a]
Down syndrome	[Massey 2006, Xavier 2009, Zipursky 2003]

usual finding; monocytes may also be present i18.15. In the bone marrow, the blast count is variable and in some cases is less than the otherwise required 20% [Chan 1997, Wong 2009b, Xue 1994]. Blasts with distinctive, long, thin Auer rods with tapered ends are characteristic and may even be seen in mature neutrophils and eosinophils i18.16, i18.17. Additional distinctive findings include salmon-colored cytoplasm with a rim of basophilia in maturing granulocytes, and dysplastic features of the mature granulocytes, including pseudo Pelger-Huët nuclei and nuclear/cytoplasmic dyssynchrony i18.18 [Nakamura 1997]. The bone marrow core biopsy is hypercellular with evidence of granulocytic maturation i18.19 [Nakamura 1997].

AML with t(8;21) may be associated with systemic mastocytosis i18.20, i18.21. In some cases the mastocytosis may be occult at diagnosis, becoming more apparent and predominant after successful therapeutic reduction of the acute leukemia i18.22, i18.23.

Immunophenotypically, blasts express typical immature (CD34, CD117) and myeloid markers [CD13, CD33, myeloperoxidase (MPO)]. Expression of particular aberrant markers (CD19, CD56, TdT) may serve as key flow cytometric clues to this diagnosis [Chen 2008, Hurwitz 1992, Khalidi 1998, Khoury 2003, Kozlov 2005, Tiacci 2004, Valbuena 2006]. Diminished CD19 and positive CD56 expression on the leukemic blasts may suggest an accompanying underlying *KIT* activating mutation in AML with t(8;21) [De 2007]. By immunohistochemistry, OCT2 and BOB1 are not reported to associate with the known PAX5 expression [Gibson 2006].

Patients with de novo AML with t(8;21) have a relatively favorable prognosis [Mrozek 2008a]. t(8;21) AML may

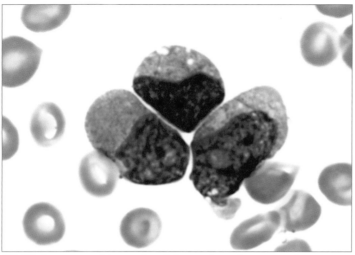

i18.16 *Long, tapered Auer rods and abnormal cytoplasmic granulation are evident in this bone marrow aspirate smear from a patient with acute myeloid leukemia and t(8;21). (Wright)*

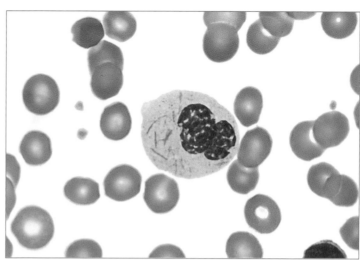

i18.17 *This neutrophil from a case of acute myeloid leukemia with t(8;21) shows Auer rods within the cytoplasm. (Wright)*

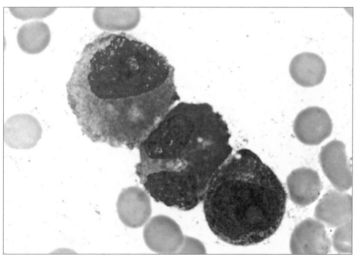

i18.18 *This bone marrow aspirate smear from a patient with acute myeloid leukemia and t(8;21) shows abnormal salmon-colored cytoplasmic granulation with a rim of basophilia, a morphologic feature of this genetic type of AML. (Wright)*

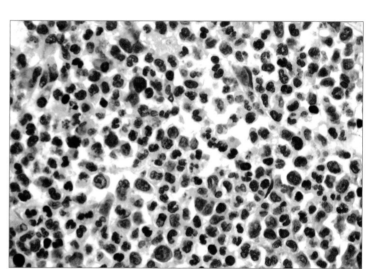

i18.19 *Substantial maturation is evident in this bone marrow core biopsy section from a patient with acute myeloid leukemia and t(8;21). (H&E)*

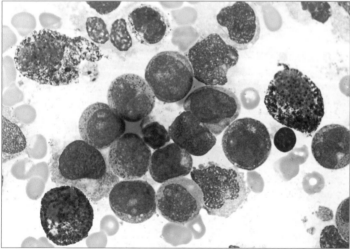

i18.20 *Systemic mastocytosis was evident in conjunction with acute myeloid leukemia associated with t(8;21) in this bone marrow aspirate smear. Note features of acute myeloid leukemia with t(8;21) as well as numerous mast cells. (Wright)*

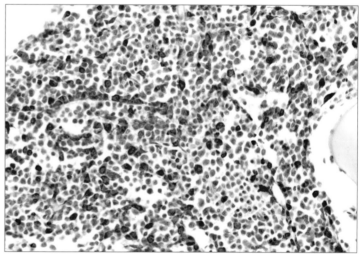

i18.21 *This bone marrow core biopsy section from a patient with concurrent acute myeloid leukemia with t(8;21) and systemic mastocytosis shows numerous admixed mast cells. (immunoperoxidase for tryptase)*

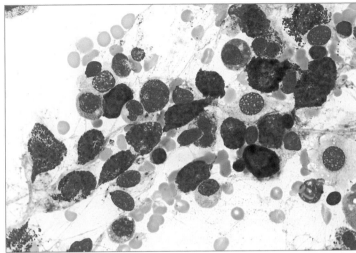

i18.22 *This bone marrow aspirate smear is taken following chemotherapy for acute myeloid leukemia with t(8;21) and associated systemic mastocytosis. The AML is in remission, but mast cells persist and are markedly increased. (Wright)*

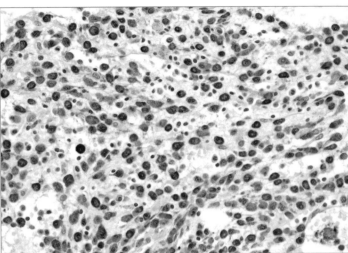

i18.23 *A striking persistence of tryptase-positive mast cells is evident in this core biopsy from a case of acute myeloid leukemia with t(8;21) and associated systemic mastocytosis. Chemotherapy effectively eradicated the AML, while systemic mastocytosis persists. (immunoperoxidase for tryptase)*

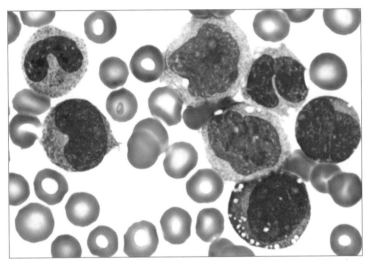

i18.24 *Monoblasts and promonocytes predominate in this peripheral blood smear from a patient with marked leukocytosis and inv(16). (Wright)*

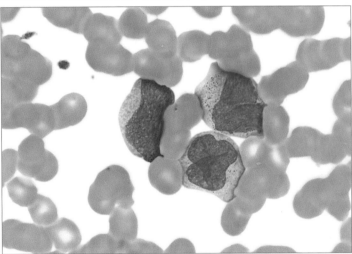

i18.25 *Circulating leukemic cells with a myelomonocytic appearance characterize this case of AML with inv(16). (Wright)*

also occur after previous chemotherapy (therapy-related) or in blast phase of chronic myelogenous leukemia (CML) [Arber 2002, Gustafson 2009, Yin 2004]. Frequent secondary cytogenetic aberrations include loss of a sex chromosome (–Y in men and –X in women) and deletion 9q [Kuchenbauer 2006, Mrozek 2008a]. *KIT* activating mutations have been identified in t(8;21) and confer an inferior overall survival [Boissel 2006, Cairoli 2006, Paschka 2006, Schnittger 2006]. *FLT3* mutations are seen in 4%-12% of AML with t(8;21), although only a minority are of the internal tandem duplication type tied most definitively to prognosis in cytogenetically normal cases (see **[18.8]** "Prognostic Factors in AML," p 417) [Boissel 2006, Care 2003, Shimada 2006, Sritana 2008]. Nevertheless, some reports suggest that *FLT3* mutation is an adverse prognostic finding in AML with t(8;21) [Boissel 2006].

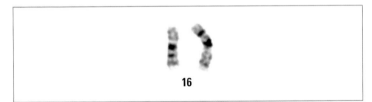

f18.4 *Normal (left) and abnormal (right) chromosome 16 illustrate inv(16) (p13.1;q22).*

AML with inv(16)/t(16;16)(p13.1;q22); CBFB-MYH11

AML with inv(16)/t(16;16) is defined by the translocation and/or molecular fusion of *CBFB* and *MYH11* regardless of blast count **f18.4**. Clues and confirmatory tests are listed in **t18.5**. Morphologically, this type of AML most often appears as a subtype of acute myelomonocytic leukemia with abnormal eosinophils.

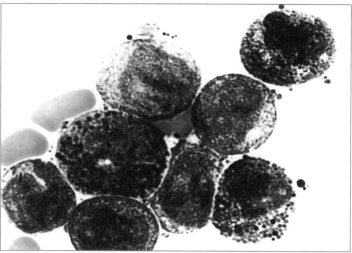

i18.26 *Numerous eosinophils with admixed aberrant basophilic granules are evident in this bone marrow aspirate smear from a patient with acute myeloid leukemia and inv(16). (Wright)*

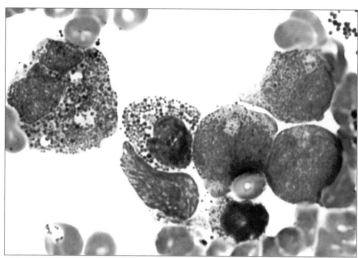

i18.27 *Numerous eosinophils with aberrant cytoplasmic granulation are evident in this bone marrow aspirate smear from a patient with acute myeloid leukemia and inv(16). (Wright)*

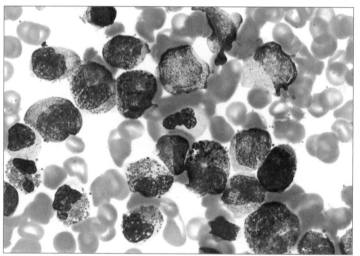

i18.28 *Significant maturation with relatively low numbers of myeloblasts, monoblasts, and promonocytes is evident on this bone marrow aspirate smear in acute myeloid leukemia with inv(16). Note predominance of eosinophils and maturing myeloid cells. (Wright)*

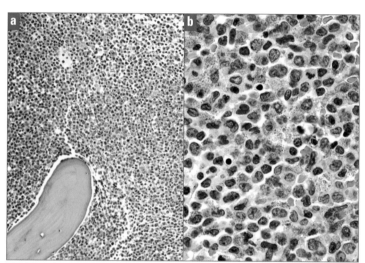

i18.29 *This composite of low and high magnification of a bone marrow core biopsy section from a patient with acute myeloid leukemia and inv(16) shows numerous eosinophils in conjunction with myelomonocytic cells showing abundant cytoplasm. (H&E)*

The peripheral blood abnormalities are variable, but leukocytosis, anemia, and thrombocytopenia are common. Monocytic cells are abundant with variable numbers of monoblasts, myeloblasts, and promonocytes i18.24, i18.25. The abnormal eosinophils (described below) are generally inconspicuous or absent in the blood.

The bone marrow is hypercellular with a variable blast count. The morphologic features show a spectrum of mature and immature monocytic cells and myeloblasts. The monocytic and granulocytic components are confirmed by positive nonspecific esterase and myeloperoxidase cytochemical stains, respectively. In addition, the bone marrow contains abnormal eosinophils with mixed eosinophilic and basophilic granules i18.26, i18.27. The abnormal basophil granules within these eosinophils lack both

myeloperoxidase and toluidine blue reactivity, distinguishing them from basophil granules. Significant maturation may be evident with relatively low numbers of blasts i18.28. Both maturation and significant eosinophilia are evident on bone marrow biopsy sections i18.29.

Immunophenotypically, AML with inv(16)/t(16;16) reveals distinct populations corresponding to the admixture of blasts, granulocytes, and monocytic cells. An immunohistochemical antibody stain (AH107) against the CBFB-MYH11 fusion protein may aid in the diagnosis [McKenna 2009, Zhao 2006].

Patients with AML with inv(16)/t(16;16) have a favorable prognosis similar to t(8;21). The inv(16) may occur rarely after previous chemotherapy or in blast phase of CML [Merzianu 2005, Wu 2006]. *KIT* mutations are present in ~30% of patients, the significance of which is unclear [Paschka 2006].

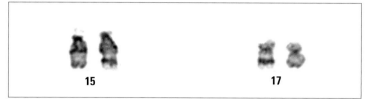

f18.5 *Partial karyotype showing chromosomes 15 and 17 illustrates t(15;17) (q22;q21). The abnormal chromosome of each pair is on the right. (Giemsa trypsin Wright)*

Activating mutations in *NRAS, KRAS, KIT,* or *FLT3* are seen in ~70% of cases [Boissel 2006, Valk 2004].

APL with t(15;17)(q22;q21); PML-RARA

AML with t(15;17)(q22;q21)/*PML-RARA* (aka APL) is a distinct clinicopathologic entity defined by the presence of the *PML-RARA* fusion, regardless of blast count **f18.5**, **f18.6**, **t18.5** [Arber 2008a]. Because of the propensity for life-threatening coagulopathy, it is imperative that cases of APL be rapidly identified [Lock 2004, Stein 2009]. This can be accomplished with a myeloperoxidase cytochemical stain, antibody against the PML protein, or FISH **f18.6**.

Two typical morphologic variants of APL are recognized (hypergranular and microgranular), plus a third variant that is quite rare (hyperbasophilic). Hypergranular APL often presents with peripheral leukopenia with rare, if any, circulating promyelocytes, while the bone marrow is typically packed with abnormal, hypergranular promyelocytes **i18.30**, **i18.31**, **i18.32**. Occasional/rare cells packed with Auer rods are noted **i18.33** [Bennett 2000]. There is little to no maturation beyond the promyelocyte stage. These hypergranular promyelocytes are intensely myeloperoxidase or Sudan black B positive, a very useful feature in the rapid diagnosis of APL **i18.34**. On

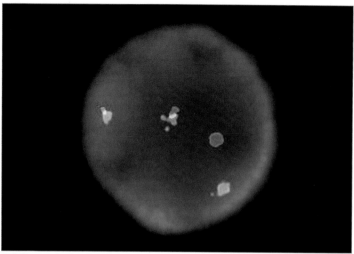

f18.6 *Dual color dual fusion probe set for PML and RARA shows the classic abnormal fusion pattern. Note 2 fused signals, one red signal and one green signal, indicating PML-RARA fusion characteristic of acute promyelocytic leukemia.*

bone marrow core biopsy sections, APL cells show moderate amounts of eosinophilic cytoplasm **i18.35**. Because of the degree of maturation, CD34 is characteristically negative **i18.36**.

Microgranular APL is morphologically distinct from the hypergranular variant in both nuclear and cytoplasmic features. Microgranular promyelocytes exhibit marked nuclear irregularities including reniform, lobulated, and monocyte-like nuclei, while the cytoplasm shows subtle often inconspicuous granulation **i18.37**, **i18.38**, **i18.39**. The rare hyperbasophilic variant is characterized by nuclear irregularity and basophilic cytoplasm; features overlap with microgranular APL **i18.40**. It is essential to distinguish microgranular APL from a true monocytic leukemia **i18.41**.

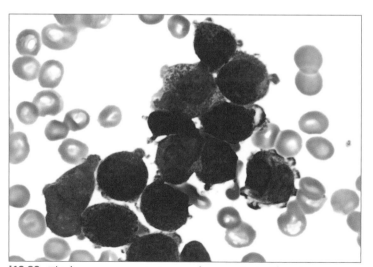

i18.30 *This bone marrow aspirate smear from a patient with acute promyelocytic leukemia shows many hypergranular promyelocytes, which are blast equivalents in only this AML subtype. (Wright)*

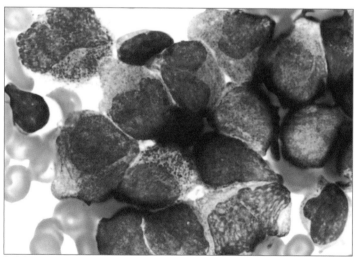

i18.31 *This bone marrow aspirate smear from a patient with acute promyelocytic leukemia shows variable nuclear irregularity in conjunction with moderate amounts of hypergranular cytoplasm. (Wright)*

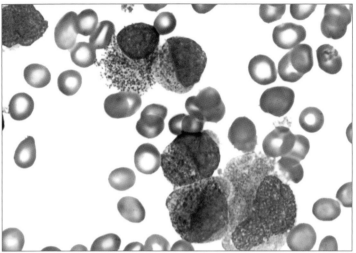

i18.32 *Intense cytoplasmic granulation, especially in the upper left cell, is evident on this bone marrow aspirate smear from a patient with acute promyelocytic leukemia. (Wright)*

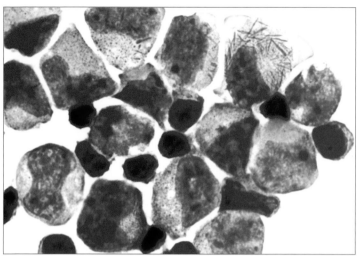

i18.33 *Numerous Auer rods are present within the cytoplasm of acute promyelocytic leukemia cells on this cytospin preparation. (Wright)*

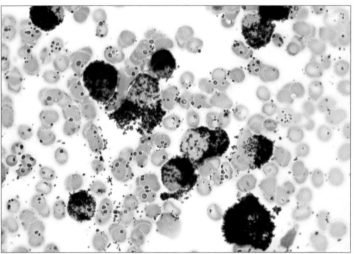

i18.34 *Cytochemical staining for myeloperoxidase shows intense uniform positivity in acute promyelocytic leukemia. (myeloperoxidase cytochemical stain)*

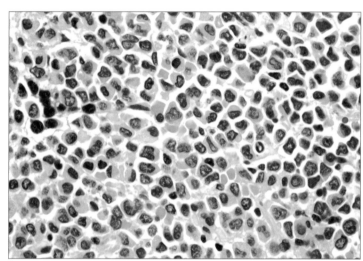

i18.35 *Little evidence of maturation beyond the promyelocyte state is evident in this bone marrow core biopsy section from a patient with acute promyelocytic leukemia. Note relative uniformity of the leukemic population and moderate to abundant amounts of eosinophilic cytoplasm. (H&E)*

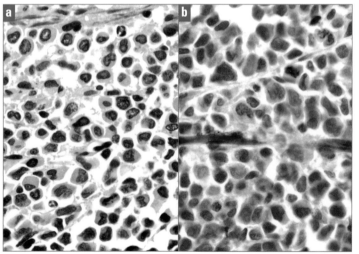

i18.36 *This composite highlights the morphologic features **a** and usual absence of CD34 staining **b** in this case of acute promyelocytic leukemia. Note CD34 positivity of only blood vessels. (H&E and immunoperoxidase for CD34)*

Cytochemically, both the hypergranular and microgranular APL cases show intense myeloperoxidase and Sudan black B positivity in the leukemic cells i18.42. This marked degree of staining is quite compelling for a diagnosis of APL and is very useful in distinguishing APL from morphologically similar disorders.

Immunophenotypically, hypergranular and microgranular APL show some similarities but also key differences. The hypergranular variant is typically CD34 negative, HLA-DR negative, with bright CD33, whereas the microgranular variant is often CD34 positive with aberrant CD2 expression (90%) [Edwards 1999, Kaleem 2003, Lin 2004, Paietta 2003]. The lack of CD34 and HLA-DR is not specific for APL, thus complete reliance on flow cytometric immunophenotyping to diagnose APL is to be avoided [Moon 2007, Oelschlaegel 2009].

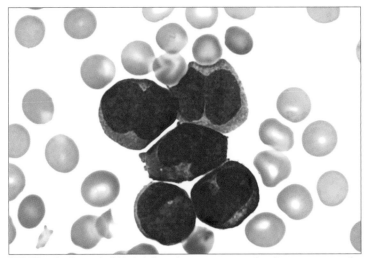

i18.37 *The distinctly folded, sliding plate appearance of nuclei in microgranular acute promyelocytic leukemia is evident in this peripheral blood smear. Note marked leukocytosis. (Wright)*

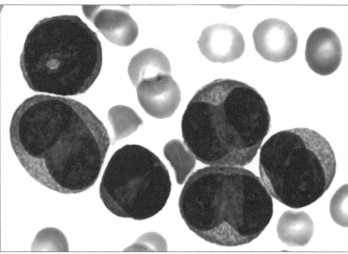

i18.38 *The distinctive nuclear features of microgranular acute promyelocytic leukemia are evident on high magnification of this peripheral blood smear. Note marked leukocytosis. (Wright)*

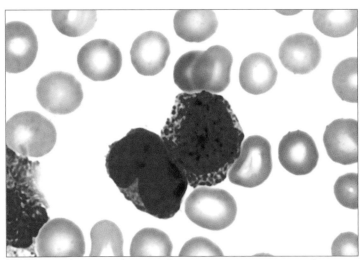

i18.39 *Rare hypergranular promyelocytes are present in microgranular acute promyelocytic leukemia in blood. (Wright)*

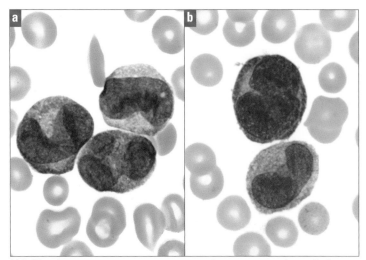

i18.40 *This composite compares microgranular acute promyelocytic leukemia* **a** *with the basophilic variant of acute promyelocytic leukemia* **b**. *(Wright)*

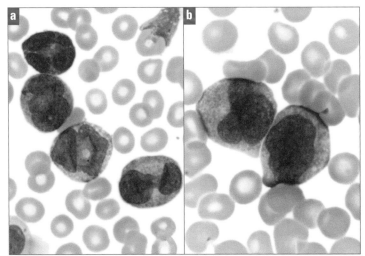

i18.41 *This composite compares microgranular acute promyelocytic leukemia* **a** *with acute monocytic leukemia* **b**. *Note the differences in nuclear configuration and the greater amounts of cytoplasm in acute monocytic leukemia. (Wright)*

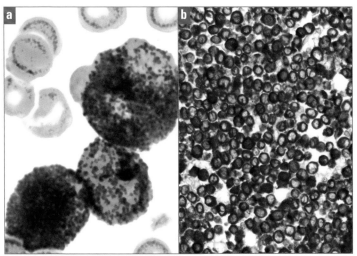

i18.42 *Intense myeloperoxidase positivity, characteristic of all types of acute promyelocytic leukemia, can be identified by either cytochemical stain* **a** *or immunoperoxidase stain* **b**. *(myeloperoxidase cytochemical and immunoperoxidase stains)*

t18.6 Characteristics of AML with Variant *RARA* Translocations

Variant Partners	Comments
ZBTB16 (11q23)	Morphologic differences from classic APL: blasts with regular nuclei, increased Pelger-Huët-like neutrophils; ATRA resistant
NUMA1 (11q13)	ATRA-sensitive
NPM1 (5q35)	Morphologic differences: no Auer rods
	Predominantly hypergranular
	ATRA-sensitive
STAT5B (17q11.2)	ATRA-resistant
PRKAR1A (17q23-24)	Single case report
	Cryptic fusion
	Typical APL: hypergranular, morphology, and immunophenotype

AML = acute myeloid leukemia; APL = acute promyelocytic leukemia;
ATRA = all trans retinoic acid

References: [Arnould 1999, Bennett 2000, Catalano 2007, Chen 1993, Redner 1996, Sainty 2000, Wells 1997]

The differential diagnostic considerations vary between hypergranular and microgranular APL largely due to their different cytologic appearances. A wave of granulocytic recovery after transient agranulocytosis, G-CSF therapy, or any other prominent promyelocyte population can mimic hypergranular APL. Key cytologic factors in granulocytic recovery include prominent paranuclear hofs (Golgi regions), round nuclei, and absence of Auer rods [Harris 1994, Innes 1987]. In addition, CD117 and CD11b expression may aid in distinguishing APL from a benign process [Rizzatti 2002]. As noted above, the microgranular variant of APL may be mistaken for acute monocytic leukemia (AMoL); however, the typical bilobed (sliding plate) appearance of microgranular APL is not seen in AMoL (see i18.41). Striking uniform myeloperoxidase cytochemical activity in the leukemic cells also indicates APL, while greater amounts of cytoplasm and nonspecific esterase positivity characterize monocytic leukemias (see i18.42).

Patients with de novo t(15;17) have a favorable prognosis. t(15;17) AML may also arise after previous chemotherapy or in blast phase of CML [Beaumont 2003, Chung 2008, Hasan 2008, Pulsoni 2002]. Occasionally the molecular fusion is present but is cytogenetically and/or FISH cryptic requiring PCR-based confirmation [Wang 2009, Wong 2009a]. *FLT3* mutations are detected in 30%-40% of APL cases and may be associated with shorter survival times [Callens 2005].

Acute Myeloid Leukemias with Variant RARA Translocations

Occasionally, a case will exhibit many features suggestive of APL but lack the t(15;17) translocation; alternative translocation partners for *RARA* on chromosome 17 have been noted in these cases **t18.6**. Morphologic differences

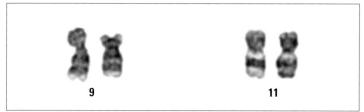

f18.7 *Partial karyotype showing chromosomes 9 and 11 illustrates t(9;11) (p22;q23). The abnormal chromosome of each pair is on the right. (Giemsa trypsin Wright)*

from classic APL include less prominent nuclear bilobation, absence of Auer rods, and pelgeroid neutrophils. The responsiveness of these variants with ATRA varies **t18.6**.

AML with t(9;11)(p22;q23); MLLT3-MLL

In the WHO 2008 classification, AML with t(9;11) is the only translocation involving the *MLL* gene included as a distinct biologic subtype **f18.7** [Arber 2008a]. Clues and confirmatory tests in AML with t(9;11) are detailed in **t18.5**.

In the peripheral blood and bone marrow, AML with t(9;11) manifests as a proliferation of monoblasts and/or promonocytes (blasts/blast equivalents ≥20%) **i18.43**, **i18.44**. Full monocytic differentiation is rarely evident. **t18.4** delineates the key morphologic, cytochemical, and immunophenotypic features of monoblasts and promonocytes **i18.45**. Prominent nonspecific esterase (NSE) cytochemical positivity and negative/weak MPO in the blasts is a key clue to the diagnosis (see **i18.14**).

Immunophenotyping reveals monocytic differentiation typified by CD36/CD64 coexpression, weak CD4, bright CD33, strong HLA-DR, variable (often negative) CD14,

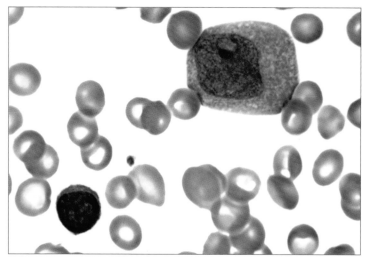

i18.43 *This peripheral blood smear shows profound pancytopenia and a rare circulating monoblast. (Wright)*

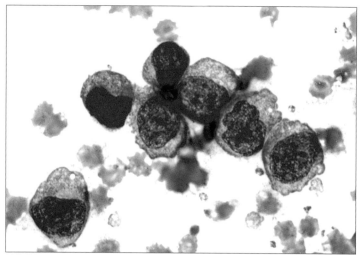

i18.44 *This bone marrow aspirate smear illustrates acute monocytic leukemia and t(9;11). Note predominance of monoblasts and promonocytes (blast equivalents). (Wright)*

while both CD34 and CD117 are typically negative [Dunphy 2007, Krasinskas 1998, Xu 2006b].

AML with t(9;11) is associated with an intermediate prognosis and reportedly fares better than AMLs with other *MLL* translocation partners [Balgobind 2009, Mrozek 1997]. AMLs with *MLL* rearrangements other than t(9;11) are diagnosed as AML, not otherwise specified, or as therapy-related leukemia with t(v;11q23) in the setting of prior cytotoxic treatment. If the cytogenetics reveal t(2;11)(p21;q23) or t(11;16)(q23;p13), these should be diagnosed as AML with myelodysplasia-related changes [Arber 2008a].

AML with Variant MLL Translocations

Although >60 fusion partner genes are known for *MLL*, the more common translocations in AML include 6q27 (*MLLT4*), 10p12 (*MLLT10*), 19p13.1 (*ELL*), and 19p13.3 (*MLLT1*), all resulting in fusion genes [Martineau 1998, Meyer 2009, Moorman 1998]. AML with *MLL* abnormalities accounts for ~3% of all AML [Schoch 2003]. In neonates, acute monoblastic leukemias frequently harbor MLL translocations, and overall survival may depend on the translocation partner [Balgobind 2009]. Given that the *MLL* gene is not invariably involved when abnormalities of 11q23 are detected by conventional cytogenetics and that *MLL* rearrangements (including those resulting from *MLL* partial tandem duplication) may be missed by standard cytogenetics, molecular or FISH techniques may be necessary to identify and verify an *MLL* abnormality [Abdou 2002, Caligiuri 1998, Mathew 1999, Watanabe 2003]. Since 11q23 is a topoisomerase II cleavage site, it has been experimentally demonstrated that topoisomerase II inhibitors (eg, etoposide) increase chromosomal recombination events involving this locus (see "Therapy-Related AML," p 403) [Bueno 2009, Chatterjee 1990, Le 2009, Libura 2005]. *MLL* amplification in AML is associated with poor outcome. *MLL*-rearranged leukemias often cause

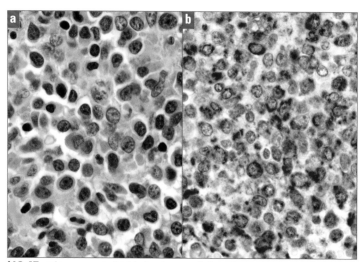

i18.45 *This composite highlights the morphologic features of acute monocytic leukemia in bone marrow core biopsy sections **a**, while strongly positive CD68 is noted, compatible with monocytic lineage differentiation **b**. (H&E and immunoperoxidase for CD68)*

high-level expression of Homeobox genes such as *HOXA9* [Faber 2009, Roth 2009].

AML with t(6;9)(p23;q34); DEK-NUP214

AML with t(6;9)(p23;q34) is rare and estimated to comprise approximately 1% of all adult and pediatric AML cases **f18.8** [Byrd 2002, Slovak 2000]. Detailed clues and confirmatory tests in this type of AML are shown in **t18.5** [Alsabeh 1997, Slovak 2006]. The CBC exhibits findings of bone marrow failure (ie, thrombocytopenia, neutropenia, anemia), circulating blasts, and often basophilia. The blasts may contain Auer rods and be cytochemically positive for myeloperoxidase and/or nonspecific esterase, thus exhibiting hybrid myeloid and monocytic features [Arber 2008a]. The bone marrow is hypercellular with ≥20% blasts. Background trilineage

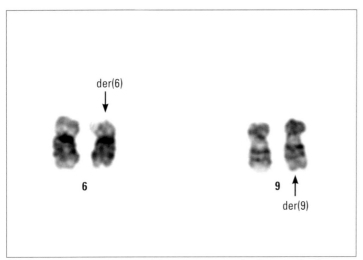

f18.8 *G-banded Wright-stained chromosomes 6 and 9 illustrate t(6;9) (p23;q34). The abnormal chromosome of each pair is on the right.*

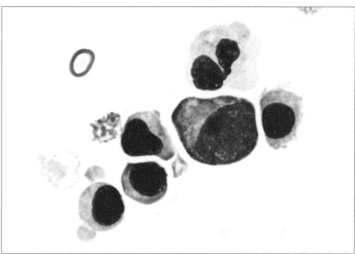

i18.46 *This cytospin smear in acute myeloid leukemia and t(6;9) shows a myeloblast with fine granules in association with dysplastic neutrophils. (Wright)*

dysplasia is common as is basophilia **i18.46**, **i18.47** [Oyarzo 2004, Pearson 1985, Slovak 2006]. Increased ring sideroblasts may be seen [Alsabeh 1997, Slovak 2006]. CD34 and CD117 are generally positive on the blasts with a subset expressing TdT.

The t(6;9) tends to be the sole cytogenetically evident, although easily overlooked, abnormality, which results in the formation of a chimeric fusion gene *DEK-NUP214* (*NUP214* once known as *CAN*) [Soekarman 1992, von Lindern 1992]. This resultant oncoprotein is likely to work together with other cryptic genetic aberrations to ultimately contribute to the development of AML [Deguchi 2002].

Up to 80% of t(6;9) AML cases may have an internal tandem duplication mutation of the tyrosine kinase *FLT3*, which may play a key role in leukoemogenesis by impeding normal cellular proliferation [Oyarzo 2004, Parcells 2006, Thiede 2002]. Increased global protein synthesis specifically in t(6;9) myeloid cells as a result of increased translation may be a mechanism underlying leukemogenesis [Ageberg 2008].

Patients with t(6;9) AML have an overall poor prognosis (5-year survival estimate in adults is 9%) [Slovak 2006]. Higher WBC counts predict shorter overall survival, while higher bone marrow blast counts predict shorter disease-free survival [Slovak 2006]. Allogeneic stem cell transplant may improve overall survival [Slovak 2006].

AML with inv(3)(q21q26.2) or t(3;3)(q21;q26.2); RPN1-EVI1

Rarely, a case of AML will bear either the inv(3) (q21;q26.2) or the t(3;3)(q21;q26.2), both of which generate fusion of *RPN1* and *EVI1* **t18.5**. The latter gene codes for a transcription factor and is itself transcriptionally complex, with alternate forms that include exons spliced in from an upstream gene *MDS1*. The fusion with *RPN1* causes aberrant expression of *EVI1* and disturbs the normal

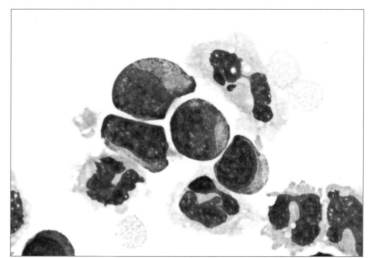

i18.47 *This bone marrow aspirate smear in acute myeloid leukemia and t(6;9) shows myeloblasts with fine cytoplasmic granules. (Wright) (courtesy J Mooney, MD)*

topographic relationship with *MDS1* [Martinelli 2003, Nucifora 1997]. The morphologic hallmark of these cases is the presence of conspicuously atypical megakaryocytes (usually small in size with monolobated or bilobated nuclei) in a background of multilineage dysplasia. A similar picture is present in the peripheral blood, with notably prominent platelet-associated abnormalities (including giant, hypogranular forms and circulating megakaryocytic nuclei) in a background of granulocytic dysplasia [Jotterand Bellomo 1992]. *EVI1* also serves as a translocation partner with genes other than *RPN1*, in which case the process is not considered to fall within this specific biologic subtype. AML with *RPN1-EVI1* is a highly aggressive disease with a median survival of only 5.5 months, though response to alternate treatment regimens may be better [Raza 2004, Testoni 1999]. It is to be hoped that wider recognition of the entity, facilitated by its specific

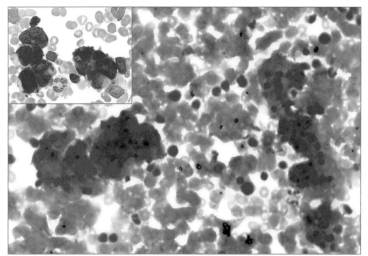

i18.48 *This bone marrow aspirate smear composite is from 2 patients with acute megakaryoblastic leukemia and t(1;22). Note prominent clumping of blasts (right). (Wright) (courtesy A Vendrell, MD)*

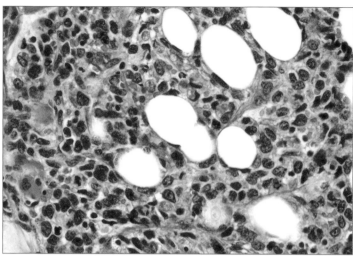

i18.49 *This bone marrow core biopsy section from a patient with acute megakaryoblastic leukemia and t(1;22) shows numerous blasts as well as differentiating megakaryocytic cells as evidenced by enlarging overall cells size and moderate to abundant amounts of eosinophilic cytoplasm. (H&E) (courtesy S Geaghan, MD)*

inclusion in the WHO 2008 system, may foster more effective therapies.

AML with t(1;22)(p13;q13); RBM15-MKL1

AML with t(1;22)(p13;q13) is an exceedingly rare diagnosis (<1% of cases) that should be considered only in children <3 years of age; most commonly, presentation is in infancy **t18.5**. The t(1;22) involves *RBM15* and *MKL1*. The latter gene is named for its association with megakaryoblastic leukemia and encodes a protein involved in chromatin organization, while RBM15 regulates c-myc; the fusion event may disturb both of these activities [Mercher 2001, Niu 2009]. As befits an AML involving *MKL1*, this is a megakaryoblastic leukemia, and these blasts may show distinct clumping on aspirate smears and are often mixed with micromega-karyocytes **i18.48, i18.49, i18.50** [Duchayne 2003]. Other clues to the possible presence of this subtype are organomegaly, the lack of significant erythroid or granulocytic dysplasia, and the presence of bone marrow fibrosis [Paredes-Aguilera 2003, Ribeiro 1993]. The fibrosis is often so extensive as to suggest a differential diagnosis of metastatic disease, an impression heightened by the relatively cohesive nature of the megakaryoblasts. Given a megakaryoblastic proliferation in an infant, it is also prudent to completely exclude a diagnosis of Down syndrome and its associated myeloid proliferations [Hama 2008]. The importance of recognizing the t(1;22) subtype as a distinct diagnostic entity is underscored by studies showing a significant survival advantage with intensive chemotherapy [Duchayne 2003].

AML with Mutated NPM1 and CEBPA

Several recurrent gene mutations now share the stage with the well-established translocations described above. The WHO 2008 scheme endorses mutations in 3 genes (*NPM1*, *CEBPA*, and *FLT3*) as especially diagnostically or

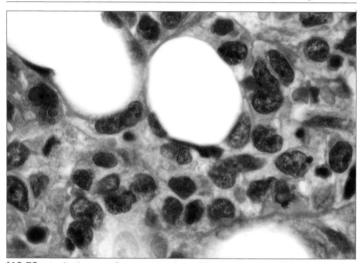

i18.50 *On high magnification, megakaryoblasts and minimally maturing megakaryocytes are evident on this bone marrow core biopsy section from a patient with acute megakaryoblastic leukemia and t(1;22). (H&E) (courtesy S Geaghan, MD)*

prognostically significant. However, the inclusion of these gene mutations has occasioned a good deal of strenuous debate, centering on a fundamental (almost philosophical) question: at what point does a genetic aberration tied to a given biologic behavior cease to be simply a prognostic factor and instead become definitional of a specific subtype of AML? *FLT3*, for example, is associated with a relatively poor prognosis but is found in a wide array of otherwise well-defined AML subtypes, such as APL. For this reason, the WHO relegates *FLT3* mutation status to a prognostic factor rather than a diagnostic subgroup. In contrast, *NPM1* and *CEBPA* mutations define specific subtypes of AML, though these entities are only provisional categories. We will adhere to this scheme and discuss *NPM1* and *CEBPA* here as biologic subtypes of AML, while reserving consideration of *FLT3* for the subsequent section on prognostic factors.

AML with Mutations of NPM1

NPM1 mutations are frequent in karyotypically normal AML, occurring in between 50% and 60% of such cases [Falini 2005]. *NPM1* encodes the protein nucleophosmin, which appears to function primarily as a shuttle for other proteins between the nucleus and the cytoplasm. It may also play a role in cell cycle control and in the regulation of centromere duplication to facilitate orderly mitosis [Falini 2007, Tsou 2006, Yu 2006, Yun 2003]. *NPM1* mutations are typically insertions of variable length that produce a frameshift sufficient to alter the nuclear localization sequence, leading to aberrant accumulation of the protein in the cytoplasm **t18.5**. Though immunohisto-chemical techniques may be applied to detect this abnormal cytoplasmic nucleophosmin, direct PCR amplification of the affected region with sizing by capillary electrophoresis is widely available in molecular diagnostic laboratories [Konoplev 2009, Luo 2010]. *NPM1* mutations have been especially associated with AML showing monocytic differentiation and absence of CD34 expression. Although neither feature is completely sensitive or specific for predicating an *NPM1* mutation, the fact that up to 90% of acute monocytic leukemias have mutated *NPM1* provides a powerful diagnostic clue [Schnittger 2005]. Mutated *NPM1* is associated with a good prognosis with one exceptionally important caveat: *NPM1* mutations are rather frequently (ie, 40%) present in tandem with *FLT3* mutations, in which case the adverse prognostic effect of the *FLT3* mutation essentially negates the otherwise beneficial behavior associated with the *NPM1* mutation [Baldus 2007, Schlenk 2008]. Thus, testing for *NPM1* should always be performed together with *FLT3* analysis.

AML with CEPBA Mutations

Mutations of the CCAAT/enhancer binding protein α (*CEBPA*) gene define the second provisional subtype of AML with gene mutations. *CEBPA* encodes a transcription factor essential for granulocytic maturation [Koschmieder 2009]. Mutations occurring in AML cluster in the N-terminal and C-terminal regions, inducing frameshift and missense mutations, respectively, that presumably contribute to leukemogenesis by interfering with the protein's contribution to terminal differentiation. *CEBPA* mutations are somewhat less common than *NPM1* mutations, and are present in between 15% and 20% of cytogenetically normal cases—most commonly, but not exclusively, in cases with the morphologic features of AML with or without maturation [see **18.7** "AML, Not Otherwise Specified (NOS)," p 408] [Baldus 2007]. Mutated *CEBPA* in isolation confers a relatively good prognosis, though recent data suggest that this effect is limited to only those cases that carry biallelic *CEBPA* mutations [Bienz 2005, Frohling 2004, Ho 2009, Pabst 2009, Schlenk 2008, Wouters 2009].

Diagnostic Strategies for Molecular Assessment in AML

The inclusion of *NPM1* and *CEBPA* mutation status in the AML classification scheme presents a challenge to the diagnostician. In contrast to conventional cytogenetics and flow cytometric immunophenotyping, which are routinely performed in newly diagnosed cases of AML, molecular analysis for gene mutations represents a new frontier. When should this specialized testing be ordered? The best answer, as of this writing, is, in cytogenetically normal cases *and/or* when, after consultation with the clinical team, it is determined that gene mutation status will provide information useful in patient management. The prognostic significance of *NPM1*, *CEBPA* (and *FLT3*) mutations is clearly established in cytogenetically normal cases [Mrozek 2007]. In other situations, including AML with myelodysplasia-related changes and cytogenetically abnormal cases that do not fulfill criteria for AML with myelodysplasia-related changes, the significance of these gene mutations remains less certain. However, our understanding of gene mutations is constantly evolving, with recent data demonstrating that *NPM1* mutation status may carry similar prognostic connotations even in karyotypically abnormal AML [Haferlach 2009a]. While, in general, strict adherence to the WHO classification scheme is desirable, communication with clinicians on a case-by-case basis is essential to its rational application in this area. Thus, at large research institutions with multiple treatment protocols and studies, maximum effort in all cases (even those carrying cytogenetic abnormalities or myelodysplasia-related changes) to identify these and other mutations might indeed be indicated. In contrast, such efforts might be excessive in an elderly or infirm patient ineligible for aggressive treatment options. It is likely that diagnostic strategies employing these gene mutations will continue to evolve as further studies more clearly define their impact in the full spectrum of morphologic subtypes of AML.

[18.6.2] Clinical Biologic Subtypes of AML

AML with Myelodysplasia-Related Changes

AML with myelodysplasia-related changes is a broad category that may be invoked by clinical setting, genetic abnormality, or morphologic findings [Arber 2008b]. Specifically, these cases of AML satisfy one or more of the following criteria:

1. the patient has a history of previously diagnosed MDS or MDS/MPN overlap syndrome
2. cytogenetic abnormalities associated with MDS are present **t18.7**, **f18.9**
3. there is multilineage dysplasia, defined for this purpose as dysplasia involving at least half of the cells in 2 separate bone marrow lineages **i18.51**, **i18.52**, **i18.53**, **i18.54**

t18.7 Cytogenetic Abnormalities Sufficient to Diagnose AML with Myelodysplasia-Related Changes*

Complex karyotype (≥3 unrelated abnormalities, none of which is included in the AML with recurrent cytogenetic abnormalities subgroup); such cases should be classified in the appropriate cytogenetic group

−7/del(7q)

−5/del(5q)

i(17q)/t(17p)

−13/del(13q)

del(11q)

del(12p)/t(12p)

del(9q)

idic(X)(q13)

t(11;16)(q23;p13.3)*

t(3;21)(q26.2;q22.1)*

t(1;3)(p36.3;q21.1)

t(2;11)(p21;q23)

t(5;12)(q33;p12)

t(5;7)(q33;q11.2)

t(5;17)(q33;p13)

t(5;10)(q33;q21)

t(3;5)(q25;q34)

*Patients with a diagnosis of AML with myelodysplasia-related changes should not have a history of prior cytotoxic therapy; in such a case, the "therapy-related myeloid neoplasm" category takes precedence over any MDS-related changes, and the disease should be classified as such; t(11;16)(q23;p13.3) and t(3;21)(q26.2;q22.1) occur in therapy-related cases with particular frequency

Reference: [Arber 2008a]

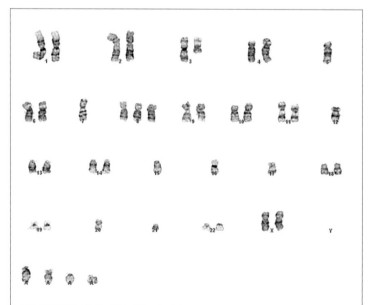

f18.9 This karyogram shows a complex karyotype including monosomy of many chromosomes as well as multiple marker chromosomes. The abnormal chromosomes are on the right. (Giemsa trypsin Wright)

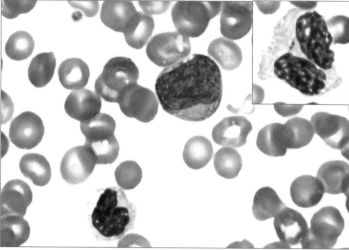

i18.51 This peripheral blood smear shows profound pancytopenia, a circulating blast, and dysplastic neutrophils. (Wright)

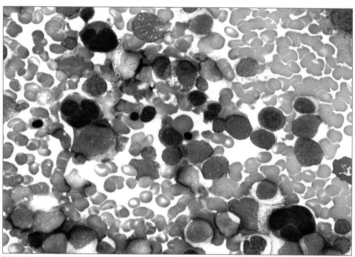

i18.52 This bone marrow aspirate smear in acute myeloid leukemia with myelodysplasia-related changes shows highly abnormal multinucleated erythroid precursors, increased myeloblasts, and dysplastic maturing granulocytic cells. (Wright)

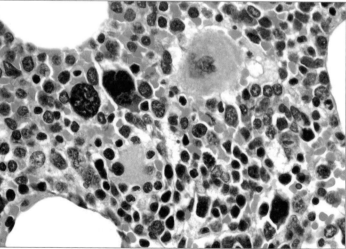

i18.53 This bone marrow core biopsy in acute myeloid leukemia with myelodysplasia-related changes shows highly atypical multinucleated erythroid cells in the approximate size range of megakaryocytes. Note increased blasts and dysplastic megakaryocytes. (H&E)

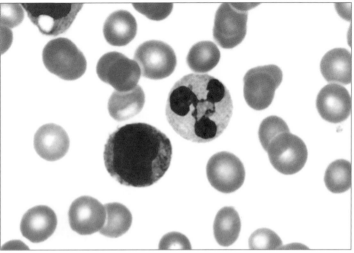

i18.54 *In this case of acute myeloid leukemia, the mature neutrophils exhibit features of myelokathexis with exceedingly long, thin interlobar strands. (Wright)*

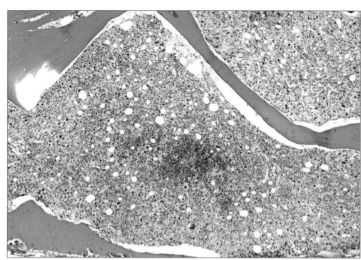

i18.55 *This bone marrow core biopsy section is from an elderly female with new onset of pancytopenia. Note hypercellularity, lymphoid aggregate, and increased megakaryocytes. (H&E)*

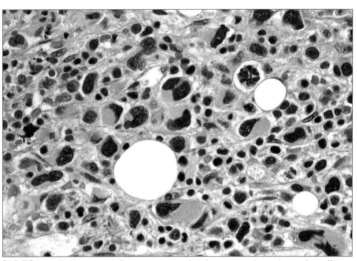

i18.56 *On higher magnification, tremendously increased numbers of small dysplastic megakaryocytes are evident on this bone marrow core biopsy section in acute myeloid leukemia with myelodysplasia-related changes (see **i18.55**). (H&E)*

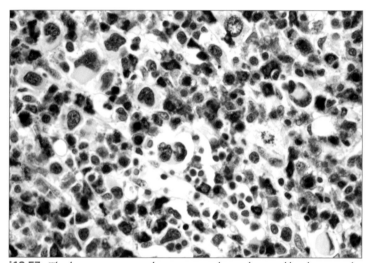

i18.57 *This bone marrow core biopsy section shows abnormal localization of myeloperoxidase-positive immature granulocytic cells in acute myeloid leukemia with myelodysplasia-related changes. (immunoperoxidase for myeloperoxidase)*

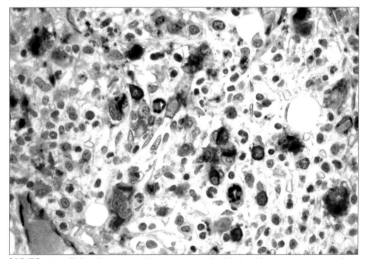

i18.58 *Small dysplastic megakaryocytes are highlighted by immunoperoxidase staining for CD31 in acute myeloid leukemia with myelodysplasia-related changes. (immunoperoxidase for CD31)*

Morphologic and immunohistochemical assessment of bone marrow core biopsies can be used to enumerate immature cells and assess for multilineage dysplasia **i18.55**, **i18.56**, **i18.57**, **i18.58** [Ngo 2008].

In addition, these cases by definition lack the clinical history (eg, prior cytotoxic therapy) and genetic abnormalities [eg, t(15;17)] that would identify them as belonging to other specific biologic subtypes of AML. However, there is a minor exception to this rule: some cases of AML with myelodysplasia-related changes will also carry mutated *NPM1* or *CEBPA*, which, as described above, could theoretically place them into the provisional categories reserved for cases with such mutations. Because the prognostic significance of *NPM1* and *CEBPA* mutations is unclear in the setting of myelodysplasia-related changes, the WHO 2008 classification recommends that these rare

t18.8 Comparison of Clinicopathologic Features of 2 Types of Therapy-Related Myeloid Neoplasms*

Feature	Secondary to Alkylating Agent Therapy[†]	Secondary to Topoisomerase II Inhibitor Therapy
Therapy	Alkylating agents or radiotherapy induce permanent genetic abnormalities Benzene exposure also linked to AML	Epipodophyllotoxins and related agents that inhibit DNA-topoisomerase II
Susceptibility	Linked to polymorphisms in genes involved in detoxification or major DNA repair pathways	11q23 is cleavage site for topoisomerase II; double-stranded DNA cleavage; repair blocked by inhibitor Repair defects linked to polymorphisms in genes that detoxify drugs
Latent period	2-11 years; shorter for patients with higher cumulative alkylating agent dose	Brief, <1-3 years
Blood	Myelodysplastic phase characterized by severe cytopenias, trilineage dysplasia, and basophilia	Abrupt onset of cytopenias in most cases; some cases have short cytopenic "prodrome" phase Leukocytosis common
Bone marrow	Usually hypercellular, but may be hypocellular Fibrosis common Multilineage dysplasia common; variable blast percentage Cases may fulfill criteria for MDS, MDS/MPN, or AML	Hypercellular Most cases acute monocytic leukemia Occasional cases of AML with t(8;21), acute promyelocytic leukemia, and AML with inv(16)
Cytogenetics/molecular	−5/del(5q), −7/del(7q) (multistep leukemogenesis) Complex karyotypic abnormalities frequent Rare translocations (of type found in de novo AML) Cooperating Class I and Class II mutations	Balanced 11q23 translocations in most cases Balanced 21q22 translocation, t(15;17), and inv(16) in occasional cases
Response to therapy	Poor response to conventional antileukemic therapy Expression of multidrug resistance-associated proteins and drug efflux	Good achievement of complete remission; relapse frequent especially in 11q23-associated cases
Survival	Poor Worse than de novo AML with comparable features	Variable; poor in 11q23 group Somewhat better survival for t-AML with translocations compared to chromosomal loss, but worse than de novo cases with same translocations

*t-AMLs, t-MDS, and t-MDS/MPN merged in WHO classification; alkylating agent type t-AML merged with topoisomerase II inhibitor group, since most patients have received both types of therapeutic agents [Vardiman 2008a]
[†]Radiation/radiotherapy also leukemogenic; may also occur after either autologous stem cell or bone marrow transplantation [Beauchamp-Nicoud 2003, Smith 2003]; rarely reported after G-CSF for stem cell donor [Hsia 2008]
AML = acute myeloid leukemia; MDS= myelodysplastic syndrome; MPN = myeloproliferative neoplasm; t- = therapy-related

References: [Czader 2009, Knight 2009, Pedersen-Bjergaard 2008, Rund 2005, Seedhouse 2007, Vardiman 2008a]

cases be assigned to the MDS-related category, with a note appended to the diagnostic line identifying the coexisting mutation. Cases of AML with myelodysplasia-related changes have a generally poor prognosis, though this may be primarily attributable to the frequent presence of high-risk cytogenetic abnormalities rather than history or morphology *per se,* as suggested by recent authors [Wandt 2008]. However, in comparison to AML, NOS, cases of AML with MDS-related changes have a significantly worse overall survival [Weinberg 2009].

Therapy-Related AML

One clinical setting that automatically triggers a specific subclassification of AML is a history of prior cytotoxic chemotherapy and/or radiation treatment [Vardiman 2008a]. Agents that have been implicated are listed in t18.1. There are 2 broad categories of therapy-related myeloid neoplasms: those that follow treatment with alkylating agents and those that follow agents directed against the enzyme topoisomerase II. Although in both cases, AML arises following direct DNA damage induced by the therapeutic agent, the genetic and clinical features of the resulting processes are quite different, as summarized in t18.8 [Czader 2009, Knight 2009, Pedersen-Bjergaard 2008, Rund 2005, Seedhouse 2007, Vardiman 2008a]. Because chemotherapeutic regimens often include both alkylating agents and topoisomerase II inhibitors, the WHO 2008 recommendation is to group all therapy-related myeloid neoplasms (t-AMLs) together rather

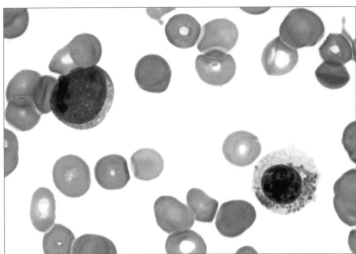

i18.59 *This peripheral blood smear is from a patient who developed therapy-related acute myeloid leukemia. Note profound cytopenias and striking red blood cell pathology. (Wright)*

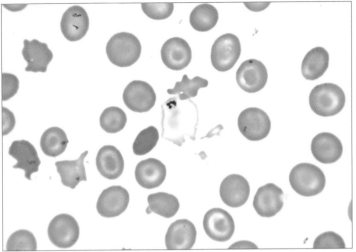

i18.60 *This peripheral blood smear shows a therapy-related myeloid neoplasm. Note profound cytopenias, circulating myeloblasts, and markedly atypical eosinophil. (Wright)*

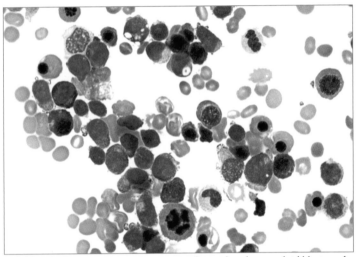

i18.61 *This bone marrow aspirate smear shows abundant myeloid blasts and abnormal erythroid cells in a therapy-related acute myeloid leukemia. (Wright)*

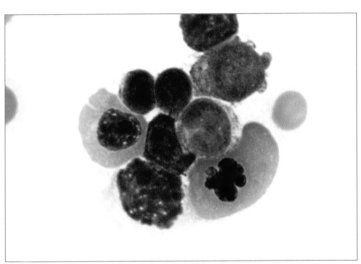

i18.62 *Both dysplastic erythroid and granulocytic lineage cells are evident on this bone marrow aspirate smear from a patient with therapy-related acute myeloid leukemia. (Wright)*

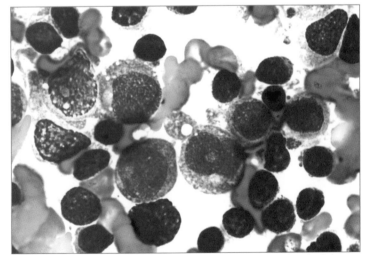

i18.63 *This bone marrow aspirate smear shows an admixture of residual chronic lymphocytic leukemia and concurrent therapy-related acute myeloid leukemia. Note abundant small lymphocytes and associated increased blasts. (Wright)*

than specifying subtypes [Vardiman 2008a]. Furthermore, therapy-related cases with the morphologic and clinical features of myelodysplastic syndrome or MDS/MPN overlap syndromes share the poor prognosis of therapy-related cases with features of acute leukemia. For this reason, all such processes are grouped together as "therapy-related myeloid neoplasms," regardless of blast count [Czader 2009, Vardiman 2008a]. Multilineage dysplasia is frequently noted in cases of t-myeloid neoplasms, and persistence of the primary neoplasm may be noted in conjunction with t-AML **i18.59, i18.60, i18.61, i18.62, i18.63, i18.64, i18.65, i18.66, i18.67, i18.68, i18.69, i18.70.** Fibrosis is common in t-myeloid neoplasms **i18.71, i18.72** [Czader 2009, Vardiman 2008a].

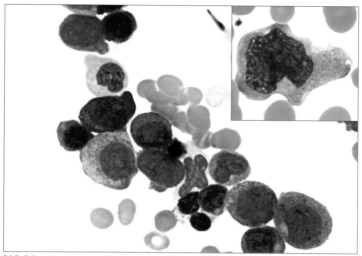

i18.64 *This bone marrow aspirate smear composite shows prominent monoblastic features in this case of therapy-related acute myeloid leukemia linked to topoisomerase II inhibitor therapy. (Wright)*

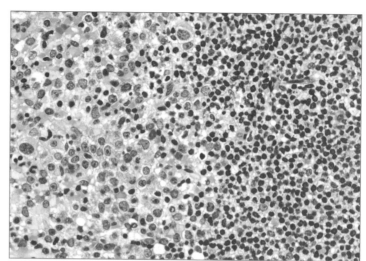

i18.65 *This bone marrow core biopsy section shows side-by-side therapy-related acute myeloid leukemia **a** with residual chronic lymphocytic leukemia **b**. (H&E)*

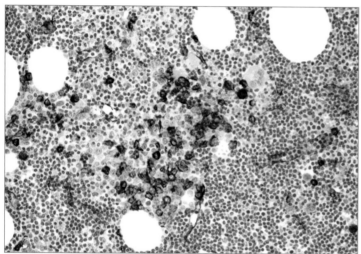

i18.66 *Immunoperoxidase staining for CD34 shows markedly increased myeloblasts in the area of therapy-related acute myeloid leukemia, while the portion of the bone marrow effaced by persistent chronic lymphocytic leukemia shows CD34 positivity only in blood vessels (see **i18.65**). (immunoperoxidase for CD34)*

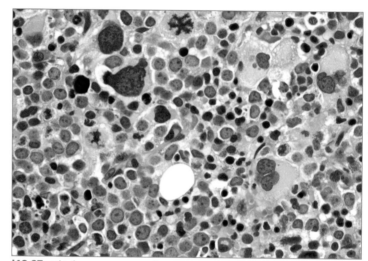

i18.67 *This bone marrow core biopsy section from a case of therapy-related acute myeloid leukemia shows markedly increased blasts in conjunction with increased and dysplastic megakaryocytes. (H&E)*

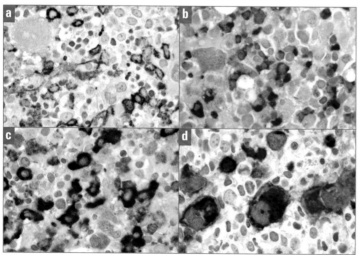

i18.68 *Composite of therapy related-acute myeloid leukemia shows increased myeloblasts **a**, disrupted erythroid colonies **b**, abnormal localization of immature granulocytic cells **c**, and increased and dysplastic megakaryocytes **d**. (immunoperoxidase for CD34, hemoglobin A, myeloperoxidase, and CD42b)*

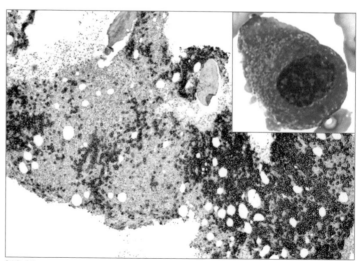

i18.69 *Residual myeloma is readily apparent by immunohistochemical staining for CD138, with persistence of highly atypical plasma cells on bone marrow aspirate smear (inset). Areas not effaced by residual myeloma were effaced by therapy-related acute myeloid leukemia. (immunoperoxidase for CD138 and Wright)*

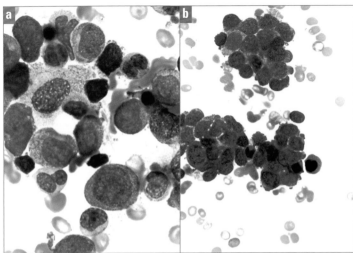

i18.70 *This composite of therapy-related acute myeloid leukemia following therapy for Ewing sarcoma shows myeloid leukemia* **a**, *and admixed clusters of metastatic Ewing sarcoma on the bone marrow aspirate smear* **b**. *(Wright)*

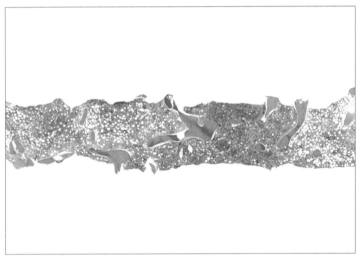

i18.71 *This low magnification of bone marrow core biopsy section illustrates a therapy-related myeloid neoplasm with irregular areas of hypercellularity and fibrosis. (H&E)*

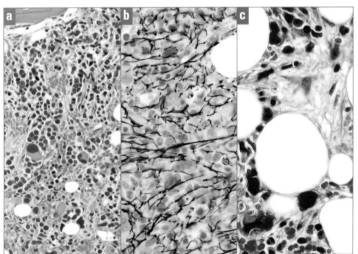

i18.72 *This composite of fibrotic therapy-related acute myeloid leukemia shows the morphologic features on high magnification* **a**, *the prominent reticulin fibrosis* **b**, *and the collagen fibrosis* **c** *(see* **i18.71***). Collagen fibrosis is unusual in therapy-related myeloid neoplasms. (H&E, reticulin, and trichrome)*

Down Syndrome-Associated AML and Transient Abnormal Myelopoiesis

Perhaps the paradigmatic example of AML that is defined by the clinical setting in which it arises is myeloid leukemia associated with Down syndrome, which is very often the sequela to an unusual phenomenon, specific to neonates with Down syndrome, called "transient abnormal myelopoiesis" (TAM, aka transient myeloproliferative disorder) [Baumann 2008]. Immunophenotypically, morphologically, and clinically, TAM is essentially indistinguishable from acute myeloid leukemia, but it shows the unique and mysterious property of spontaneous regression **i18.73, i18.74, i18.75, i18.76**. The incidence of TAM is quite high in Down syndrome, occurring in at least 1 in 10 neonates. The true incidence could be even higher, since differential counts on the CBCs of apparently healthy newborns with Down syndrome may not be routinely obtained. In addition, TAM can occur in utero, in which case it may cause fetal hydrops and spontaneous abortion. If series of both in utero and neonatal cases are combined, it is estimated that perhaps 20% of conceptions with trisomy 21 that reach at least late-term gestation experience TAM [Zipursky 2003]. The natural history of TAM is spontaneous hematologic remission, though approximately 20% of patients succumb before this occurs to associated morbidities, including cardiopulmonary failure in the setting of ascites, and fatal progressive hepatic fibrosis secondary to the leukemic infiltration and cytokine secretion [Massey 2006, Zipursky 2003]. Some 20% of patients with TAM later develop a non-remitting myeloid leukemia associated with Down syndrome (MLADS), which is usually megakaryoblastic in nature and occurs before the age of 4 **i18.77, i18.78, i18.79,**

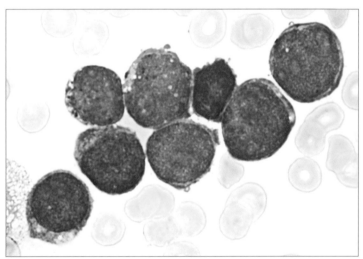

i18.73 *This peripheral blood smear is from a premature infant with Down syndrome, illustrating a marked leukocytosis with a predominance of blasts characteristic of transient abnormal myelopoiesis. (Wright) (courtesy R McKenna, MD)*

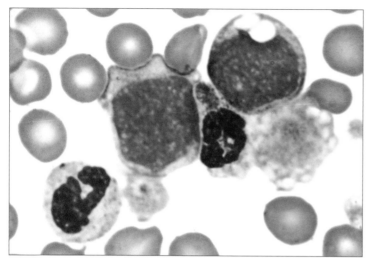

i18.74 *Both megakaryoblasts and differentiating megakaryocytes are evident in this peripheral blood smear from a Down syndrome neonate with transient abnormal myelopoiesis. Note large megakaryocyte fragments. (Wright)*

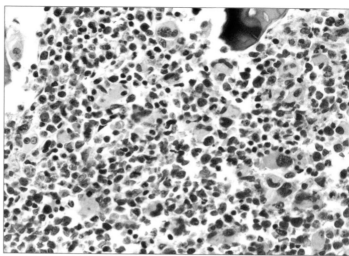

i18.75 *This bone marrow core biopsy is from a 4-week-old Down syndrome baby with transient abnormal myelopoiesis. Note increased immature cells and markedly increased small abnormal megakaryocytes. (H&E)*

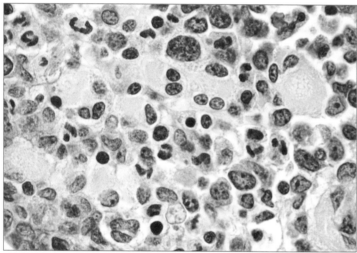

i18.76 *This bone marrow core biopsy section is from a 4-week-old Down syndrome infant with transient abnormal myelopoiesis. At high magnification, a marked increase in immature blastic cells is evident in conjunction with abnormal megakaryocytes. (H&E)*

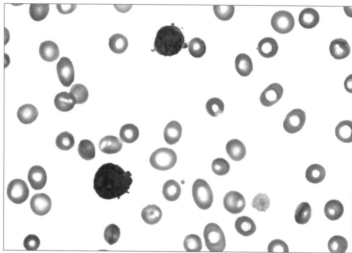

i18.77 *This peripheral blood smear is from a 22-month-old Down syndrome baby with acute megakaryoblastic leukemia. Note profound pancytopenia, circulating megakaryoblasts, and dysplastic platelet. (Wright)*

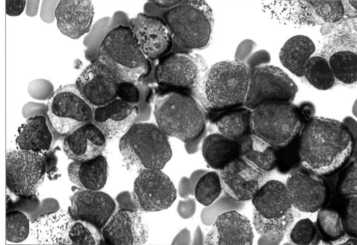

i18.78 *This bone marrow aspirate smear shows Down syndrome-associated acute megakaryoblastic leukemia. (Wright)*

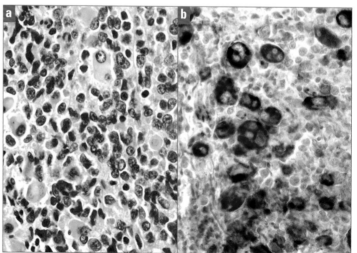

i18.79 *This composite of Down syndrome-associated acute megakaryoblastic leukemia shows a comparison of the morphologic features **a** in conjunction with the markedly increased megakaryocytic component highlighted by CD31. (H&E and immunoperoxidase for CD31)*

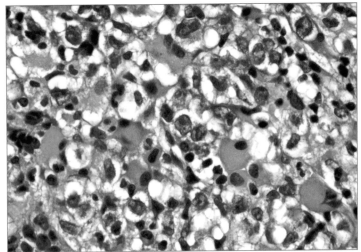

i18.80 *Both blasts and small dysplastic megakaryocytes characterize this case of Down syndrome-associated acute megakaryoblastic leukemia. (H&E) (courtesy S Peiper, MD)*

i18.80 [Hitzler 2007]. The megakaryoblasts seen in MLADS are largely indistinguishable from TAM; however, they have been shown to harbor more complex cytogenetic abnormalities compared to blasts from TAM [Massey 2006]. MLADS is extremely chemosensitive with an overall survival in excess of 80% [Creutzig 2005, Webb 2005, Xavier 2009]. The diagnostic distinction of TAM from MLADS depends largely on the clinical setting, with the former occurring exclusively in neonates and, by definition, resolving by 3 months of age. MLADS includes a phase of disease with the features of myelodysplastic syndrome, which usually precedes the onset of more pronounced blastemia. Because of this close temporal and prognostic relationship, both of these disease states (MDS-like and AML-like) fall under the umbrella term MLADS without regard to blast percentage. TAM and MLADS are further compared in **t18.5**. See **sidebar 18.1** for further discussion of the significance of *GATA1* mutations in these processes.

[18.7]   AML, Not Otherwise Specified (NOS)

Despite attempts to utilize a biologic-based classification of AML to the greatest extent possible, the 2008 WHO classification has included 11 subtypes of AML, not otherwise specified (NOS) [Arber 2008c, Vardiman 2009]. A lineage-based system is used to subclassify those cases of AML that lack any specific AML-defining biologic characteristic. Consequently, the AML, NOS category is reserved for cases that fulfill general criteria for AML but *lack:* a) an AML recurrent cytogenetic or molecular abnormality, b) a link to prior chemotherapy, c) multilineage dysplasia involving the majority of cells, d) MDS-type cytogenetic abnormalities, e) an association with Down syndrome, or f) a history of MDS or MDS/MPN

[sidebar 18.1]   *GATA1*, Down Syndrome, and Myeloid Leukemia

Myeloid leukemia associated with Down syndrome (MLADS) in the pediatric age group is overwhelmingly megakaryoblastic in nature, as is transient abnormal myelopoiesis (TAM) described further in "Down Syndrome-Associated AML and Transient Abnormal Myelopoiesis," p 406. Interestingly, both processes harbor acquired mutations in *GATA1*, a gene on the short arm of the X chromosome that encodes a transcription factor. *GATA1* mutations seem to be surprisingly specific for these settings. The GATA family of proteins contain zinc finger domains that bind specific DNA sequences. In fact, the name "GATA" is derived from the key portion of the sequence recognized: G-A-T-A [Bates 2008]. *GATA1* also binds a series of partner proteins, including the endearingly named "friend of *GATA1*" (FOG1) [Hamlett 2008, Johnson 2007]. Depending on the partner protein in the complex, *GATA1* can act as an activator or repressor of transcription at its target sites, many of which bear upon erythroid and megakaryocytic differentiation. DS-associated *GATA1* mutations introduce early stop codons that result in the utilization of an alternative downstream start site and, consequently, the production of a shorter GATA1 protein lacking the N-terminal domain necessary for proper regulation of its transcriptional targets [Xavier 2009].

GATA1 mutations alone do not produce acute leukemia, a point underscored by the existence of a family cohort with an inherited mutation similar to those seen in Down syndrome. These individuals do not develop TAM or leukemia [Hollanda 2006]. Thus, there is not only a special propensity to develop acquired *GATA1* mutations in the setting of trisomy 21, but also a specific leukemogenic effect directly dependent on the presence of the extra chromosome 21. Some investigators have implicated *RUNX1* in this regard [Hitzler 2007]. The gene encoding the *RUNX1* transcription factor is present in the Down syndrome critical region on chromosome 21, and RUNX1 physically associates with GATA1 [Elagib 2007]. *RUNX1* is also a key player in translocations that define certain types of AML and ALL, though its connection with DS-associated processes remains at present circumstantial and controversial [Xu 2006a].

Another unexplained mystery in these cases is why some, but only some, TAM progresses to MLADS. Researchers have analyzed, via microarray, blasts from TAM and from the subsequent MLADS, and found that, despite being largely immunophenotypically and morphologically similar, they form 2 distinct groups at the level of gene expression [Lightfoot 2004]. In other words, there appears to be a progression, with many gene pathways affected, that underlies the reappearance and the aggressive behavior of the *GATA1*+ clone [Roy 2009]. This contention is also supported by the observation that blasts in MLADS have often acquired cytogenetic abnormalities in addition to the constitutional trisomy 21 [Forestier 2008, Massey 2006]. Similarly, while 12% of TAM had detectable telomerase activity, this number increases to 52% when considering cases of MLADS [Holt 2002]. Further investigation of TAM and MLADS will likely yield additional insights into both the similarities and the differences between these unique disorders.

[Arber 2008c]. Although up to 1/3 of AML cases currently fall into AML, NOS, it is likely that this proportion will steadily decline as more biologic entities are defined by molecular genetic studies.

The fairly complex lineage and degree of maturation-based classification criteria for AML, NOS cases and their key features and associations are delineated in **t18.9** [Arber 2008c, Barbaric 2007, Bene 2001, Dunphy 2004, Haferlach 2009b, Hama 2008, Kaleem 2001, Malinge 2008, Oki 2006]. Each subtype will be briefly reviewed and illustrated to complement the information in **t18.9**.

t18.9 Acute Myeloid Leukemia, Not Otherwise Specified (AML, NOS)

Type	Typical Features	Other/Comments
AML with minimal differentiation	Predominance of agranular blasts Lineage of blasts *not* apparent by morphology or cytochemistry	Myeloid lineage confirmed by imunophenotyping; aberrant features common Cytogenetic abnormalities common; if MDS-related cytogenetic abnormalitiy, classify case as AML with MDS-related change No recurrent cytogenetic abnormalities; poor prognosis
AML without maturation	Blasts ≥90%; blasts exhibit myeloid features by morphology (granules, Auer rods) and/or cytochemistry (MPO+)	Myeloid lineage confirmed by flow cytometric immunophenotyping, aberrant features common No recurrent cytogenetic abnormalities
AML with maturation	≥20% blasts in blood or bone marrow ≥10% maturing granulocytic lineage cells <20% monocytic cells	Myeloid antigens expressed; occasional aberrant features Key differential diagnostic considerations are RAEB-2 and AMML No recurrent cytogenetic abnormalities
AMML	Blasts and blast equivalents (promonocytes) ≥20% in blood or bone marrow ≥20% maturing granulocytic lineage cells ≥20% monocytic lineage cells Cytochemically stains MPO+ and NSE+	Myelomonocytic lineage confirmed by flow cytometry; aberrant features common No recurrent cytogenetic abnormalities Monocytosis common Blood picture may closely resemble CMML Key differential diagnoses include CMML, AMoL and AML with maturation, and microgranular APL
AMML t(8;16) (p11;p13)	Fulfills AMML criteria Ingestion of erythrocytes by myelomonocytic blasts	Disruption and fusion of *MYST3* (8p11) and *CREBBP* (16p13) Rare AML subtype, <0.5% de novo AML (see text) and <2% t-AML DIC, extramedullary disease including CNS infiltration common
Acute monocytic leukemia, 2 types	≥80% monocytic lineage cells ≤20% neutrophilic lineage cells If monoblasts predominate, termed *acute monoblastic leukemia*; if promonocytes predominate, termed *acute monocytic leukemia* NSE+ in majority of cells	Monocytic lineage confirmed by immunophenotyping; aberrant features common Extramedullary lesions common (CNS, skin, gingiva) Key differential diagnosis includes CMML, microgranular APL, AMML
Acute erythroid leukemia, 2 types	Erythroleukemia consists of ≥50 erythroid cells and ≥20% myeloblasts (percent based on non-erythroid cells)	Dysplasia often prominent; if ≥50% in 2 lineages, designation of AML with MDS-related changes should be used; if MDS-related cytogenetic features present, should be called AML with MDS-related changes Must also distinguish from RAEB and non-neoplastic disorders
	Pure erythroid leukemia ≥80% erythroblasts	Erythroid lineage must be confirmed by immunophenotyping; CD45–; may be CD36+ If MDS-related cytogenetic abnormalities detected, should be classified as AML for MDS-related changes Differential diagnosis includes Burkitt leukemia, megaloblastic anemia, and other acute leukemias
Acute megakaryo-blastic leukemia	≥20% blasts in blood or bone marrow >50% of blasts are megakaryoblasts Clumps (pseudometastasis) Variable cytological features Pure megakaryoblastic vs multilineage Fibrosis common Micromegakaryocytes not included in blast percentage	Maturation of megakaryocytic lineage may be present Megakaryocytic lineage confirmed by immunophenotyping (CD61+, CD41+, CD42b+); may also be CD36+ Down syndrome associated cases excluded Differential diagnoses include APMF, metastatic lesions, MPN
Acute basophilic leukemia	AML with primary basophilic differentiation Coarse basophilic granules (toluidine blue, Alcian blue positive)	Immunophenotyping to confirm basophilic differentiation (CD123+, CD203c+, CD9+) Must exclude *BCR-ABL1* cases and t(6;9) cases Key differential diagnosis is mast cell leukemia
Acute panmyelosis with myelofibrosis	≥20% myeloid blasts Proliferation of all hematopoietic lineages Fibrosis Absent or minimal splenomegaly	Immunohistochemical staining to confirm increased myeloblasts and other lineage involvement If MDS-related cytogenetic features detected, should be classified as AML with MDS-related changes If dysplasia ≥50% of 2 lineages classify as AML with MDS-related changes Differential diagnoses include acute megakaryoblastic leukemia, primary myelofibrosis, post polycythemic PV, metastatic lesions

*These AML cases *lack* any distinctive clinical (ie, not therapy-related), morphologic (ie, multilineage dysplasia), or molecular/genetic features to allow inclusion in biologic categories

AEL = acute erythroblastic leukemia; AML = acute myeloid leukemia; AMML = acute myelomonocytic leukemia; AMoL = acute monocytic leukemia; APL = acute promyelocytic leukemia; APMF = acute panmyelosis with myelofibrosis; CMML = chronic myelomonocytic leukemia; CNS = central nervous system; DIC = disseminated intravascular coagulation; MDS = myelodysplastic syndrome; MPN = myeloproliferative neoplasm; MPO = myeloperoxidase; NSE = nonspecific esterase; RAEB = refractory anemia with excess blasts

References: [Arber 2008c, Barbaric 2007, Bene 2001, Dunphy 2004, Haferlach 2009b, Hama 2008, Kaleem 2001, Malinge 2008, Oki 2006]

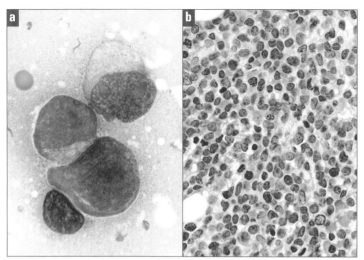

i18.81 *Acute myeloid leukemia with minimal differentiation is illustrated in this composite, showing the appearance on bone marrow aspirate smear **a** and bone marrow core biopsy sections **b**. There were no convincing morphologic or cytochemical features to document myeloid lineage differentiation. (Wright and H&E)*

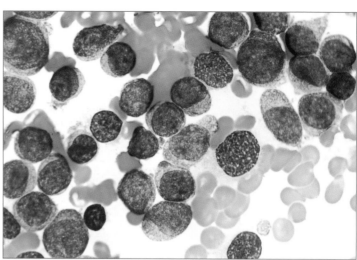

i18.82 *This bone marrow aspirate smear is from a patient with acute myeloid leukemia without maturation. Note predominance of blasts with little evidence of differentiation. (Wright)*

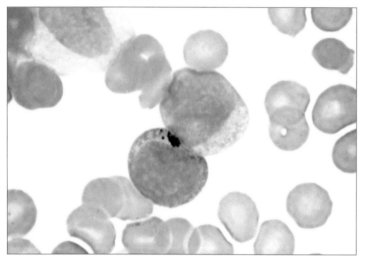

i18.83 *Confirmation of myeloid lineage differentiation is evidenced by scant myeloperoxidase positivity in this case of myeloid leukemia without maturation. (myeloperoxidase cytochemical stain)*

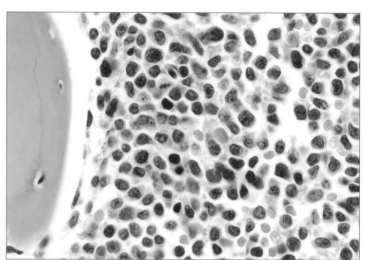

i18.84 *This bone marrow core biopsy section from a patient with acute myeloid leukemia without maturation shows a striking predominance of blasts with moderate amounts of cytoplasm. (H&E)*

[18.7.1]   **AML with Minimal Differentiation**

Agranular, lineage-indeterminant blasts predominate in this AML, NOS subtype, and flow cytometric immuno-phenotyping is required for delineation of myeloid lineage **i18.81** [Arber 2008c, Barbaric 2007, Bene 2001, Kaleem 2001]. There are no recurrent cytogenetic abnormalities, and prognosis is poor.

[18.7.2]   **AML without Maturation**

Myeloid lineage blasts, based on morphologic and cytochemical properties, predominate in this AML, NOS subtype **i18.82**, **i18.83**, **i18.84**. The blast percentage exceeds 90%, and there is no significant maturation of these leukemia cells.

[18.7.3]   **AML with Maturation**

The designation "with maturation" is applied to AML cases (≥20% blast threshold met) in which at least 10% of cells are promyelocytes, myelocytes, metamyelocytes, or neutrophils **i18.85**, **i18.86**. However, a significant monocytic component is *not* present. Although dysplasia is common in AML with maturation, both the extent of dysplasia and the cytogenetic findings cannot fulfill AML with MDS-related changes criteria (see "AML with Myelodysplasia-Related Changes," p 400).

[18.7.4]   **Acute Myelomonocytic Leukemia (AMML)**

Blasts and promonocytes must be at least 20%, and substantial granulocytic and monocytic lineage involvement must be present to justify a diagnosis of acute myelomonocytic leukemia (AMML) **t18.9**, **i18.87**, **i18.88**. Both

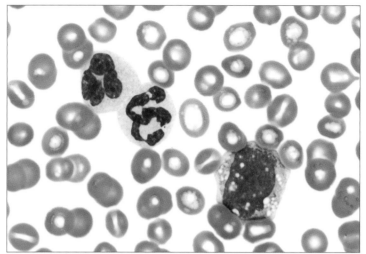

i18.85 *This peripheral blood smear of acute myeloid leukemia with maturation shows circulating dysplastic neutrophils. (Wright)*

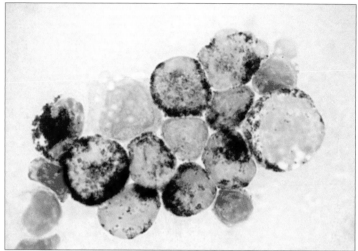

i18.86 *A wide spectrum of intensity of myeloperoxidase staining characterizes acute myeloid leukemia with maturation. (myeloperoxidase cytochemical stain)*

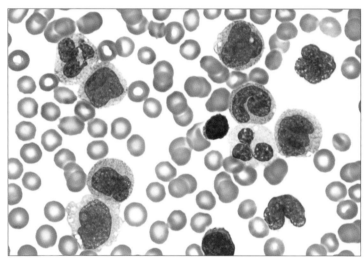

i18.87 *Both myeloid and monocytic differentiation are evident in this peripheral blood smear of acute myelomonocytic leukemia characterized by marked leukocytosis, anemia, and thrombocytopenia. Note dysplastic neutrophil and promonocytes. (Wright)*

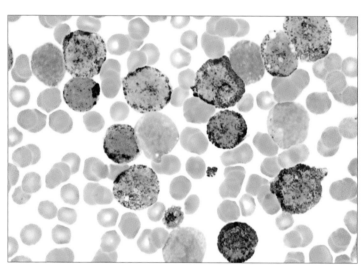

i18.88 *Moderate amounts of myeloperoxidase cytochemical staining are evident within a subset of the blasts in this case of acute myelomonocytic leukemia. Note the admixed monoblasts are myeloperoxidase negative. (myeloperoxidase cytochemical stain)*

cytochemical staining and flow cytometric immunophenotyping are useful in confirming the dual lineage involvement in AMML i18.88. Careful attention to promonocyte enumeration is key to distinguishing AMML from CMML t18.4, i18.13. Similarly, both strong uniform myeloperoxidase positivity and confirmation of *PML-RARA* fusion are critical in distinguishing AMML from microgranular APL.

AMML with t(8;16)(p11;p13); MYST3-CREBBP

A very rare subtype of AMML has distinctive genetic and morphologic features. Cases of AML with t(8;16)(p11;p13) show prominent erythrophagocytosis by blasts, prominent cytoplasmic granulation, and frequent extramedullary disease t18.5, i18.89, i18.90 [Haferlach 2009b]. Cytochemical nonspecific esterase and myeloperoxidase positivity are present, supporting a granulocytic and monocytic lineage despite the

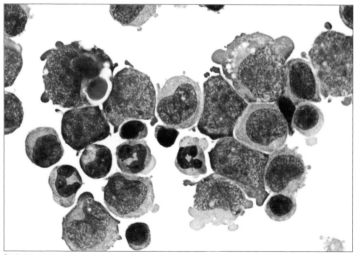

i18.89 *This cytospin smear is from a patient with acute myeloid leukemia and t(8;16). Note erythrophagocytosis by blasts. (Wright)*

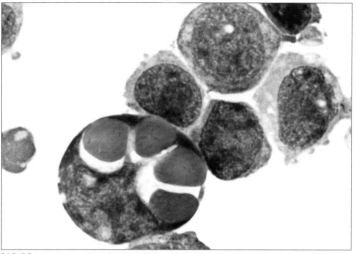

i18.90 *Ingestion of multiple red blood cells by a leukemic blast is evident on the cytospin smear from a patient with acute myelomonocytic leukemia and t(8;16).*

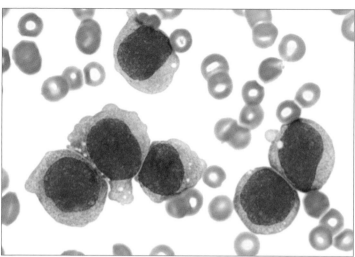

i18.91 *This peripheral blood smear illustrates the typical cytologic features of acute monoblastic leukemia. Note that virtually all nuclei are oval to round in shape and there is little evidence of monocytic maturation. (Wright)*

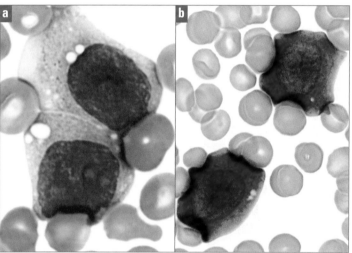

i18.92 *This composite illustrates the cytologic and cytochemical features of acute monoblastic leukemia. Note strong nonspecific esterase positivity **b**. (Wright and nonspecific esterase cytochemical stain)*

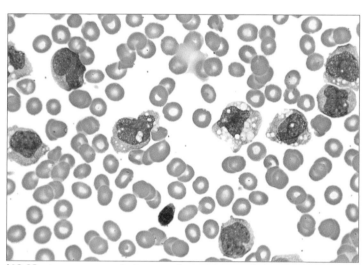

i18.93 *Acute monocytic leukemia with maturation including atypical monocytes is evident in this peripheral blood smear from a patient with marked leukocytosis and profound anemia and thrombocytopenia. (Wright) (courtesy T Keith, MD)*

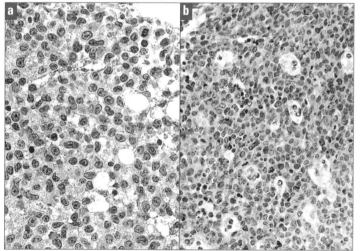

i18.94 *This composite illustrates the features of acute monocytic leukemia on bone marrow core biopsy sections. Note widely spaced nuclei due to abundant amounts of cytoplasm, homogeneous uniform cell infiltrates, and increased tingible body macrophages. (H&E)*

more monocytoid appearance of the blasts. The incidence of t(8;16) is low (0.2%-0.4% of de novo AML) [Haferlach 2009b, Mitelman 1992]. These patients have a poor prognosis [Becher 1988, Bernasconi 2000, Haferlach 2009b, Heim 1987, Velloso 1996].

[18.7.5]   **Acute Monocytic Leukemias**

Immature monocytic cells predominate in this AML, NOS type; 2 subtypes are designated based on whether monoblasts predominate (ie, acute monoblastic leukemia) or minimally more differentiated blast equivalent promonocytes predominate (ie, acute monocytic leukemia) **t18.9**, **i18.91**, **i18.92**, **i18.93**, **i18.94**. Very rare acute monocytic leukemias can exhibit histiocytic differentiation [Boeckx 2007, Esteve 1995]. Both cytochemical nonspecific esterase staining and flow cytometric immunophenotyping can be used to document monocytic differentiation, but nonspecific

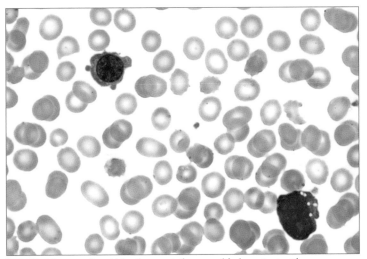

i18.95 *This peripheral blood smear is from an elderly patient with pancytopenia. Note circulating erythroblasts. (Wright)*

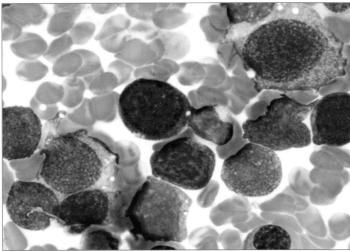

i18.96 *This bone marrow aspirate smear shows acute erythroid leukemia with increased myeloblasts and erythroblasts. (Wright)*

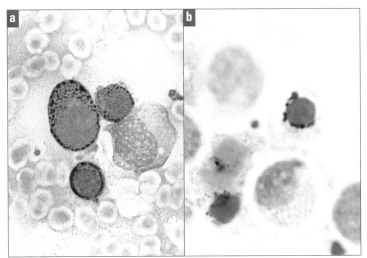

i18.97 *This composite illustrates abnormal PAS positivity in dysplastic erythroid cells **a** and ring sideroblasts **b** in acute erythroid leukemia. (Periodic acid-Schiff and Prussian blue)*

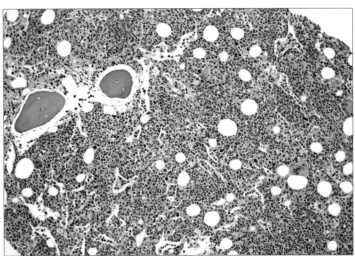

i18.98 *This bone marrow core biopsy section from a patient with acute erythroid leukemia shows hypercellularity. Areas of dark blue are erythroid, while areas that are slightly more eosinophilic are myeloid infiltrates. (H&E)*

esterase stains may be negative or weak in up to 20% of cases [Arber 2008c, Dunphy 2004]. Extramedullary disease is common in acute monoblastic/monocytic leukemias. Key differential diagnostic considerations include CMML, microgranular APL, and AMML.

[18.7.6]   **Acute Erythroid Leukemia**

The acute erythroid leukemias are further divided into 2 subtypes. In cases designated as "erythroleukemia," both a myeloblast component (≥20% of non-erythroid cells) and an erythroid component (≥50% of all cells) are present, while the term "pure erythroid leukemia" is reserved for cases with ≥80% erythroblasts with little, if any, granulocytic lineage involvement i18.95, i18.96, i18.97, i18.98, i18.99, i18.100, i18.101, i18.102, i18.103 [Arber 2008c]. Dysplasia is common in erythroleukemia, but it must be ≤50% of the lineage cells. If ≥50% of

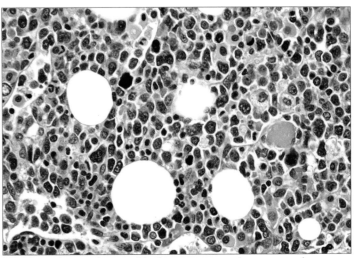

i18.99 *High magnification of this bone marrow core biopsy section from a patient with acute erythroid leukemia shows abundant immature erythroid and myeloid lineage cells. (H&E)*

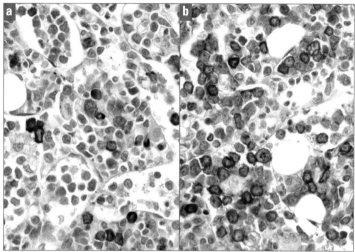

i18.100 *This composite of immunohistochemical stains from a case of acute erythroid leukemia shows increased myeloblasts by CD34 staining* **a** *and numerous erythroblasts by CD117 staining* **b**. *(immunoperoxidase for CD34 and CD117)*

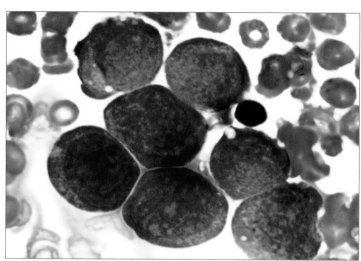

i18.101 *This bone marrow aspirate smear in acute pure erythroid leukemia shows an overwhelming predominance of erythroblasts. (Wright)*

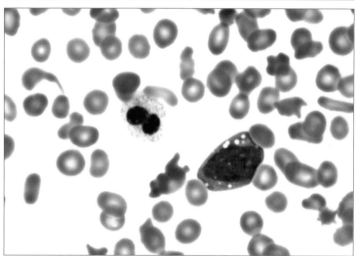

i18.102 *Both abnormal erythroblasts, marked anisopoikilocytosis, and dysplastic neutrophils are evident in the peripheral blood in a patient with acute erythroid leukemia. (Wright)*

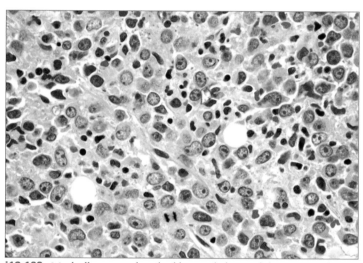

i18.103 *Markedly increased erythroblasts with dispersed chromatin and oblong nucleoli efface this bone marrow core biopsy section in acute pure erythroid leukemia. (H&E)*

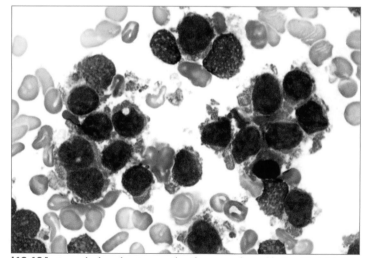

i18.104 *A marked predominance of uniform megakaryoblasts with striking cytoplasmic blebbing is evident on this bone marrow aspirate smear from a 15-month-old male with acute megakaryoblastic leukemia not related to Down syndrome. (Wright)*

cells in at least 2 lineages are dysplastic, a diagnosis of AML with MDS-related changes is warranted. The diagnosis of pure erythroid leukemia is challenging because erythroblasts can closely resemble Burkitt leukemia, acute megakaryoblastic leukemia, and other neoplasms. Immunophenotyping is essential in lineage delineation i18.101.

[18.7.7] **Acute Megakaryoblastic Leukemia**

The diagnosis of acute megakaryoblastic leukemia can be uniquely challenging because of the frequent assocation with fibrosis, which can preclude aspiration for morphology and flow cytometric immunophenotyping t18.9. Consequently, immuno-histochemical stains are often required to help confirm both the minimal 20% blast percentage necessary for a diagnosis of AML and to confirm that at least 50% of the blasts are megakaryo-cytic i18.104, i18.105, i18.106, i18.107, i18.108, i18.109, i18.110, i18.111

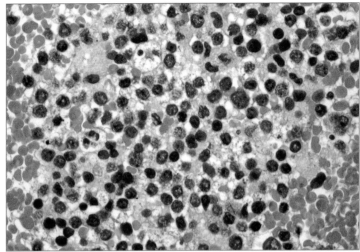

i18.105 *This bone marrow clot section is effaced by megakaryoblasts in this 15-month-old male with acute megakaryoblastic leukemia not related to Down syndrome. (H&E)*

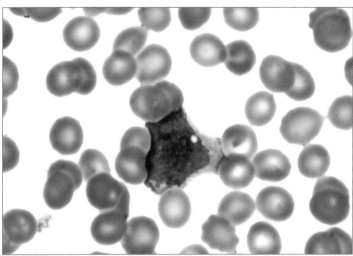

i18.106 *This circulating megakaryoblast is nondescript and megakaryoblastic lineage is not apparent. (Wright)*

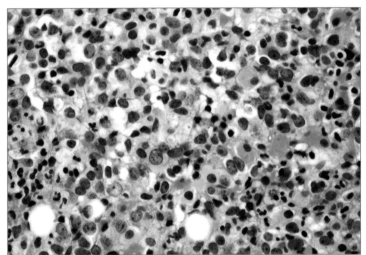

i18.107 *Markedly increased immature megakaryocytic lineage cells are evident in this bone marrow core biopsy section from an adult with acute megakaryoblastic leukemia. (H&E)*

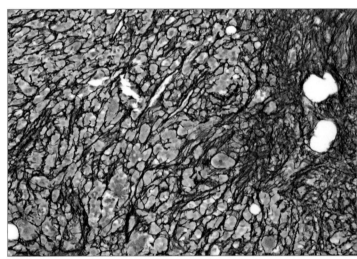

i18.108 *Striking bone marrow fibrosis is evident in this bone marrow core biopsy section of acute megakaryoblastic leukemia. (reticulin)*

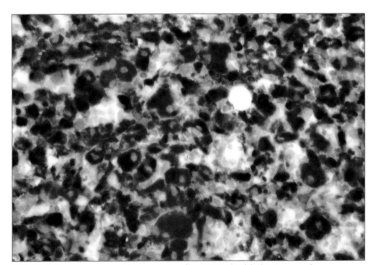

i18.109 *Immunoperoxidase staining for CD61 highlights tremendous numbers of megakaryocytic cells on this bone marrow core biopsy section of acute megakaryoblastic leukemia. (immunoperoxidase for CD61)*

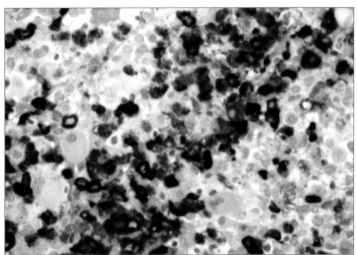

i18.110 *Admixed immature granulocytic cells are highlighted by myeloperoxidase staining in this bone marrow core biopsy section in acute megakaryoblastic leukemia (see **i18.109**). (myeloperoxidase cytochemical stain)*

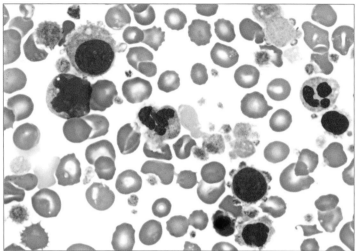

i18.111 *Both circulating megakaryoblasts and more differentiated megakaryocytic lineage cells are evident in this peripheral blood smear from a patient with a high-grade megakaryocytic neoplasm. Note tremendously enlarged and agranular circulating megakaryocyte fragments. (Wright)*

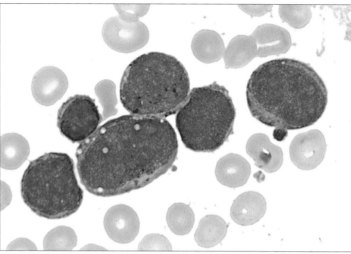

i18.112 *This bone marrow aspirate smear shows acute basophilic leukemia. (Wright) (courtesy R McKenna, MD)*

[Arber 2008c]. As emphasized, early differentiating megakaryocytic lineage cells and dysplastic megakaryocytes such as micromegakaryocytes are not included in the blast percentage i18.107, i18.111. Similarly, cases of acute megakaryoblastic leukemia linked to biologic genetic features such as Down syndrome or t(1;22) are not included in this AML, NOS category.

Acute megakaryoblastic leukemia is more common in children than adults. Pediatric cases of this leukemia show a similar favorable outcome regardless of whether or not they are linked to Down syndrome [Hama 2008]. Outcome in adults is unfavorable [Oki 2006].

The differential diagnosis of acute megakaryoblastic leukemia includes other acute leukemias as well as diverse disorders associated with bone marrow fibrosis, including chronic myeloproliferative neoplasms and metastatic lesions.

[18.7.8] **Acute Basophilic Leukemia**

De novo acute leukemias that exhibit basophilic differentiation are very uncommon and must be distinguished from *BCR-ABL1*-related disorders such as basophilic blast phase of chronic myelogenous leukemia t18.9, i18.112, i18.113. Genetic testing is essential in making this distinction as well as in identifying cases of AML with t(6;9), which are excluded from this AML, NOS group. Basophilic differentiation is best determined by either metachromatic staining (toluidine blue and alcian blue positivity) or by flow cytometric immuno-phenotyping to exclude mast cell leukemia and other myeloid lineage leukemias, as well as to provide support for basophilic lineage differentiation (CD123+, CD203c+, CD9+) [Arber 2008c]. Electron microscopy can also be used to identify theta granules [Peterson 1991, Shvidel 2003].

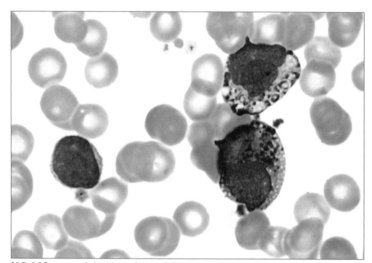

i18.113 *Basophilic blast phase of chronic myelogenous leukemia is evident in this bone marrow aspirate smear. (Wright)*

[18.7.9] **Acute Panmyelosis with Myelofibrosis**

The diagnosis of this rare subtype of AML, NOS, is problematic both because of the obligatory myelofibrosis and because diagnostic requirements include confirmation that blasts exceed 20% and documentation of expanded myeloid, erythroid, and megakaryocytic populations in a bone marrow that is typically inaspirable t18.9, i18.114, i18.115 [Arber 2008c, Orazi 2005, Thiele 2004]. There is a heavy reliance on immunohisto-chemical staining to establish this diagnosis i18.115.

The potential overlap with myeloproliferative neoplasms is substantial. Therefore, cases of acute panmyelosis with myelofibrosis (APMF) must exhibit an acute onset, lack significant splenomegaly, and lack teardrop erythrocytes. Confirmation of an AML-defining blast threshold by immunohistochemical staining for CD34 is critical in distinguishing APMF from myelodysplasia with fibrosis i18.115

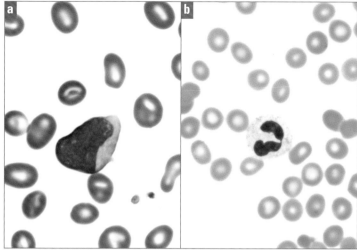

i18.114 *This peripheral blood smear composite is from a 56-year-old male with acute panmyelosis with myelofibrosis. The patient did not have spleno-megaly. This peripheral blood smear composite shows a circulating myeloblast, a dysplastic neutrophil, and profound cytopenias. (Wright)*

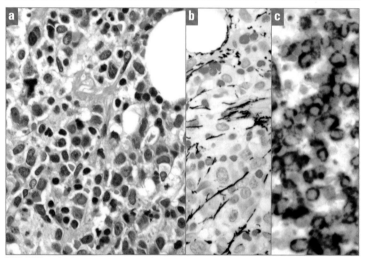

i18.115 *This bone marrow core biopsy composite from a patient with acute panmyelosis with myelofibrosis shows increased immature myeloid lineage cells and abnormal megakaryocytes **a**, while increased fibrosis **b** and markedly increased blasts are evident **c**. (H&E, reticulin, and immunoperoxidase for CD34).*

(see **t16.12**). Estimation of the extent of lineage dysplasia is important to distinguish APMF from AML with MDS-related changes. Finally, a metastatic lesion must be excluded by morphologic and immunohistochemical assessment.

[18.8] Prognostic Factors in AML

[18.8.1] Cytogenetics

Pretreatment conventional cytogenetic studies identify an acquired clonal abnormality in approximately 50%-60% of patients with de novo AML, of which 10%-20% are complex (≥3 chromosomal aberrations). In approximately 40%-50% of cases, no karyotypic abnormality is detected using typical banding techniques, yielding an AML with normal karyotype [Byrd 2002, Cheng 2009, Grimwade 1999, 2001, Mrozek 2004, Slovak 2000]. Molecular

t18.10 Prognostic Risk of Cytogenetic Abnormalities in Patients <60 Years with De Novo AML

Prognostic Risk Group	Cytogenetic Finding
Favorable	t(15;17)(q22;q21)
	t(8;21)(q22;q22)
	inv(16)(p13;q22)/t(16;16)(p13;q22)
Intermediate	Normal karyotype
	t(9;11)(p22;q23)*
	del(7q), del(9q)*
	−Y, +11, +13, +21
Unfavorable	Complex karyotype†
	inv(3)(q21;q26)/t(3;3)
	t(6;9)(p23;q34)‡
	−5, −7

*Some may classify as unfavorable
†≥3 chromosomal abnormalities
‡In intermediate risk group in [Byrd 2002]
AML = acute myeloid leukemia

References: [Breems 2008, Byrd 2002, Cheng 2009, Dohner 2010, Farag 2006, Grimwade 1999, Grimwade 2001, Kelly 2009, Kolitz 2004, Mrozek 2004, 2008a, Schlenk 2004, Slovak 2000, Weinberg 2010]

(submicroscopic) characterization of the karyotypically normal AMLs is an area of active investigation (see [18.8.2] "Molecular Genetics").

Based on several large studies, a cytogenetic risk stratification system has been proposed for AML that categorizes specific karyotypic abnormalities as favorable, intermediate, or unfavorable **t18.10** [Breems 2008, Byrd 2002, Cheng 2009, Dohner 2010, Farag 2006, Grimwade 1999, 2001, Kelly 2009, Kolitz 2004, Mrozek 2004, 2008a, Schlenk 2004, Slovak 2000]. These data may be used to stratify therapy [Kolitz 2004]. The majority of large studies agree that the AML patients with t(15;17), inv(16)/t(16;16), or t(8;21) have a favorable prognosis compared with those that have a complex karyotype and monosomy 7 [Mrozek 2008a]. Of note, while additional chromosomal changes with t(8;21), inv(16)/t(16;16), or t(15;17) may be seen, these have not been generally shown to affect prognosis [Byrd 2002, Kelly 2009, Schlenk 2004]. *FLT3* mutations may occur in t(8;21) and inv(16), and although not well established, may suggest an adverse prognosis [Boissel 2006]. A monosomal karyotype in AML may portend a particularly unfavorable prognosis [Breems 2008, Weinberg 2010].

In patients ≥60 years with de novo AML, the significance of some of cytogenetic risk groups may differ from younger patients. A very complex karyotype, defined as ≥5 chromosomal abnormalities, is associated with an unfavorable risk in the older age group, are non-complex karyotypes showing a rare aberration such as trisomy 4, abnormalities of 3q, t(6;9)(p23;q34), and double minutes [Farag 2006, Grimwade 2001].

[18.8.2] Molecular Genetics

In addition to the gene mutations (*NPM1* and *CEBPA*) that currently define provisional biologic subtypes of AML (see [18.6] "Biologic Subtypes of AML," p 385), there is an ever-expanding catalogue of additional genetic alterations that occur in significant numbers in AML of various subtypes. These include mutations (eg, *TET2*, *MLL*, *KRAS*, *NRAS*, *WT1*) and alterations in gene expression levels (eg, *BAALC*, *ERG*, *MN1*, *EVI1*, *MN1*, *PRAME*, *MLL*, *WT1*, *RHAMM*) [Abdel-Wahab 2009, Baldus 2007, Gaidzik 2008, Paschka 2008b, Santamaria 2009, Schlenk 2008].

As mentioned in [18.6] "Biologic Subtypes of AML", *KIT* mutations are particularly associated with a relatively adverse prognosis in the core binding factor AMLs [t(8;21) and inv(16)/t(16;16)] [Cairoli 2006, Care 2003, Paschka 2006]. In general, these alterations contribute to leukemogenesis and carry prognostic significance, but, in contrast to *NPM1* and *CEBPA* mutations, they do not presently define distinct biologic or clinical entities. Scoring systems incorporating many of these alterations have been developed and appear to be useful in predicting prognosis [Santamaria 2009]. A major challenge in the coming years will be the rational and cost-effective implementation of such "multivariate" molecular assays.

Standing out from this "alphabet soup" is *FLT3*, which encodes a membrane-bound receptor tyrosine kinase. Activating *FLT3* mutations occur in 2 forms, only 1 of which is at present incontrovertibly significant for AML prognosis. So-called internal tandem duplications (ITD) affecting the juxtamembrane portion of the protein correlate with poor prognosis, an association that has been particularly documented in karyotypically normal cases [Kottaridis 2001, Schlenk 2008, Stirewalt 2003, Zwaan 2003]. In contrast, the significance of mutations affecting the tyrosine kinase domain (TKD) of the protein is controversial, with recent data suggesting that *FLT3*-TKD mutations may impact prognosis, though perhaps differently, in distinct subtypes of AML [Bacher 2008, Frohling 2002, Mead 2007, Whitman 2008, Yanada 2005]. Clinical trials are currently evaluating the pharmacologic effectiveness of specific FLT3 inhibitors [Sanz 2009a]. As of this writing, a few general observations may be made about the clinical situations in which *FLT3* analysis is indicated. First, *FLT3* *must* be examined in all cases submitted for *NPM1* mutation analysis, since an *FLT3* mutation in an *NPM1*-mutated case drastically reduces the beneficial prognosis otherwise associated with the latter finding. Second, because *FLT3*-ITD status is among the strongest independent prognostic factors in cytogenetically normal AML, molecular analysis for alterations at this location is eminently defensible. Third, given the burgeoning interest in targeted anti-*FLT3* therapy, the practicing pathologist may find him- or herself fielding requests for *FLT3* mutation analysis for a wide array of AML subtypes. In such a situation, the diagnostician should remain cognizant of the fact that

t18.11 Potential Immunophenotypic Markers with Prognostic Significance in AML at Diagnosis

Marker	Prognostic Significance
CD25	Adverse overall and relapse-free survival
CD15	Favorable prognosis
CD7	Controversial; lower complete remission rate; adverse prognosis in several studies
CD11b	Adverse prognosis
CD56	Lower complete remission rate
Expression of lymphoid antigens	Lower complete remission rate (adults)
	No prognostic significance (majority of pediatric patients)
Leukemia-associated phenotype (LAP) (aberrant/ asynchronous antigen profile patterns)	Lower complete remission rate; adverse prognosis
Early clearance of peripheral blasts	Better disease-free survival

References: [Al-Mawali 2009b, Casasnovas 1998, Del Poeta 1995, Lacombe 2009, Mason 2006, Smith 1992, Terwijn 2009]

the exact prognostic significance of *FLT3* mutations may be variable or undocumented in the context of these distinct AML subtypes.

[18.8.3] Flow Cytometry

Aside from the fact that certain immunophenotypic profiles tend to "track" with specific AML categories, certain aberrant immunophenotypic findings have prognostic significance. These distinctive immunophenotypic features are also useful in the assessment for minimal residual disease. Potential predictive markers in AML diagnosis are listed in t18.11 [Al-Mawali 2009b, Casasnovas 1998, Del Poeta 1995, Lacombe 2009, Mason 2006, Smith 1992, Terwijn 2009].

The prognostic value of immunophenotyping in AML is controversial [Bradstock 1993, Ball 1991]. Many of the studies have been small, single-institution studies, with few results being confirmed in large clinical trials. The different results likely stem from a variety of technical, analytic, and population-based factors. In particular, how the blast population is gated and the cut-off point (or percentage) for selection of antigen positivity is problematic.

[18.8.4] Other Prognostic Factors

Additional prognostic factors delineated in various AML outcome studies in adults include age, WBC, de novo vs secondary AML, performance status, and rapidity in the

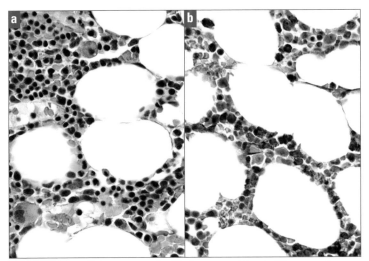

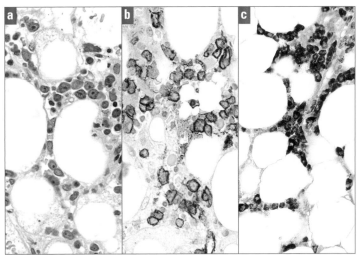

i18.116 *Hypocellular acute myeloid leukemia is evident in this composite illustrating morphologic features* **a** *and markedly increased immunophenotypic blasts* **b**. *(H&E and immunoperoxidase for CD34)*

i18.117 *This composite highlights the morphologic and immunohistochemical features of hypocellular acute myeloid leukemia* **a**, *characterized by increased CD34+ blasts* **b** *that are myeloperoxidase positive* **c**. *(H&E and immunoperoxidase for CD34 and myeloperoxidase)*

clearance of blasts from either blood or bone marrow [Derolf 2009, Dohner 2010, Hussein 2008, Lacombe 2009, Wheatley 2009]. Although overall survival in adults with AML has improved over time, the survival time for advanced elderly patients (≥80 years) with AML has not improved [Derolf 2009]. Improved survival times for children with AML have also been noted, although factors predictive of inferior survival include age >16 years, non-white ethnicity, absence of a related donor, WBC ≥100 × 10⁹/L, and adverse karyotype [Lange 2008].

[18.9] Diagnostic Pitfalls in AML Diagnosis

[18.9.1] Low Blast Count AML

AMLs with t(8;21), inv(16)/t(16;16), or t(15;17) as described earlier and in **t18.5** may be diagnosed when the blast count is <20% **i18.15**, **i18.28**. Clues to identifying these low blast count AML cases include severe peripheral cytopenias with variable numbers of blasts, Auer rods, abnormal salmon-colored granules and/or abnormal eosinophil precursors, or distinctive flow cytometric studies. All of these features are associated with the more overt AMLs with these same cytogenetic abnormalities **t18.5**. Cytogenetic studies are essential in confirming the AML-defining translocations and excluding other differential diagnostic considerations.

[18.9.2] Hypocellular AML

Rare cases of AML present in a markedly hypocellular bone marrow **i18.116**, **i18.117**. Causes of this uniquely reduced cellularity are unknown. The key challenge in these cases is to document that blasts exceed the 20% threshold. Further subclassification may or may not be feasible. Distinction from hypocellular MDS, hypocellular hairy cell leukemia, and

aplastic anemia can usually be achieved by the integration of morphology and immunohistochemical stains **i18.117**.

[18.9.3] AML with Necrosis

The delineation of lineage and stage of maturation is uniquely challenging in extensively necrotic specimens. Bone marrow aspirate smears may contain insufficient intact cells for adequate assessment. Similarly, both flow cytometric immunophenotyping and conventional karyotyping are frequently unsuccessful due to low viability and paucicellularity. The successful diagnosis of extensively necrotic AML is most often achieved by serial sectioning of generous core biopsy sections and extensive immunohistochemical assessment **i18.118**, **i18.119**, **i18.120**. Distinction from other necrotic bone marrow infiltrates rests largely with comprehensive immunohistochemical staining. However, blood smears should be reviewed for evidenced of circulating viable neoplastic cells that could be assessed for lineage and stage of maturation by flow cytometric techniques.

[18.9.4] AML with Fibrosis

Fibrosis is a defining feature of APMF and is highly characteristic of acute megakaryoblastic leukemia and therapy-related myeloid neoplasms. Beyond these specific AML subtypes, mild to moderate reticulin fibrosis can be encountered in almost any other AML subtype. In light of the inaspirability of these fibrotic bone marrows, definitive diagnosis of AML often relies upon immunohistochemical assessment of good quality bone marrow core biopsy sections to confirm by estimate that CD34+ blasts are ≥20% and to confirm myeloid lineage by CD33, MPO, and other myeloid antigen expression **i18.121**, **i18.122**. CD117 staining is also useful in delineating immature myeloid and some monocytic cells. Distinction from other fibrotic neoplastic and

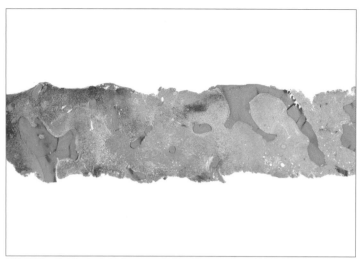

i18.118 *This low magnification of a bone marrow core biopsy section is extensively necrotic in this patient with massive relapse of acute myeloid leukemia following bone marrow bone transplantation. (H&E)*

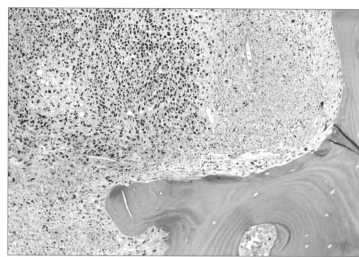

i18.119 *Necrotic acute myeloid leukemia is highlighted on higher magnification of this bone marrow core biopsy section. The necrotic areas are eosinophilic (right), while scattered collections of intact leukemia cells are evident (left). (H&E)*

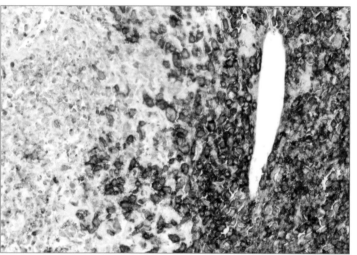

i18.120 *Necrotic acute myeloid leukemia is highlighted by immunoperoxidase staining for CD43 in the focally viable areas. (immunoperoxidase for CD43)*

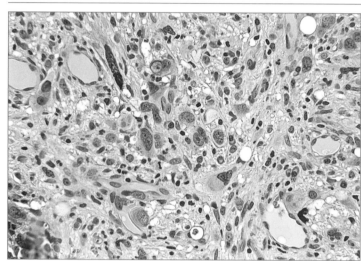

i18.121 *This bone marrow core biopsy section shows prominent fibrosis in association with acute myeloid leukemia. Note spindling of cells reflecting fibrosis. (H&E)*

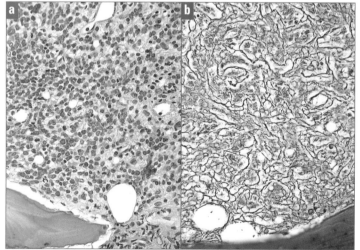

i18.122 *A predominance of blasts is evident on H&E stain **a**, while strikingly increased reticulin fibers are highlighted **b** in acute myeloid leukemia with fibrosis. (H&E and reticulin)*

non-neoplastic disorders is achieved largely through immunohistochemical studies (see **t16.12**).

[18.9.5] **Myeloid Proliferations with Abundant Erythroid Cells**

Myeloid proliferations with abundant erythroid cells can generate a challenging set of differential diagnostic possibilities, including both benign and malignant processes **t18.12** [Arber 2008c, Morice 2005, Tso 2009, Vardiman 2008b]. Arriving at the correct diagnosis most often requires the assimilation of a substantial amount of data, including hematologic indices, morphology, additional laboratory studies (eg, vitamin B_{12}, folate, and zinc levels), and genetics. In cases that are clearly malignant, adherence to the diagnostic criteria for each myeloid neoplasm category will lead to the correct WHO 2008 subclassification [Vardiman 2008b]. By convention, erythroblasts

t18.12 Differential Diagnostic Possibilities for Myeloid Proliferations with Abundant Erythroid Cells

Diagnostic Possibility	Comments/Bone Marrow Features
Acute erythroid leukemia:	≥50% erythroid cells
pure erythroid type	≥80% erythroblasts
erythroleukemia (erythroid/myeloid)	Myeloblasts ≥20% of non-erythroid cells
Myelodysplastic syndrome	<20% myeloblasts; variable erythroid percentage (see Chapter 16)
AML with myelodysplasia-related changes	≥20% blasts; ≥50% of dysplastic cells in at least 2 lineages
AML, NOS, with increased erythroid precursors	≤50% erythroid lineage cells
Polycythemia vera	Erythroid predominance with complete maturation; minimal/no dysplasia
	Blasts not increased
	Peripheral erythrocytosis
	Low erythropoietin level
	Increased megakaryocytes, usually hyperlobated
	Bone marrow hypercellularity with megakaryocyte abnormalities
	JAK2 V617F mutation positive in 95% of cases
Non-neoplastic erythroid proliferations:	
megaloblastic anemia	Erythroid hyperplasia with left shift, sieve-like chromatin, giant metamyelocytes (see Chapter 6)
florid hemolytic anemia	Erythroid hyperplasia with intact maturation; nuclear budding, multinucleation (see Chapter 6)
florid erythroid regeneration post chemotherapy	Intact maturation, minimal dysplastic change (mainly seen in most mature cells)
recombinant erythropoietin administration	Erythroid hyperplasia with left shift (see Chapter 35)
congenital dyserythropoietic anemia	Ineffective erythropoiesis, marked dyserythopoiesis; multinucleation (see Chapter 6)
Tumors mimicking erythroblasts:	Immunophenotypic studies reveal lineage
Burkitt/ other lymphoma types	
metastatic tumors	
other acute leukemias	
myeloma	

AML = acute myeloid leukemia; NOS = not otherwise specified

References: [Arber 2008c, Morice 2005, Tso 2009, Vardiman 2008b]

should predominate in acute erythroid leukemia, while myelodysplasia tends to show an admixture of all stages of erythroid maturation i18.96, i18.101 (see Chapter 16). Distinguishing high-grade myelodysplasia with abundant erythroid cells (≥50%) from AML with MDS-related changes or acute erythroid leukemia hinges on the percent of non-erythroid cells that are myeloblasts. Clinical heterogeneity is well-described in acute erythroleukemia; many patients may not require the urgent therapy needed in other settings of acute leukemia (ie, clinically more akin to MDS). In such scenarios it is prudent to communicate with the submitting physician regarding the diagnostic criteria utilized and the clinical heterogeneity of cases with ≥50% erythroid lineage cells that fulfill AML criteria.

Megaloblastoid change is a frequent dysplastic morphologic feature in myeloid malignancies. Without other types of overt dysplasia, an increase in blasts, or Auer rods, megaloblastic anemia must remain in the differential diagnosis. Genetic studies are often helpful in addition to serum vitamin B$_{12}$, folate, and methylmalonic acid levels (see Chapter 6).

[18.9.6] **G-CSF Therapy**

Therapeutic doses of recombinant G-CSF or granulocyte macrophage colony-stimulating factor (GM-CSF) act similarly and may induce a variety of cellular changes (eg, transient increases in peripheral blood or bone marrow blasts and/or neutrophil dysplasia) that may mimic a myeloid neoplasm (see **t10.6**) [Meyerson 1998]. Consequently, it is essential that the diagnostician have information about cytokine therapy as part of routine bone marrow examination. In de novo presentations of bone marrow left-shifted myeloid hyperplasia and increased blasts, but *lacking* definitive dysplasia, Auer rods, or abnormal karyotype, one should

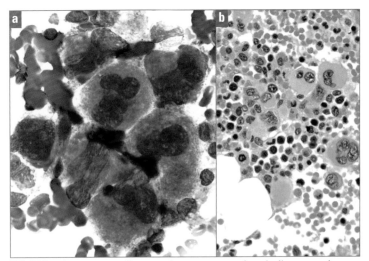

i18.123 *This composite illustrates the appearance of markedly increased benign megakaryocytes on a bone marrow aspirate smear* **a** *and bone marrow clot section* **b** *in this abnormal megakaryocytic proliferation following induction chemotherapy for acute myeloid leukemia and t(11q23). (Wright and H&E)*

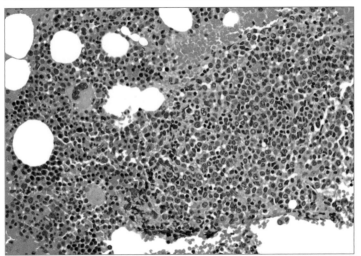

i18.124 *This bone marrow clot section is from a patient with early relapse of acute promyelocytic leukemia in which only half (right side) of the particle is effaced by recurrent leukemia. (H&E)*

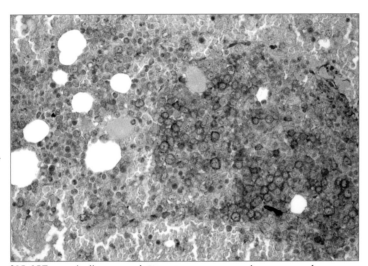

i18.125 *Markedly increased CD117 positive promyelocytes are evident in a distinct zoning pattern in this bone marrow clot section from a patient with early relapse of acute promyelocytic leukemia(see* **i18.124**). *(immunoperoxidase for CD117)*

exercise extreme caution prior to diagnosing a myeloid malignancy. A reactive process such as CSF effect, infection, or paraneoplastic phenomenon secondary to an underlying solid tumor must be ruled out.

[18.10] Minimal Residual Disease, Post-Therapy Changes, and Relapse

Minimal residual disease monitoring in AML by either flow cytometric immunophenotyping or molecular techniques can potentially improve assessment of ongoing treatment response and ultimately improve outcomes [Al-Mawali 2009a]. Established minimum residual disease (MRD) assays include PCR amplification of known genetic aberrations or flow cytometric detection of aberrant immunophenotypes [Kern 2008, Shook 2009]. Quantitative PCR assessment of APL is addressed in Chapter 36.

Flow cytometric immunophenotyping may attain a sensitivity of aberrant cell detection of 10^{-4} compared with the traditional techniques of morphology (1%-5%) and cytogenetics (1%-5%) (see Chapter 36). The sensitivity of detection of MRD by molecular techniques is in the range of 10^{-5}.

Several published reports indicate that the detection of MRD is a valuable tool in predicting relapse [Feller 2004, San Miguel 1997, 2001, Venditti 2002]. The lack of flow cytometric detection of leukemic cells after induction chemotherapy may argue against early AML relapse, and a threshold of ≤0.15% residual leukemic cells post induction and post consolidation therapy predicts for better overall survival (see Chapter 36 for more details) [Al-Mawali 2009a, Drach 1992].

The morphologic spectrum of bone marrow features during induction chemotherapy is detailed in Chapter 35. Distinctive post-therapy findings in AML include striking non-neoplastic dysplastic megakaryocytic proliferations and ATRA-induced morphologically abnormal maturing promyelocytes in APL **i18.123** [Rosenthal 1991, Tohyama 2003]. Relapse of AML is generally characterized by a marked decline in cell counts in blood, variable numbers of circulating blasts, and variable extent of bone marrow effacement **i18.124, i18.125**. These relapsed AMLs generally exhibit similar morphologic, immunophenotypic, and genetic features to the original leukemia, although clonal evolution may occur. Rare AML patients develop therapy-related secondary AML, creating a unique diagnostic challenge. In general, the characteristic morphologic and cytogenetic features of t-AML will be distinct from those of the original leukemia.

[18.11] Differential Diagnosis of AML

Depending upon the lineages involved and the extent of maturation, the differential diagnosis of AML is diverse.

The primary differential diagnostic considerations for specific AML subtypes have been included earlier in the discussion of specific AML subtypes. Similarly, the differential diagnosis of hypocellular, fibrotic, and necrotic AML is included in [18.9] "Diagnostic Pitfalls in AML Diagnosis," p 419. Because myeloid neoplasms with abundant erythroid lineage cells are particularly problematic, an earlier section focuses on the differential diagnosis of these erythroid predominant lesions. For AML, definitive diagnosis hinges on accurate blast enumeration to allow distinction from high-grade MDS and MDS/MPN. The diagnostician must be aware that a diagnosis of AML is warranted in cases with ≤20% blasts if an AML-defining translocation is identified (see "Low Blast Count AML," p 419). Transformations into AML by other myeloid neoplasms must also be recognized. This is best achieved when comprehensive clinical information is readily available. Previous bone marrow specimens should be compared systematically to current specimens to clarify issues of transformation of an underlying hematologic disorder such as MDS, MPN, and MDS/MPN. Auer rods are for the most part indicative of AML, but they may be present in rare patients with MDS (see Chapter 16). However, Auer rod-like inclusions have also been noted in lymphomas and myeloma (see i23.20) [Groom 1991, Hutter 2009].

Morphologic look-alikes of myeloid blasts include granular ALL, blastic plasmacytoid dendritic cell neoplasm, aggressive NK cell leukemia, myeloma, and lymphomas [Groom 1991, Pitman 2007]. Although bone marrow core biopsy section morphology generally allows distinction, the bone marrow aspirate smear appearance of rhabdomyosarcoma, neuroblastoma, medulloblastoma, and other metastatic lesions can closely mimic acute leukemia (see Chapter 29) [Chen 2004, Etzell 2006]. Even immunophenotypic overlap between metastatic lesions and AML has been noted [Etzell 2006].

A systematic evaluation including cytochemical stains and immunophenotyping can aid in these distinctions. Benign disorders that can mimic selected AML subtypes include megaloblastic anemia, G-CSF therapy, arsenic toxicity, and other toxic bone marrow insults.

[18.12] Components of the Diagnostic Interpretation

The components of the diagnostic interpretation of AML must include information regarding blast/blast equivalent enumeration, lineages involved, extent of maturation, and extent of dysplastic features of all lineages. The integration of molecular genetic information is also essential. t18.13 provides tips and strategies for this process.

t18.13 Diagnosis of AML: Key Tips/Strategies

Parameter	WHO Criteria	Comments/Tips/Caveats
Percent blasts/blast equivalents	≥20% for AML (blast threshold based on percentage of non-erythroid cells for AML subtypes with ≥50% erythroid cells in BM)	20% threshold may be met in blood or BM
		Difficult to count blasts on inaspirable specimens
		Promyelocytes are blast equivalents *only* for APL
	Threshold < 20% for genetically defined AML [eg, t(8;21), t(15;17), inv(16)]	Promonocytes are always blast equivalents
		Erythroblasts are blast equivalents *only* in acute pure erythroid leukemia
	Myeloblast threshold may not be reached in acute pure erythroid leukemia due to marked preponderance of erythroblasts (≥80%)	Distinction from MDS and MDS/MPN based largely on blast percentage and genotype
		Flow cytometry is not a substitute for morphology in determining blast percent; not all blasts are CD34+
Lineage of blasts	Must confirm lineage of immature cells by morphology, cytochemistry, and/or IP	Morphology, cytochemical stains, and multicolor flow cytometric IP integrated into myeloid lineage determination and exclusion of ALL
	Most relevant to AML, NOS classification for acute myelomonocytic, monocytic, megakaryoblastic leukemias	May have to rely on IHC staining on core biopsy for inaspirable specimens
Cytogenetics/ FISH/molecular	Biologic parameters are integral part of WHO classification of AML	Recurrent cytogenetic abnormalities that define AML subtypes include t(8;21), t(15;17), inv(16), t(9;11), t(6;9), inv(3), t(1;22)
	A specific cytogenetic or molecular finding defines many AML subtypes	Molecular abnormalities that define AML subtypes include *NPM1* and *CEBPA* mutations

ALL = acute lymphoblastic leukemia; AML = acute myeloid leukemia; AML, NOS = AML, not otherwise specified; APL = acute promyelocytic leukemia; BM = bone marrow; FISH = fluorescence in situ hybridization; IHC = immunohistochemistry; IP = immunophenotype; MDS = myelodysplastic syndrome; MPN = myeloproliferative neoplasm

[18.13] Clues and Caveats

1. Clinical, morphologic, cytochemical, immunophenotypic, and molecular genetic features should all be integrated into AML diagnosis.
2. Hematopoietic failure (anemia, neutropenia, and thrombocytopenia) is an expected feature of all types of acute myeloid leukemia; the WBC count is highly variable.
3. Exceptions to the 20% threshold for AML diagnosis include cases with AML-defining cytogenetic abnormalities [(eg, t(8;21), t(15;17), and inv(16)] and acute erythroid leukemia.
4. Promyelocytes are blast equivalents only in APL.
5. Promonocytes (blast equivalents) have slightly folded nuclei, dispersed chromatin, nucleoli, and moderate amounts of basophilic cytoplasm.
6. Promonocyte enumeration is critical in the distinction between acute and chronic monocytic leukemias.
7. Erythroblasts are included in the blast percentage only in cases of acute "pure" erythroid leukemia.
8. Maturing megakaryocytic lineage cells and micromegakaryocytes are *not* blast equivalents.
9. Rapid diagnosis of APL is imperative due to risk of hemorrhage.
10. Classic hypergranular APL is usually associated with a very low WBC, while marked leukocytosis is typical in microgranular APL.
11. Flow cytometric immunophenotyping is not the optimal modality to diagnose APL; morphology and cytochemistry are superior for diagnosis, which should be confirmed by genetic testing.
12. The biologic classification of AML includes cases defined by specific cytogenetic or molecular features, as well as cases defined by clinical parameters: underlying Down syndrome, prior chemotherapy, or antecedent myeloid neoplasm (eg, myelodysplasia).
13. Therapy-related disorders include cases of AML, myelodysplasia, and hybrid myelodysplastic/myeloproliferative diseases, but, due to similarities in outcome, these subtypes are merged into the single category of therapy-related myeloid neoplasms.
14. Down syndrome-associated neoplasms include transient abnormal myelopoiesis (spontaneously regressing neonatal disorder) and myeloid leukemia associated with Down syndrome (typically acute megakaryoblastic leukemia in ≤4-year-old child).
15. Transient abnormal myelopoiesis and Down syndrome-associated acute megakaryoblastic leukemia can be morphologically indistinguishable.

16. Distinctive morphologic clues to AML with t(8;21) include low blast count, long, tapered Auer rods, and salmon-colored cytoplasmic granulation with a rim of basophilia.
17. Distinctive morphologic clues to AML with inv(16) include increased bone marrow eosinophils with mixed eosinophil/basophil granules.
18. Distinctive clues to APL include marked leukopenia, profound thrombocytopenia, hypergranular promyelocytes, stacks of Auer rods, maturation block at promyelocyte stage, intense myeloperoxidase positivity, and coagulopathy.
19. Distinctive morphologic and CBC features of microgranular APL include leukocytosis, folded (sliding plate) nuclei, rare hypergranular promyelocytes, maturation block at promyelocyte stage, intense myeloperoxidase positivity, and coagulopathy.
20. There is substantial morphologic overlap between microgranular APL and acute monocytic/myelomonocytic leukemias.
21. Three different scenarios are used to classify a case as AML with MDS-related changes:
    a. History of MDS or MDS/MPN (but not linked to antecedent therapy)
    b. MDS-associated cytogenetic abnormality
    c. Multilineage (at least 2 lineages) dysplasia involving at least 50% of cells in each affected lineage.
22. The lack of nonspecific esterase positivity does *not* exclude a diagnosis of acute monocytic/myelomonocytic leukemia if morphology and flow cytometric immunophenotyping support the diagnosis.
23. Recurrent AML-defining cytogenetic abnormalities prevail over other findings in AML classification, although therapy-related myeloid neoplasm with an AML-defining cytogenetic abnormality should be classified as therapy-related AML with t(15;17), etc.
24. If a case of AML has complex cytogenetic abnormalities that include an AML-defining cytogenetic abnormality [eg, t(8;21), t(15;17), etc.], it should be classified within the AML-defining cytogenetic abnormality group.

[18.14] References

Abdel-Wahab O, Mullally A, Hedvat C, et al [2009] Genetic characterization of TET1, TET2, and TET3 alterations in myeloid malignancies. *Blood* 114:144-147.

Abdou SM, Jadayel DM, Min T, et al [2002] Incidence of MLL rearrangement in acute myeloid leukemia, and a CALM-AF10 fusion in M4 type acute myeloblastic leukemia. *Leuk Lymphoma* 43:89-95.

Ades L, Chevret S, De Botton S, et al [2005] Outcome of acute promyelocytic leukemia treated with all trans retinoic acid and chemotherapy in elderly patients: the European group experience. *Leukemia* 19:230-233.

Ageberg M, Drott K, Olofsson T, et al [2008] Identification of a novel and myeloid specific role of the leukemia-associated fusion protein DEK-NUP214 leading to increased protein synthesis. *Genes Chromosomes Cancer* 47:276-287.

Al-Mawali A, Gillis D, Lewis I [2009a] The role of multiparameter flow cytometry for detection of minimal residual disease in acute myeloid leukemia. *Am J Clin Pathol* 131:16-26.

Al-Mawali A, To LB, Gillis D, et al [2009b] The presence of leukaemia-associated phenotypes is an independent predictor of induction failure in acute myeloid leukaemia. *Int J Lab Hematol* 31:61-68.

Alsabeh R, Brynes RK, Slovak ML, Arber DA [1997] Acute myeloid leukemia with t(6;9)(p23;q34): association with myelodysplasia, basophilia, and initial CD34 negative immunophenotype. *Am J Clin Pathol* 107:430-437.

Alter BP, Giri N, Savage SA, Rosenberg PS [2009] Cancer in dyskeratosis congenita. *Blood* 113:6549-6557.

Arber D, Brunning R, Le Beau M, et al [2008a] Acute myeloid leukaemia with recurrent genetic abnormalities. In: Swerdlow S, Campo E, Harris N, et al, eds. *WHO Classification of Tumours: Pathology and Genetics: Tumours of Haematopoietic and Lymphoid Tissues.* Lyon, France: IARC Press; 110-123.

Arber D, Brunning R, Orazi A, et al [2008b] Acute myeloid leukaemia with myelodysplasia-related changes. In: Swerdlow S, Campo E, Harris N, et al, eds. *WHO Classification of Tumours: Pathology and Genetics: Tumours of Haematopoietic and Lymphoid Tissues.* Lyon, France: IARC Press; 124-126.

Arber D, Brunning R, Orazi A, et al [2008c] Acute myeloid leukemia, not otherwise specified. In: Swerdlow S, Campo E, Harris N, et al, eds. *WHO Classification of Tumours: Pathology and Genetics: Tumours of Haematopoietic and Lymphoid Tissues.* Lyon, France: IARC Press; 130-139.

Arber DA, Slovak ML, Popplewell L, et al [2002] Therapy-related acute myeloid leukemia/myelodysplasia with balanced 21q22 translocations. *Am J Clin Pathol* 117:306-313.

Arbuthnot C, Wilde JT [2006] Haemostatic problems in acute promyelocytic leukaemia. *Blood Rev* 20:289-297.

Arnould C, Philippe C, Bourdon V, et al [1999] The signal transducer and activator of transcription STAT5b gene is a new partner of retinoic acid receptor α in acute promyelocytic-like leukaemia. *Hum Mol Genet* 8:1741-1749.

Bacher U, Haferlach C, Kern W, et al [2008] Prognostic relevance of FLT3-TKD mutations in AML: the combination matters—an analysis of 3082 patients. *Blood* 111:2527-2537.

Baldus CD, Mrozek K, Marcucci G, Bloomfield CD [2007] Clinical outcome of de novo acute myeloid leukaemia patients with normal cytogenetics is affected by molecular genetic alterations: a concise review. *Br J Haematol* 137:387-400.

Balgobind BV, Raimondi SC, Harbott J, et al [2009] Novel prognostic subgroups in childhood 11q23/MLL-rearranged acute myeloid leukemia: results of an international retrospective study. *Blood* 114:2489-2496.

Ball ED, Davis RB, Griffin JD, et al [1991] Prognostic value of lymphocyte surface markers in acute myeloid leukemia. *Blood* 77:2242-2250.

Barbaric D, Alonzo TA, Gerbing RB, et al [2007] Minimally differentiated acute myeloid leukemia (FAB AML-M0) is associated with an adverse outcome in children: a report from the Children's Oncology Group, studies CCG-2891 and CCG-2961. *Blood* 109:2314-2321.

Bates DL, Chen Y, Kim G, et al [2008] Crystal structures of multiple GATA zinc fingers bound to DNA reveal new insights into DNA recognition and self-association by GATA. *J Mol Biol* 381:1292-1306.

Baumann I, Niemeyer C, Brunning R, et al [2008] Myeloid proliferations related to Down syndrome. In: Swerdlow S, Campo E, Harris N, et al, eds. *WHO Classification of Tumours: Pathology and Genetics: Tumours of Haematopoietic and Lymphoid Tissues.* Lyon, France: IARC Press; 142-144.

Beauchamp-Nicoud A, Feneux D, Bayle C, et al [2003] Therapy-related myelodysplasia and/or acute myeloid leukaemia after autologous haematopoietic progenitor cell transplantation in a prospective single centre cohort of 221 patients. *Br J Haematol* 122:109-117.

Beaumont M, Sanz M, Carli PM, et al [2003] Therapy-related acute promyelocytic leukemia. *J Clin Oncol* 21:2123-2137.

Becher R, Haas OA, Graeven U, et al [1988] Translocation t(8;16) in acute monocytic leukemia. *Cancer Genet Cytogenet* 34:265-271.

Becker H, Marcucci G, Maharry K, et al [2010] Favorable prognostic impact of NPM1 mutations in older patients with cytogenetically normal de novo acute myeloid leukemia and associated gene- and microRNA-expression signatures: a Cancer and Leukemia Group B study. *J Clin Oncol* 28:596-604.

Belson M, Kingsley B, Holmes A [2007] Risk factors for acute leukemia in children: a review. *Environ Health Perspect* 115:138-145.

Bene MC, Bernier M, Casasnovas RO, et al [2001] Acute myeloid leukaemia M0: haematological, immunophenotypic and cytogenetic characteristics and their prognostic significance: an analysis in 241 patients. *Br J Haematol* 113:737-745.

Bennett JM, Catovsky D, Daniel MT, et al [2000] Hypergranular promyelocytic leukemia: correlation between morphology and chromosomal translocations including t(15;17) and t(11;17). *Leukemia* 14:1197-1200.

Bernasconi P, Orlandi E, Cavigliano P, et al [2000] Translocation (8;16) in a patient with acute myelomonocytic leukemia, occurring after treatment with fludarabine for a low-grade non-Hodgkin's lymphoma. *Haematologica* 85:1087-1091.

Bhatia S, Robison LL, Oberlin O, et al [1996] Breast cancer and other second neoplasms after childhood Hodgkin's disease. *N Engl J Med* 334:745-751.

Bienz M, Ludwig M, Leibundgut EO, et al [2005] Risk assessment in patients with acute myeloid leukemia and a normal karyotype. *Clin Cancer Res* 11:1416-1424.

Boeckx N, Renard M, Uyttebroeck A [2007] Acute monocytic leukaemia with histiocytic features. *Br J Haematol* 137:2.

Boissel N, Leroy H, Brethon B, et al [2006] Incidence and prognostic impact of c-Kit, FLT3, and Ras gene mutations in core binding factor acute myeloid leukemia (CBF-AML). *Leukemia* 20:965-970.

Bradstock KF [1993] The diagnostic and prognostic value of immunophenotyping in acute leukemia. *Pathology* 25:367-374.

Breems DA, Van Putten WL, De Greef GE, et al [2008] Monosomal karyotype in acute myeloid leukemia: a better indicator of poor prognosis than a complex karyotype. *J Clin Oncol* 26:4791-4797.

Bueno C, Catalina P, Melen GJ, et al [2009] Etoposide induces MLL rearrangements and other chromosomal abnormalities in human embryonic stem cells. *Carcinogenesis* 30:1628-1637.

Burroughs L, Woolfrey A, Shimamura A [2009] Shwachman-Diamond syndrome: a review of the clinical presentation, molecular pathogenesis, diagnosis, and treatment. *Hematol Oncol Clin North Am* 23:233-248.

Byrd JC, Mrozek K, Dodge RK, et al [2002] Pretreatment cytogenetic abnormalities are predictive of induction success, cumulative incidence of relapse, and overall survival in adult patients with de novo acute myeloid leukemia: results from Cancer and Leukemia Group B (CALGB 8461). *Blood* 100:4325-4336.

Cairoli R, Beghini A, Grillo G, et al [2006] Prognostic impact of c-KIT mutations in core binding factor leukemias: an Italian retrospective study. *Blood* 107:3463-3468.

Caligiuri MA, Strout MP, Lawrence D, et al [1998] Rearrangement of ALL1 (MLL) in acute myeloid leukemia with normal cytogenetics. *Cancer Res* 58:55-59.

Callens C, Chevret S, Cayuela JM, et al [2005] Prognostic implication of FLT3 and Ras gene mutations in patients with acute promyelocytic leukemia (APL): a retrospective study from the European APL Group. *Leukemia* 19:1153-1160.

Care RS, Valk PJ, Goodeve AC, et al [2003] Incidence and prognosis of c-KIT and FLT3 mutations in core binding factor (CBF) acute myeloid leukaemias. *Br J Haematol* 121:775-777.

Casasnovas RO, Campos L, Mugneret F, et al [1998] Immunophenotypic patterns and cytogenetic anomalies in acute non-lymphoblastic leukemia subtypes: a prospective study of 432 patients. *Leukemia* 12:34-43.

Catalano A, Dawson MA, Somana K, et al [2007] The PRKAR1A gene is fused to RARA in a new variant acute promyelocytic leukemia. *Blood* 110:4073-4076.

Chan GC, Wang WC, Raimondi SC, et al [1997] Myelodysplastic syndrome in children: differentiation from acute myeloid leukemia with a low blast count. *Leukemia* 11:206-211.

Chang H, Yi QL [2006] Acute myeloid leukemia with pseudo-Chediak-Higashi anomaly exhibits a specific immunophenotype with CD2 expression. *Am J Clin Pathol* 125:791-794.

Chatterjee S, Trivedi D, Petzold SJ, Berger NA [1990] Mechanism of epipodophyllotoxin-induced cell death in poly(adenosine diphosphate-ribose) synthesis-deficient V79 Chinese hamster cell lines. *Cancer Res* 50:2713-2718.

Chen L, Shah HO, Lin JH [2004] Alveolar rhabdomyosarcoma with concurrent metastases to bone marrow and lymph nodes simulating acute hematologic malignancy. *J Pediatr Hematol Oncol* 26:696-697.

Chen SW, Li CF, Chuang SS, et al [2008] Aberrant co-expression of CD19 and CD56 as surrogate markers of acute myeloid leukemias with t(8;21) in Taiwan. *Int J Lab Hematol* 30:133-138.

Chen Z, Brand NJ, Chen A, et al [1993] Fusion between a novel Kruppel-like zinc finger gene and the retinoic acid receptor-α locus due to a variant t(11;17) translocation associated with acute promyelocytic leukaemia. *Embo J* 12:1161-1167.

Cheng Y, Wang Y, Wang H, et al [2009] Cytogenetic profile of de novo acute myeloid leukemia: a study based on 1432 patients in a single institution of China. *Leukemia* 23:1801-1806.

Chi Y, Lindgren V, Quigley S, Gaitonde S [2008] Acute myelogenous leukemia with t(6;9)(p23;q34) and marrow basophilia: an overview. *Arch Pathol Lab Med* 132:1835-1837.

Chung HJ, Chi HS, Cho YU, et al [2008] Promyelocytic blast crisis of chronic myeloid leukemia during imatinib treatment. *Ann Clin Lab Sci* 38:283-286.

Cimino G, Papa G, Tura S, et al [1991] Second primary cancer following Hodgkin's disease: updated results of an Italian multicentric study. *J Clin Oncol* 9:432-437.

Creutzig U, Reinhardt D, Diekamp S, et al [2005] AML patients with Down syndrome have a high cure rate with AML-BFM therapy with reduced dose intensity. *Leukemia* 19:1355-1360.

Czader M, Orazi A [2009] Therapy-related myeloid neoplasms. *Am J Clin Pathol* 132:410-425.

Dale DC, Cottle TE, Fier CJ, et al [2003] Severe chronic neutropenia: treatment and follow-up of patients in the Severe Chronic Neutropenia International Registry. *Am J Hematol* 72:82-93.

De J, Zanjani R, Hibbard M, Davis BH [2007] Immunophenotypic profile predictive of KIT activating mutations in AML1-ETO leukemia. *Am J Clin Pathol* 128:550-557.

de Botton S, Coiteux V, Chevret S, et al [2004] Outcome of childhood acute promyelocytic leukemia with all-trans-retinoic acid and chemotherapy. *J Clin Oncol* 22:1404-1412.

Deguchi K, Gilliland DG [2002] Cooperativity between mutations in tyrosine kinases and in hematopoietic transcription factors in AML. *Leukemia* 16:740-744.

Del Poeta G, Stasi R, Venditti A, et al [1995] CD7 expression in acute myeloid leukemia. *Leuk Lymphoma* 17:111-119.

Derolf AR, Kristinsson SY, Andersson TM, et al [2009] Improved patient survival for acute myeloid leukemia: a population-based study of 9729 patients diagnosed in Sweden between 1973 and 2005. *Blood* 113:3666-3672.

Deschler B, Lubbert M [2006] Acute myeloid leukemia: epidemiology and etiology. *Cancer* 107:2099-2107.

Dohner H, Estey EH, Amadori S, et al [2010] Diagnosis and management of acute myeloid leukemia in adults: recommendations from an international expert panel, on behalf of the European LeukemiaNet. *Blood* 115:453-474.

Donadieu J, Leblanc T, Bader Meunier B, et al [2005] Analysis of risk factors for myelodysplasias, leukemias and death from infection among patients with congenital neutropenia. Experience of the French Severe Chronic Neutropenia Study Group. *Haematologica* 90:45-53.

Downing JR [2003] The core-binding factor leukemias: lessons learned from murine models. *Curr Opin Genet Dev* 13:48-54.

Doyle D [2009] Notoriety to respectability: a short history of arsenic prior to its present day use in haematology. *Br J Haematol* 145:309-317.

Duchayne E, Fenneteau O, Pages MP, et al [2003] Acute megakaryoblastic leukaemia: a national clinical and biological study of 53 adult and childhood cases by the Groupe Francais d'Hematologie Cellulaire (GFHC). *Leuk Lymphoma* 44:49-58.

Dufour A, Schneider F, Metzeler KH, et al [2010] Acute myeloid leukemia with biallelic CEBPA gene mutations and normal karyotype represents a distinct genetic entity associated with a favorable clinical outcome. *J Clin Oncol* 28:570-577.

Dunphy CH, Orton SO, Mantell J [2004] Relative contributions of enzyme cytochemistry and flow cytometric immunophenotyping to the evaluation of acute myeloid leukemias with a monocytic component and of flow cytometric immunophenotyping to the evaluation of absolute monocytoses. *Am J Clin Pathol* 122:865-874.

Dunphy CH, Tang W [2007] The value of CD64 expression in distinguishing acute myeloid leukemia with monocytic differentiation from other subtypes of acute myeloid leukemia: a flow cytometric analysis of 64 cases. *Arch Pathol Lab Med* 131:748-754.

Edwards RH, Wasik MA, Finan J, et al [1999] Evidence for early hematopoietic progenitor cell involvement in acute promyelocytic leukemia. *Am J Clin Pathol* 112:819-827.

Elagib KE, Goldfarb AN [2007] Regulation of *RUNX1* transcriptional function by *GATA1*. *Crit Rev Eukaryot Gene Expr* 17:271-280.

Esteve J, Rozman M, Campo E, et al [1995] Leukemia after true histiocytic lymphoma: another type of acute monocytic leukemia with histiocytic differentiation (AML-M5c)? *Leukemia* 9:1389-1391.

Etzell JE, Keet C, McDonald W, Banerjee A [2006] Medulloblastoma simulating acute myeloid leukemia: case report with a review of "myeloid antigen" expression in nonhematopoietic tissues and tumors. *J Pediatr Hematol Oncol* 28:703-710.

Faber J, Krivtsov AV, Stubbs MC, et al [2009] HOXA9 is required for survival in human MLL-rearranged acute leukemias. *Blood* 113:2375-2385.

Falini B, Mecucci C, Tiacci E, et al [2005] Cytoplasmic nucleophosmin in acute myelogenous leukemia with a normal karyotype. *N Engl J Med* 352:254-266.

Falini B, Nicoletti I, Martelli MF, Mecucci C [2007] Acute myeloid leukemia carrying cytoplasmic/mutated nucleophosmin (NPMc+ AML): biologic and clinical features. *Blood* 109:874-885.

Farag SS, Archer KJ, Mrozek K, et al [2006] Pretreatment cytogenetics add to other prognostic factors predicting complete remission and long-term outcome in patients 60 years of age or older with acute myeloid leukemia: results from Cancer and Leukemia Group B 8461. *Blood* 108:63-73.

Felix CA [1998] Secondary leukemias induced by topoisomerase-targeted drugs. *Biochim Biophys Acta* 1400:233-255.

Feller N, van der Pol MA, van Stijn A, et al [2004] MRD parameters using immunophenotypic detection methods are highly reliable in predicting survival in acute myeloid leukaemia. *Leukemia* 18:1380-1390.

Foley R, Soamboonsrup P, Carter RF, et al [2001] CD34+ acute promyelocytic leukemia is associated with leukocytosis, microgranular/hypogranular morphology, expression of CD2 and bcr3 isoform. *Am J Hematol* 67:34-41.

Forestier E, Izraeli S, Beverloo B, et al [2008] Cytogenetic features of acute lymphoblastic and myeloid leukemias in pediatric patients with Down syndrome: an iBFM-SG study. *Blood* 111:1575-1583.

Freedman MH, Alter BP [2002] Risk of myelodysplastic syndrome and acute myeloid leukemia in congenital neutropenias. *Semin Hematol* 39:128-133.

Frohling S, Schlenk RF, Breitruck J, et al [2002] Prognostic significance of activating FLT3 mutations in younger adults (16-60 years) with acute myeloid leukemia and normal cytogenetics: a study of the AML Study Group Ulm. *Blood* 100:4372-4380.

Frohling S, Schlenk RF, Stolze I, et al [2004] CEBPA mutations in younger adults with acute myeloid leukemia and normal cytogenetics: prognostic relevance and analysis of cooperating mutations. *J Clin Oncol* 22:624-633.

Gaidzik V, Dohner K [2008] Prognostic implications of gene mutations in acute myeloid leukemia with normal cytogenetics. *Semin Oncol* 35:346-355.

Gamerdinger U, Teigler-Schlegel A, Pils S, et al [2003] Cryptic chromosomal aberrations leading to an AML1/ETO rearrangement are frequently caused by small insertions. *Genes Chromosomes Cancer* 36:261-272.

Geddis AE [2009] Congenital amegakaryocytic thrombocytopenia and thrombo-cytopenia with absent radii. *Hematol Oncol Clin North Am* 23:321-331.

Gibson SE, Dong HY, Advani AS, Hsi ED [2006] Expression of the B cell-associated transcription factors PAX5, OCT-2, and BOB.1 in acute myeloid leukemia: associations with B-cell antigen expression and myelomonocytic maturation. *Am J Clin Pathol* 126:916-924.

Gomis F, Sanz J, Sempere A, et al [2004] Immunofluorescent analysis with the anti-PML monoclonal antibody PG-M3 for rapid and accurate genetic diagnosis of acute promyelocytic leukemia. *Ann Hematol* 83:687-690.

Green AM, Kupfer GM [2009] Fanconi anemia. *Hematol Oncol Clin North Am* 23:193-214.

Grimwade D [1999] The pathogenesis of acute promyelocytic leukaemia: evaluation of the role of molecular diagnosis and monitoring in the management of the disease. *Br J Haematol* 106:591-613.

Grimwade D, Walker H, Harrison G, et al [2001] The predictive value of hierar-chical cytogenetic classification in older adults with acute myeloid leukemia (AML): analysis of 1065 patients entered into the United Kingdom Medical Research Council AML11 trial. *Blood* 98:1312-1320.

Grisolano JL, O'Neal J, Cain J, Tomasson MH [2003] An activated receptor tyrosine kinase, TEL/PDGFbetaR, cooperates with AML1/ETO to induce acute myeloid leukemia in mice. *Proc Natl Acad Sci USA* 100:9506-9511.

Groom DA, Wong D, Brynes RK, Macaulay LK [1991] Auer rod-like inclusions in circulating lymphoma cells. *Am J Clin Pathol* 96:111-115.

Gurney JG, Severson RK, Davis S, Robison LL [1995] Incidence of cancer in children in the United States. Sex-, race-, and 1-year age-specific rates by histologic type. *Cancer* 75:2186-2195.

Gustafson SA, Lin P, Chen SS, et al [2009] Therapy-related acute myeloid leukemia with t(8;21)(q22;q22) shares many features with de novo acute myeloid leukemia with t(8;21)(q22;q22) but does not have a favorable outcome. *Am J Clin Pathol* 131:647-655.

Haferlach C, Mecucci C, Schnittger S, et al [2009a] AML with mutated NPM1 carrying a normal or aberrant karyotype show overlapping biologic, pathologic, immunophenotypic, and prognostic features. *Blood* 114:3024-3032.

Haferlach T, Kohlmann A, Klein HU, et al [2009b] AML with translocation t(8;16)(p11;p13) demonstrates unique cytomorphological, cytogenetic, molecular and prognostic features. *Leukemia* 23:934-943.

Hama A, Yagasaki H, Takahashi Y, et al [2008] Acute megakaryoblastic leukaemia (AMKL) in children: a comparison of AMKL with and without Down syndrome. *Br J Haematol* 140:552-561.

Hamlett I, Draper J, Strouboulis J, et al [2008] Characterization of megakaryocyte GATA1-interacting proteins: the corepressor ETO2 and GATA1 interact to regulate terminal megakaryocyte maturation. *Blood* 112:2738-2749.

Harris AC, Todd WM, Hackney MH, Ben-Ezra J [1994] Bone marrow changes associated with recombinant granulocyte-macrophage and granulocyte colony-stimulating factors. Discrimination of granulocytic regeneration. *Arch Pathol Lab Med* 118:624-629.

Hasan SK, Mays AN, Ottone T, et al [2008] Molecular analysis of t(15;17) genomic breakpoints in secondary acute promyelocytic leukemia arising after treatment of multiple sclerosis. *Blood* 112:3383-3390.

Heim S, Avanzi GC, Billstrom R, et al [1987] A new specific chromosomal rearrangement, t(8;16)(p11;p13), in acute monocytic leukaemia. *Br J Haematol* 66:323-326.

Helbling D, Mueller BU, Timchenko NA, et al [2005] CBFB-SMMHC is correlated with increased calreticulin expression and suppresses the granulocytic differentiation factor CEBPA in AML with inv(16). *Blood* 106:1369-1375.

Hijiya N, Ness KK, Ribeiro RC, Hudson MM [2009] Acute leukemia as a secondary malignancy in children and adolescents: current findings and issues. *Cancer* 115:23-35.

Hitzler JK [2007] Acute megakaryoblastic leukemia in Down syndrome. *Pediatr Blood Cancer* 49:1066-1069.

Ho PA, Alonzo TA, Gerbing RB, et al [2009] Prevalence and prognostic implications of CEBPA mutations in pediatric acute myeloid leukemia (AML): a report from the Children's Oncology Group. *Blood* 113:6558-6566.

Hollanda LM, Lima CS, Cunha AF, et al [2006] An inherited mutation leading to production of only the short isoform of *GATA1* is associated with impaired erythropoiesis. *Nat Genet* 38:807-812.

Holt SE, Brown EJ, Zipursky A [2002] Telomerase and the benign and malignant megakaryoblastic leukemias of Down syndrome. *J Pediatr Hematol Oncol* 24:14-17.

Hsia CC, Linenberger M, Howson-Jan K, et al [2008] Acute myeloid leukemia in a healthy hematopoietic stem cell donor following past exposure to a short course of G-CSF. *Bone Marrow Transplant* 42:431-432.

Huang L, Abruzzo LV, Valbuena JR, et al [2006] Acute myeloid leukemia associated with variant t(8;21) detected by conventional cytogenetic and molecular studies: a report of 4 cases and review of the literature. *Am J Clin Pathol* 125:267-272.

Hung D, St Heaps L, Benson W, et al [2007] Deletion of 3'CBFbeta in an inv(16)(p13;lq22) ascertained by fluorescence in situ hybridization and reverse-transcriptase polymerase chain reaction. *Cancer Genet Cytogenet* 172:92-94.

Hurwitz CA, Raimondi SC, Head D, et al [1992] Distinctive immunophenotypic features of t(8;21)(q22;q22) acute myeloblastic leukemia in children. *Blood* 80:3182-3188.

Hussein K, Jahagirdar B, Gupta P, et al [2008] Day 14 bone marrow biopsy in predicting complete remission and survival in acute myeloid leukemia. *Am J Hematol* 83:446-450.

Hutter G, Nowak D, Blau IW, Thiel E [2009] Auer rod-like intracytoplasmic inclusions in multiple myeloma. A case report and review of the literature. *Int J Lab Hematol* 31:236-240.

Innes DJ, Jr, Hess CE, Bertholf MF, Wade P [1987] Promyelocyte morphology. Differentiation of acute promyelocytic leukemia from benign myeloid prolif-erations. *Am J Clin Pathol* 88:725-729.

Ito S, Ishida Y, Oyake T, et al [2004] Clinical and biological significance of CD56 antigen expression in acute promyelocytic leukemia. *Leuk Lymphoma* 45:1783-1789.

Johnson KD, Boyer ME, Kang JA, et al [2007] Friend of *GATA1*-independent transcriptional repression: a novel mode of *GATA1* function. *Blood* 109:5230-5233.

Jotterand Bellomo M, Parlier V, Muhlematter D, et al [1992] Three new cases of chromosome 3 rearrangement in bands q21 and q26 with abnormal thrombopoiesis bring further evidence to the existence of a 3q21q26 syndrome. *Cancer Genet Cytogenet* 59:138-160.

Kaito K, Katayama T, Masuoka H, et al [2005] CD2+ acute promyelocytic leukemia is associated with leukocytosis, variant morphology and poorer prognosis. *Clin Lab Haematol* 27:307-311.

Kaleem Z, Crawford E, Pathan MH, et al [2003] Flow cytometric analysis of acute leukemias. Diagnostic utility and critical analysis of data. *Arch Pathol Lab Med* 127:42-48.

Kaleem Z, White G [2001] Diagnostic criteria for minimally differentiated acute myeloid leukemia (AML-M0). Evaluation and a proposal. *Am J Clin Pathol* 115:876-884.

Kelaidi C, Chevret S, De Botton S, et al [2009] Improved outcome of acute promyelocytic leukemia with high WBC counts over the last 15 years: the European APL Group experience. *J Clin Oncol* 27:2668-2676.

Kelly MJ, Meloni-Ehrig AM, Manley PE, Altura RA [2009] Poor outcome in a pediatric patient with acute myeloid leukemia associated with a variant t(8;21) and trisomy 6. *Cancer Genet Cytogenet* 189:48-52.

Kern W, Haferlach C, Haferlach T, Schnittger S [2008] Monitoring of minimal residual disease in acute myeloid leukemia. *Cancer* 112:4-16.

Khalidi HS, Medeiros LJ, Chang KL, et al [1998] The immunophenotype of adult acute myeloid leukemia: high frequency of lymphoid antigen expression and comparison of immunophenotype, French-American-British classification, and karyotypic abnormalities. *Am J Clin Pathol* 109:211-220.

Khoury H, Dalal BI, Nevill TJ, et al [2003] Acute myelogenous leukemia with t(8;21)—identification of a specific immunophenotype. *Leuk Lymphoma* 44:1713-1718.

Knight JA, Skol AD, Shinde A, et al [2009] Genome-wide association study to identify novel loci associated with therapy-related myeloid leukemia susceptibility. *Blood* 113:5575-5582.

Kolitz JE, George SL, Dodge RK, et al [2004] Dose escalation studies of cytarabine, daunorubicin, and etoposide with and without multidrug resistance modulation with PSC-833 in untreated adults with acute myeloid leukemia younger than 60 years: final induction results of Cancer and Leukemia Group B Study 9621. *J Clin Oncol* 22:4290-4301.

Konoplev S, Huang X, Drabkin HA, et al [2009] Cytoplasmic localization of nucleophosmin in bone marrow blasts of acute myeloid leukemia patients is not completely concordant with NPM1 mutation and is not predictive of prognosis. *Cancer* 115:4737-4744.

Koschmieder S, Halmos B, Levantini E, Tenen DG [2009] Dysregulation of the C/EBPalpha differentiation pathway in human cancer. *J Clin Oncol* 27:619-628.

Kottaridis PD, Gale RE, Frew ME, et al [2001] The presence of a FLT3 internal tandem duplication in patients with acute myeloid leukemia (AML) adds important prognostic information to cytogenetic risk group and response to the first cycle of chemotherapy: analysis of 854 patients from the United Kingdom Medical Research Council AML 10 and 12 trials. *Blood* 98:1752-1759.

Kozlov I, Beason K, Yu C, Hughson M [2005] CD79a expression in acute myeloid leukemia t(8;21) and the importance of cytogenetics in the diagnosis of leukemias with immunophenotypic ambiguity. *Cancer Genet Cytogenet* 163:62-67.

Krasinskas AM, Wasik MA, Kamoun M, et al [1998] The usefulness of CD64, other monocyte-associated antigens, and CD45 gating in the subclassification of acute myeloid leukemias with monocytic differentiation. *Am J Clin Pathol* 110:797-805.

Kuchenbauer F, Schnittger S, Look T, et al [2006] Identification of additional cytogenetic and molecular genetic abnormalities in acute myeloid leukaemia with t(8;21)/AML1-ETO. *Br J Haematol* 134:616-619.

Kussick SJ, Stirewalt DL, Yi HS, et al [2004] A distinctive nuclear morphology in acute myeloid leukemia is strongly associated with loss of HLA-DR expression and FLT3 internal tandem duplication. *Leukemia* 18:1591-1598.

Lacombe F, Arnoulet C, Maynadie M, et al [2009] Early clearance of peripheral blasts measured by flow cytometry during the first week of AML induction therapy as a new independent prognostic factor: a GOELAMS study. *Leukemia* 23:350-357.

Lange BJ, Smith FO, Feusner J, et al [2008] Outcomes in CCG-2961, a children's oncology group phase 3 trial for untreated pediatric acute myeloid leukemia: a report from the children's oncology group. *Blood* 111:1044-1053.

Le Deley MC, Suzan F, Cutuli B, et al [2007] Anthracyclines, mitoxantrone, radiotherapy, and granulocyte colony-stimulating factor: risk factors for leukemia and myelodysplastic syndrome after breast cancer. *J Clin Oncol* 25:292-300.

Le H, Singh S, Shih SJ, et al [2009] Rearrangements of the MLL gene are influenced by DNA secondary structure, potentially mediated by topoisomerase II binding. *Genes Chromosomes Cancer* 48:806-815.

Lee JJ, Cho D, Chung IJ, et al [2003] CD34 expression is associated with poor clinical outcome in patients with acute promyelocytic leukemia. *Am J Hematol* 73:149-153.

Leone G, Pagano L, Ben-Yehuda D, Voso MT [2007] Therapy-related leukemia and myelodysplasia: susceptibility and incidence. *Haematologica* 92:1389-1398.

Leroy H, de Botton S, Grardel-Duflos N, et al [2005] Prognostic value of real-time quantitative PCR (RQ-PCR) in AML with t(8;21). *Leukemia* 19:367-372.

Leu L, Mohassel L [2009] Arsenic trioxide as first-line treatment for acute promyelocytic leukemia. *Am J Health Syst Pharm* 66:1913-1918.

Libura J, Slater DJ, Felix CA, Richardson C [2005] Therapy-related acute myeloid leukemia-like MLL rearrangements are induced by etoposide in primary human CD34+ cells and remain stable after clonal expansion. *Blood* 105:2124-2131.

Lightfoot J, Hitzler JK, Zipursky A, et al [2004] Distinct gene signatures of transient and acute megakaryoblastic leukemia in Down syndrome. *Leukemia* 18:1617-1623.

Lin P, Hao S, Medeiros LJ, et al [2004] Expression of CD2 in acute promyelocytic leukemia correlates with short form of PML-RARalpha transcripts and poorer prognosis. *Am J Clin Pathol* 121:402-407.

Lipton JM [2006] Diamond blackfan anemia: new paradigms for a "not so pure" inherited red cell aplasia. *Semin Hematol* 43:167-177.

Lock RJ, Virgo PF, Kitchen C, Evely RS [2004] Rapid diagnosis and characterization of acute promyelocytic leukaemia in routine laboratory practice. *Clin Lab Haematol* 26:101-106.

Luo J, Qi C, Xu W, et al [2010] Cytoplasmic expression of nucleophosmin accurately predicts mutation in the nucleophosmin gene in patients with acute myeloid leukemia and normal karyotype. *Am J Clin Pathol* 133:34-40.

Malinge S, Ragu C, Della-Valle V, et al [2008] Activating mutations in human acute megakaryoblastic leukemia. *Blood* 112:4220-4226.

Marcucci G, Caligiuri MA, Bloomfield CD [2003] Core binding factor (CBF) acute myeloid leukemia: is molecular monitoring by RT-PCR useful clinically? *Eur J Haematol* 71:143-154.

Marcucci G, Mrozek K, Ruppert AS, et al [2005] Prognostic factors and outcome of core binding factor acute myeloid leukemia patients with t(8;21) differ from those of patients with inv(16): a Cancer and Leukemia Group B study. *J Clin Oncol* 23:5705-5717.

Martineau M, Berger R, Lillington DM, et al [1998] The t(6;11)(q27;q23) translocation in acute leukemia: a laboratory and clinical study of 30 cases. EU Concerted Action 11q23 Workshop participants. *Leukemia* 12:788-791.

Martinelli G, Ottaviani E, Buonamici S, et al [2003] Association of 3q21q26 syndrome with different RPN1/EVI1 fusion transcripts. *Haematologica* 88:1221-1228.

Mason KD, Juneja SK, Szer J [2006] The immunophenotype of acute myeloid leukemia: is there a relationship with prognosis? *Blood Rev* 20:71-82.

Massey GV, Zipursky A, Chang MN, et al [2006] A prospective study of the natural history of transient leukemia (TL) in neonates with Down syndrome (DS): Children's Oncology Group (COG) study POG-9481. *Blood* 107:4606-4613.

Mathew S, Behm F, Dalton J, Raimondi S [1999] Comparison of cytogenetics, Southern blotting, and fluorescence in situ hybridization as methods for detecting MLL gene rearrangements in children with acute leukemia and with 11q23 abnormalities. *Leukemia* 13:1713-1720.

McKenna M, Arnold C, Catherwood MA, et al [2009] Myeloid sarcoma of the small bowel associated with a CBFbeta/MYH11 fusion and inv(16)(p13q22): a case report. *J Clin Pathol* 62:757-759.

Mead AJ, Linch DC, Hills RK, et al [2007] FLT3 tyrosine kinase domain mutations are biologically distinct from and have a significantly more favorable prognosis than FLT3 internal tandem duplications in patients with acute myeloid leukemia. *Blood* 110:1262-1270.

Mercher T, Coniat MB, Monni R, et al [2001] Involvement of a human gene related to the Drosophila spen gene in the recurrent t(1;22) translocation of acute megakaryocytic leukemia. *Proc Natl Acad Sci USA* 98:5776-5779.

Merzianu M, Medeiros LJ, Cortes J, et al [2005] inv(16)(p13q22) in chronic myelogenous leukemia in blast phase: a clinicopathologic, cytogenetic, and molecular study of 5 cases. *Am J Clin Pathol* 124:807-814.

Meyer C, Kowarz E, Hofmann J, et al [2009] New insights to the MLL recombinome of acute leukemias. *Leukemia* 23:1490-1499.

Meyerson HJ, Farhi DC, Rosenthal NS [1998] Transient increase in blasts mimicking acute leukemia and progressing myelodysplasia in patients receiving growth factor. *Am J Clin Pathol* 109:675-681.

Mitelman F, Heim S [1992] Quantitative acute leukemia cytogenetics. *Genes Chromosomes Cancer* 5:57-66.

Miyoshi H, Kozu T, Shimizu K, et al [1993] The t(8;21) translocation in acute myeloid leukemia results in production of an AML1-MTG8 fusion transcript. *Embo J* 12:2715-2721.

Mohamedbhai S, Pule M, Conn B, et al [2008] Acute promyelocytic leukaemia presenting with a myeloid sarcoma of the tongue. *Br J Haematol* 141:565.

Moon H, Lee S, Huh J, Chung WS [2007] Characteristics of acute myeloid leukemia without HLA-DR expression. *Korean J Lab Med* 27:313-317.

Moorman AV, Hagemeijer A, Charrin C, et al [1998] The translocations, t(11;19)(q23;p13.1) and t(11;19)(q23;p13.3): a cytogenetic and clinical profile of 53 patients. European 11q23 Workshop participants. *Leukemia* 12:805-810.

Morice WG, Rodriguez FJ, Hoyer JD, Kurtin PJ [2005] Diffuse large B-cell lymphoma with distinctive patterns of splenic and bone marrow involvement: clinicopathologic features of 2 cases. *Mod Pathol* 18:495-502.

Mrozek K, Bloomfield CD [2008a] Clinical significance of the most common chromosome translocations in adult acute myeloid leukemia. *J Natl Cancer Inst Monogr* 52-57.

Mrozek K, Heerema NA, Bloomfield CD [2004] Cytogenetics in acute leukemia. *Blood Rev* 18:115-136.

Mrozek K, Heinonen K, Lawrence D, et al [1997] Adult patients with de novo acute myeloid leukemia and t(9;11)(p22;q23) have a superior outcome to patients with other translocations involving band 11q23: a cancer and leukemia group B study. *Blood* 90:4532-4538.

Mrozek K, Marcucci G, Paschka P, et al [2007] Clinical relevance of mutations and gene-expression changes in adult acute myeloid leukemia with normal cytogenetics: are we ready for a prognostically prioritized molecular classification? *Blood* 109:431-448.

Mrozek K, Marcucci G, Paschka P, Bloomfield CD [2008b] Advances in molecular genetics and treatment of core-binding factor acute myeloid leukemia. *Curr Opin Oncol* 20:711-718.

Mrozek K, Prior TW, Edwards C, et al [2001] Comparison of cytogenetic and molecular genetic detection of t(8;21) and inv(16) in a prospective series of adults with de novo acute myeloid leukemia: a Cancer and Leukemia Group B Study. *J Clin Oncol* 19:2482-2492.

Mueller BU, Pabst T, Fos J, et al [2006] ATRA resolves the differentiation block in t(15;17) acute myeloid leukemia by restoring PU.1 expression. *Blood* 107:3330-3338.

Nakamura H, Kuriyama K, Sadamori N, et al [1997] Morphological subtyping of acute myeloid leukemia with maturation (AML-M2): homogeneous pink-colored cytoplasm of mature neutrophils is most characteristic of AML-M2 with t(8;21). *Leukemia* 11:651-655.

Natelson EA [2007] Benzene exposure and refractory sideroblastic erythropoiesis: is there an association? *Am J Med Sci* 334:356-360.

Ngo NT, Lampert IA, Naresh KN [2008] Bone marrow trephine findings in acute myeloid leukaemia with multilineage dysplasia. *Br J Haematol* 140:279-286.

Niu C, Zhang J, Breslin P, et al [2009] c-Myc is a target of RNA-binding motif protein 15 in the regulation of adult hematopoietic stem cell and megakaryocyte development. *Blood* 114:2087-2096.

Nucifora G [1997] The EVI1 gene in myeloid leukemia. *Leukemia* 11:2022-2031.

Oelschlaegel U, Mohr B, Schaich M, et al [2009] HLA-DRneg patients without acute promyelocytic leukemia show distinct immunophenotypic, genetic, molecular, and cytomorphologic characteristics compared to acute promyelocytic leukemia. *Cytometry B Clin Cytom* 76:321-327.

Oki Y, Kantarjian HM, Zhou X, et al [2006] Adult acute megakaryocytic leukemia: an analysis of 37 patients treated at M.D. Anderson Cancer Center. *Blood* 107:880-884.

Okumura AJ, Peterson LF, Okumura F, et al [2008] t(8;21)(q22;q22) Fusion proteins preferentially bind to duplicated AML1/RUNX1 DNA-binding sequences to differentially regulate gene expression. *Blood* 112:1392-1401.

Orazi A, O'Malley DP, Jiang J, et al [2005] Acute panmyelosis with myelofibrosis: an entity distinct from acute megakaryoblastic leukemia. *Mod Pathol* 18:603-614.

Oyarzo MP, Lin P, Glassman A, et al [2004] Acute myeloid leukemia with t(6;9)(p23;q34) is associated with dysplasia and a high frequency of flt3 gene mutations. *Am J Clin Pathol* 122:348-358.

Pabst T, Eyholzer M, Fos J, Mueller BU [2009] Heterogeneity within AML with CEBPA mutations; only CEBPA double mutations, but not single CEBPA mutations are associated with favourable prognosis. *Br J Cancer* 100:1343-1346.

Paietta E [2003] Expression of cell-surface antigens in acute promyelocytic leukaemia. *Best Pract Res Clin Haematol* 16:369-385.

Parcells BW, Ikeda AK, Simms-Waldrip T, et al [2006] FMS-like tyrosine kinase 3 in normal hematopoiesis and acute myeloid leukemia. *Stem Cells* 24:1174-1184.

Paredes-Aguilera R, Romero-Guzman L, Lopez-Santiago N, Trejo RA [2003] Biology, clinical, and hematologic features of acute megakaryoblastic leukemia in children. *Am J Hematol* 73:71-80.

Paschka P [2008a] Core binding factor acute myeloid leukemia. *Semin Oncol* 35:410-417.

Paschka P, Marcucci G, Ruppert AS, et al [2006] Adverse prognostic significance of KIT mutations in adult acute myeloid leukemia with inv(16) and t(8;21): a Cancer and Leukemia Group B Study. *J Clin Oncol* 24:3904-3911.

Paschka P, Marcucci G, Ruppert AS, et al [2008b] Wilms' tumor 1 gene mutations independently predict poor outcome in adults with cytogenetically normal acute myeloid leukemia: a cancer and leukemia group B study. *J Clin Oncol* 26:4595-4602.

Patt DA, Duan Z, Fang S, et al [2007] Acute myeloid leukemia after adjuvant breast cancer therapy in older women: understanding risk. *J Clin Oncol* 25:3871-3876.

Pearson MG, Vardiman JW, Le Beau MM, et al [1985] Increased numbers of marrow basophils may be associated with a t(6;9) in ANLL. *Am J Hematol* 18:393-403.

Pedersen-Bjergaard J, Andersen MK, Andersen MT, Christiansen DH [2008] Genetics of therapy-related myelodysplasia and acute myeloid leukemia. *Leukemia* 22:240-248.

Peterson LC, Parkin JL, Arthur DC, Brunning RD [1991] Acute basophilic leukemia. A clinical, morphologic, and cytogenetic study of 8 cases. *Am J Clin Pathol* 96:160-170.

Pitman SD, Huang Q [2007] Granular acute lymphoblastic leukemia: a case report and literature review. *Am J Hematol* 82:834-837.

Pulsoni A, Pagano L, Lo Coco F, et al [2002] Clinicobiological features and outcome of acute promyelocytic leukemia occurring as a second tumor: the GIMEMA experience. *Blood* 100:1972-1976.

Ravandi F, Estey E, Jones D, et al [2009] Effective treatment of acute promyelocytic leukemia with all-trans-retinoic acid, arsenic trioxide, and gemtuzumab ozogamicin. *J Clin Oncol* 27:504-510.

Raza A, Buonamici S, Lisak L, et al [2004] Arsenic trioxide and thalidomide combination produces multi-lineage hematological responses in myelodysplastic syndromes patients, particularly in those with high pre-therapy EVI1 expression. *Leuk Res* 28:791-803.

Redner RL, Rush EA, Faas S, et al [1996] The t(5;17) variant of acute promyelocytic leukemia expresses a nucleophosmin-retinoic acid receptor fusion. *Blood* 87:882-886.

Ribeiro RC, Oliveira MS, Fairclough D, et al [1993] Acute megakaryoblastic leukemia in children and adolescents: a retrospective analysis of 24 cases. *Leuk Lymphoma* 10:299-306.

Rizzatti EG, Garcia AB, Portieres FL, et al [2002] Expression of CD117 and CD11b in bone marrow can differentiate acute promyelocytic leukemia from recovering benign myeloid proliferation. *Am J Clin Pathol* 118:31-37.

Rosenberg PS, Alter BP, Ebell W [2008a] Cancer risks in Fanconi anemia: findings from the German Fanconi Anemia Registry. *Haematologica* 93:511-517.

Rosenberg PS, Alter BP, Link DC, et al [2008b] Neutrophil elastase mutations and risk of leukaemia in severe congenital neutropenia. *Br J Haematol* 140:210-213.

Rosenthal NS, Farhi DC [1991] Dysmegakaryopoiesis resembling acute megakaryoblastic leukemia in treated acute myeloid leukemia. *Am J Clin Pathol* 95:556-560.

Roth JJ, Crist RC, Buchberg AM [2009] Might as well face it: MLL's addicted to HOX. *Blood* 113:2372-2373.

Rowe D, Cotterill SJ, Ross FM, et al [2000] Cytogenetically cryptic AML1—ETO and CBFbeta—MYH11 gene rearrangements: incidence in 412 cases of acute myeloid leukaemia. *Br J Haematol* 111:1051-1056.

Roy A, Roberts I, Norton A, Vyas P [2009] Acute megakaryoblastic leukaemia (AMKL) and transient myeloproliferative disorder (TMD) in Down syndrome: a multi-step model of myeloid leukaemogenesis. *Br J Haematol* 147:3-12.

Rund D, Krichevsky S, Bar-Cohen S, et al [2005] Therapy-related leukemia: clinical characteristics and analysis of new molecular risk factors in 96 adult patients. *Leukemia* 19:1919-1928.

Sainty D, Liso V, Cantu-Rajnoldi A, et al [2000] A new morphologic classification system for acute promyelocytic leukemia distinguishes cases with underlying PLZF/RARA gene rearrangements. Group Francais de Cytogenetique Hematologique, UK Cancer Cytogenetics Group and BIOMED 1 European Community-Concerted Action "Molecular Cytogenetic Diagnosis in Haematological Malignancies. *Blood* 96:1287-1296.

San Miguel JF, Martinez A, Macedo A, et al [1997] Immunophenotyping investigation of minimal residual disease is a useful approach for predicting relapse in acute myeloid leukemia patients. *Blood* 90:2465-2470.

San Miguel JF, Vidriales MB, Lopez-Berges C, et al [2001] Early immunophenotypical evaluation of minimal residual disease in acute myeloid leukemia identifies different patient risk groups and may contribute to postinduction treatment stratification. *Blood* 98:1746-1751.

Santamaria CM, Chillon MC, Garcia-Sanz R, et al [2009] Molecular stratification model for prognosis in cytogenetically normal acute myeloid leukemia. *Blood* 114:148-152.

Sanz M, Burnett A, Lo-Coco F, Lowenberg B [2009a] FLT3 inhibition as a targeted therapy for acute myeloid leukemia. *Curr Opin Oncol* 21:594-600.

Sanz MA, Grimwade D, Tallman MS, et al [2009b] Management of acute promyelocytic leukemia: recommendations from an expert panel on behalf of the European LeukemiaNet. *Blood* 113:1875-1891.

Schlenk RF, Benner A, Krauter J, et al [2004] Individual patient data-based meta-analysis of patients aged 16-60 years with core binding factor acute myeloid leukemia: a survey of the German Acute Myeloid Leukemia Intergroup. *J Clin Oncol* 22:3741-3750.

Schlenk RF, Dohner K, Krauter J, et al [2008] Mutations and treatment outcome in cytogenetically normal acute myeloid leukemia. *N Engl J Med* 358:1909-1918.

Schnittger S, Kohl TM, Haferlach T, et al [2006] KIT-D816 mutations in AML1-ETO-positive AML are associated with impaired event-free and overall survival. *Blood* 107:1791-1799.

Schnittger S, Schoch C, Kern W, et al [2005] Nucleophosmin gene mutations are predictors of favorable prognosis in acute myelogenous leukemia with a normal karyotype. *Blood* 106:3733-3739.

Schoch C, Schnittger S, Klaus M, et al [2003] AML with 11q23/MLL abnormalities as defined by the WHO classification: incidence, partner chromosomes, FAB subtype, age distribution, and prognostic impact in an unselected series of 1897 cytogenetically analyzed AML cases. *Blood* 102:2395-2402.

Seedhouse C, Russell N [2007] Advances in the understanding of susceptibility to treatment-related acute myeloid leukaemia. *Br J Haematol* 137:513-529.

Shimada A, Taki T, Tabuchi K, et al [2006] KIT mutations, and not FLT3 internal tandem duplication, are strongly associated with a poor prognosis in pediatric acute myeloid leukemia with t(8;21): a study of the Japanese Childhood AML Cooperative Study Group. *Blood* 107:1806-1809.

Shook D, Coustan-Smith E, Ribeiro RC, et al [2009] Minimal residual disease quantitation in acute myeloid leukemia. *Clin Lymphoma Myeloma* 9Suppl3:S281-285.

Shvidel L, Shaft D, Stark B, et al [2003] Acute basophilic leukaemia: 8 unsuspected new cases diagnosed by electron microscopy. *Br J Haematol* 120:774-781.

Slovak ML, Gundacker H, Bloomfield CD, et al [2006] A retrospective study of 69 patients with t(6;9)(p23;q34) AML emphasizes the need for a prospective, multicenter initiative for rare "poor prognosis" myeloid malignancies. *Leukemia* 20:1295-1297.

Slovak ML, Kopecky KJ, Cassileth PA, et al [2000] Karyotypic analysis predicts outcome of preremission and postremission therapy in adult acute myeloid leukemia: a Southwest Oncology Group/Eastern Cooperative Oncology Group Study. *Blood* 96:4075-4083.

Smith FO, Lampkin BC, Versteeg C, et al [1992] Expression of lymphoid-associated cell surface antigens by childhood acute myeloid leukemia cells lacks prognostic significance. *Blood* 79:2415-2422.

Smith SM, Le Beau MM, Huo D, et al [2003] Clinical-cytogenetic associations in 306 patients with therapy-related myelodysplasia and myeloid leukemia: the University of Chicago series. *Blood* 102:43-52.

Soekarman D, von Lindern M, van der Plas DC, et al [1992] DEK-CAN rearrangement in translocation (6;9)(p23;q34). *Leukemia* 6:489-494.

Speck NA, Gilliland DG [2002] Core-binding factors in haematopoiesis and leukaemia. *Nat Rev Cancer* 2:502-513.

Spencer DV, Cavalier M, Kalpatthi R, Quigley DI [2007] Inverted and deleted chromosome 16 with deletion of 3'CBFB identified by fluorescence in situ hybridization. *Cancer Genet Cytogenet* 179:82-84.

Sritana N, Auewarakul CU [2008] KIT and FLT3 receptor tyrosine kinase mutations in acute myeloid leukemia with favorable cytogenetics: 2 novel mutations and selective occurrence in leukemia subtypes and age groups. *Exp Mol Pathol* 85:227-231.

Stankova J, Mitchell D, Bernard C, et al [2006] Atypical presentation of acute promyelocytic leukaemia. *Br J Haematol* 132:379-380.

Stein E, McMahon B, Kwaan H, et al [2009] The coagulopathy of acute promyelocytic leukaemia revisited. *Best Pract Res Clin Haematol* 22:153-163.

Stirewalt DL, Radich JP [2003] The role of FLT3 in haematopoietic malignancies. *Nat Rev Cancer* 3:650-665.

Tallman MS, Altman JK [2009] How I treat acute promyelocytic leukemia. *Blood* 114:5126-5135.

Terwijn M, Feller N, van Rhenen A, et al [2009] Interleukin-2 receptor α-chain (CD25) expression on leukaemic blasts is predictive for outcome and level of residual disease in AML. *Eur J Cancer* 45:1692-1699.

Testoni N, Borsaru G, Martinelli G, et al [1999] 3q21 and 3q26 cytogenetic abnormalities in acute myeloblastic leukemia: biological and clinical features. *Haematologica* 84:690-694.

Thiede C, Steudel C, Mohr B, et al [2002] Analysis of FLT3-activating mutations in 979 patients with acute myelogenous leukemia: association with FAB subtypes and identification of subgroups with poor prognosis. *Blood* 99:4326-4335.

Thiele J, Kvasnicka HM, Zerhusen G, et al [2004] Acute panmyelosis with myelofibrosis: a clinicopathological study on 46 patients including histochemistry of bone marrow biopsies and follow-up. *Ann Hematol* 83:513-521.

Tiacci E, Pileri S, Orleth A, et al [2004] PAX5 expression in acute leukemias: higher B-lineage specificity than CD79a and selective association with t(8;21)-acute myelogenous leukemia. *Cancer Res* 64:7399-7404.

Tohyama K, Shiga S, Fujimoto H, et al [2003] Automated analysis of differentiation-induced leukemic cells during all-trans retinoic acid therapy of acute promyelocytic leukemia. *Arch Pathol Lab Med* 127:e4-10.

Tso AC, Kumaran TO, Bain BJ [2009] Case 41. A misdiagnosis of erythroleukemia. *Leuk Lymphoma* 50:1030-1032.

Tsou MF, Stearns T [2006] Controlling centrosome number: licenses and blocks. *Curr Opin Cell Biol* 18:74-78.

Valbuena JR, Medeiros LJ, Rassidakis GZ, et al [2006] Expression of B cell-specific activator protein/PAX5 in acute myeloid leukemia with t(8;21)(q22;q22). *Am J Clin Pathol* 126:235-240.

Valk PJ, Bowen DT, Frew ME, et al [2004] Second hit mutations in the RTK/RAS signaling pathway in acute myeloid leukemia with inv(16). *Haematologica* 89:106.

Van Maele-Fabry G, Duhayon S, Lison D [2007] A systematic review of myeloid leukemias and occupational pesticide exposure. *Cancer Causes Control* 18:457-478.

Vardiman J, Arber D, Brunning R, et al [2008a] Therapy-related myeloid neoplasms. In: Swerdlow S, Campo E, Harris N, et al, eds. *WHO Classification of Tumours: Pathology and Genetics: Tumours of Haematopoietic and Lymphoid Tissues.* Lyon, France: IARC Press; 127-129.

Vardiman J, Brunning R, Arber D, et al [2008b] Introduction and overview of the classification of the myeloid neoplasms. In: Swerdlow S, Campo E, Harris N, et al, eds. *WHO Classification of Tumours: Pathology and Genetics: Tumours of Haematopoietic and Lymphoid Tissues.* Lyon, France: IARC Press; 18-30.

Vardiman JW, Thiele J, Arber DA, et al [2009] The 2008 revision of the WHO classification of myeloid neoplasms and acute leukemia: rationale and important changes. *Blood* 114:937-951.

Velloso ER, Mecucci C, Michaux L, et al [1996] Translocation t(8;16)(p11;p13) in acute non-lymphocytic leukemia: report on 2 new cases and review of the literature. *Leuk Lymphoma* 21:137-142.

Venditti A, Tamburini A, Buccisano F, et al [2002] Clinical relevance of minimal residual disease detection in adult acute myeloid leukemia. *J Hematother Stem Cell Res* 11:349-357.

Vineis P, Alavanja M, Buffler P, et al [2004] Tobacco and cancer: recent epidemiological evidence. *J Natl Cancer Inst* 96:99-106.

von Lindern M, Fornerod M, Soekarman N, et al [1992] Translocation t(6;9) in acute non-lymphocytic leukaemia results in the formation of a DEK-CAN fusion gene. *Baillieres Clin Haematol* 5:857-879.

Wandt H, Schakel U, Kroschinsky F, et al [2008] MLD according to the WHO classification in AML has no correlation with age and no independent prognostic relevance as analyzed in 1766 patients. *Blood* 111:1855-1861.

Wang HY, Ding J, Vasef MA, Wilson KS [2009] A bcr3/short form PML-RARalpha transcript in an acute promyelocytic leukemia resulted from a derivative chromosome 17 due to submicroscopic insertion of the PML gene into the RARalpha locus. *Am J Clin Pathol* 131:64-71.

Wang ZY, Chen Z [2008] Acute promyelocytic leukemia: from highly fatal to highly curable. *Blood* 111:2505-2515.

Watanabe N, Kobayashi H, Ichiji O, et al [2003] Cryptic insertion and translocation or nondividing leukemic cells disclosed by FISH analysis in infant acute leukemia with discrepant molecular and cytogenetic findings. *Leukemia* 17:876-882.

Webb DK [2005] Optimizing therapy for myeloid disorders of Down syndrome. *Br J Haematol* 131:3-7.

Weinberg OK, Seetharam M, Ren L, et al [2009] Clinical characterization of acute myeloid leukemia with myelodysplasia-related changes as defined by the 2008 WHO classification system. *Blood* 113:1906-1908.

Weinberg O, Seetharam M, Ren L, et al [2010] Acute myeloid leukemia (AML) with monosomal karyotype is characterized by absence of *NPM1* and *FLT3* mutations, worse clinical outcome and usually falls within AML with myelodysplasia-related changes (MRC). *Mod Pathol* 23:328A.

Weisser M, Haferlach C, Hiddemann W, Schnittger S [2007] The quality of molecular response to chemotherapy is predictive for the outcome of AML1-ETO-positive AML and is independent of pretreatment risk factors. *Leukemia* 21:1177-1182.

Wells RA, Catzavelos C, Kamel-Reid S [1997] Fusion of retinoic acid receptor α to NuMA, the nuclear mitotic apparatus protein, by a variant translocation in acute promyelocytic leukaemia. *Nat Genet* 17:109-113.

Wheatley K, Brookes CL, Howman AJ, et al [2009] Prognostic factor analysis of the survival of elderly patients with AML in the MRC AML11 and LRF AML14 trials. *Br J Haematol* 145:598-605.

Whitman SP, Ruppert AS, Radmacher MD, et al [2008] FLT3 D835/I836 mutations are associated with poor disease-free survival and a distinct gene-expression signature among younger adults with de novo cytogenetically normal acute myeloid leukemia lacking FLT3 internal tandem duplications. *Blood* 111:1552-1559.

Wong KF, Chow E, Siu LL, Wong WS [2009a] Acute promyelocytic leukaemia with cryptic PML-RARA fusion. *Br J Haematol* 145:2.

Wong KF, Siu LL, Wong WS [2009b] Aleukaemic acute myeloid leukaemia with t(8;21)(q22;q22). *Br J Haematol* 146:345.

Wouters BJ, Lowenberg B, Erpelinck-Verschueren CA, et al [2009] Double CEBPA mutations, but not single CEBPA mutations, define a subgroup of acute myeloid leukemia with a distinctive gene expression profile that is uniquely associated with a favorable outcome. *Blood* 113:3088-3091.

Wu Y, Slovak ML, Snyder DS, Arber DA [2006] Coexistence of inversion 16 and the Philadelphia chromosome in acute and chronic myeloid leukemias : report of 6 cases and review of literature. *Am J Clin Pathol* 125:260-266.

Xavier AC, Ge Y, Taub JW [2009] Down syndrome and malignancies: a unique clinical relationship: a paper from the 2008 william beaumont hospital symposium on molecular pathology. *J Mol Diagn* 11:371-380.

Xu G, Kanezaki R, Toki T, et al [2006a] Physical association of the patient-specific GATA1 mutants with RUNX1 in acute megakaryoblastic leukemia accompanying Down syndrome. *Leukemia* 20:1002-1008.

Xu W, Zhou HF, Fan L, et al [2008] Trisomy 22 as the sole abnormality is an important marker for the diagnosis of acute myeloid leukemia with inversion 16. *Onkologie* 31:440-444.

Xu Y, McKenna RW, Wilson KS, et al [2006b] Immunophenotypic identification of acute myeloid leukemia with monocytic differentiation. *Leukemia* 20:1321-1324.

Xue Y, Yu F, Zhou Z, et al [1994] Translocation (8;21) in oligoblastic leukemia: is this a true myelodysplastic syndrome? *Leuk Res* 18:761-765.

Yanada M, Matsuo K, Suzuki T, et al [2005] Prognostic significance of FLT3 internal tandem duplication and tyrosine kinase domain mutations for acute myeloid leukemia: a meta-analysis. *Leukemia* 19:1345-1349.

Yeasmin S, Nakayama K, Ishibashi M, et al [2008] Therapy-related myelodysplasia and acute myeloid leukemia following paclitaxel- and carboplatin-based chemotherapy in an ovarian cancer patient: a case report and literature review. *Int J Gynecol Cancer* 18:1371-1376.

Yin CC, Medeiros LJ, Glassman AB, Lin P [2004] t(8;21)(q22,q22) in blast phase of chronic myelogenous leukemia. *Am J Clin Pathol* 121:836-842.

Yu Y, Maggi LB, Jr, Brady SN, et al [2006] Nucleophosmin is essential for ribosomal protein L5 nuclear export. *Mol Cell Biol* 26:3798-3809.

Yun JP, Chew EC, Liew CT, et al [2003] Nucleophosmin/B23 is a proliferate shuttle protein associated with nuclear matrix. *J Cell Biochem* 90:1140-1148.

Zhao W, Claxton DF, Medeiros LJ, et al [2006] Immunohistochemical analysis of CBFbeta-SMMHC protein reveals a unique nuclear localization in acute myeloid leukemia with inv(16)(p13q22). *Am J Surg Pathol* 30:1436-1444.

Zipursky A [2003] Transient leukaemia—a benign form of leukaemia in newborn infants with trisomy 21. *Br J Haematol* 120:930-938.

Zwaan CM, Meshinchi S, Radich JP, et al [2003] FLT3 internal tandem duplication in 234 children with acute myeloid leukemia: prognostic significance and relation to cellular drug resistance. *Blood* 102:2387-2394.

CHAPTER

Blastic Plasmacytoid Dendritic Cell Neoplasms in Bone Marrow

Kaaren Reichard, MD

B lastic plasmacytoid dendritic cell neoplasm (BPDCN) is an entity recently renamed based on cell culture experimental evidence indicating the plasmacytoid dendritic cell (pDC) as the putative cell of origin [Facchetti 2008]. Heretofore, this entity was known as blastic natural killer cell lymphoma (2001 WHO) and has been reported on using a wide variety of names, including agranular CD4+/CD56+ hematodermic tumor, primary cutaneous CD4+/CD56+ hematolymphoid neoplasm, etc t19.1 [Brody 1995, Chaperot 2001, Feuillard 2002, Herling 2003, Jacob 2003, Khoury 2002, Kimura 2001, Petrella 1999, 2002]. These varying terminologies reflect the typical BPDCN clinical presentation (hematodermic), its cytologic appearance (agrawnular and blastic), and previously thought cell of origin (natural killer [NK] cell).

Dendritic cells play a critical role in maintaining the immune system. One of their main functions is the presentation of antigens to T cells [Douagi 2009, Lipscomb 2002]. Two dendritic cell subsets include the plasmacytoid dendritic cell (pDC, DC2) and the myeloid dendritic cell (mDC, DC1). mDCs initiate a primary T-cell response, thereby potentiating acquired immunity, while pDCs in contrast produce large amounts of type 1 interferons contributing to their predominant antiviral innate immunity [Cao 2009]. Developmental pathways for human pDCs and mDCs remain enigmatic [Liu 2009]. However, mDCs and pDCs may originate from either common lymphoid or common myeloid precursors [Ishikawa 2007, Kadowaki 2009]. A putative developmental and maturational sequence of the pDC and mDC is presented in Chapter 1 (f1.3, p 9).

[19.1] Definition and Epidemiology

Blastic plasmacytoid dendritic cell neoplasm is a high-grade malignancy derived from pDCs [Facchetti 2008]. It is a distinct clinicopathologic entity characterized by typical involvement of skin and/or bone marrow [Chaperot 2001, Feuillard 2002, Petrella 1999]. This neoplasm may be referred to as "lineage negative" and, as such, is a diagnosis of exclusion [Garnache-Ottou 2009, Herling 2007, Jacob 2003, Reichard 2005]. BPDCN is a rare entity, the exact incidence of which is difficult to determine with certainty.

[19.2] Pathogenetic Mechanisms

To date, BPDCN is not known to be associated with Epstein-Barr virus infection or other viral etiology, but does exhibit some recurring cytogenetic abnormalities t19.2. The cytogenetic findings in BPDCN are generally complex, consisting of heterogeneous structural and numerical abnormalities. Alterations of 5q, 6q, chromosome 9, 12p, and

t19.1 Previous Terminologies for Blastic Plasmacytoid Dendritic Cell Neoplasm

Acute agranular CD4+ NK-cell leukemia

Primary cutaneous CD4+/CD56+ blastic hematolymphoid neoplasm

Agranular CD4+/CD56+ blastic NK cell leukemia/lymphoma

DC2 precursor acute leukemia

CD56+/TdT+ blastic NK cell tumor of skin

CD4+/CD56+ acute leukemia

Agranular CD4+/CD56+ hematodermic tumor

"Lineage negative" early plasmacytoid dendritic cell leukemia/lymphoma

DC2-related CD4+/CD56+ blastic tumor of skin

References: [Brody 1995, Chaperot 2001, Feuillard 2002, Herling 2003, Jacob 2003, Khoury 2002, Kimura 2001, Petrella 1999, 2002]

t19.2 Features of Blastic Plasmacytoid Dendritic Cell Neoplasm

Incidence	Very rare
Epidemiology	Male:female ratio of ~3:1
Clinical features	Disease of the elderly; rare pediatric cases
Morphology	"Lymphoblast-like," occasional cytoplasmic vacuoles or pseudopods, agranular
Blood/bone marrow	Involvement may be subtle to florid
Cytochemistry	Myeloperoxidase and non-specific esterase negative
Immunophenotype	Positive for CD4, CD56, CD123, TCL-1, BDCA-2, BDCA-4, CD2AP
	Exclusion of B-, T-, myelomonocytic and NK lineage
	Markers seen occasionally: TdT (may be weak and subset of cells), CD2, CD5, CD7, CD33, CD36, CD68, and CD99
	Epstein-Barr virus negative
Genetics	Complex karyotype
	Recurring abnormalities of 5q, 6q, chromosome 9, 12p, 13q
	T-cell receptor and B-cell IGH@ germline
Outcome	Resistant to conventional chemotherapy
	Aggressive clinical course
	Medial survival of 12-16 months

NK = natural killer

13q have been reported to be recurrent [Leroux 2002]. Recent gene expression profiling studies in conjunction with comparative genomic hybridization demonstrate that BPDCN is characterized by deletions of chromosomes 4q, 9, and 13 [Dijkman 2007, Jardin 2009]. Interestingly, high expression levels of pDC-related genes were also noted, providing further evidence for the pDC as the cell of origin.

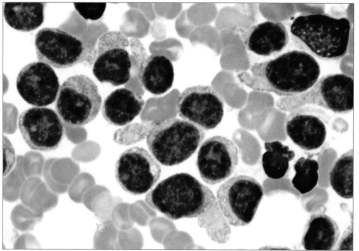

i19.1 *Typical cytologic features of blastic plasmacytoid dendritic cell neoplasm in bone marrow aspirate smear: small to intermediate size cells, fine, yet somewhat condensed chromatin, inconspicuous nucleoli and scant cytoplasm. (Wright)*

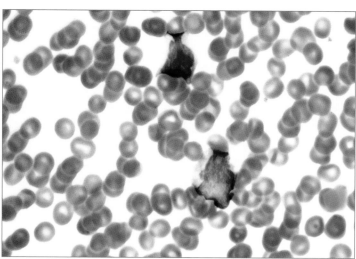

i19.2 *Circulating plasmacytoid dendritic cells in the peripheral blood showing morphologic overlap with lymphoblastic leukemia. (Wright)*

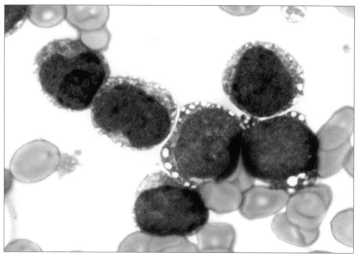

i19.3 *Blastic plasmacytoid dendritic cell neoplasm in a bone marrow aspirate smear exhibiting circumferential cytoplasmic vacuolization, so-called "pearl necklace" appearance. (Wright)*

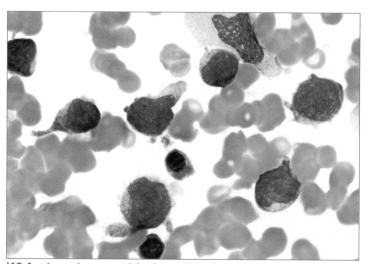

i19.4 *Blastic plasmacytoid dendritic cell neoplasm in a bone marrow aspirate smear exhibiting pseudopod-like morphology. (Wright)*

[19.3] ## Classification

Both cytology and immunophenotypic studies are essential in the diagnosis of BPDCN **t19.2**. The cytologic features are predominantly "lymphoblast-like," including small to intermediate size, fine chromatin, inconspicuous nucleoli, and scant cytoplasm **i19.1**, **i19.2**. On occasion, the cytoplasm harbors small vacuoles that encircle the nucleus (so-called "pearl necklace") **i19.3** or shows a pseudopod-like tail extension **i19.4**. In some cases the tumor cells exhibit features of myeloid/monocytic blasts with more abundant cytoplasm and prominent nucleoli **i19.5**; however, cytoplasmic granules should not be seen.

In early involvement of the bone marrow, BPDCN shows a nonparatrabecular nodular or, less commonly, a patchy interstitial infiltration pattern. Such lesions may be morphologically occult; therefore immunophenotypic studies are

prudent. In late stage disease, generally at relapse or disease progression, BPDCN effaces the marrow with only rare foci of residual hematopoietic elements **i19.6**. In such instances, the neoplastic cells circulate in the peripheral blood, and there is associated anemia and thrombocytopenia.

Immunophenotyping is essential in identifying the tumor cells as plasmacytoid dendritic cells (positive for CD4, CD56, CD123, TCL-1, BDCA-2, BDCA-4, CD2AP) **t19.2 i19.7**, **i19.8** [Garnache-Ottou 2009, Jaye 2006, Marafioti 2008, Pilichowska 2007]. CD22 may be detected on BPDCN with the s-HLC-1–specific antibody clone [Reineks 2009]. Blastic morphologic mimics should be excluded by specific lineage assessment (B-, T-, NK-, and myelomonocytic lineage) **t19.3**. Taken individually, many of the pDC markers listed herein are not specific to BPDCN. For example, CD4 is seen on monocytic cells, CD56 on aberrant myeloid cells, NK tumors, and plasma cell myeloma,

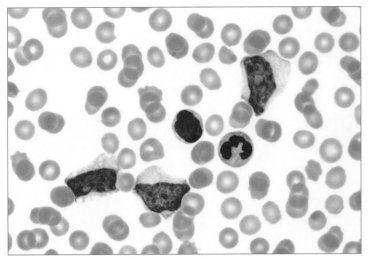

i19.5 *Blastic plasmacytoid dendritic cells in the peripheral blood exhibiting more abundant cytoplasm and occasional nucleoli mimicking a blastic myeloid process. (Wright)*

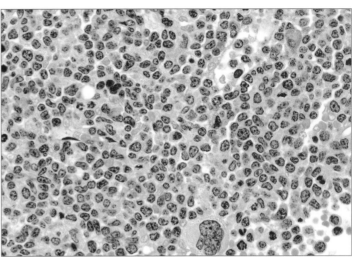

i19.6 *Bone marrow core biopsy nearly completely effaced by blastic plasmacytoid dendritic cell neoplasm. A rare residual megakaryocyte is visible. (H&E)*

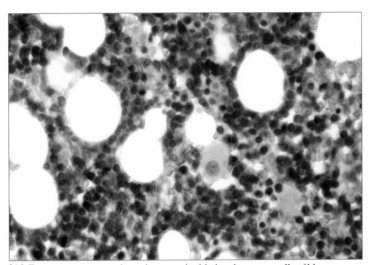

i19.7 *CD123 immunohistochemistry highlights the tumor cells of blastic plasmacytoid dendritic cell neoplasm in the bone marrow. A residual megakaryocyte is negative. (immunohistochemistry for CD123)*

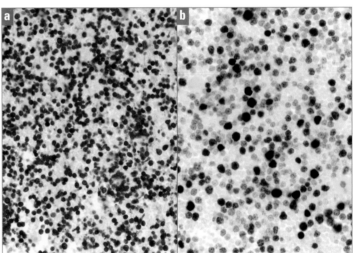

i19.8 *TCL-1 expression is prominent in this case of blastic plasmacytoid dendritic cell neoplasm in the bone marrow **a**; Ki-67 immunostain reveals an increased proliferation rate consistent with a blastic process **b**. (immunohistochemistry for TCL-1 and Ki-67)*

---

t19.3 Diagnostic Strategies to Distinguish Blastic Plasmacytoid Dendritic Cell Neoplasm from Morphologic Mimics

Lymphoblastic leukemia	B-lineage	CD19, CD20, CD79a, strong and uniform TdT, strong CD34
	T-lineage	CD1a, CD3, CD4 and/or CD8, TCR+, strong CD34
Acute myeloid leukemia	Clinical	May form subcutaneous nodules in 15% of cases, but generally florid marrow involvement at presentation
	Immunophenotype	Uniform expression of myeloid markers CD13, CD33 and/or monocytic markers CD36/CD64, CD14
	Cytochemistry	MPO+ or NSE+ (for monocytic)
Aggressive NK leukemia/lymphoma	EBER+, cytotoxic granule +	
Blastic mantle cell lymphoma	B-cell markers positive, surface light chain restricted, cyclin D1+	
Myeloid neoplasm with plasmacytoid dendritic cell nodules/proliferation	pDC nodules may be clonally related to myeloid neoplasm	

EBER = Epstein-Barr virus–encoded small RNAs; MPO = myeloperoxidase; NK = natural killer; NSE = nonspecific esterase (α-naphthyl butyrate esterase); pDC = plasmacytoid dendritic cell; TCR = T-cell receptor rearrangement; TdT = terminal deoxynucleotidyl transferase

References: [Chen 2003, Garnache-Ottou 2009, Herling 2007, Petrella 2004, Reichard 2005]

CD123 on some acute myeloid leukemias, and TCL-1 in T-cell prolymphocytic leukemia (T-PLL). CD123 is the interleukin 3 receptor α chain and is expressed on >90% of BPDCN cases. CD123, however, is also present on various other potential differential diagnostic mimics, including acute myeloid leukemia (all types except acute megakaryoblastic) and B-cell lymphoblastic leukemia (aka precursor B-cell acute lymphoblastic leukemia [ALL]) [Garnache-Ottou 2009, Munoz 2001]. The pattern of CD123 expression in some myelomonocytic leukemias is reported to be dim, in contrast to the strong positivity in BPDCN [Herling 2003]. T-cell leukemia-1 (TCL-1) is an Akt kinase regulator with normal expression limited to plasmacytoid dendritic cells and B cells. In tumors, TCL-1 is a molecular hallmark of T-PLL and is also seen in some B-cell lymphomas and rare cases of precursor T-cell ALL [Herling 2004]. TCL-1 is consistently negative in cases of CD123+ myelomonocytic leukemias, which can be helpful in diagnostically difficult cases [Herling 2003, Petrella 2004]. Therefore, only when these markers are seen *in aggregate* and without evidence of another lineage origin may the diagnosis of BPDCN be made with confidence. Other immunohistochemical markers that are seen in subsets of normal pDCs may be detected on occasion on BPDCN and include TdT (may be weak) (~40%-50%), CD2, CD7, CD33, and CD68 [Herling 2007].

Cytogenetic studies should be pursued in all cases to ensure that a recurring abnormality more characteristic of a non-BPDCN disorder (eg, *BCR-ABL1* fusion, *MLL* rearrangement) is not present.

[19.4] Differential Diagnosis and Diagnostic Strategies

Blastic plasmacytoid dendritic cell neoplasm must be distinguished from other blastic neoplasms and aggressive leukemias t19.3, i19.9 [Garnache-Ottou 2009, Herling 2007, Petrella 2004, Reichard 2005]. Such distinction can be made using an integrated approach of morphology, cytochemistry, immunophenotyping, cytogenetics, and molecular studies. Morphologically, one may encounter certain clues to the diagnosis of BPDCN (eg, cutaneous neoplasm with cytoplasmic pseudopods or pearl necklace distribution of vacuoles in the cytoplasm) but these are rarely encountered and, as individual findings, are nonspecific.

Distinction of BPDCN from lymphoblastic leukemia/lymphoma can be achieved most readily with immunophenotypic studies. The latter will demonstrate B- or T-cell associated markers and often markers of immaturity (strong CD34 and strong, uniform TdT). Although BPDCN may express CD2, CD5, or CD7 on occasion (generally at low levels), CD3, CD1a, and CD34 are invariably absent. TdT is not as helpful in distinguishing between lymphoblastic

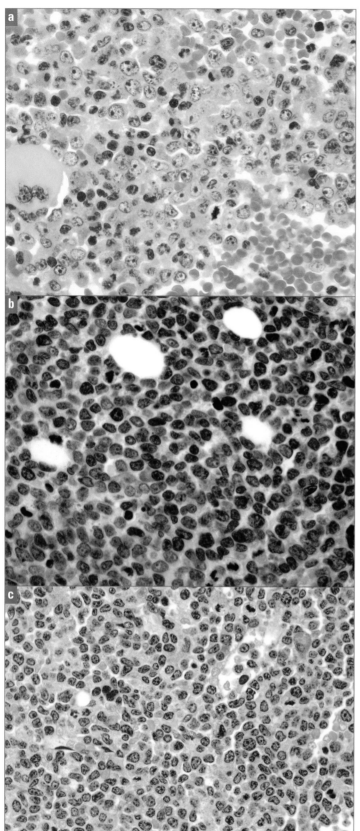

i19.9 *Blastic-appearing processes in the bone marrow requiring distinction from blastic plasmacytoid dendritic cell neoplasm: acute myeloid leukemia* **a**, *lymphoblastic leukemia* **b**, *blastic plasmacytoid dendritic cell neoplasm (BPDCN)* **c**. *The morphologic resemblance of BPDCN to lymphoblastic leukemia is evident in this composite photograph. (H&E)*

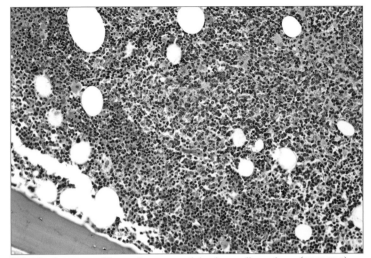

i19.10 *Concurrent blastic plasmacytoid dendritic cell neoplasm (BPDCN) and essential thrombocythemia in a bone marrow core biopsy. The BPDCN forms a vaguely nodular focus (upper right). (H&E)*

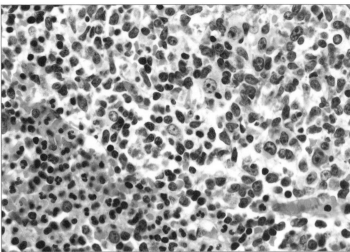

i19.11 *Higher-magnification image of concurrent BPDCN and essential thrombocythemia in a bone marrow core biopsy (see **i19.10**). The BPDCN forms a vaguely nodular focus (upper right). Note cytologic feature of the blastic plasmacytoid dendritic cells. (H&E)*

leukemias and BPDCN, as it is present in approximately 50% of BPDCN cases. However, TdT may be of weaker intensity and be present in only a subset of tumor cells in BPDCN.

Distinction of BPDCN from immature myeloid processes may be difficult, but extensive immunophenotypic and cytochemical findings are generally sufficient **t19.3**. Myeloperoxidase or nonspecific esterase positivity excludes the diagnosis of BPDCN.

Also in the differential diagnosis of a high-grade blastic malignancy with lymphoblast-like morphology are aggressive T-cell/NK cell processes. Epstein-Barr virus positivity is very useful in this regard, as it excludes BPDCN as a diagnostic consideration.

If the aforementioned differential diagnostic possibilities appear excluded, then assessing for CD123, TCL-1, and BDCA-2 provide further support for the diagnosis of BPDCN in this immunophenotypic context.

Occasionally, collections of plasmacytoid dendritic cells (pDCs) are seen in association with a myeloid neoplasm (most commonly chronic myelomonocytic leukemia) (see Chapter 17). These collections of plasmacytoid monocytes or "interferon-producing cells" occur in bone marrow and nodal sites. They may even be clonally related to the myeloid tumor [Vermi 2004]. These nodular pDC proliferations have been argued to represent an "intermediate stage of differentiation" between normal and frankly leukemic pDCs [Chen 2003]. In some cases, these nodules look very blastic and atypical. BPDCN may also occur concurrently with a myeloid disorder **i19.10**, **i19.11**.

t19.4 Components of the Diagnostic Interpretation of Blastic Neoplasms in Bone Marrow

Determine blastic morphology in blood and marrow

Perform extensive immunophenotyping with flow cytometry and/or immunohistochemistry to evaluate for B-, T-, NK- and myeloid lineages

Supplement immunoprofile with CD123, TCL-1, and BDCA-2 if a CD4+CD56+ "lineage-negative" process is encountered

Perform cytochemical studies (MPO and NSE) to definitively exclude myeloid and monocytic lineage as available

In bone marrow (and extramedullary sites), be careful to evaluate background cellular process for presence of an associated myeloid disorder, in cases with pDC nodular collections

MPO = myeloperoxidase; NSE = nonspecific esterase; pDC = plasmacytoid dendritic cell

[19.5] Components of the Diagnostic Interpretation

Blastic plasmacytoid dendritic cell neoplasm is a rare but distinctive entity that involves bone marrow in ~20%-40% of cases at presentation but >90% at relapse. Key points to assist in its distinction from other blastic-appearing lesions involve use of immunophenotyping and often cytogenetics. **t19.4** suggests an approach to the workup of these lesions.

[19.6] Clues and Caveats

1. BPDCN is rare and a diagnosis of exclusion.
2. BPDCN morphology and bone marrow infiltration pattern mimic acute leukemia of all types, but mainly lymphoblastic leukemia.

3. BPDCNs are derived from pDCs, which are important mediators in innate immunity.

4. BPDCNs display characteristic cutaneous and/or blood/ marrow involvement (so-called hematodermic).

5. The classic immunophenotypic profile of BPDCNs is CD4+, CD56+, HLA-DR+, CD123+, TCL-1+, and BDCA-2+.

6. T-cell (CD2, CD5, CD7) or myeloid-associated antigens (CD33) may be detected in a small fraction of cases.

7. Rare cases are CD56–.

8. Highly aggressive despite initial response to therapy (median survival ~12 months)

9. BPDCNs may occur prior, concurrent, or subsequent to myeloid, particularly myelomonocytic, neoplasms.

10. Nodular collections of pDCs (aka plasmacytoid monocytes or interferon-producing cells) are common in myeloid disorders, particularly myelodysplasia and chronic myelomonocytic leukemia.

[19.7] References

Brody JP, Allen S, Schulman P, et al [1995] Acute agranular CD4+ natural killer cell leukemia. Comprehensive clinicopathologic studies including virologic and in vitro culture with inducing agents. *Cancer* 75:2474-2483.

Cao W [2009] Molecular characterization of human plasmacytoid dendritic cells. *J Clin Immunol* 29:257-264.

Chaperot L, Bendriss N, Manches O, et al [2001] Identification of a leukemic counterpart of the plasmacytoid dendritic cells. *Blood* 97:3210-3217.

Chen YC, Chou JM, Ketterling RP, et al [2003] Histologic and immunohistochemical study of bone marrow monocytic nodules in 21 cases with myelodysplasia. *Am J Clin Pathol* 120:874-881.

Dijkman R, van Doorn R, Szuhai K, et al [2007] Gene-expression profiling and array-based CGH classify CD4+CD56+ hematodermic neoplasm and cutaneous myelomonocytic leukemia as distinct disease entities. *Blood* 109:1720-1727.

Douagi I, Gujer C, Sundling C, et al [2009] Human B cell responses to TLR ligands are differentially modulated by myeloid and plasmacytoid dendritic cells. *J Immunol* 182:1991-2001.

Facchetti F, Jones D, Petrella T [2008] Blastic plasmacytoid dendritic cell neoplasm. In: Swerdlow S, Campo E, Harris N, et al, eds. *WHO Classification of Tumours: Pathology & Genetics: Tumours of Haematopoietic and Lymphoid Tissues*. Lyon, France: IARC Press; 145-147.

Feuillard J, Jacob MC, Valensi F, et al [2002] Clinical and biologic features of CD4+CD56+ malignancies. *Blood* 99:1556-1563.

Garnache-Ottou F, Feuillard J, Ferrand C, et al [2009] Extended diagnostic criteria for plasmacytoid dendritic cell leukaemia. *Br J Haematol* 145:624-636.

Herling M, Jones D [2007] CD4+/CD56+ hematodermic tumor: the features of an evolving entity and its relationship to dendritic cells. *Am J Clin Pathol* 127:687-700.

Herling M, Khoury JD, Washington LT, et al [2004] A systematic approach to diagnosis of mature T-cell leukemias reveals heterogeneity among WHO categories. *Blood* 104:328-335.

Herling M, Teitell MA, Shen RR, et al [2003] TCL1 expression in plasmacytoid dendritic cells (DC2s) and the related CD4+ CD56+ blastic tumors of skin. *Blood* 101:5007-5009.

Ishikawa F, Niiro H, Iino T, et al [2007] The developmental program of human dendritic cells is operated independently of conventional myeloid and lymphoid pathways. *Blood* 110:3591-3660.

Jacob MC, Chaperot L, Mossuz P, et al [2003] CD4+ CD56+ lineage negative malignancies: a new entity developed from malignant early plasmacytoid dendritic cells. *Haematologica* 88:941-955.

Jardin F, Callanan M, Penther D, et al [2009] Recurrent genomic aberrations combined with deletions of various tumour suppressor genes may deregulate the G1/S transition in CD4+CD56+ haematodermic neoplasms and contribute to the aggressiveness of the disease. *Leukemia* 23:698-707.

Jaye DL, Geigerman CM, Herling M, et al [2006] Expression of the plasmacytoid dendritic cell marker BDCA-2 supports a spectrum of maturation among CD4+ CD56+ hematodermic neoplasms. *Mod Pathol* 19:1555-1562.

Kadowaki N [2009] The divergence and interplay between pDC and mDC in humans. *Front Biosci* 14:808-817.

Khoury JD, Medeiros LJ, Manning JT, et al [2002] CD56(+) TdT(+) blastic natural killer cell tumor of the skin: a primitive systemic malignancy related to myelomonocytic leukemia. *Cancer* 94:2401-2408.

Kimura S, Kakazu N, Kuroda J, et al [2001] Agranular CD4+CD56+ blastic natural killer leukemia/lymphoma. *Ann Hematol* 80:228-231.

Leroux D, Mugneret F, Callanan M, et al [2002] CD4+, CD56+ DC2 acute leukemia is characterized by recurrent clonal chromosomal changes affecting 6 major targets: a study of 21 cases by the Groupe Français de Cytogénétique Hématologique. *Blood* 99:4154-4159.

Lipscomb MF, Masten BJ [2002] Dendritic cells: immune regulators in health and disease. *Physiol Rev* 82:97-130.

Liu K, Victora GD, Schwickert TA, et al [2009] In vivo analysis of dendritic cell development and homeostasis. *Science* 324:392-397.

Marafioti T, Paterson JC, Ballabio E, et al [2008] Novel markers of normal and neoplastic human plasmacytoid dendritic cells. *Blood* 111:3778-3792.

Munoz L, Nomdedeu JF, Lopez O, et al [2001] Interleukin-3 receptor α chain (CD123) is widely expressed in hematologic malignancies. *Haematologica* 86:1261-1269.

Petrella T, Comeau MR, Maynadie M, et al [2002] Agranular CD4+ CD56+ hematodermic neoplasm (blastic NK-cell lymphoma) originates from a population of CD56+ precursor cells related to plasmacytoid monocytes. *Am J Surg Pathol* 26:852-862.

Petrella T, Dalac S, Maynadie M, et al [1999] CD4+ CD56+ cutaneous neoplasms: a distinct hematological entity? *Am J Surg Pathol* 23:137-146.

Petrella T, Meijer CJ, Dalac S, et al [2004] TCL1 and CLA expression in agranular CD4/CD56 hematodermic neoplasms (blastic NK-cell lymphomas) and leukemia cutis. *Am J Clin Pathol* 122:307-313.

Pilichowska ME, Fleming MD, Pinkus JL, Pinkus GS [2007] CD4+/CD56+ hematodermic neoplasm ("blastic natural killer cell lymphoma"): neoplastic cells express the immature dendritic cell marker BDCA-2 and produce interferon. *Am J Clin Pathol* 128:445-453.

Reichard KK, Burks EJ, Foucar MK, et al [2005] CD4(+) CD56(+) lineage-negative malignancies are rare tumors of plasmacytoid dendritic cells. *Am J Surg Pathol* 29:1274-1283.

Reineks EZ, Osei ES, Rosenberg A, et al [2009] CD22 expression on blastic plasmacytoid dendritic cell neoplasms and reactivity of anti-CD22 antibodies to peripheral blood dendritic cells. *Cytometry B Clin Cytom* 76B:237-248.

Vermi W, Facchetti F, Rosati S, et al [2004] Nodal and extranodal tumor-forming accumulation of plasmacytoid monocytes/interferon-producing cells associated with myeloid disorders. *Am J Surg Pathol* 28:585-595.

Acute Leukemias of Ambiguous Lineage

David Czuchlewski, MD

Since 1845, when Bennett and Virchow first described acute leukemia, diagnosis has involved the application of morphologic, cytochemical, immunophenotypic, and genetic techniques of steadily increasing complexity to characterize a population of leukemic blasts [Degos 2001]. One of the most fundamental obligations of the diagnostic hematopathologist is to assign a lineage to a given acute leukemia, allowing prognostic expectations and optimal treatment to be matched to the particular identity of the blasts. In some cases, however, the disease process refuses to cooperate with this project of subcategorization. Such "acute leukemias of ambiguous lineage" are rare, but they present a significant diagnostic challenge and, by their very oddity, offer important insights into the process of leukemogenesis itself.

[20.1] Definition of Acute Leukemias of Ambiguous Lineage

Historically, the concept of acute leukemia of ambiguous lineage has been considerably confused by definitional and nosological issues. One fundamental stumbling block has been the very frequent (~20%) coexpression on blasts of markers that are considered, in other contexts, to be characteristic of separate and distinct lineages [Cruse 2005, El-Sissy 2006, Thalhammer-Scherrer 2002]. This "cross-lineage" antigen expression may be seen, for example, in the routine identification of B-cell markers such as PAX5 and CD19 on myeloid blasts with the t(8;21)(q22;q22), or in the expression of CD2 by the majority of myeloid blasts with inv(16)(p13.1q22) or t(16;16)(p13.1;q22) [Adriaansen 1993, He 2008, Hurwitz 1992, Kita 1992, Kozlov 2005, Tiacci 2004, Weir 2001]. Yet, as every other aspect of these cells' biology and behavior is consistent with acute myeloid leukemia (AML), the expression of these unexpected antigens is considered to be anomalous behavior by a myeloid clone, rather that indicative of fundamental ambiguity in the lineage of derivation. The first important concept to appreciate when considering acute leukemias of ambiguous lineage is: *not all cross-lineage antigen expression defines a leukemic clone as ambiguous in its lineage.*

Given this, one is immediately prompted to ask, "Then *how much* cross-lineage antigen expression is sufficient to consider a case truly ambiguous?" This question has provoked a great deal of disagreement, both in the literature and in historical classification schemes. The 2001 World Health Organization (WHO) classification, for example, endorsed the European Group for the Immunological Characterization of Acute Leukemias (EGIL) scoring system, which assigned different "weights" to the expression of different antigens [Bene 1995], but many editions of the 2001 WHO book included

t20.1 WHO 2008 Criteria for Assigning >1 Lineage to a Single Blast Population

Assign myeloid lineage if	MPO positive (by flow, IPOX, or cytochemistry)
	or
	2 or more of the following: NSE, CD11c, CD14, CD64, lysozyme (ie, monocytic differentiation)
Assign T-cell lineage if	Cytoplasmic CD3*
	or
	Surface CD3
Assign B-cell lineage if	*Strong* CD19 with strong expression of *1* of the following (CD79a, cytoplasmic CD22, CD10)
	or
	Weak CD19 with strong expression of *2* of the following (CD79a, cytoplasmic CD22, CD10)[†]

*Monoclonal antibodies to CD3 ε chain, typically via flow cytometry, must be used; IPOX with polyclonal CD3 antibodies may also detect CD3 ζ chain, which is not T-cell specific and may be present in NK cells
[†]WHO does allow B lineage to be assigned if CD19 is negative; however, as CD79a and CD10 lack B-lineage specificity on their own, as a general rule B lineage should *almost never* be diagnosed without at least weak CD19 expression
MPO = myeloperoxidase; NSE = nonspecific esterase; WHO = World Health Organization

an unfortunate misprint in the description of the threshold score necessary to assign a given lineage [Bagg 2007]. Many "acute leukemias of ambiguous lineage" described in the literature were diagnosed as such using variable and even less stringent criteria, complicating our understanding of the phenomenon.

The current 2008 WHO classification proposes a comparatively strict and specific set of criteria that must be fulfilled before making the diagnosis of acute leukemia of ambiguous lineage [Borowitz 2008]. These criteria, which take into account much of the prognostic and pathophysiologic data discussed herein, are summarized in t20.1 and presented in algorithmic form in f20.1, f20.2, f20.3. Essentially, there are 3 ways to arrive at a firm diagnostic multilineage phenotype for a single population of blasts:
1. Identify myeloid lineage through expression of myeloperoxidase or multiple monocytic markers
2. Identify T-cell lineage through expression of cytoplasmic CD3 (or surface CD3)
3. Identify B-cell lineage through expression of CD19 in concert with other markers

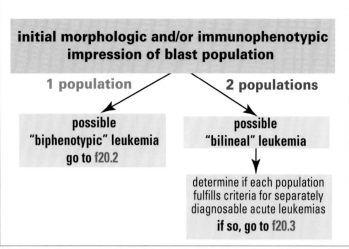

f20.1 *Initial recognition of possible acute leukemia of ambiguous lineage.*

When 2 of the aforementioned conditions are simultaneously satisfied, the resulting overlap in immunophenotype justifies a diagnosis of acute leukemia of ambiguous lineage.

As illustrated in **f20.1**, there are 2 ways in which a population of leukemic cells can be ambiguous in lineage:

1. A single population coexpressing the ambiguous markers (ie, "biphenotypic" leukemia)
2. Two distinct populations, each of which is diagnosable as a distinct acute leukemia (ie, "bilineage" or "bilineal" leukemia) **i20.1, i20.2, i20.3**

In addition, when leukemic blasts do not satisfy *any* of the preceding criteria for a particular lineage, they are by definition ambiguous in lineage; great care must be exercised, however, to avoid misdiagnosing a leukemia of other rare derivation, or even a nonhematopoietic tumor, as such a truly undifferentiated leukemia.

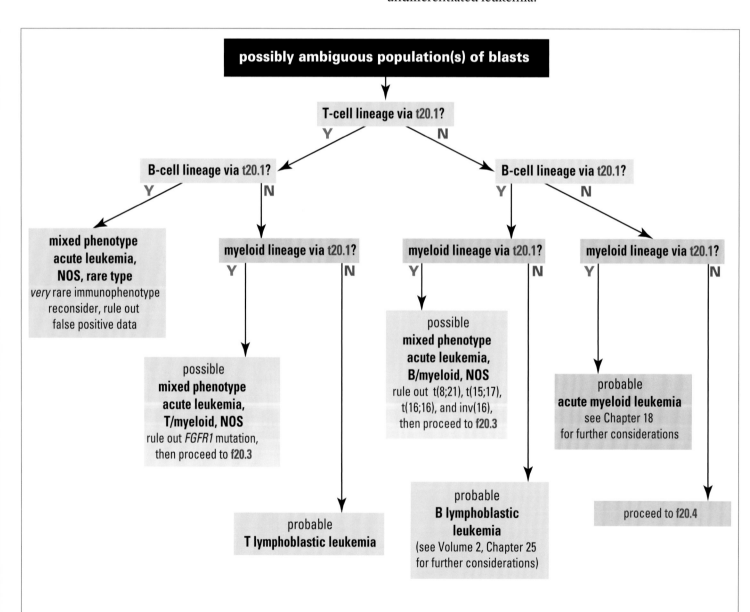

f20.2 *Assessment of a single population of possibly ambiguous blasts.*

While the definition of acute leukemia of ambiguous lineage is now relatively more specific, it remains by necessity a diagnosis of exclusion. Thus, if a leukemia fulfills the criteria for another diagnostic entity (eg, chronic myelogenous leukemia [CML] in blast phase), then the more specific entity takes precedence over the ambiguous phenotype. A complete strategy for navigating the complex definitional requirements is presented in [20.3] "Diagnostic Considerations for Acute Leukemias of Ambiguous Lineage."

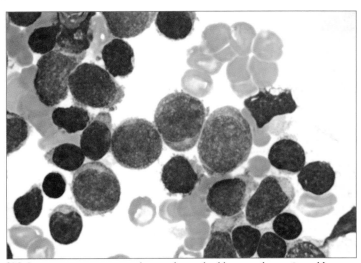

i20.1 Bone marrow aspirate shows a dimorphic blast population. Some blasts are lymphoid in character, with relatively smooth chromatin and smaller size, while others are larger with slightly more open chromatin, imparting a myeloid appearance. As depicted in f20.1, this finding raises the possibility of a bilineal leukemia.

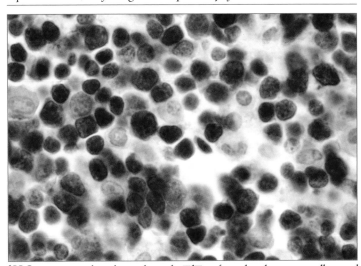

i20.2 An immunohistochemical stain for TdT performed on the same case illustrated in i20.1 shows that the smaller blasts are strongly TdT positive. Flow cytometry also identified strong expression of CD79a and CD19, confirming B-cell phenotype as required in f20.1.

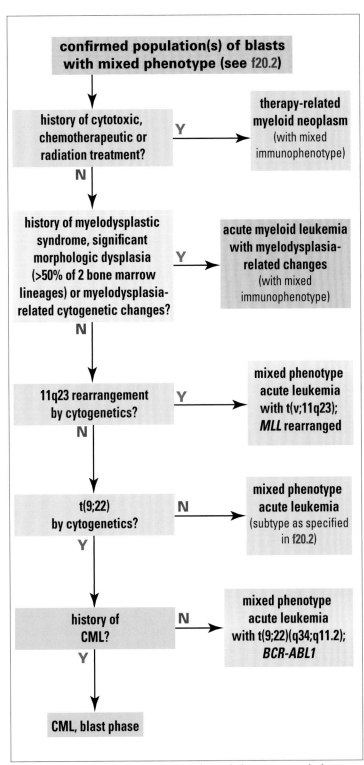

f20.3 Specific entities to rule out confirmed mixed phenotype acute leukemia

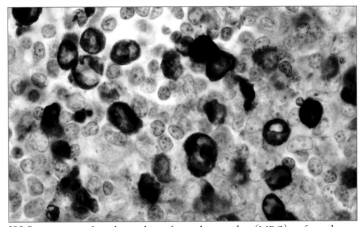

i20.3 An immunohistochemical stain for myeloperoxidase (MPO) performed on the same case illustrated in i21.1 and i20.2 shows that a subset of the larger blasts express MPO, satisfying the criteria for myeloid lineage set forth in f20.1. The blasts were found to harbor the t(9;22), and the 18-year-old patient did not have a history of chronic myelogenous leukemia. Therefore the final diagnosis, according to f20.3, is mixed phenotype acute leukemia with t(9;22)(q34;q11.2); BCR-ABL1.

[20.2] Morphology of Acute Leukemias of Ambiguous Lineage

Since the definition of acute leukemia of ambiguous lineage rests on immunophenotypic data, there are no morphologic clues specifically associated with the diagnosis. In general, however, there are 2 situations in which morphology may be the first indication of an ambiguous lineage.

1. 2 distinct populations of blasts are present, often including some smaller and lymphoid in appearance and some larger and more myeloid in appearance
2. Blasts are completely morphologically uninformative, with convincing features of neither lymphoid nor myeloid derivation

Importantly, in both situations, the leukemia will turn out, in the vast majority of cases, to be a "garden variety" entity upon full immunophenotyping. At best, these morphologic features only prompt the pathologist to specifically consider (and usually exclude) an ambiguous phenotype by the methodical application of ancillary techniques.

[20.3] Diagnostic Considerations for Acute Leukemias of Ambiguous Lineage

The most important diagnostic consideration when entertaining a diagnosis of acute leukemias of ambiguous lineage is maintaining an awareness of the rarity of the entity. Acute leukemias of ambiguous lineage are thought to account for 3%-5% of all cases of acute leukemia [Bagg 2007, Han 2007, Killick 1999, Thalhammer-Scherrer 2002], and, as discussed earlier ([20.1] "Definition of Acute Leukemias of Ambiguous Lineage," p 441), even this number is almost certainly falsely inflated by past imprecision in rendering the diagnosis. Given the infrequency of bona fide cases of acute leukemia of ambiguous lineage, the best overall strategy for pursuing this diagnosis is to assume that a case in fact will fall short of true lineage ambiguity, and then endeavor to prove the opposite.

The initial step in diagnosing an acute leukemia of ambiguous lineage is the recognition of possible mixed phenotype. This may occur to the pathologist on encountering morphologic characteristics that do not seem to support definitive lineage or after initial immunophenotypic analysis, which should be broad enough to screen for mixed phenotype by including at least CD19, cytoplasmic CD3, and myeloperoxidase (MPO). As seen in f20.1, if there is a single apparently ambiguous population, then a "biphenotypic" acute leukemia becomes a possibility; if 2 separate blast populations are present, then a "bilineal" process may be at work. In the case of a bilineal process, a mixed phenotype acute leukemia is present when each blast population is separately diagnostic of different lineage-specific acute leukemias, with the caveat that the usual numeric criteria (>20% blasts for AML) do not apply. The next step in cases of apparent biphenotypic nature, rigorous application of

the WHO 2008 criteria for lineage assignment, is detailed in f20.2 and t20.1.

If no lineage can be assigned at all according to t20.1, an acute undifferentiated leukemia becomes a leading contender in the differential diagnosis. However, this entity *cannot* be established simply by application of the criteria in t20.1. Nonhematopoietic neoplasms, NK-cell leukemias, and even some myeloid processes such as acute erythroid leukemia, acute megakaryoblastic leukemia, and blastic plasmacytoid dendritic cell neoplasm may all fail to express the necessary lineage markers listed in t20.1. Rhabdomyosarcoma in particular is infamous for masquerading as an acute leukemia and should be ruled out, along with the other entities mentioned, before establishing a diagnosis of acute undifferentiated leukemia [Chen 2004, Naithani 2007, Shinkoda 2009].

Very occasionally, an acute leukemia will fail to express the required antigens in t20.1, and yet will express "nondefinitive" antigens that hint at lineages (eg, a neoplasm that shows no B-cell markers, is CD3– and MPO–, but positive for CD7, CD5, CD13, and CD33). Such cases should *not* be considered "acute undifferentiated leukemias," because there is an apparent attempt at differentiation, albeit contradictory and/or insufficient for definitive lineage assignment. The term "acute unclassifiable leukemia" is recommended in this case, and the diagnosis would necessitate a long comment detailing the documented immunophenotype and the reasoning behind the diagnostic conundrum. The WHO suggests that lack of an assignable lineage based on the criteria in t20.1, in combination with expression of *no more* than one "nondefinitive" antigen (eg, CD13) for any given lineage, could be called "acute undifferentiated leukemia," while similar neoplasms with *more* than one suggestive antigen in each of more than one lineage should be considered "acute unclassifiable leukemias." This rather confusing area is schematically outlined in f20.4.

If myeloid lineage is established in the absence of B- or T-cell antigen expression that meets the threshold in t20.1, the diagnostic algorithm should revert to a workup for AML. However, in this situation some thought should be given to the reasons why mixed phenotype leukemia was considered in the first place, because the specific pattern of cross-lineage antigen expression in AML is often a clue to the underlying genetic lesion. AML with t(8;21) is typically positive for B-cell antigens (and CD56+) [He 2008, Hurwitz 1992, Kita 1992, Kozlov 2005, Tiacci 2004, Weir 2001], while AML with t(16;16) or inv(16) typically expresses CD2 [Adriaansen 1993, Weir 2001]. AML with t(15;17) may also show cross-lineage expression [Chapiro 2006, Weir 2001]. Similarly, if working through f20.2 leads to a probable acute lymphoblastic leukemia, an *MLL* rearrangement may be responsible for the cross-lineage antigen expression [Weir 2001].

Two specific destinations within f20.2 deserve special comment. First, if B- and T-cell lineages are simultaneously confirmed, the case may be best classified as "mixed phenotype acute leukemia, NOS, rare type." However, mixed B/T leukemias are so vanishingly rare that prudence demands a careful review

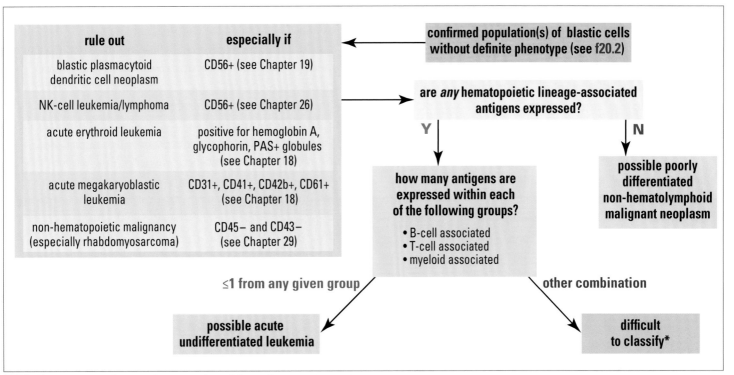

f20.4 *Diagnostic considerations for cases without definitive lineage assignment.*
*These leukemias are difficult to classify in an algorithmic format. The final diagnosis must be based on the specific patterns of antigen expression on a case-by-case basis. Thus, for example, a CD34+ CD13+ CD33+ MPO– leukemia would be classified by many as acute myeloid leukemia with minimal differentiation. However, the addition of CD5 and CD7 (without cytoplasmic CD3) to this immunophenotype would instead favor an acute unclassifiable leukemia.

of factors that may contribute to false-positive immunophenotypic data, including unsatisfactory immunohistochemical controls and inadequate flow cytometric gating and/or color compensation [Costa 2008]. Second, if isolated T-lineage specificity is present, then the case is overwhelmingly likely to be an acute lymphoblastic leukemia of T-cell derivation. However, NK-cells may also express cytoplasmic (but not surface) CD3. Thus, given an acute leukemia of apparent T-cell derivation, consideration should still be given to the possibility of an NK-cell lymphoblastic leukemia/lymphoma, especially if the NK-cell associated antigen CD56 is coexpressed [Morice 2007]. If NK lineage is a significant possibility, molecular studies for T-cell receptor (TCR) γ gene rearrangement should be undertaken. A clonal TCR rearrangement excludes NK lineage; if TCR is germline, then both T and NK lineages remain possible, but specialized flow cytometric analysis for CD94, CD161, and killer immunoglobulin receptors (KIRs) (see **sidebar 26.1**) may permit discrimination between these entities. Blastic plasmacytoid dendritic cell neoplasm (CD4 and CD56 positive) is another differential diagnostic consideration for an apparent T-lymphoblastic leukemia that is not quite "behaving" immunophentypically.

Finally, if the algorithm presented in **f20.2** leads to a probable bona fide mixed phenotype acute leukemia, still further analysis is necessary before the diagnosis is confirmed. In the presence of *FGFR1* mutation or certain recurrent abnormalities [t(15;17), t(8;21), t(16;16), inv(16)], the genetic lesions essentially abrogate the significance of the mixed phenotype and dictate that the case

be assigned to the category relevant to the specific genetic finding. Also, as noted earlier, certain clinical histories or genetic lesions will modify the final diagnosis even in a case of acute leukemia of truly ambiguous lineage. **f20.3** demonstrates these decision points, which relate to prior chemotherapy, myelodysplasia, *MLL* rearrangement, *BCR-ABL1* fusion, and documented prior history of CML.

[20.4] Lineage Switching in Acute Leukemia

As if the diagnosis of acute leukemia of ambiguous lineage were not intricate enough, follow-up of these neoplasms is also fraught with unusual complications. Although it is not uncommon for expression of antigens to change and shift in any hematopoietic neoplasm after treatment and relapse or recurrence, the acute leukemias of ambiguous lineage (especially those with *MLL* rearrangements or *BCR-ABL1*) may have a special propensity to undergo dramatic immunophenotypic evolution [Langebrake 2005, Pui 1991]. The change may take the form of biphenotypic to bilineal transformation, bilineal to biphenotypic transformation, or transformation from ambiguous lineage to outright AML or acute lymphoblastic leukemia (ALL) [Derwich 2009].

The diagnostic pathologist should be aware of the mutability of these cases so that follow-up studies may be appropriately broad. Specifically, immunophenotypic analysis should not be so abbreviated or narrow that a dramatic shift in antigen expression could obscure the recognition of residual blasts.

[20.5] Prognostic and Therapeutic Significance of Ambiguous Phenotype

The algorithms presented in this chapter are sufficiently onerous that the diagnostician may understandably wonder to what purpose such effort is expended. In general, recognition of ambiguous lineage is important because it has been thought to confer a poor prognosis [Lee 2008, Weir 2007]. Other data, however, suggest that mixed phenotype leukemias may not differ prognostically from AML [Lee 2007, Rubnitz 2009]. At least one study demonstrated no prognostic difference between biphenotypic acute leukemia and lineage definitive acute leukemia in children, but significantly inferior prognosis for biphenotypic cases in patients older than 15 years of age [Killick 1999]. Mixed phenotypic acute leukemia with the t(9;22) has a particularly bad prognosis, even when compared with other acute leukemias of ambiguous lineage. However, the prognosis may not in fact be worse than Philadelphia chromosome positive ALL [Killick 1999]. Similarly, the frequency of unfavorable karyotypic findings in cases of mixed phenotype acute leukemia, B/myeloid, may in fact independently explain the poor outcome of many such cases [Legrand 1998]. More definitive conclusions have been hindered by both the rarity of the disease and historical definitional inconsistency.

Acute leukemias of ambiguous lineage represent a significant challenge to the treating physician, as at least 2 distinct treatment options (ie, directed against myeloid or lymphoid disease) are equally defensible [Aribi 2007, Killick 1999]. Data are sparse regarding optimal direction of treatment, with some studies showing no significant difference between myeloid- and lymphoid-oriented treatment [Aribi 2007]. "Hybrid" or sequential approaches have also been advocated [Rubnitz 2009, Velangi 2006], but combined myeloid/lymphoid induction may increase mortality [Killick 1999]. Unfortunately, predictors of response in this situation have not been identified. Some reports suggest that imatinib therapy may be beneficial in the setting of mixed phenotypic acute leukemia with the t(9;22) [Saitoh 2006]. In difficult cases, one might be tempted to pursue T-cell receptor or immunoglobulin gene rearrangement analysis to provide an additional hint regarding lineage and treatment response, but in fact such results should be interpreted with caution, since rearrangements are often detectable even in unambiguous myeloid clones [Adriaansen 1991, Chapiro 2006, Meleshko 2005].

[20.6] Ambiguous Immunophenotypes and Pathways of Hematopoietic Differentiation

Although this chapter is devoted to the currently accepted diagnostic strategies for acute leukemias of ambiguous lineage, a discussion of the topic would be incomplete without at least a brief consideration of the larger significance of cross-lineage antigen expression and lineage ambiguity. Although it is theoretically possible that lineage ambiguity could arise through a process of "loss of control" or arbitrary "aberrant behavior" within the chaotic milieu of the leukemic blast, at least 4 lines of evidence indicate that this cannot be entirely the case. First, the occurrence of reproducible patterns of cross-lineage antigen expression in the presence of certain molecular-level derangements [eg, B-cell lineage expression with the t(8;21), ambiguous lineage in the presence of the t(6;14)(q25;q32), or changes in CD19 expression in the presence of KIT mutations] suggests that cross-lineage antigen expression may be driven by specific regulatory pathways [De 2007, Georgy 2008, He 2008]. Second, the expression of the aberrant antigens can be shown in some cases to confer pro-proliferative properties on the blasts [Anderson 2007]. Third, gene expression profiling has shown that most acute leukemias of ambiguous lineage do not naturally cluster with the expression patterns of either AML or ALL, arguing that there are consistent large-scale molecular differences between lineage ambiguous and unambiguous acute leukemias [Rubnitz 2009]. Fourth, the hypothesis that cross-lineage antigen expression is random cannot account for the near complete absence of cases showing overlap between lymphoid and megakaryocytic or erythroid phenotypes [Luc 2008]. Indeed, the exclusion of such hybrids suggests that cross-lineage antigen expression reflects fundamental pathways of hematopoietic differentiation. For a further discussion of lineage commitment and the significance of immunophenotypic ambiguity, please see **sidebar 1.1**.

[20.7] Clues and Caveats

1. Definition of acute leukemia of ambiguous lineage has been historically inconsistent.
2. Not all cross-lineage antigen expression defines a leukemic clone as ambiguous in lineage.
3. The 2008 WHO classification includes specific criteria that must be fulfilled in the diagnosis of acute leukemia of ambiguous lineage.
4. Acute leukemia of ambiguous lineage may be either biphenotypic (single population) or bilineal (2 populations).
5. Morphology cannot predict lineage ambiguity, but mixed populations of blasts or blasts that are difficult to classify may suggest the possibility of a mixed phenotype.
6. Initial flow cytometric or immunohistochemical panels should include at least CD19 and cytoplasmic CD3 to screen for lineage ambiguity. Similarly, MPO is assessed via flow, immunohistochemistry, or cytochemistry.
7. Failure to identify definitive lineage does not automatically establish a diagnosis of acute undifferentiated leukemia, as many other specific entities must be ruled out.
8. Some acute leukemias that fail to demonstrate definitive lineage by WHO criteria, but which nevertheless show some suggestion of lineage commitment in that they express multiple lineage-associated antigens, may be considered acute unclassifiable leukemias.

9. If mixed phenotype is established to the satisfaction of WHO criteria, additional parameters to be investigated include: *FGFR1* mutation, t(15;17), t(8;21), t(16;16), inv(16), *MLL* rearrangement, prior chemotherapy, myelodysplasia-related changes, *BCR-ABL1* fusion, and prior history of CML. These findings either prevent or add modifiers to the diagnosis of outright acute leukemia of ambiguous lineage.

10. Acute leukemias of ambiguous lineage can show significant evolution in immunophenotype during and after treatment.

11. Lineage ambiguity may be a poor prognostic factor, and it complicates treatment decisions regarding optimal chemotherapy.

12. Acute leukemias of ambiguous lineage offer insight into early pathways of differentiation in precursor cells.

[20.8] References

Adriaansen HJ, Soeting PW, Wolvers-Tettero IL, van Dongen JJ [1991] Immunoglobulin and T-cell receptor gene rearrangements in acute non-lymphocytic leukemias: analysis of 54 cases and a review of the literature. *Leukemia* 5:744-751.

Adriaansen HJ, te Boekhorst PA, Hagemeijer AM, et al [1993] Acute myeloid leukemia M4 with bone marrow eosinophilia (M4Eo) and inv(16)(p13q22) exhibits a specific immunophenotype with CD2 expression. *Blood* 81:3043-3051.

Anderson K, Rusterholz C, Mansson R, et al [2007] Ectopic expression of PAX5 promotes maintenance of biphenotypic myeloid progenitors coexpressing myeloid and B-cell lineage-associated genes. *Blood* 109:3697-3705.

Aribi A, Bueso-Ramos C, Estey E, et al [2007] Biphenotypic acute leukaemia: a case series. *Br J Haematol* 138:213-216.

Bagg A [2007] Lineage ambiguity, infidelity, and promiscuity in immunophenotypically complex acute leukemias: genetic and morphologic correlates. *Am J Clin Pathol* 128:545-548.

Bene MC, Castoldi G, Knapp W, et al [1995] Proposals for the immunological classification of acute leukemias: European Group for the Immunological Characterization of Leukemias (EGIL). *Leukemia* 9:1783-1786.

Borowitz M, Bene M-C, Harris N, et al [2008] Acute leukaemias of ambiguous lineage. In: Swerdlow S, Campo E, Harris N, et al, eds. *WHO Classification of Tumours: Pathology and Genetics: Tumours of Haematopoietic and Lymphoid Tissues.* Lyon, France: IARC Press;150-155.

Chapiro E, Delabesse E, Asnafi V, et al [2006] Expression of T-lineage-affiliated transcripts and TCR rearrangements in acute promyelocytic leukemia: implications for the cellular target of 17. *Blood* 108:3484-3493.

Chen L, Shah HO, Lin JH [2004] Alveolar rhabdomyosarcoma with concurrent metastases to bone marrow and lymph nodes simulating acute hematologic malignancy. *J Pediatr Hematol Oncol* 26:696-697.

Costa ES, Thiago LS, Otazu IB, et al [2008] An uncommon case of childhood biphenotypic precursor-B/T acute lymphoblastic leukemia. *Pediatr Blood Cancer* 50:941-942.

Cruse JM, Lewis RE, Pierce S, et al [2005] Aberrant expression of CD7, CD56, and CD79a antigens in acute myeloid leukemias. *Exp Mol Pathol* 79:39-41.

De J, Zanjani R, Hibbard M, Davis BH [2007] Immunophenotypic profile predictive of KIT activating mutations in AML1-ETO leukemia. *Am J Clin Pathol* 128:550-557.

Degos L [2001] John Hughes Bennett, Rudolph Virchow, and Alfred Donne: the first description of leukemia. *Hematol J* 2:1.

Derwich K, Sedek L, Meyer C, et al [2009] Infant acute bilineal leukemia. *Leuk Res* (epub ahead of press).

El-Sissy AH, El-Mashari MA, Bassuni WY, El-Swaayed AF [2006] Aberrant lymphoid antigen expression in acute myeloid leukemia in Saudi Arabia. *J Egypt Natl Canc Inst* 18:244-249.

Georgy M, Yonescu R, Griffin CA, Batista DA [2008] Acute mixed lineage leukemia and a t(6;14)(q25;q32) in 2 adults. *Cancer Genet Cytogenet* 185:28-31.

Han X, Bueso-Ramos CE [2007] Precursor T-cell acute lymphoblastic leukemia/ lymphoblastic lymphoma and acute biphenotypic leukemias. *Am J Clin Pathol* 127:528-544.

He G, Wu D, Sun A, et al [2008] B-lymphoid and myeloid lineages biphenotypic acute leukemia with t(8;21)(q22;q22). *Int J Hematol* 87:132-136.

Hurwitz CA, Raimondi SC, Head D, et al [1992] Distinctive immunophenotypic features of t(8;21)(q22;q22) acute myeloblastic leukemia in children. *Blood* 1992;80:3182-3188.

Killick S, Matutes E, Powles RL, et al [1999] Outcome of biphenotypic acute leukemia. *Haematologica* 84:699-706.

Kita K, Nakase K, Miwa H, et al [1992] Phenotypical characteristics of acute myelocytic leukemia associated with the t(8;21)(q22;q22) chromosomal abnormality: frequent expression of immature B-cell antigen CD19 together with stem cell antigen CD34. *Blood* 80:470-477.

Kozlov I, Beason K, Yu C, Hughson M [2005] CD79a expression in acute myeloid leukemia t(8;21) and the importance of cytogenetics in the diagnosis of leukemias with immunophenotypic ambiguity. *Cancer Genet Cytogenet* 163:62-67.

Langebrake C, Brinkmann I, Teigler-Schlegel A, et al [2005] Immunophenotypic differences between diagnosis and relapse in childhood AML: implications for MRD monitoring. *Cytometry B Clin Cytom* 63:1-9.

Lee JH, Min YH, Chung CW, et al [2008] Prognostic implications of the immunophenotype in biphenotypic acute leukemia. *Leuk Lymphoma* 49:700-709.

Lee MY, Tan TD, Feng AC [2007] Clinicopathologic analysis of acute myeloid leukemia in a single institution: biphenotypic acute myeloid leukemia may not be an aggressive subtype. *J Chin Med Assoc* 70:269-273.

Legrand O, Perrot JY, Simonin G, et al [1998] Adult biphenotypic acute leukaemia: an entity with poor prognosis which is related to unfavourable cytogenetics and P-glycoprotein over-expression. *Br J Haematol* 100:147-155.

Luc S, Buza-Vidas N, Jacobsen SE [2008] Delineating the cellular pathways of hematopoietic lineage commitment. *Semin Immunol* 20:213-220.

Meleshko AN, Lipay NV, Stasevich IV, Potapnev MP [2005] Rearrangements of IgH, TCRD and TCRG genes as clonality marker of childhood acute lymphoblastic leukemia. *Exp Oncol* 27:319-324.

Morice WG [2007] The immunophenotypic attributes of NK cells and NK-cell lineage lymphoproliferative disorders. *Am J Clin Pathol* 127:881-886.

Naithani R, Kumar R, Mahapatra M, et al [2007] Pelvic alveolar rhabdomyosarcoma with bone marrow involvement misdiagnosed as acute myeloid leukemia. *Pediatr Hematol Oncol* 24:153-155.

Pui CH, Raimondi SC, Head DR, et al [1991] Characterization of childhood acute leukemia with multiple myeloid and lymphoid markers at diagnosis and at relapse. *Blood* 78:1327-1337.

Rubnitz JE, Onciu M, Pounds S, et al [2009] Acute mixed lineage leukemia in children: the experience of St Jude Children's Research Hospital. *Blood* (epub ahead of press).

Saitoh T, Matsushima T, Iriuchishima H, et al [2006] Presentation of extramedullary Philadelphia chromosome-positive biphenotypic acute leukemia as testicular mass: response to imatinib-combined chemotherapy. *Leuk Lymphoma* 47:2667-2669.

Shinkoda Y, Nagatoshi Y, Fukano R, et al [2009] Rhabdomyosarcoma masquerading as acute leukemia. *Pediatr Blood Cancer* 52:286-287.

Thalhammer-Scherrer R, Mitterbauer G, Simonitsch I, et al [2002] The immunophenotype of 325 adult acute leukemias: relationship to morphologic and molecular classification and proposal for a minimal screening program highly predictive for lineage discrimination. *Am J Clin Pathol* 117:380-389.

Tiacci E, Pileri S, Orleth A, et al [2004] PAX5 expression in acute leukemias: higher B-lineage specificity than CD79a and selective association with t(8;21)-acute myelogenous leukemia. *Cancer Res* 64:7399-7404.

Velangi MR, Reid MM, Sen S, et al [2006] Hybrid chemotherapy in 2 children with acute leukemia of ambiguous lineage. *Pediatr Blood Cancer* 46:833.

Weir EG, Ali Ansari-Lari M, Batista DA, et al [2007] Acute bilineal leukemia: a rare disease with poor outcome. *Leukemia* 21:2264-2270.

Weir EG, Borowitz MJ [2001] Flow cytometry in the diagnosis of acute leukemia. *Semin Hematol* 38:124-138.

APPENDIX

1 Normal Mean Red Blood Cell Indices in the Normal Fetus

Parameter (Units)	Weeks of Gestation			
	18-22	23-26	27-29	>30
RBC count[†] ($\times 10^{12}$/L)	2.8	3.1	3.5	3.8
Hemoglobin (g/dL)	14[‡]/11.7[†]	14.5[‡]/12.2[†]	15-16[‡]/12.9[†]	16.5-18[‡]/13.6[†]
Hematocrit (%)	40%/37%	43%/38.6%	44%-47%/41%	48%-54%/44%
MCV (fL)	122/131	120-116/125	115-113/119	113-105/114
MCH (pg)[†]	40.5	40-39	39	38-36
nRBC[§] ($\times 10^6$/μL)[¶]	2.11	0.99	1.08	1.31

*Given the ranges in these values depending on the source, individual data points should be interpreted within the context of your particular institution keeping in my mind that minor differences are likely observed due to type of instrumentation utilized, how the specimen was obtained (capillary vs venous specimen), ethnic and/or environmental variation (eg, high altitude)

[†]Data from [Christensen 2009]

[‡]Data from [Forestier 1991] (obtained from a Coulter S plus II instrument)

[§]Data extrapolated from [Forestier 1991] after correction of total while blood count for nRBCs

[¶]Elevated circulating fetal nRBCs is a sign of significant intrauterine stress [Hermansen 2001]

CBC = complete blood count; MCHC = mean cell hemoglobin concentration; MCV = mean cell volume; nRBC = nucleated red blood cell; RBC = red blood cell

References: [Christensen 2009, Forestier 1991, Hermansen 2001]

2 Normal CBC Parameters, Birth to 1 Year*

Parameter (Units)	Age				
	Birth (at term)	1 week	1 month	6 months	1 year
RBC count ($\times 10^{12}$/L)	3.9-5.5[†]	3.9-6.3[†]	3.0-5.4	3.1-4.5	4.0-5.2
Hemoglobin (g/dL)	13.5-19.5	13.5-21.5	10.0-18.0	9.5-13.5	11.5-15.5
Hematocrit (%)	42%-65%	42%-66%	31%-55%	29%-41%	33%-39%
MCV (fL)	98-118	88-126	85-123	74-108	70-86
MCHC (g/dL)	30-36	28-38	29-37	30-36	30-36
Reticulocyte (%)	1.8%-4.6%	0.2%-0.8%	0-1%	0-1%	0-2%
WBC ($\times 10^9$/L)	~15-30	5.0-21	5.0-19.5	6.0-17.5	6.0-17.5
ANC ($\times 10^9$/L)	~7-28	1.5-10	1.0-9.0	1.0-8.5	1.5-8.5
ALC ($\times 10^9$/L)	2.0-11	2.0-17	2.5-16.5	4.0-13.5	4.0-10.5
Platelet ($\times 10^9$/L)	235-341	279-397	271-415	316-414	236-392

*Adapted from a number of sources; numbers represent the mean ±2 standard deviations, and/or should encompass 95% of normal individuals; although data has been gleaned from diverse sources, individual ranges are derived from single sources to maintain the validity of the statistical distributions; it is vital to remember that normal ranges should be established for each individual laboratory, as variation is expected due to differing patient populations, preanalytic variables, and analytic methodology

[†]Expect many nucleated red blood cells at birth, diminishing rapidly in number by 1 week of age

ALC = absolute lymphocyte count; ANL = absolute neutrophil count; CBC = complete blood count; MCHC = mean cell hemoglobin concentration; MCV = mean cell volume; nRBC = nucleated red blood cell; RBC = red blood cell

References: [Brugnara 2003, de Alarcon 2005, Foucar 2008, Kjeldsberg 2010]

appendix

3 Normal CBC Parameters, Children*

Age	RBC (× 10¹²/L)	Hemoglobin (g/dL)	Hematocrit (%)	MCV (fL)	MCHC (g/dL)	WBC (× 10⁹/L)	ANC (× 10⁹/L)	ALC (× 10⁹/L)	Platelet (× 10⁹/L)
1	3.7-5.3	10.5-13.5	33%-39%	70-86	30-36	6.0-17.5	1.5-8.5	4.0-10.5	
2						6.0-17.0	1.5-8.5	3.0-9.5	
3	3.9-5.3	11.5-13.5	34%-40%	75-87					
4						5.5-15.5	1.5-8.5	2.0-8.0	
5									
6						5.0-14.5	1.5-8.0	1.5-7.0	
7									
8	4.0-5.2	11.5-15.5	35%-45%	77-95		4.5-13.5	1.5-8.0	1.5-6.8	
9					31-37				~150-400
10						4.5-13.5	1.8-8.0	1.5-6.5	
11									
12									
13									
14	F 4.1-5.1	F 12-16	F 36%-46%	F 78-102					
15	M 4.5-5.3	M 13-16	M 37%-49%	M 78-98					
16						4.5-13.0	1.8-8.0	1.2-5.2	
17									

*Adapted from a number of sources; numbers represent the mean ±2 standard deviations and/or should encompass 95% of normal individuals; although data have been gleaned from diverse sources, individual ranges are derived from single sources to maintain the validity of the statistical distributions

It is vital to remember that normal ranges should be established for each individual laboratory, as variation is expected due to differing patient populations, preanalytic variables, and analytic methodology

ALC = absolute lymphocyte count; ANC = absolute neutrophil count; CBC = complete blood count; F = female; M = male; MCHC = mean corpuscular hemoglobin concentration; MCV = mean corpuscular volume; RBC = red blood cell count; WBC = white blood cell count

References: [Brugnara 2003, Foucar 2008, Kjeldsberg 2010]

4 Normal CBC Parameters, Adults*

Parameter	Average Normal Range[†]
Hemoglobin (g/dL)	F: ~12-15.5 M: ~13-17.5
Hematocrit (%)	F: 36-46 M: 40-51
RBC (× 10¹²/L)	F: 3.9-5.0 M: 4.4-5.8
MCV (fL)	82-99
MCH (pg)	27.0-33.5
MCHC (g/dL)	32-35.6
WBC (× 10⁹/L)	4.1-10.2
Platelet (× 10⁹/L)	~150-400

*It is vital to remember that normal ranges should be established for each individual laboratory, as variation is expected due to differing patient populations, preanalytic variables, and analytic methodology

CBC = complete blood count; MCHC = mean corpuscular hemoglobin concentration; MCV = mean corpuscular volume; RBC = red blood cell count; WBC = white blood cell count

References: [Bick 1993, NORIP 2010, Perkins 2003, Ryan 2006]

5 Normal Bone Marrow Differential Counts

Cell Type	Normal Range (%)
Myeloblasts	0-3%*
Promyelocytes	1%-8%
Myelocytes	10%-15%
Metamyelocytes	10%-15%
Band/neutrophils	12%-25%
Eosinophils and precursors	1%-5%
Basophils and precursors	0-1%
Monocytes	0-2%
Erythroblasts	0-2%
Other erythroid elements	15%-25%
Lymphocytes	10%-15%[†]
Plasma cells	0-1%

*Percent myeloblasts higher in pediatric specimens (3%-4%), lower in specimens from adults, especially elderly (0%-1%)
[†]Percent lymphocytes higher in specimens from young children due to abundant hematogones (benign lymphocyte precursor cells)

References: [Bain 1996, Wickramasinghe 2007]

appendix

6 Age-Related Normal Values in Bone Marrow

Age	% Cellularity	% Granulocyte	% Erythroid	% Lymphocytes	Comments
Newborn	80%-100%	40%-50%	40%	10%-20%	High EPO at birth; drops dramatically after birth Hematogones may be prominent*
1-3 months	80%-100%	50%-60%	5%-10%	30%-50%	Dramatic decline in erythroid precursors until EPO production resumes at 3-4 months Abundant lymphocytes with many hematogones*
Child	60%-80%	50%-60%	20%	20%-30%	Variable number of hematogones*; more numerous in young children
Adult (30-70 yrs)	40%-70%	50%-70%	20%-25%	10%-15%	Cellularity fairly stable throughout most of adulthood
Elderly (>70 yrs)	<25%	50%-70%	20%-25%	10%-15%	Decline in cellularity in elderly may be linked to a reduction in bone volume with subsequent increase in volume of the hematopoietic cavity

*Hematogones are normal B lymphocyte precursor cells (see Volume 1, Chapter 2)
EPO = erythropoietin

References: [Bain 1996, Friebert 1998, Gulati 1988, Hartsock 1965, Rimsza 2004, Trimoreau 1997, Wickramasinghe 2007, Zutter 1998]

7 Sample Procedure for General Bone Marrow Histologic Processing

I. Specimen is received in AZF fixative* and left for 2 hours (minimum) or overnight (maximum)
II. Remove from AZF fixative
   1) Clot specimen
      A. Label cassette with accession number and patient's last name
      B. Fold embedding bag around clot, place in cassette, and wash in running tap water for 5 minutes
   2) Biopsy specimen
      A. Place in embedding bag
      B. Immerse the embedding bag in rapid decalcification solution† for 30 minutes
      C. After decalcification, fold embedding bag and place in cassette labeled with accession number
      D. Wash in running tap water for 3 minutes
III. Place cassettes in basket along with the other surgical specimens grossed to be processed overnight

*Acetic zinc formalin; Newcomer Supply, Middleton, WI
†Decal Stat; Decal Chemical, Tallman, NY

8 Sample Procedures for Cytochemical and Special Stains Important in the Analysis of Bone Marrow Specimens

I. Myeloperoxidase (p a6)

II. Nonspecific esterase (p a7)

III. Prussian blue (p a9)

IV. Reticulin (p a10)

V. Trichrome (p a11)

I. Myeloperoxidase

  1) Preparation

    A. Myeloperoxidase fixative

      1. Formaldehyde (CH_2O) 37% 10 mL

      2. Absolute ethyl alcohol (CH_3CH_2OH) 90 mL

      3. Shelf life is 1 year

      4. Stored in safety hood in hematology at room temperature

    B. Incubation mixture

      1. Mix in safety hood in hematology

      2. To a clean, dry 200 mL beaker, add 100 mL of 80% ethyl alcohol (37.5 mL 80% EtOH + 62.5 mL distilled water); mix for 15 minutes

      3. To the alcohol, add 0.30 gs benzidine dihydrochloride; mix until granules dissolve.
Warning: Benzidine dihydrochloride is a highly toxic substance that may cause cancer or inheritable genetic damage. It is very toxic by inhalation, by contact with skin, and if swallowed. Wear suitable protective clothing, gloves, and eye-face protection when handling this substance. Wear a mask and protective glasses when weighing the dry material, and wear gloves and use the safety hood when staining smears.

      4. Add 1 mL $ZnSO_4\cdot7\,H_2O$.

        a. Prepared by adding 3.8 g $ZnSO_4$ + 100 mL DI H_2O

        b. Mix for 15 minutes

        c. Store at room temperature

        d. Date with an expiration date of 1 year

      5. Add 1.0 g sodium acetate; mix for 15 minutes

      6. Add 0.7 mL 3% hydrogen peroxide (dilute 30% hydrogen peroxide 1:10); mix 15 minutes

      7. Add 1.5 mL 1.0 N sodium hydroxide (NaOH); mix 15 minutes

      8. Add 0.20 g safranin O stain; mix 15 minutes

      9. Filter and store in tightly stoppered brown bottle

      10. Date with an expiration date of 1 year

  2) Quality control

    A. Prepare peripheral blood thin smears from a fresh EDTA tube with at least a mild neutrophilia

    B. Mature neutrophils should be MPO+

    C. If the mature neutrophils do not stain as anticipated, then:

      1. Recheck the reagents for outdating

      2. Repeat the procedure with fresh control smears

  3) Technical procedure

    A. Fix smear(s) for each patient and control in myeloperoxidase fixative; fix for 60 seconds

    B. Rinse in running tap water for 15-20 seconds

    C. Blot off excess water and air dry

    D. Fix smears in incubation mixture for 30 seconds

    E. Rinse in running tap water for 5-10 seconds

    F. Air dry

    G. Dip slides in xylene

    H. Coverslip

II. Nonspecific esterase
1) Preparation
A. Acetone-formalin fixative stock solution
1. Sodium phosphate diabasic anyhdrous (Na_2HPO_4) 0.1 g
2. Potassium phosphate monobasic (KH_2PO_4) 0.5 g
3. Distilled water 150 mL
4. Formaldehyde 37% 125 mL
5. Acetone 225 mL
6. Completely dissolve sodium phosphate and potassium phosphate in the distilled water
7. Add the formaldehyde, followed by the acetone
8. Adjust to pH 6.6

B. 0.2 M phosphate buffer
1. Stock sodium phosphate monobasic
   a. Measure sodium phosphate monobasic (NaH_2PO_4) 28 g
   b. Dissolve in distilled water 900 mL
   c. Pour into a graduated cylinder and adjust the volume to 1,000 mL with distilled water
2. Stock sodium phosphate dibasic
   a. Measure sodium phosphate dibasic (Na_2HPO_4) 28 g
   b. Dissolve sodium phosphate diabasic in slightly warmed distilled water 900 mL
   c. Pour into a graduated cylinder and adjust the volume to 1,000 mL with distilled water
3. Working buffer
   a. Stock sodium phosphate monobasic (stock NaH_2PO_4) 625 mL
   b. Stock sodium phosphate dibasic (stock Na_2HPO_4) 375 mL
   c. Combine the solutions above and adjust the pH to 6.6
   d. Store in refrigerator
   e. Date with an expiration date of 1 year

C. Pararosanilin stock solution
1. Pararosanilin hydrochloride 1.0 g
2. Distilled water 20 mL
3. Hydrochloric acid (HCl) 5 mL
4. With moderate heat and stirring, dissolve the pararosanilin in the distilled water
5. Add HCl and allow to cool
6. Store solution in refrigerator
7. Date with an expiration date of 1 year

D. Sodium nitrite 4%
1. Sodium nitrite ($NaNO_2$) 0.2 g
2. Distilled water 5 mL
3. Make this solution fresh each time and use only once

E. α-naphthyl butyrate
1. Butyrate ($C_{14}H_{14}O_2$) is a liquid; allow it to come to room temperature before aliquoting
2. Dispense 40 μL into multiple vials
3. Label and date the vials
4. Store in a freezer until ready to use

F. Sodium fluoride
1. Sodium fluoride (NaF) 0.03 g
2. Working buffer 0.2 M phosphate buffer 20 mL
3. Measure out multiple aliquots of sodium fluoride solution
4. Label, date and store in refrigerator

G. Gill hematoxylin #3
H. Ethylene glycol monoethyl ether
I. Ammonia water

2) **Technical procedure**
   A. Measure out 100 mL of working buffer solution; adjust pH to 6.6 and set aside
   B. Fix smears in cold acetone-formalin fixative solution for 30 seconds
       1. Wash for 2 minutes in tap water
       2. Rinse in distilled water
       3. Allow smears to air dry for 15 minutes
   C. Prepare working solution of sodium nitrite solution; set aside
   D. Place fixed smears in 2 Coplin jars
       1. Mark 1 jar "with fluoride"
       2. Mark 1 jar "without fluoride"
       3. Pre-warm in 37°C oven for 15 minutes
   E. Add 1.0 mL of ethylene glycol monoethyl ether to an aliquot of α-naphthyl butyrate (40 μL); mix and set aside
   F. Add 2.0 mL stock pararosanilin to 2.0 mL working sodium nitrite solution
       1. Mix and time for one minute
       2. The solution should be amber in color with many fine bubbles
   G. At exactly one minute, add the above solution (step F) to 100 mL of working buffer solution
       1. Mix and adjust the pH to 6.3; *this is a critical step: the pH value is very important*
   H. Work quickly through the next steps; have all materials ready
       1. Add the substrate, α naphthyl butyrate, which was mixed with ethylene glycol monoethyl ether in step E to the above buffer solution
           a. The solution will become cloudy
           b. Mix well, then filter with coarse paper into a flask
           c. Repeat filtration with fine filter paper to obtain a clear wheat-amber colored solution
           d. Note: this step should be done rather quickly, in 5 minutes or less
       2. In Coplin jar with smears marked "with fluoride":
           a. Measure out 20 mL of the above solution
           b. Mix with 0.03 g of sodium fluoride; stir
           c. Add this solution to the Coplin jar with smears marked "with fluoride"
       3. In Coplin jar with smears marked "without fluoride"
           a. Pour remaining solution into Coplin jar with smears not requiring fluoride inhibition
           b. Incubate both sets of slides in the 37°C oven for 60 minutes
       4. After the incubation period, wash all of the smears in tap water and check the stain quality with the microscope
           a. If additional staining time is necessary, return the smears to the appropriate solutions and stain with heat for an additional 30 minutes
           b. Keep repeating this step until desired result is obtained
       5. Counterstain with Gill hematoxylin #3 for 5 minutes; wash smears gently in distilled water
       6. Blue smears in ammonia water, rinse in distilled water and mount with aqueous mounting media

III. Prussian blue

1) Preparation
   - A. Potassium ferrocyanide 10% (part A)
     1. Distilled water 250 mL
     2. Potassium ferrocyanide ($K_4[Fe(CN)_6] \cdot 3H_2O$) (yellow) 25 g
        *Caution: Potassium ferrocyanide is slightly irritating to eyes and skin. In case of contact, wash thoroughly. If swallowed, take 2-4 glasses of water, induce vomiting, and seek medical attention. **Note:** Cyanide is not digested in this form, and therefore is not a hazard.*
   - B. Hydrochloric acid 20% (part B)
     1. Distilled water 200 mL
     2. Hydrochloric acid (HCl) 50 mL
        Danger: Hydrochloric acid causes burns, may be fatal if swallowed. Avoid contact. Do not breathe vapors. Wash thoroughly for 15 minutes after contact, and seek medical attention.
   - C. Working iron solution
     1. Hydrochloric acid 20% (part B) 15 mL
     2. Potassium ferrocyanide 10% (part A) 15 mL
     3. Combine in order just before use
   - D. Aluminum sulfate 5%
     1. Distilled water 450 mL
     2. Aluminum sulfate $[Al_2(SO_4)_3]$ 22.5 g
   - E. Nuclear fast red
     1. Nuclear fast red 0.45 g
        Caution: Nuclear fast red may cause irritation; after contact, wash thoroughly for 15 minutes and seek medical attention. If swallowed, induce vomiting and seek medical attention.
     2. 5% aluminum sulfate 450 mL
     3. Dissolve with heat, cool, filter, and add one thymol crystal
        Caution: Thymol may cause irritation. After contact, wash thoroughly for 15 minutes and seek medical attention. If swallowed, drink large quantities of water. Do not induce vomiting. Seek medical attention.
   - F. Alkalinized hydrogen peroxide
     1. Hydrogen peroxide (H_2O_2) 30% 45 mL
        Warning: Hydrogen peroxide is a strong oxidizer and combustible when dry. In case of contact, wash for 15 minutes in running water and seek medical attention. If swallowed, give 2 glasses of water, induce vomiting, and seek medical attention.
     2. Ammonium hydroxide (NH_4OH) 1% 5 mL
        Danger: Ammonium hydroxide causes burns. May be fatal if swallowed. Avoid contact with eyes, skin or clothing. Do not breathe vapors. Wash thoroughly in running water for 15 minutes after contact and seek medical attention.

2) Technical procedure
   - A. Deparaffinize, clear, and hydrate to distilled water
   - B. Incubate in working iron solution 30 minutes
   - C. Rinse with distilled water, 2 times
   - D. Incubate in nuclear fast red solution, 10 minutes
   - E. Rinse with distilled water
   - F. Dehydrate
   - G. Clear
   - H. Mount with a solvent-based resin

IV. Reticulin

1) Preparation

A. Ammoniacal silver solution

1. Use acid-clean glassware
2. Combine 10 mL of silver nitrate ($AgNO_3$) solution 20% and 2.5 mL of a 10% aqueous solution of potassium hydroxide (KOH 1.0 g dissolved in distilled water 10 mL)
3. Add 50% ammonia water (ammonium hydroxide [NH_4OH] 20 mL and distilled water 10 mL) drop by drop, while shaking the container or using magnetic stirrer continuously, until solution becomes just cloudy in color
4. Dilute the solution with distilled water to twice its volume
5. Filter with double filter paper

B. Potassium permanganate 0.5% solution

1. Potassium permanganate ($KMnO_4$) 0.2 g
2. Dissolve in distilled water 50 mL

C. Potassium metabisulfite 2% solution

1. Potassium metabisulfite ($K_2S_2O_2$) 1 g
2. Dissolve in distilled water 50 mL

D. Ferric ammonium sulfate 2% solution

1. Ferric ammonium sulfate [$NH_4Fe(SO_4)_2 \cdot 12H_2O$] 1 g
2. Dissolve in distilled water 50 mL

E. Formalin 20% solution

1. Formaldehyde solution (CH_2O) 10 mL
2. Dissolve in distilled water 40 mL

F. Gold chloride (AuCl) 0.2% solution

1. Stock gold chloride solution 10 mL
2. Dissolve in distilled water 40 mL
3. Filter before use

G. Sodium thiosulfate solution 2%

1. Sodium thiosulfate ($Na_2S_2O_3$) 1 g
2. Dissolve in distilled water 50 mL

2) Technical procedure

A. Xylene for 10 minutes

B. Perform slow dips through absolute alcohol ×2 changes
1. 95% alcohol
2. 80% alcohol

C. Wash in running tap water for 3 minutes

D. Rinse in distilled water and place slides on glass rack

E. Oxidize by flooding with 0.5% aqueous solution of potassium permanganate for 1 minute

F. Rinse in tap water 2 minute

G. Differentiate by flooding with 2% aqueous solution of potassium metabisulfite for 1 minute

H. Wash in tap water for 2 minutes

I. Sensitize by flooding with 2% solution of ferric ammonium sulfate for 1 minute

J. Wash in tap water for 2 minutes, followed with 2 changes of distilled water, 30 seconds each

K. Impregnate in the silver solution for 1 minute

L. Rinse in distilled water for 20 seconds

M. Reduce in 20% formalin for 3 minutes

N. Wash in tap water for 5 minutes

O. Tone in Coplin jar containing 0.2% solution of gold chloride for 10 minutes

P. Rinse in distilled water

Q. Reduce toning in a 2% solution of potassium metabisulfite for 1 minute

R. Fix in 2% solution of sodium thiosulfate for 1 minute

S. Wash in tap water 5 minutes

T. Dehydrate and mount in Permount

V. Trichrome

1) **Preparation**
   A. Bouin fixative
   1. Picric acid, saturated aqueous solution 750 mL
   2. 37%-40% formaldehyde 250 mL
   3. Glacial acetic acid 50 mL
   B. Mayers alum hematoxylin (Sigma Diagnostics catalog #MHS-32)
   C. Masson solution
   1. Aqueous acid fuchsin 2.3% 15 mL
   2. Aqueous ponceau xylidine 0.7% 45 mL
   3. Glacial acetic acid (CH_3COOH) 0.5 mL
   D. Phosphotungstic acid 5%
   1. Phosphotungstic acid 5 g
   2. Distilled water 100 mL
   E. Light green 2%
   1. Light green 5 g
   2. Distilled water 250 mL
   3. Glacial acetic acid 2 mL
   F. Acetic water 0.5%
   1. Glacial acetic acid (CH_3COOH) 1 mL
   2. Distilled water 100 mL

2) **Technical procedure**
   A. Deparaffinize and hydrate to distilled water
   B. If tissue is formalin fixed
   1. Incubate in Bouin fixative for 1 hour in oven at 56°C
   2. Allow slides to cool, then wash in tap water until yellow color is removed
   3. Rinse in distilled water
   C. Stain in Mayer hematoxylin for 10 minutes
   D. Wash in tap water for 5 minutes
   E. Rinse in distilled water
   F. Stain in Masson solution for 1 minute
   G. Place in phosphotungstic acid 5% for 2 minutes
   H. Drain
   I. Stain in light green 2% for 3 minutes
   J. Rinse in distilled water
   K. Place in acetic water 0.5% for 30 seconds
   L. Dehydrate
   M. Clear
   N. Mount

9 Selected Cluster of Differentiation (CD) Antigens Useful in Diagnostic Hematopathology

appendix

CD#	Full Name(s)*	Normal Expression	Selected Diagnostic Utility in Appropriate Context†
CD1a	T-cell surface glycoprotein CD1A T-cell surface antigen T6/Leu-6 HTA1 thymocyte antigen	Cortical thymocytes Dendritic cells Langerhans cells	Identification of maturing T cells Identification of precursor dendritic cells Identification of Langerhans cells
CD2	T-cell surface antigen CD2 T-cell surface antigen T11/Leu-5 LFA-2 LFA-3 receptor Erythrocyte receptor Rosette receptor	T cells NK cells	Identification of T cells and NK-cells Aberrant loss may suggest T-cell lymphoma If expressed in acute myeloid leukemia may suggest inv(16)/t(16;16)
CD3	T-cell surface glycoprotein CD3 (δ chain/ε chain/γ chain)	Pan T-cell	Identification of T cells Aberrant loss may suggest T-cell lymphoma NK cells show cytoplasmic, but not cell surface, CD3
CD4	T-cell surface glycoprotein CD4 T-cell surface antigen T4/Leu-3	Helper T-cell Monocytes Macrophages Dendritic cells	Identification of T-cell subset Severely skewed CD4/CD8 ratio may suggest T-cell lymphoma, HIV, classical Hodgkin lymphoma, reactive process CD4+/CD8+ seen in immature T cells, some malignant T cells, progressively transformed germinal centers, nodular lymphocyte predominant Hodgkin lymphoma CD4–/CD8– T cells may be neoplastic, reactive (especially γ-δ T cells), or may be increased in autoimmune lymphoproliferative syndrome Present in blastic plasmacytoid dendritic cell neoplasm
CD5	T-cell surface glycoprotein CD5 Lymphocyte glycoprotein T1/Leu-1	T cells Minor subset naive B cells	Identification of T-cell subset Aberrant loss may suggest T-cell lymphoma Abnormally expressed by B cells in some B-cell lymphomas
CD7	T-cell antigen CD7 Gp40 T-cell leukemia antigen Tp41 Leu-9	Some hematopoietic stem cells T cells Monocytes NK cells	Identification of T cells Aberrant loss may suggest T-cell lymphoma Reactive T cells may show loss of CD7, especially in setting of cutaneous pathology
CD8	T-cell surface glycoprotein CD8 α chain/β chain T-lymphocyte differentiation antigen T8/Leu-2 Lyt-2 Lyt-3	Cytotoxic T cells Some NK cells	Identification of T-cell/NK cell subsets Severely skewed CD4/CD8 ratio may suggest T-cell lymphoma, HIV, classical Hodgkin lymphoma, reactive process CD4+/CD8+ seen in immature T cells, some malignant T cells, progressively transformed germinal centers, nodular lymphocyte predominant Hodgkin lymphoma CD4–/CD8– T cells may be neoplastic or reactive (especially γ-δ T cells) or may be increased in autoimmune lymphoproliferative syndrome
CD10	Neprilysin EC 3.4.24.11 Neutral endopeptidase NEP Enkephalinase Common acute lymphocytic leukemia antigen CALLA	Pre-B and pre-T cells Germinal center B cells Some neutrophils	Present in acute lymphoblastic leukemia/lymphoma (B>T) CD10– B-ALL should raise possibility of 11q23 rearrangement Identification of hematogones Identification both normal and neoplastic germinal center B cells Present in angioimmunoblastic T-cell lymphoma

*First name listed is most commonly accepted; table is continued on next page
†"Selected Diagnostic Utility" is intended to highlight important applications of the given immunophenotypic marker. It is *not* an exhaustive list of all diagnostic contingencies involving these antigens.

References: [Kipps 2006, UniProt 2010]

CD#	Full Name(s)*	Normal Expression	Selected Diagnostic Utility in Appropriate Context†
CD11c	Integrin α-X Leukocyte adhesion glycoprotein p150,95 α chain Leukocyte adhesion receptor p150,95 Leu M5	Monocytes Macrophages Neutrophils NK cells Some B cells Some T cells	Strongly positive in hairy cell leukemia
CD13	Aminopeptidase N EC 3.4.11.2 Microsomal aminopeptidase Gp150	Myeloid cells Osteoclasts	Identification of myeloid cells
CD14	Monocyte differentiation antigen CD14 Myeloid cell-specific leucine-rich glycoprotein LPS receptor	Monocytes Dendritic cells	Identification of monocytic cells
CD15	Sialyl Lewis sLE	Neutrophils Eosinophils Monocytes	Identification of Reed-Sternberg cells Positive in some CMV-infected cells
CD19	B-lymphocyte antigen CD19 B-lymphocyte surface antigen B4 Leu-12	B cells	Identification of pan B-cell lineage Present on B cells before acquisition of CD20 If expressed in acute myeloid leukemia may suggest t(8;21)
CD20	B-lymphocyte antigen CD20 Membrane-spanning 4-domains subfamily A member 1 B-lymphocyte surface antigen B1 Leu-16 Bp35	B cells	Identification of B cells Use with caution in patients treated with rituximab Abnormally bright in hairy cell leukemia Abnormally dim in chronic lymphocytic leukemia/small lymphocytic lymphoma
CD22	B-cell receptor CD22 Sialic acid-binding Ig-like lectin 2 Siglec-2 Leu-14 B-lymphocyte cell adhesion molecule BL-CAM	B cells	Identification of B cells Abnormally dim in chronic lymphocytic leukemia/small lymphocytic lymphoma
CD23	Low affinity immunoglobulin ε Fc receptor Lymphocyte IgE receptor Fc-epsilon-RII BLAST-2	Naïve B cells Monocytes Some T cells Follicular dendritic cells NK cells Platelets	Typically present on B cells in chronic lymphocytic leukemia/small lymphocytic lymphoma Identification of follicular dendritic cells
CD25	Interleukin-2 receptor α chain IL-2 receptor α subunit p55 Tac antigen	Activated B cells and T cells Early myeloid cells	Present in hairy cell leukemia, but usually not hairy cell leukemia-variant Present in adult T-cell leukemia/lymphoma

*First name listed is most commonly accepted; table is continued from previous page
†"Selected Diagnostic Utility" is intended to highlight important applications of the given immunophenotypic marker. It is *not* an exhaustive list of all diagnostic contingencies involving these antigens.

References: [Kipps 2006, UniProt 2010]

appendix

CD#	Full Name(s)*	Normal Expression	Selected Diagnostic Utility in Appropriate Context[†]
CD30	Tumor necrosis factor receptor superfamily member 8 CD30L receptor Lymphocyte activation antigen CD30 Ki-1	Activated B cells, T cells and NK cells Monocytes	Identification of activated B cells and T cells Present in Reed-Sternberg cells Present in anaplastic large cell lymphoma
CD33	Myeloid cell surface antigen CD33 Sialic acid-binding Ig-like lectin 3 Siglec-3 Gp67	Mature/maturing myelomonocytic cells	Identification of myeloid cells
CD34	Hematopoietic progenitor cell antigen CD34	Hematopoietic stem cells	Identification of blasts (though not all blasts will be CD34+) Acute myeloid leukemia without CD34 should raise the possibility of acute promyelocytic leukemia B-ALL without CD34 should raise possibility of t(1;19)
CD38	ADP-ribosyl cyclase 1 EC 3.2.2.5 Cyclic ADP-ribose hydrolase 1 Lymphocyte differentiation antigen CD38 Acute lymphoblastic leukemia cells antigen CD38 T10	Plasma cells Early or activated B cells and T cells Monocytes NK cells Myeloid progenitors	Identification of plasma cells or activated B cells Identification of hematogones and blasts
CD42b	Platelet glycoprotein Ib α chain GP-Ib α GPIbA GPIb-α	Platelets Megakaryocytes	Identification of megakaryocytic cells
CD43	Leukosialin Leucocyte sialoglycoprotein Sialophorin Galactoglycoprotein GalGp	T cells Neutrophils Macrophages Monocytes NK cells Platelets Activated B cells (weak) Plasma cells Hematopoietic stem cells	Identification of T cells Abnormally expressed in some B-cell lymphomas (especially useful in some cases of marginal zone B-cell lymphoma) Alternative to CD45 in identifying hematopoietic lineage in poorly-differentiated processes
CD45	Leukocyte common antigen LCA T200 EC 3.1.3.48	All hematopoietic cells (except red blood cells)	Identification of general hematopoietic lineage, especially in poorly differentiated processes Negative in Reed-Sternberg cells CD45RO is isoform expressed on cortical thymocytes and effector T cells CD45RA is isoform expressed on medullary thymocytes May be weak or negative in plasma cells and lymphoblasts
CD56	Neural cell adhesion molecule 1 NCAM-1 N-CAM-1	NK cells Some activated T cells	Identification of NK cells Implication of malignancy plasma cells in plasma cell myeloma, some cases of monoclonal gammopathy of undetermined significance Present in blastic plasmacytoid dendritic cell neoplasm Present in some T-cell lymphoma subtypes
CD57	Sulfated glucuronic acid complex Leu-7 HNK-1	NK cells Some activated T cells Rare activated B cells	Identification of cytotoxic/large granular lymphocytes CD57+ T cells form rosettes around L&H cells in nodular lymphocyte predominant Hodgkin lymphoma

*First name listed is most commonly accepted; table is continued from previous page

[†]"Selected Diagnostic Utility" is intended to highlight important applications of the given immunophenotypic marker. It is *not* an exhaustive list of all diagnostic contingencies involving these antigens.

References: [Kipps 2006, UniProt 2010]

CD#	Full Name(s)*	Normal Expression	Selected Diagnostic Utility in Appropriate Context[†]
CD61	Integrin β-3 Platelet membrane glycoprotein IIIa GP IIIa	Platelets Megakaryocytes Monocytes Macrophages Some B cells	Identification of megakaryocytic cells
CD64	High affinity immunoglobulin γ Fc receptor I Fc-gamma RI FcRI IgG Fc receptor I	Monocytes Macrophages Activated neutrophils	Identification of monocytic cells
CD68	Macrosialin Gp110	Monocytes Macrophages Dendritic cells Granulocytes Osteoclasts Mast cells Activated lymphocytes Myeloid progenitors	Identification of macrophages
CD79a	B-cell antigen receptor complex associated protein α-chain Ig-α MB-1 membrane glycoprotein Surface-IgM-associated protein Membrane-bound immunoglobulin associated protein	B cells Plasma cells	Identification of B cells and plasma cells (present on B cells before acquisition of CD20)
CD103	Integrin α-E Mucosal lymphocyte-1 antigen HML-1	1%-2% of circulating lymphocytes	Present in hairy cell leukemia, but usually not in splenic marginal zone lymphoma
CD117	Mast/stem cell growth factor receptor EC 2.7.1.112 SCFR Proto-oncogene tyrosine-protein kinase KIT c-KIT	Hematopoietic progenitors Mast cells Some NK-cells	Identification of blasts Identification of early erythroid progenitors Identification of mast cells
CD123	Interleukin-3 receptor α chain IL-3R-α	Pluripotent stem cells Committed hematopoietic progenitor cells Plasmacytoid dendritic cells	Present in blastic plasmacytoid dendritic cell neoplasm Present in hairy cell leukemia
CD138	Syndecan-1 SYND1	Pre-B/immature B cells Plasma cells	Identification of plasma cells
CD163	Scavenger receptor cysteine-rich type 1 protein M130 CD163 antigen Hemoglobin scavenger receptor	Monocytes Macrophages	Very sensitive and specific marker for monocytic/histiocytic lineage

*First name listed is most commonly accepted; table is continued from previous page
[†]"Selected Diagnostic Utility" is intended to highlight important applications of the given immunophenotypic marker. It is *not* an exhaustive list of all diagnostic contingencies involving these antigens.

References: [Kipps 2006, UniProt 2010]

appendix

10 Common Recurring Cytogenetic Abnormalities in Myeloid Neoplasms

Hematologic Abnormality	Cytogenetic Finding(s)	Gene(s) Involved	Other Diseases with Similar Cytogenetic Findings	Primary Prognosis/Notes
Acute Myeloid Leukemia (AML)				
AML	t(8;21)(q22;q22)	*RUNX1-RUNX1T1*	None	Favorable
	t(15;17)(q22;q12) or t(v;17)	*PML-RARA* v=5q35 *(NPM)* v=11q23 *(ZBTB16)* v=11q13 *(NUMA1)* v=17q11.2 *(STAT5B)*		Favorable *ZBTB16-RARA* and *STAT5B-RARA* are ATRA resistant
	inv(16)(p13;q22) or t(16;16)(p13;q22)	*CBFB-MYH11*		Favorable
	inv(3)(q21;q26) or t(3;3)(q21;q26)	*RPN1-EVI1*	MDS	Unfavorable; marked megakaryocytic dysplasia
	t(8;16)(p11;p13)	*MYST3-CREBBP*		Prominent hemophagocytosis
	t(6;9)(p23;q34)	*DEK-NUP214*		Unfavorable; bone marrow and peripheral blood basophilia
	t(1;22)(p13;q13)	*RBM15-MKL1*		An acute megakaryoblastic leukemia
	t(9;11)(p22;q23)	*MLLT3-MLL*		Intermediate risk group
Myeloproliferative Neoplasms				
CML	t(9;22)(q34;q11) *or* t(9;22;v)	*BCR-ABL1*	De novo AML, ALL	5% of cases cryptic Accelerated phase may show additional Ph, +8, i(17)(q10), +19, +21
PV	+8, +9, del(13q), del(20q), gain 1q	Various	MDS, AML	
ET	+8, +9,del(13q),del (20q), gain 1q			
PMF	+8, del(13q),del(20q), gain 1q, del(12p), monosomy7/del(7q) and der(6)(1;6)(q21-23;p21.3)			Abnormal karyotype in PMF not prognostic
Myelodysplastic Syndrome				
	+8, −Y, del(20q)	Various	Presence of these abnormalities alone, without evidence of dysplasia, is not sufficient for a diagnosis of MDS; these findings are present in other myeloid processes Loss of 1 Y chromosome may also be age-related	
	Unbalanced: −7 or del(7q), −5 or del(5q), i(17q) OR t(17p), −13 *or* del(13q), del(11q), del(12p) *or* t(12p), del(9q), idic(X)(q13) Balanced: t(11;16)(q23;p13.3) t(3;21)(q26.2;q22.1) t(1;3)(p36.3;q21.2) t(2 ;11)(p21;q23) inv(3)(q21;q26.2) t(6;9)(p23;q34)		These abnormalities are considered presumptive evidence of MDS when present with persistent cytopenias, even in the absence of dysplasia; many of these abnormalities are also seen in other myeloid disorders, including AML, underscoring the necessity of a complete and systematic evaluation of every case	

ALL = acute lymphoblastic leukemia; ATRA = all trans retinoic acid; CML = chronic myelogenous leukemia; ET = essential thrombocythemia; Ph = Philadelphia chromosome; MDS = myelodysplastic syndrome; PMF = primary myelofibrosis; PV = polycythemia vera

11 Testing Recommendations for Lymphoid Disorders

Diagnosis under Consideration	CBC with Differential	Morphology Review*	Flow Cytometry	Targeted FISH	Full Karyotyping	IGVH Mutation	Other Molecular
CLL	Y	Y	Y; include CD38, ZAP-70	S; especially in younger patients Include 11q22-23, 13q14.3, 12, 17p13 Consider t(11;14) IGH@-CCND1 if MCL is in differential	S; alert lab to possible diagnosis	S; especially in younger patients	X
Hairy cell leukemia	Y	Y	Y; include CD22, annexin1, CD11c, CD103, CD25	X	X	X	X
Possible lymphoproliferative disorder	Y	Y	Y	S; FISH based on flow results If CD5+, consider t(11;14) IGH@-CCND1 and/or CLL FISH (listed above) If CD10+, consider t(14;18) IGH@-BCL2	S; alert lab to possible diagnosis	X; not necessary if CLL excluded	S; TRG@, IGH@ may be necessary if clonality not clear-cut
T-cell large granular lymphocytic leukemia (T-LGL) (blood/BM)	Y	Y	Y	X	X	X	Y, TRG@ important to exclude reactive LGL
Other T-LPD (blood/BM)	Y	Y	Y	X	S; alert lab to possible diagnosis iso(7q) in HSTL inv(14) in T-PLL t(2;5)|p23;q35) in ALCL	X	S
Acute lymphoblastic leukemia	Y	Y	Y; comprehensive acute leukemia panel	Y; include possibly cryptic t(12;21) ETV6-RUNX1 BCR-ABL1 if cytogenetics normal	Y	X	S; possible minimal residual disease monitoring (eg, Q BCR-ABL1)
Non-Hodgkin lymphoma (any site)	Y	Y	Y	S; FISH based on flow, morphology Consider for FL, MCL, ALCL, MALT as appropriate	S; alert lab to possible diagnosis	X	TRG@, IGH@ Other in specific circumstances
Burkitt lymphoma	Y	Y	Y	S; MYC rearrangement in most cases, though diagnosis may be made without this finding (up to 10% of cases)	Y; MYC rearrangement in most cases Identify additional abnormalities	X	X
Multiple myeloma	Y	Y	Y; include CD38, CD56	Y; may include 13q14, 17p13, t(4;14), t(14;16), t(11;14), others	Y; alert lab to plasma cell dyscrasia	X	X
Hodgkin lymphoma	Y	Y	X; if morphology and IHC clear-cut, flow not contributory	X	X	X	X; (only if B-, T- NHL under consideration)

*Morphologic, hematologic review should guide all specialized testing
Y = Yes, necessary in all or almost all circumstances
S = Sometimes recommended in specific circumstances; factor in clinical issues such as patient age, co-morbidities, likelihood of therapy
X = No, not recommended; not necessary for diagnosis, but *may* be needed in selected cases to *exclude* other differential diagnostic considerations
ALCL = anaplastic large cell lymphoma; BM = bone marrow; CLL = chronic lymphocytic leukemia; HSTL = hepatosplenic γ/δ T-cell lymphoma; IHC = immunohistochemistry; MALT = mucosa-associated lymphoid tissue lymphoma; MCL = mantle cell lymphoma; NHL = non-Hodgkin lymphoma; Q = quantitative RT-PCR; T-PLL = T-cell prolymphocytic leukemia;

appendix

12 Testing Recommendations for Myeloid Disorders

Diagnosis under Consideration	CBC with Differential	Morphology Review*	Flow Cytometry	Targeted FISH	Full Karyotyping	Other Molecular (Specify)
MDS MDS/MPN	Y	Y	S; utility in detecting aberrant antigen profiles Blast quantification may not be accurate May be useful in monocytic lineage assessment	S If suboptimal cytogenetics† Consider t(9;22) *BCR-ABL1* if cytogenetics normal	Y	S *JAK2* may be helpful in some MDS/MPNs and can confirm clonality
MPN, non-CML	Y	Y	S Limited utility unless blasts substantially increased	S t(9;22) *BCR-ABL1* if CG normal *PDGFRA* rearrangement (especially if marked eosinophilia)	S Exclude t(9;22) (q34;q11.2), 5q31~33 (*PDGFRB*), 8p11(*FGFR1*) rearrangements	S *JAK2* V617F Consider *JAK2* exon 12 mutation analysis if V617F negative Consider *MPL* mutation analysis *BCR-ABL1* to exclude CML
CML	Y	Y	X in clear-cut chronic phase; Y if blasts increased (acute leukemia panel)	S t(9;22) *BCR-ABL1* if CG normal or failed†	Y	Y *JAK2* in selected circumstances Q *BCR-ABL1* for monitoring treatment response (often useful to establish baseline transcript type and level at diagnosis)
MLNE	Y	Y	S Not generally needed unless blasts increased	Y *PDGFRA* rearrangement (especially *FIP1L1-PDGFRA* via *CHIC2* deletion) Exclude t(9;22) *BCR-ABL1*	Y Exclude t(9;22) (q34;q11.2) 5q31~33 (*PDGFRB*) or 8p11 (*FGFR1*) rearrangements	S For detection of occult fusion genes
AML	Y	Y	Y Comprehensive acute leukemia panel	S t(15;17) *PML-RARA* for STAT result *CBFB* rearrangement if possible inv(16)	Y Alert lab to possible inv(16) if morphology suggestive	S *FLT3, NPM1, CEBPA* if karyotypically normal, other circumstances Q *PML-RARA*, etc in selected circumstances Other as needed

*Morphologic, hematologic review should guide all specialized testing
†Suboptimal = <20 metaphases, poor quality staining, banding, or spreading
Y = Yes, necessary in all or almost all circumstances
S = Sometimes recommended in specific circumstances; factor in clinical issues such as patient age, co-morbidities, likelihood of therapy
X = No, not recommended; not necessary for diagnosis, but *may* be needed in selected cases to *exclude* other differential diagnostic considerations
AML = acute myeloid leukemia; CML = chronic myelogenous leukemia; MDS = myelodysplastic syndrome; MDS/MPN = myelodysplastic syndrome/myeloproliferative neoplasm; MPN = myeloproliferative neoplasm; MLNE = myeloid and lymphoid neoplasm with eosinophilia and abnormalities of *PDGFRA, PDGFRB* or *FGFR1;* Q = quantitative RT-PCR

13 Practical Approach to Upfront Genetic Testing in Selected Bone Marrow Disease Processes

Disease Process	Initial Step	Subsequent Step(s)
AML	CC in all cases	If normal but there are morphologic clues of AML with maturation, FISH for *RUNX1-RUNX1T1* associated with t(8;21)(q22;q22)
		If normal and/or del(16q) but there are abnormal eosinophils, FISH or RT-PCR for *CBFB-MYH11*
		If normal, molecular testing for *FLT3*, *NPM1*, and *CEBPA* mutations
	Add FISH upfront for *PML-RARA* if t(15;17) suspected	If positive, consider RT-PCR to establish molecular fingerprint for MRD
	Add FISH for *BCR-ABL1* [t(9;22)] if background basophilia or small, mononuclear megakaryocytes	
MDS	CC	If cytogenetics suboptimal (poor quality, insufficient number of metaphases), consider FISH panel [−5/5q, −7/7q, +8, del(20q)] or at least del(5q) because of available therapy (lenalidomide)
MPN	CC	If positive for *BCR-ABL1* (ie, CML), perform RT-PCR to establish baseline level for MRD
	JAK2 V617F (PCR)	If *JAK2* V617F normal, consider *JAK2* exon 12 and/or *MPL* mutation analysis
ALL	CC	If CC normal or suboptimal, FISH for *BCR-ABL1* to exclude cryptic Philadelphia chromosome (adults/pediatric)
	FISH for cryptic *ETV6-RUNX1* [t(12;21)] (pediatric B-ALL)	
Primary eosinophilia	CC	
	Molecular for occult T-cell clone	
	FISH for *FIP1L1-PDGFRA*	
	Molecular for *KIT* D816V mutation if abnormal mast cells	
B-NHL	FISH for *CCND1-IGH@* [t(11;14)] if suspect MCL and cyclin D1 not available or equivocal	*Note: Cyclin D1 not specific for MCL; also (+) in HCL and myeloma*
	FISH for *IGH@-BCL2* [t(14;18)] if FL suspected but difficult case	Consider *IGHV* mutation status as warranted for prognosis in CLL/SLL
	CC and FISH (11q22-23, 13q14.3, 12, and 17p13) for CLL/SLL prognosis	
ENMZL	If gastric, FISH for *API2-MALT1* [t(11;18)]	*API2-MALT1* associated with *Helicobacter pylori* therapy resistance
Plasma cell myeloma	CC with IL-4 stimulation	
	FISH for del(17p), t(4;14), t(14;16) for prognosis	
T-NHL		
ALCL	CC	If normal or suboptimal in ALCL, FISH for *ALK* rearrangement with *ALK* break-apart probe
T-PLL	CC	
HSTCL	CC	If normal or suboptimal in HSTCL, FISH for 7q with centromere 7 may indirectly detect iso(7q)

ALCL = anaplastic large cell lymphoma; ALL = acute lymphoblastic leukemia; AML = acute myeloid leukemia; CC = conventional cytogenetics; CML = chronic myelogenous leukemia; ENMZL = extranodal marginal zone lymphoma; FISH = fluorescence in situ hybridization; FL = follicular lymphoma; HCL = hairy cell leukemia; HSTCL hepatosplenic T-cell lymphoma; MCL = mantle cell lymphoma; MDS = myelodysplastic syndrome; MPN = myeloproliferative neoplasm; MRD = minimum residual disease; NHL = non-Hodgkin lymphoma; SLL = small lymphocytic lymphoma; T-PLL = T-cell prolymphocytic leukemia

14 General Suggestions for Workup of Bone Marrows Obtained during or after Induction Chemotherapy

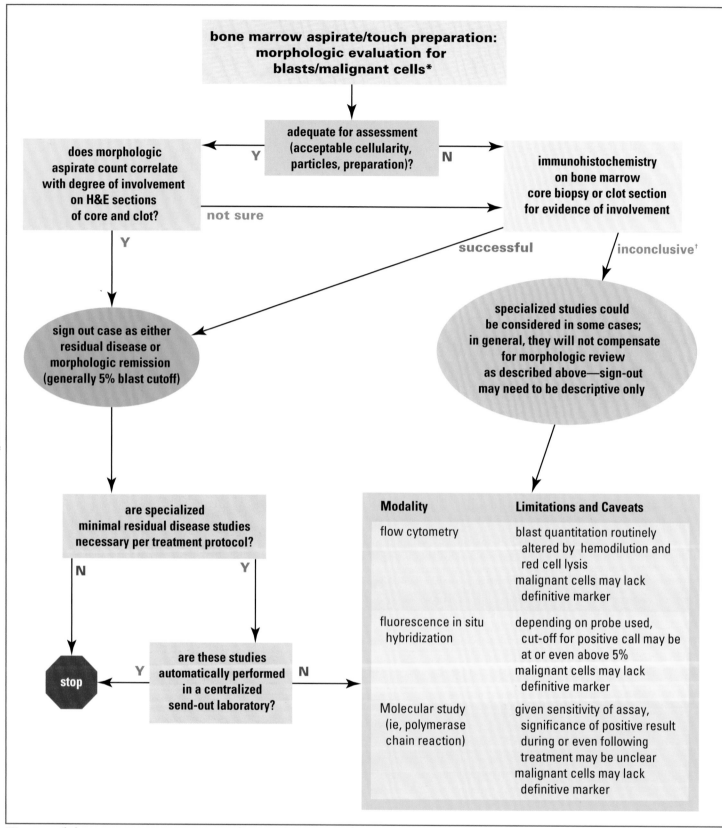

Direct morphologic comparison to pre-treatment neoplastic population is essential.

†*Inconclusive results most often arise from inadequate specimens or technical issues related to decalcification. In some cases the malignant cells may lack markers (eg, CD34) that would allow for detection. In some cases the total population of blasts may meet or exceed 5%, but the clinical setting (eg, regenerating marrow, G-CSF therapy) and lack of characteristic immunophenotypic or morphologic markers on the malignant cells render it difficult to definitively determine the relative burden of malignant cells. It may also be challenging to accurately quantitate blast percentages near the 5% threshold based only on immunohistochemistry.*

15 Examples of Integrated Bone Marrow Reports

Note: These sample reports are included to demonstrate the composition and purpose of integrated bone marrow reports. In each case, individual components of the analysis (eg, flow cytometry, cytogenetics, morphology) were signed out separately. After the completion of all studies, these integrated reports were generated by listing the separate diagnoses and comments, then adding a "final integrated diagnosis" and comment to lead off the report.

Example #1

Final integrated diagnosis
Bone marrow, aspirate and core biopsy evaluated by flow cytometric immunophenotyping, morphologic and immunohistochemical assessment, and conventional cytogenetics:
• no morphologic, immunophenotypic, or immunohistochemical evidence of multiple myeloma
• abnormal karyotype identified in 3 of 20 metaphases analyzed revealing del(11)(q13q23) (see comment)

Comment
The identification of a clonal cytogenetic abnormality in 3 of 20 metaphases in a specimen negative for evidence of residual myeloma based on morphologic, flow cytometric immunophenotypic, and immunohistochemical techniques raises the possibility of an acquired clonal abnormality in residual hematopoietic elements
Because del(11)(q23) can be found in therapy related situations, this is a clinical possibility in the current case. This cytogenetic abnormality is distinctly uncommon in multiple myeloma; the lack of evidence for residual multiple myeloma based on a multiparameter analysis, further supports the concern that this cytogenetic abnormality is present in residual hematopoietic cells.

Previous consultation reports

Hematopathology consultation

Diagnosis
Peripheral blood, bone marrow aspirate, touch preparation, clot and trephine biopsy sections:
• mild macrocytic anemia of the peripheral blood
• normocellular marrow (50%) with no significant plasma cells, consistent with multiple myeloma in morphologic remission (see comment)

Comment
The morphology examination of the marrow shows ~1% plasma cells, which are polyclonal by κ and λ light chain in situ hybridization. Flow cytometry shows <1% polyclonal plasma cells. Cytogenetics is pending. The marrow is consistent with remission status.

Diagnosis
Bone marrow aspirate; flow cytometric analysis:
no significant plasma cell population identified by flow (see comment)

Comment
There are no significant plasma cells identified by flow cytometry. Please refer to HHU-07-567 for morphologic diagnosis. Cytogenetics is pending and the result will be reported separately.

Cytogenetics consultation

Karyotype:
46,XX,del(11)(q13q23)[3]/46,XX[16]

Interpretation:
Abnormal female chromosome complement with an interstitial deletion of the long arm of chromosome 11
in 3 cells. 16 cells were female chromosome complement with no clonal abnormalities detected. Deletion 11q is a recurrent finding in AML, chronic lymphoproliferative disorder, CLL and other hematopoietic disorders.

Example #2

Final integrated diagnosis
Bone marrow aspirate; flow cytometric and cytogenetic analysis:
acute myeloid leukemia with erythrophagocytosis associated with t(8;16)(p11.2;p13.3) (see comment)

Comment
The erythrophagocytosis noted on the cytospin preparation in this case was a morphologic clue that I have seen in cases with t(8;16), which was confirmed in this case by cytogenetic testing. The proposed fusion genes involved in this translocation are *MYST3-CREBBP* [Rozman 2004]. Of importance, extramedullary disease is relatively more common in this rare subtype of AML compared to AML cases overall. Thank you for sharing this fascinating case with us.

Previous consultation reports

Hematopathology consultation

Diagnosis
Bone marrow aspirate; flow cytometric analysis:
acute myeloid leukemia (see comment)

Comment
Blasts comprise 57% of total events and express CD45, CD33, CD4, CD13, HLA-DR and CD64, consistent with acute myeloid leukemia with monocytic differentiation. In addition, the morphologic finding of erythrophagocytosis has been associated with a specific cytogenetic abnormality: t(8;16) (p11;p13). Correlation with bone marrow morphology and cytogenetic findings is necessary for further subclassification

Cytogenetics consultation

Karyotype:
46, XX, t(8;16)(p11.2;p13.3)[18]

Interpretation
Abnormal female chromosome complement with a translocation of the short arm of chromosome 8 with the short arm of chromosome 16 in all cells analyzed; 2 of these cells had non clonal aberrations, including +8; the translocation t(8;16) is a rare but recurrent finding in AML.

appendix

16 References

Bain BJ [1996] The bone marrow aspirate of healthy subjects. *Br J Haematol* 94:206-209.

Bick R [1993] *Hematology: Clinical and Laboratory Practice*. St Louis: Mosby; 1993.

Brugnara C [2003] Reference values in infancy and childhood. In: Nathan DG, Orkin SH, Ginsburg D, Look AT, eds. *Nathan and Oski's Hematology of Infancy and Childhood*. 6th ed. Philadelphia: WB Saunders; 1848-1851.

Christensen RD, Henry E, Jopling J, Wiedmeier SE [2009] The CBC: reference ranges for neonates. *Semin Perinatol* 33:3-11.

de Alarcon P, Werner E [2005] Normal values and laboratory methods. In: de Alarcon P, Werner E, eds. *Neonatal Hematology*: Cambridge University Press; 406-430.

Forestier F, Daffos F, Catherine N, et al [1991] Developmental hematopoiesis in normal human fetal blood. *Blood* 77:2360-2363.

Foucar K, Viswanatha D, Wilson C [2008] Appendix. In: King D, Gardner W, Sobin L, et al, eds. *Non-Neoplastic Disorders of Bone Marrow (AFIP fascicle)*. Washington, DC: American Registry of Pathology; 397-401.

Friebert SE, Shepardson LB, Shurin SB, et al [1998] Pediatric bone marrow cellularity: are we expecting too much? *J Pediatr Hematol Oncol* 20:439-443.

Gulati GL, Ashton JK, Hyun BH [1988] Structure and function of the bone marrow and hematopoiesis. *Hematol Oncol Clin North Am* 2:495-511.

Hartsock RJ, Smith EB, Petty CS [1965] Normal variations with aging of the amount of hematopoietic tissue in bone marrow from the anterior iliac crest: a study made from 177 cases of sudden death examined by necropsy. *Am J Clin Pathol* 43:326-331.

Hermansen MC [2001] Nucleated red blood cells in the fetus and newborn. *Arch Dis Child Fetal Neonatal Ed* 84:F211-215.

Kipps T [2006] The cluster of differentiation (CD) antigens. In: Lictman M, Beutler E, Kipps T, et al, eds. *Williams Hematology*. 7th ed. New York: McGraw-Hill; 183-199.

Kjeldsberg C, Perkins S [2010] Hematology reference values. In: Kjeldsberg C, Perkins S, eds. *Practical Diagnosis of Hematologic Disorders*. 5th ed. Chicago: ASCP Press; 919-927.

Nordic Reference Interval Project (NORIP) [2010] Available at: http://www.furst.no/norip/; accessed February 16, 2010.

Perkins S [2003] Normal blood and bone marrow values in humans. In: Greer J, Foerster J, Lukens H, et al, eds. *Wintrobe's Clinical Hematology*. 11th ed. Philadelphia: Lippincott, Williams & Wilkins; 2967-2707.

Rimsza LM, Douglas VK, Tighe P, et al [2004] Benign B-cell precursors (hematogones) are the predominant lymphoid population in the bone marrow of preterm infants. *Biol Neonate* 86:247-253.

Rozman M, Camos M, Colomer D, et al [2004] Type I MOZ/CBP (MYST3/CREBBP) is the most common chimeric transcript in acute myeloid leukemia with t(8;16)(p11;p13) translocation. *Genes Chromosomes Cancer* 40:140-145.

Ryan D [2006] Examination of the blood. In: Lictman M, Beutler E, Kipps T, et al, eds. *Williams Hematology*. 7th ed. New York: McGraw-Hill; 11-19.

Trimoreau F, Verger C, Praloran V, Denizot Y [1997] No sex-related difference in the myeloid: erythroid ratio in morphologically normal bone marrow aspirates. *Br J Haematol* 97:687.

UniProt Consortium [2010] Human cell differentiation molecules: CD nomenclature and list of entries, Release 57.15 of March 2, 2010; available at: http://www.expasy.ch/cgi-bin/lists?cdlist.txt; accessed March 15, 2010.

Wickramasinghe S [2007] Bone marrow. In: Mills S, ed. *Histology for Pathologists*. 3rd ed. Philadelphia: Lippincott Williams & Wilkins; 799-836.

Zutter MM, Hess JL. Guidelines for the diagnosis of leukemia or lymphoma in children. *Am J Clin Pathol* 109:S9-22.

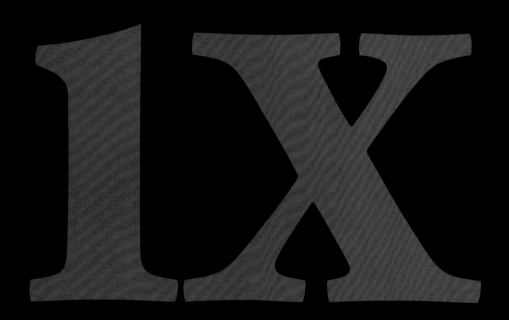

INDEX

ix

index

index

index

index

index

index

index

index

index